屡试验方集锦

Collection of Proven and Effective Prescriptions

赵德生 ◎著
By Zhao Desheng

CLEARWIND
清风出版社

屡试验方集锦

赵德生　著

责任编辑：James Calloway
封面设计：胡斌

Published by
Clearwind Press,USA
PO Box 240052, Montgomery, AL 36124, U.S.A.

本书由美国清风出版社出版

2026 年 8 月第 1 版

开本：170mm×240mm
字数：671 千字

Library of Congress Control Number
美国国会图书馆编目号码：2026944968

国际标准书号 ISBN-13：978-1-68372-874-0

前 言
Preface

作者，赵德生，出生 1951 年。

The author, Zhao Desheng, was born in 1951.

1968 年初中毕业。

He graduated from junior high school in 1968.

同年参加了丰润县赤脚医生培训班。

In the same year, he attended the barefoot doctor training class in Fengrun County.

1969 年在“唐山市军民联合新医疗法医疗站”学习针灸、推拿、穴位注射等。

In 1969, he studied acupuncture, massage, acupoint injection, and other techniques at the “Tangshan Military-Civilian Joint New Medical Therapy Station.”

1971 年由乡卫生院推荐，到丰润县五·七大学学习中医。

In 1971, recommended by the township health center, he went to the May 7th University of Fengrun County to study traditional Chinese medicine.

1973 年由乡卫生院选拔到三女河乡卫生院当医生。

In 1973, he was selected by the township health center to work as a doctor at the Sannvhe Township Health Center.

1988 年，在改革开放的大潮中，毅然决然地下海到丰润县城西医院创建“肛肠科”并个人承包。

In 1988, amidst the tide of reform and opening up, he resolutely plunged into the business world, establishing and personally contracting the “Proctology Department” at Fengrun County West Hospital.

1990 年从城西医院出来，成立了“丰润县德生诊所”。

In 1990, he left the West Hospital and established the “Fengrun County Desheng Clinic.”

1993 年创建了“丰润县结肠炎医院”后改为“唐山丰润德生医院”至今。

In 1993, he founded the “Fengrun County Colitis Hospital,” which was later renamed “Tangshan Fengrun Desheng Hospital” and remains so to this day.

2014 年 9 月因年事已高，功成勇退，将医院承包给他人经营管理，自己专心搞创作。

In September 2014, due to his advanced age and having achieved his goals, he bravely stepped down, contracting the hospital to others for management and operation, while he devoted himself entirely to writing.

本人自承包城西医院“肛肠科”以后，为了掌握形势，搜集信息，补充自己的不足，在 1989 年至 1999 年十年间，曾经订阅了《健康报》《中国医药报》《中国抗癌报》《中药科技报》《中药事业报》《中医药信息报》《中药时报》《中国中医药报》《民族医药报》《健康导报》《中医药报》等十余种报纸。

Since contracting the “Proctology Department” of the West Hospital, in order to keep abreast of the situation, collect information, and make up for his own shortcomings, he subscribed to more than a dozen newspapers between 1989 and 1999, including Health News, China Medical News, China Anti-Cancer News, Chinese Materia Medica Science and Technology News, Chinese Medicine Enterprise News, TCM Information News, Chinese Materia Medica Times, China TCM News, National Minority Medicine News, Health Guide, and TCM News.

另外还订阅了《中医学》《中药学》《河北中医》《肿瘤学》《中国医学文摘》等十余种杂志。

In addition, he also subscribed to more than a dozen magazines such as Traditional Chinese Medicine, Chinese Materia Medica, Hebei Journal of Traditional Chinese Medicine, Oncology, and Chinese Medical Digest.

每份报纸杂志看完后，自己认为有意义的片段或章节，都把它用笔勾画或剪辑下来，一直保存到现在。

After reading each newspaper and magazine, he would highlight with a pen or clip out the passages or sections he found meaningful, and has kept them all until now.

此时，我通过排选分类，可以写成多本书。

Now, by sorting and classifying them, I can compile multiple books.

其中有《趣谈古今中外医药故事》《屡试验方法集锦》《医药师之友》《古今中外养生长寿集锦》《中药鉴别》《性知识与科学》《特色医疗》《育儿经》等十余本书。

Among them are more than ten books, including Interesting Talks on Medical Stories from Ancient and Modern Times, China and Abroad, Collection of Proven Methods, Friend of Medical Professionals, Collection of Health and Longevity Practices from Ancient and Modern Times, China and Abroad, Identification of Traditional Chinese Medicine, Sexual Knowledge and Science, Characteristic Medical Treatments, and Parenting Guide.

这些文字记录了古今中外许多医药故事和前人经验技术的总结。

These writings record many medical stories from ancient and modern times, both in China and abroad, as well as summaries of the experiences and techniques of our predecessors.

再现了历史的风采。

They recreate the splendor of history.

反过来它又可以使现代人们继承和发扬我国的传统文化，又可以使人们通过过去的故事和经验得以启发，使梦笔生花。

In turn, they can enable modern people to inherit and carry forward our country’s traditional culture, and inspire people through past stories and experiences, sparking brilliant creativity.

从而演绎出新的历史喜剧，推动社会的进步和人类的发展。

Thus, they can create new historical triumphs, and promote social progress and human development.

既可以成为人们的精神食粮，又可以从中学到一些技能和启发，服务于社会。

They can not only serve as spiritual nourishment for people, but also allow them to learn skills and gain inspiration to serve society.

这是我的出发点，也是我梦想为人类做一点贡献的实际行动。

This is my starting point, and also the practical action toward my dream of making a small contribution to humanity.

为此感到欣慰。

I feel gratified by this.

如有不妥之处，敬请谅解。

Please excuse any shortcomings.

作者：赵德生

Author: Zhao Desheng

2015 年春月

Spring, 2015

唐山丰润德生医院简介

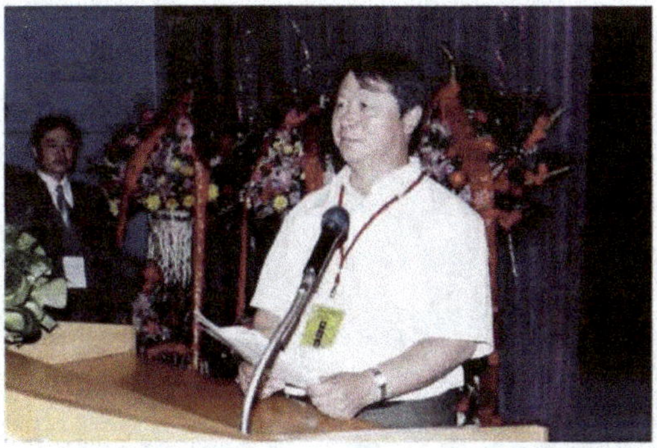

2003年，赵德生应中华中医药学会邀请，参加在北京举办的第三次代表大会并在会上发言。

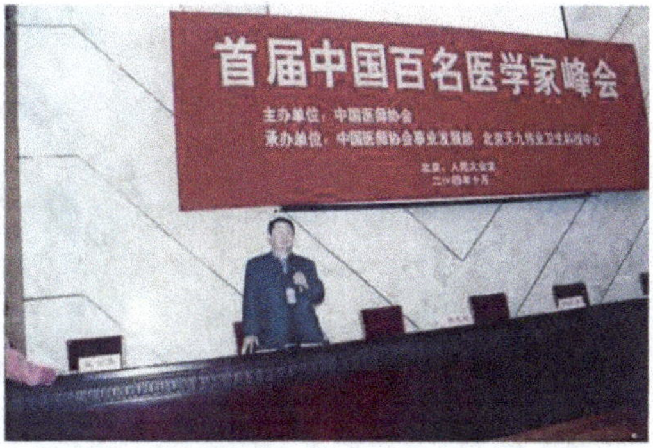

2004年，赵德生应中国医师协会邀请，参加在北京人民大会堂召开的“首届中国百名医学家峰会”，并在会上发言。

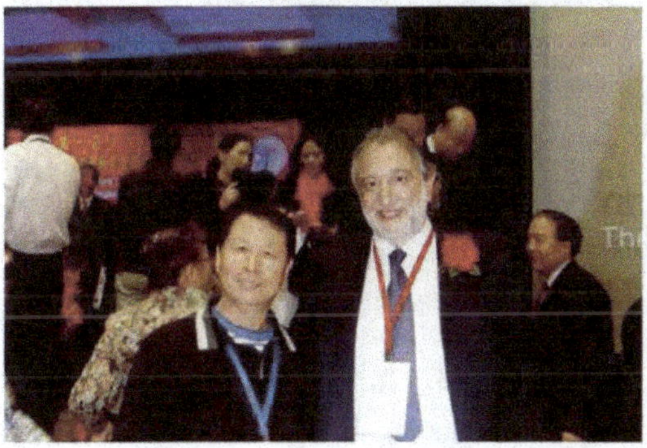

2013 年，赵德生参加在美国旧金山举办的，世界中医药大会上，与世界中医药学会秘书长合影。

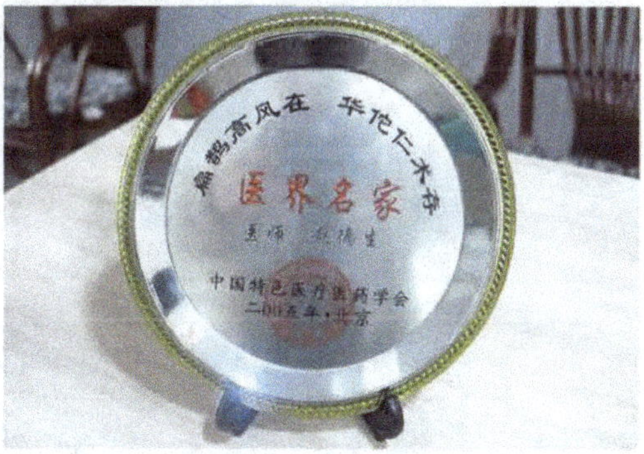

2005 年，赵德生被“中国特色医疗医药学会”授予“医界名家”称号。

唐山丰润德生医院简介

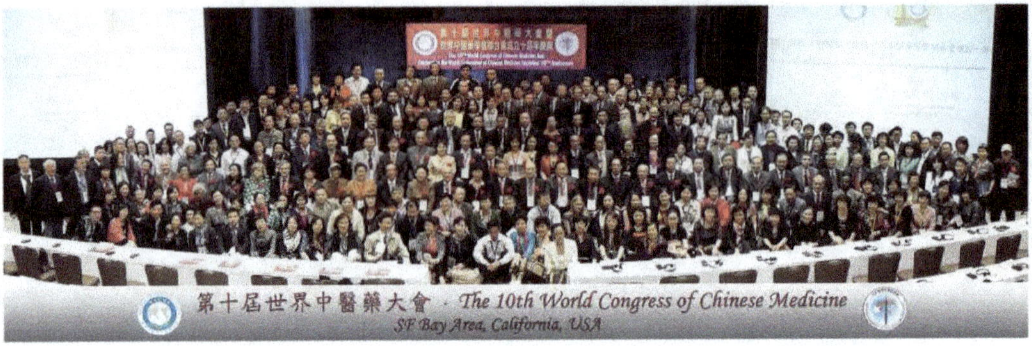

2013 年 9 月 22 日赵德生应世界中医药学会邀请
参加在美国旧金山举办的第十届世界中医药大会

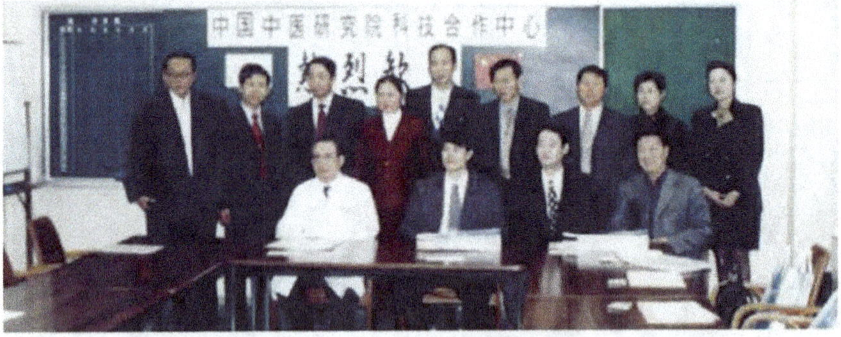

2001 年赵德生应“中国中医研究院”邀请赴日本洽谈技术合作事项

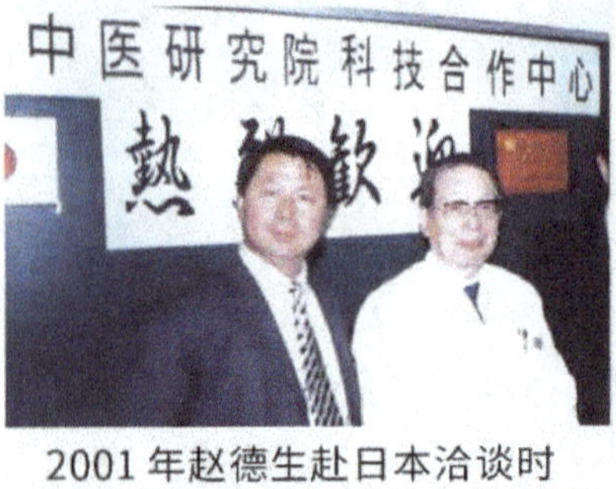

2001 年赵德生赴日本洽谈时
与日方负责人“上羽康之”合影

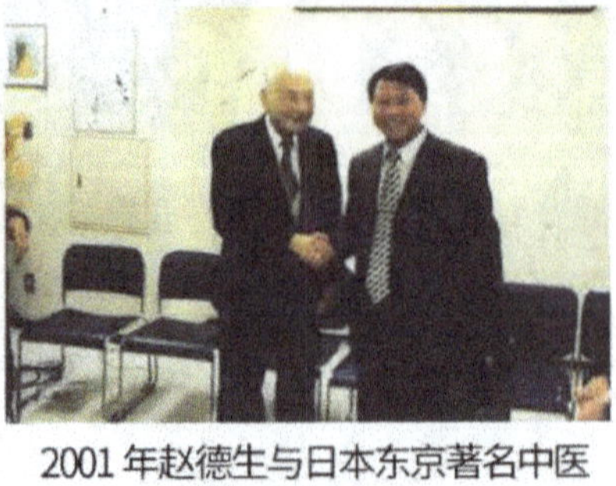

2001 年赵德生与日本东京著名中医
专家桑木崇秀先生合影

唐山丰润德生医院简介

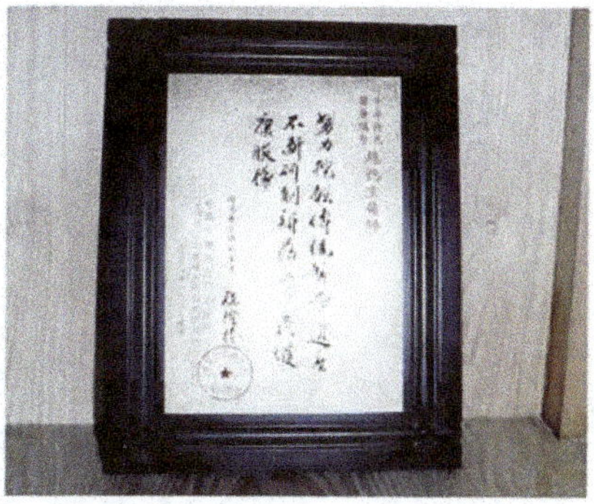

2001 年，国家卫生部副部长孙隆椿为赵德生题词：“努力挖掘传统医学遗产，不断研制新药，为人民健康服务。”

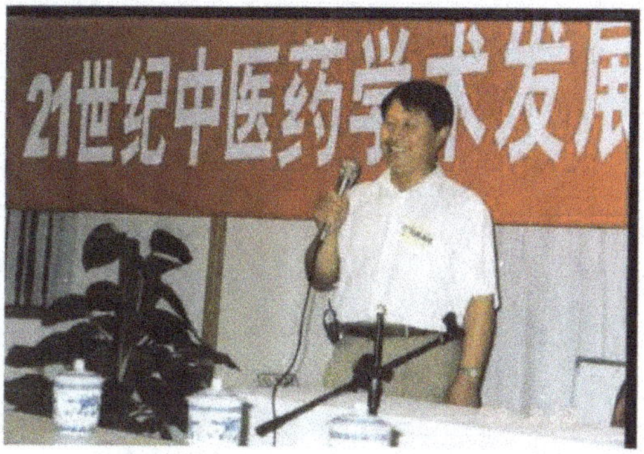

2001 年，赵德生应中国中医药学会邀请，参加在北京举办的《21 世纪中医药学术发展论坛大会》，并在会上发言。

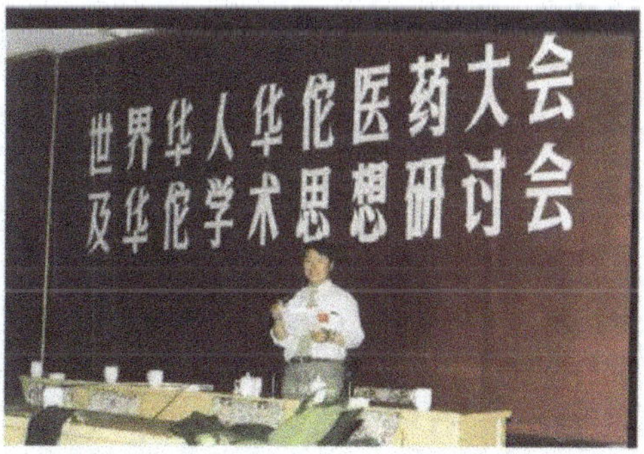

1998 年 5 月，赵德生应“世界华人华佗医药大会”邀请参会。并在医药大会上宣读论文。

1998 年 5 月，赵德生在“世界华人华佗医药大会上宣读《中医药治疗癌症 48 例疗效观察》的论文，经专家评审，获论文“一等奖”。

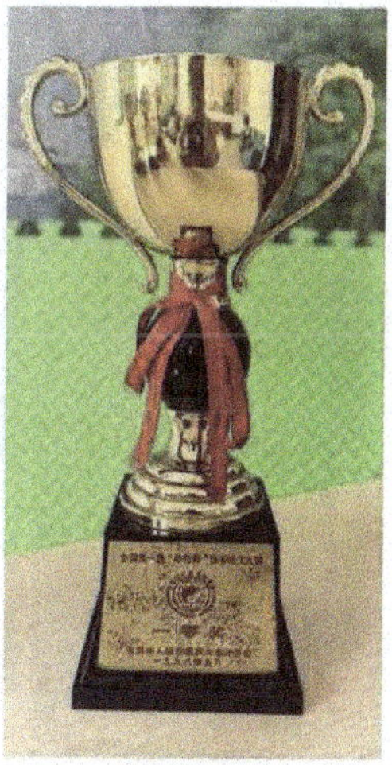

唐山丰润德生医院简介

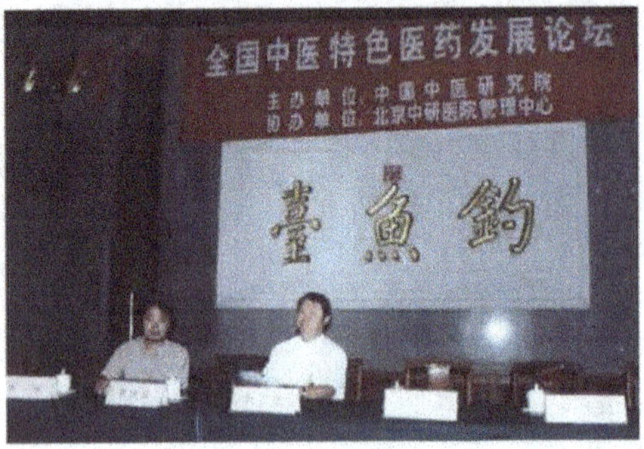

2004 年，赵德生应“中国中医研究院”邀请，参加在北京钓鱼台国宾馆召开的“全国中医特色医药发展论坛大会”应邀在会上宣读论文，并获论文“一等奖”

2004 年 6 月，赵德生撰写的论文《癌复康治疗多种癌症 68 例疗效观察》获一等奖。

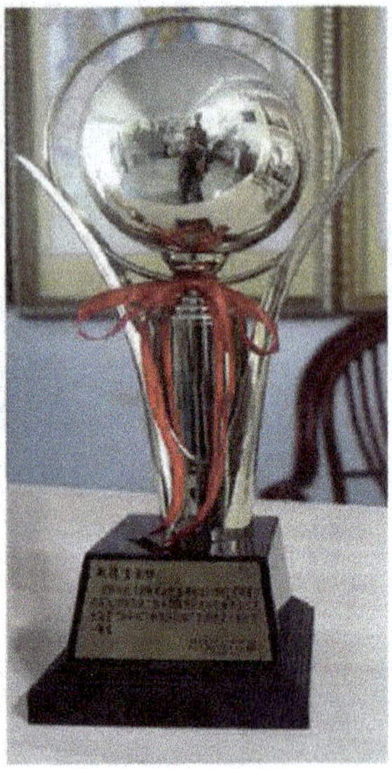

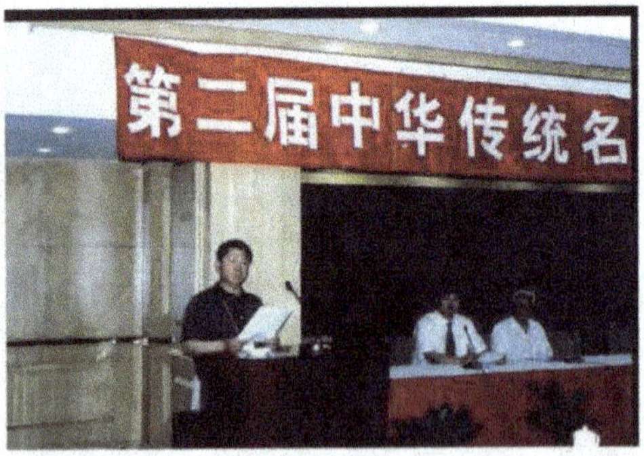

2003年，赵德生应中华医学会邀请，参加在北京人民大会堂召开的第二届中华传统名医名药论坛及中医药成果交流大会，并在会上宣读《用中医药治疗癌症的疗效观察》论文，经大会专家评审荣获金奖。（见右图）

2003 年 12 月，赵德生在第二届中华传统名医名药交流大会上宣读的《用中医中药治疗癌症 32 例疗效观察》的论文获金奖。

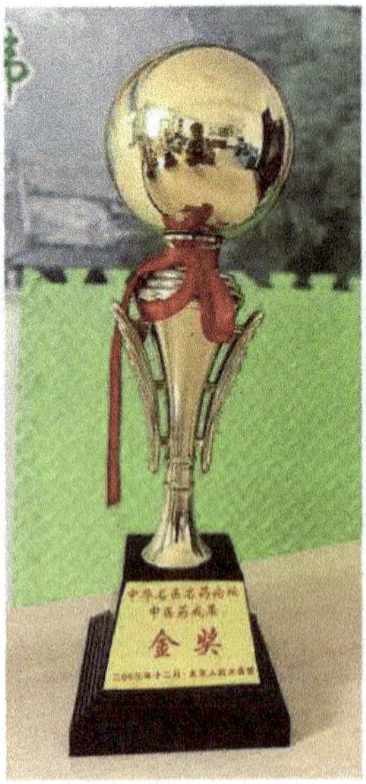

唐山丰润德生医院简介

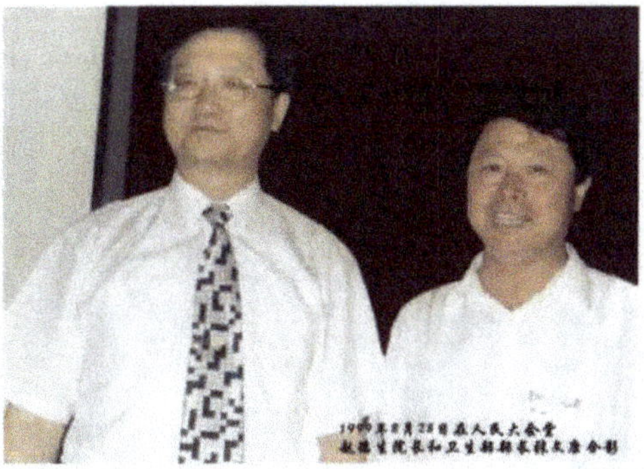

1999 年在人民大会堂召开的“ 中国民间疗法首届学术研讨会上 ”，赵德生谈到民间疗法有“ 辟谷疗法 ”“ 拜佛疗法 ”和“ 气功疗法 ”等多种民间疗法治疗癌症的。张文康部长很感兴趣，主动邀赵德生合影留念。在会下张文康部长也恳切地对赵德生说：“ 一定要在治疗癌症上下功夫，一定要研究出治疗癌症的新方法。赵德生牢记部长指示，回家以后访民间、访中医、查古书、找秘方，为落实张部长的指示，而不断的奔波和研究。”

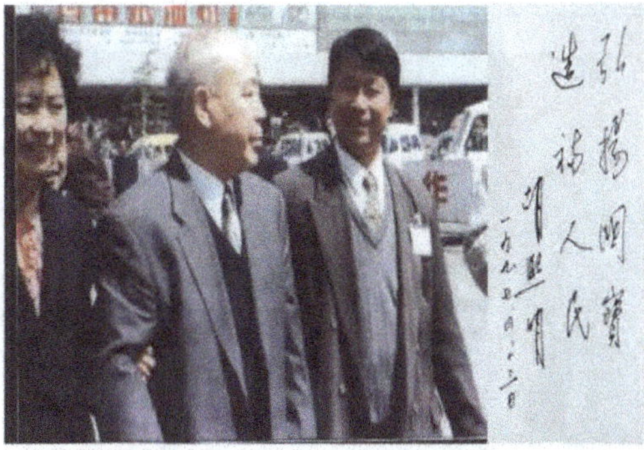

1997 年 4 月，在河南洛阳召开的“ 全国第二届专科专病学术交流大会上，赵德生又介绍了在治疗癌症方面的新进展，受到了卫生部副部长胡熙明的赞赏，并给题词：“ 弘扬国宝，造福人民。”在会议休息期间，胡部长非常恳切地对赵德生说：“ 一定要下功夫研究出治疗癌症的新药，造福人民。”为了落实胡部长的指示，赵德生不断地在多方面进行研究，探讨。

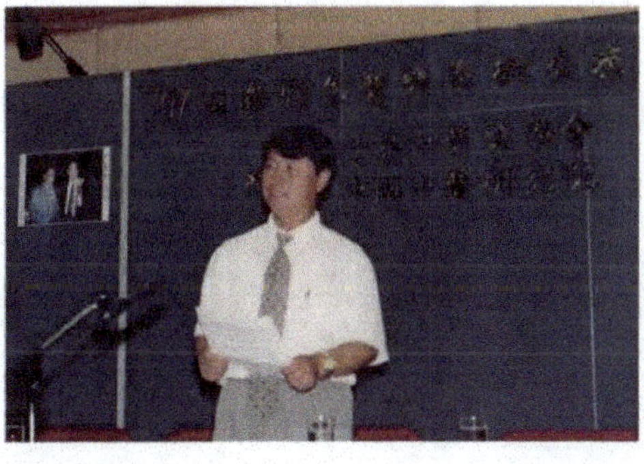

1997 年 ，赵德生应“ 世界中医药学会邀请 ”，参加在香港召开的“97 国际特色医药学术交流大会 ”并在会上宣读“ 用中医药治疗癌症的论文 ”，经专家评审荣获壹等奖。(见右侧照片）

1997 年 7 月，赵德生应世界中医药学会邀请，参加在香港举办的“ 国际特色医药学术交流大会 ”上，提交的关于治疗癌症的论文经专家评审荣获“ 世界中医药学会壹等奖 ”。

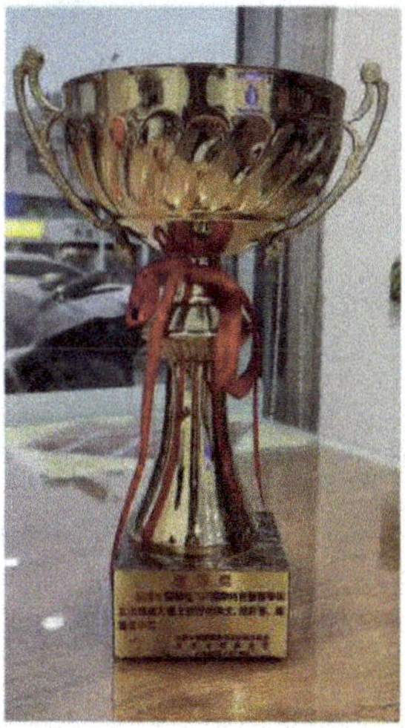

唐山丰润德生医院简介

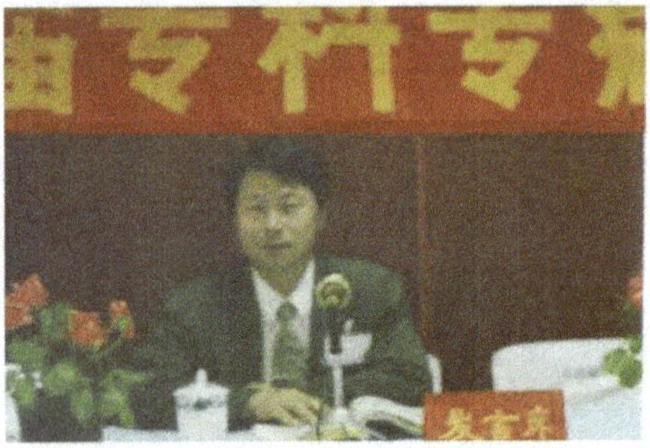

1996 年，赵德生应中华医学会邀请，参加在北京举办的“ 全国第一届专科专病学术交流大会”，并在会上发言。

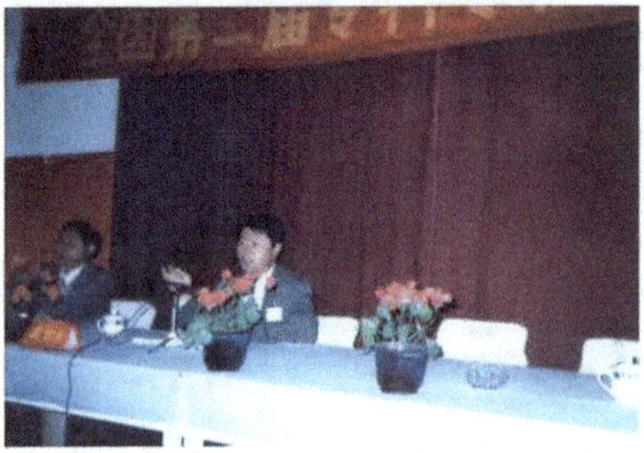

1997 年，赵德生应中华医学会邀请，参加“ 全国第二届专科专病学术交流大会，并在会上宣读论文。

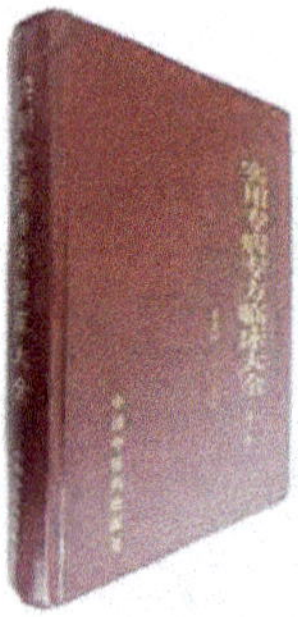

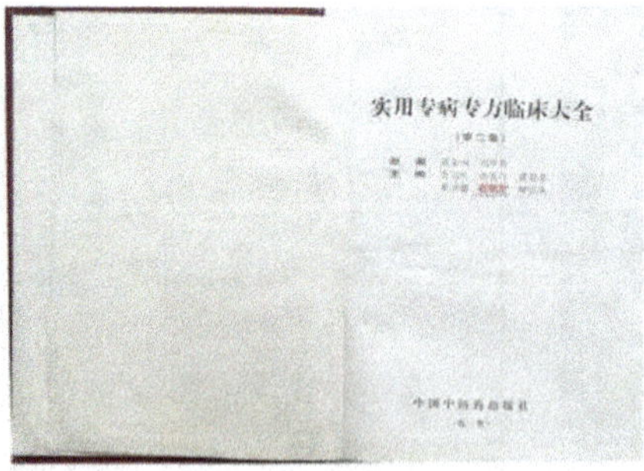

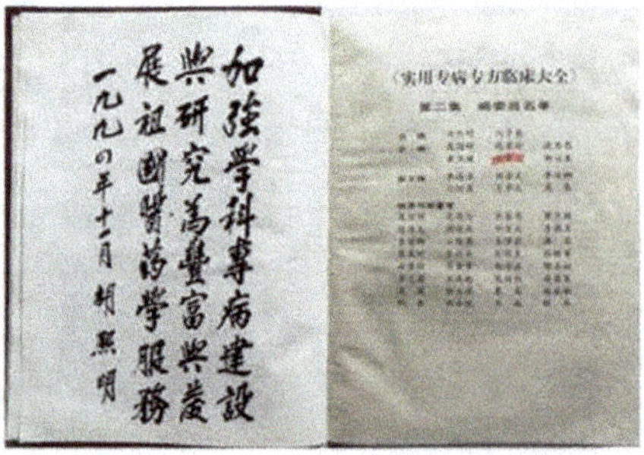

赵德生参加编写了：“1997 年在北京中国中医药出版社出版的《实用专病专方临床大全》第二集一书。以卫生部副部长胡熙明为总编，以庞国明、赵德生等为主编。

免责声明 / Disclaimer

本书内容仅供医学、药学研究、教学和参考之用，不构成任何形式的医疗诊断、治疗建议、处方建议或用药指导。书中涉及的药物、方剂、治疗方法、剂量及相关经验，可能因个体体质、病情、年龄、过敏史、既往病史、合并用药及当地医疗法规不同而产生不同效果或风险。

读者不得仅凭本书内容自行诊断疾病、购买药品、调整药物剂量、停用处方药或替代专业医疗服务。如有疾病症状、用药疑问或治疗需求，应及时咨询具有合法执业资格的医师、药师或其他专业医疗人员。

本书所载资料力求准确，但医学与药学知识不断更新，作者及出版社不保证所有信息在任何时间、任何地区均完全适用。因使用或误用本书内容所产生的任何后果，作者及出版社不承担法律责任。

The content of this book is intended for medical and pharmaceutical research, education, and general reference only. It does not constitute medical diagnosis, treatment advice, prescription advice, or medication guidance of any kind. The drugs, formulas, treatment methods, dosages, and clinical experiences discussed in this book may vary in effect and risk depending on individual constitution, medical condition, age, allergy history, prior medical history, concurrent medications, and applicable local medical regulations.

Readers should not diagnose illnesses, purchase medications, adjust dosages, discontinue prescription drugs, or replace professional medical care based solely on the content of this book. Anyone with symptoms, medication questions, or treatment needs should consult a licensed physician, pharmacist, or other qualified healthcare professional.

Although efforts have been made to ensure accuracy, medical and pharmaceutical knowledge is constantly evolving. The author and publisher do not guarantee that all information in this book is complete, current, or applicable in every situation or jurisdiction. The author and publisher shall not be held legally responsible for any consequences arising from the use or misuse of the information contained in this book.

目　录

CONTENTS

第一章　内 科

Chapter 1　Internal Medicine

第二章　胃肠病

Chapter 2　Gastrointestinal Diseases

第三章　心脑血管病

Chapter 3　Cardiovascular and Cerebrovascular Diseases

第四章　肝胆病

Chapter 4　Hepatobiliary Diseases

第五章　五官科

Chapter 5　Otorhinolaryngology and Ophthalmology

第六章　美容科

Chapter VI: Medical Aesthetics

第七章　骨病科

Chapter VII Orthopedics

第八章　泌尿科
Chapter 8　Urology Department

第九章　男科

Chapter 9　Andrology

第十章　妇科

Chapter 10　gynecology

第十一章　儿科
Chapter 11　Pediatrics

第十二章　肿瘤
Chapter 12　Tumors

第十三章　皮肤科
Chapter 13　Dermatology

第十四章　其他科
Chapter 14　Other Departments

第十五章　单味多效中药

Chapter 15　Single Herbs with Multiple Therapeutic Effects

第一章　内 科
Chapter 1　Internal Medicine

一、感 冒（8方）
I. Common Cold (8 Prescriptions)

1. 治感冒头痛、鼻塞流清涕、周身酸楚：

1.For cold-induced headache, nasal congestion with clear runny nose, and general body ache:

用生姜适量，洗净后切成厚约 0.3cm 的小片，与精盐少许相拌，再用湿草纸包好入柴火或炭火中煨，待姜片煨熟后取出并沾 40° 以上米酒，在患者太阳穴、项部、背部等处“刮痧”（即用沾酒的热姜片自上而下刮擦，用力要适中），至皮肤呈红紫色为度。

Take an appropriate amount of fresh ginger, wash it, cut it into slices about 0.3 cm thick, mix with a little refined salt, wrap in wet straw paper, and roast in a firewood or charcoal fire; after the ginger slices are roasted, take them out, dip them in rice wine of over 40% alcohol content, and perform "Gua Sha" (scraping therapy) on the patient's temples, neck, and back (i.e., scrape from top to bottom with the hot, wine-soaked ginger slices using moderate pressure) until the skin turns reddish-purple.

每日 1-2 次，一般 2 天可愈。

Apply 1–2 times daily; recovery usually occurs within 2 days.

2. 治伤风感冒、头痛鼻塞、恶风无汗：

2. For wind-cold common cold, headache, nasal congestion, aversion to wind, and absence of sweating:

取生姜40g、淡豆豉20g、葱白7根、吴茱萸3g，茶叶少许，食盐适量，入热锅内捣烂，加水250ml，煮沸取汁，趁热顿服后覆被而卧，使微汗出。

Take 40g fresh ginger, 20g fermented soybeans, 7 scallion whites, 3g Evodia fruit, a little tea leaves, and an appropriate amount of salt; mash them in a hot pan, add 250 ml water, boil, strain the juice, drink it all at once while hot, then cover up with a blanket to induce slight sweating.

不效可再服，一般2-3次可愈。

If ineffective, repeat the dose; recovery generally occurs after 2–3 administrations.

3. 治伤风咳嗽：

3. For wind-cold cough:

鲜枇杷叶数片，烤热后敷贴脐部及胸背部，每日3-4次，一般1-2天获效。

Take several fresh loquat leaves, roast them until warm, and apply to the navel, chest, and back; use 3–4 times daily, with effects typically seen within 1–2 days.

《民族医药报》1991年7月5日（唐乾利）

Ethnic Medicine News, July 5, 1991 (Tang Qianli)

4. 流行性感冒是临床上的多发病和常见病我院采用民间传统偏方治疗，收效明显，报道如下，供患者选用。

4. Influenza is a frequently occurring and common clinical disease; our hospital has adopted traditional folk remedies with remarkable results, as reported below for patients' reference.

方药：采鲜马鞭草、鲜一枝黄花各50克（儿童酌减）加水共煎，日1剂分2次服。

Prescription: Take 50g each of fresh verbena and fresh goldenrod (reduce dosage for children), decoct together in water, and take as one daily dose divided into two servings.

临床验证：该方有明显的清热、疏风、解毒、利尿作用，对流感疗效甚佳，也适用于其它类型的呼吸道感染。

Clinical verification: This prescription has significant effects of clearing heat, dispelling wind, detoxifying, and promoting diuresis; it is highly effective for influenza and also applicable to other types of respiratory tract infections.

本方无副作用，不妨一试。

This formula has no side effects and is worth trying.

上两药多生于山野，路边，采集方便，故此方具有“验、便、廉”等优点。

Both herbs grow mostly in mountains, fields, and roadsides and are easy to collect; thus, this formula possesses the advantages of being "effective, convenient, and inexpensive."

《中药科技报》1992 年 5 月 6 日（孙扬）

Chinese Materia Medica Science and Technology News, May 6, 1992 (Sun Yang)

5. 蛋酒治感冒

5. Egg Wine for Treating Colds

自古以来，蛋酒在民间都被视为治疗感冒的良药，酒能通经活络，发汗解表，蛋能滋润气血，营养机体，同时能助酒发汗又能抑制酒之发汗过度，酒又能促使蛋的营养运行到全身。

Since ancient times, egg wine has been regarded in folk tradition as an excellent remedy for colds; wine unblocks meridians and collaterals, induces sweating and releases the exterior, while eggs nourish qi and blood and nurture the body; meanwhile, eggs assist the wine in inducing sweating yet prevent excessive perspiration, and the wine helps distribute the nutrients of the egg throughout the body.

此方两药相辅相成，攻补兼施，实为妙法。

The two ingredients in this formula complement each other, combining both eliminating pathogenic factors and tonifying the body, making it truly a wonderful method.

制作鸡蛋酒时，首先应温热酒，酒的温度愈高愈好，鸡蛋则用另一个容器搅拌充分后，倒入正在煮开的酒中即可，一般 50 克酒加一个鸡蛋为一次量。

When preparing egg wine, first warm the wine—the hotter, the better—and beat the egg thoroughly in a separate container before pouring it into the boiling wine; typically, one serving consists of 50g of wine mixed with one egg.

（若不能喝白酒可用黄酒、清酒代替）据临床观察，蛋酒不仅对感冒有效，如果工作至深夜而感到疲劳不堪，喝一点蛋酒，就能够熟睡和消除疲劳。

(If strong liquor is unsuitable, yellow wine or sake may be substituted.) Clinical observation shows that egg wine is not only effective for colds but also helpful for those exhausted from working late into the night—a small amount can promote deep sleep and relieve fatigue.

《民族医药报》（成都 戴廷荣）

Ethnic Medicine News (Chengdu, Dai Tingrong)

6. 巧通感冒鼻塞

6. A Clever Way to Relieve Nasal Congestion from Colds

感冒鼻子不通气，十分难受。

Nasal congestion during a cold is extremely uncomfortable.

你可以切下生葱的葱白约 3 厘米左右，再纵切一刀，然后将有黏性的切口贴在两个鼻孔之间，约十五分钟，鼻子即可通气。

You can cut off about 3 cm of fresh scallion white, make a longitudinal cut, and place the sticky cut surface between the nostrils; in about fifteen minutes, the nasal passages will open.

也可以用脱脂棉蘸取生葱汁，分别塞入鼻孔，效果比上述的方法还显著。

Alternatively, soak absorbent cotton in fresh scallion juice and insert it into each nostril separately; this method yields even more pronounced results than the one described above.

《民族医药报》

Ethnic Medicine News

7. 大蒜穴位揉按治感冒

7. Garlic Acupoint Massage for Treating Colds

取紫皮大蒜一至两枚切成片状，将大蒜片贴在百会、太阳、风池、合谷、迎香诸穴揉按五分钟；然后用大蒜片贴脚下涌泉穴揉按 15 分钟，便可防治感冒。

Take one or two cloves of purple-skinned garlic, slice them, apply the slices to the Baihui, Taiyang, Fengchi, Hegu, and Yingxiang acupoints, and massage for five minutes; then apply garlic slices to the Yongquan acupoint on the sole of the foot and massage for 15 minutes to prevent and treat colds.

此法对感冒初期效果甚佳。

This method is highly effective in the early stage of a cold.

重感冒应配合吃药。

For severe colds, medication should be used in conjunction.

揉按后穴位表面皮肤形成大蒜薄膜，应保持四小时再洗净。

After massage, a thin film of garlic forms on the skin over the acupoints; leave it on for four hours before washing off.

此方法防治感冒效果明显，简便易掌握。

This method is obviously effective in preventing and treating colds, and is simple and easy to master.

《民族医药报》1991 年 11 月 5 日（董寿琪）

Ethnic Medicine News, November 5, 1991 (Dong Shouqi)

8. 取大蒜适量捣烂取汁，加 10 倍冷开水，滴鼻，一日 3 次，每次二、三滴，连用 3 天，有预防和治疗感冒功效。

8. Take an appropriate amount of garlic, mash it to extract the juice, dilute with ten times cooled boiled water, and instill into the nose three times daily, 2–3 drops each time, for three consecutive days; this has preventive and therapeutic effects on colds.

若感冒后头痛鼻塞、恶寒发热，可用大蒜、葱白、生姜等量，煎汤温服，出汗即愈。

If a cold is accompanied by headache, nasal congestion, chills, and fever, decoct equal amounts of garlic, scallion white, and fresh ginger in water, drink the warm decoction, and recover upon sweating.

《中药科技报》1992 年 4 月 17 日（李明）

Chinese Materia Medica Science and Technology News, April 17, 1992 (Li Ming)

二、气管炎、哮喘（58 方）
II. Bronchitis and Asthma (58 Prescriptions)

1. 南杏仁 5 克，北杏仁 5 克，清水泡软去皮，粘米粉 50 克，加冰糖及清水适量煮成稠糊食用。

1.Soak 5g southern apricot kernels and 5g northern apricot kernels in water until soft, peel them, add 50g rice flour along with rock sugar and an appropriate amount of water, and cook into a thick paste for consumption.

每日 1 次，连服 10 日。

Take once daily for 10 consecutive days.

2. 柚子一个，去皮后切成块，鸡肉 500 克切成块，加清水适量，食盐调味，隔水炖熟。

2. Peel one pomelo and cut into pieces; cut 500g chicken meat into chunks, add an appropriate amount of water, season with salt, and double-boil until cooked.

饮汤吃鸡。

Drink the soup and eat the chicken.

每周 1 次。

Use once weekly.

3. 黑芝麻 2 匙（炒熟磨细），杏仁 10 克，生姜 3 片同煎。

3. Decoct 2 spoonfuls of black sesame seeds (roasted and ground fine), 10g apricot kernels, and 3 slices of fresh ginger together.

服时加适量蜂蜜饮下。

Add an appropriate amount of honey when drinking.

10 天为一疗程。

Ten days constitute one course of treatment.

4. 淮山药 60 克，捣烂加甘蔗汁半碗，放锅中隔水炖熟服食。

4. Mash 60g Chinese yam, add half a bowl of sugarcane juice, double-boil in

a pot until cooked, and consume.

每日 1 次，连服 10 日。

Take once daily for 10 consecutive days.

5. 白果仁、甜杏仁各 100 克，胡桃仁、花生仁各 200 克，共捣烂。

5. Mash together 100g each of ginkgo nuts and sweet apricot kernels, and 200g each of walnut kernels and peanut kernels.

每日早晨取 20 克，加水 1 小碗，煮开后打鸡蛋 1 个，冰糖适量，待鸡蛋煮熟后一次服。

Each morning, take 20g of the mixture, add a small bowl of water, bring to a boil, crack in one egg and add rock sugar to taste, and consume all at once after the egg is cooked.

连服 1 个月。

Take continuously for one month.

6. 百合、莲子各 30 克，冰糖适量，加水煎煮后服用。

6. Decoct 30g each of lily bulbs and lotus seeds with an appropriate amount of rock sugar in water, and take the decoction.

每日 1 次，连服 1 个月。

Take once daily for one consecutive month.

7. 红枣 20 枚，去皮南瓜 500 克，红糖适量，加水煮烂。

7. Boil 20 red dates, 500g peeled pumpkin, and an appropriate amount of brown sugar in water until mushy.

每日分两次服用，连服一周。

Divide into two servings daily for one consecutive week.

8. 糯米 15 克，杏仁、甘草各 10 克，水煎煮后滤汁，再溶入牛皮胶 15 克。

8. Decoct 15g glutinous rice, 10g apricot kernels, and 10g licorice root in water, strain the liquid, and dissolve 15g ox-hide gelatin into it.

每日分 2 次服用。 Take in two divided doses daily.

9. 将大白萝卜挖空一半，装进适量蜂蜜，放置 3 小时后，取汁用温开水冲服。

9. Hollow out half of a large white radish, fill with an appropriate amount of

honey, let stand for 3 hours, then mix the extracted juice with warm boiled water to drink.

每日 3 次，每次 1 汤匙。

Take three times daily, one tablespoon each time.

10. 雪梨一个去皮核，加川贝母粉 10 克同蒸。

10. Peel and core one snow pear, add 10g Fritillaria cirrhosa powder, and steam together.

睡前服食，连用 10 天。

Consume before bedtime for 10 consecutive days.

《中药科技报》1993 年 4 月 29 日（刘永连）

Chinese Materia Medica Science and Technology News, April 29, 1993 (Liu Yonglian)

11. 慢性支气管炎：苦菜 30 克。

11. Chronic bronchitis: Use 30g sow thistle.

开花期间，带根采集，水煎，每日 2 次，每次 1 剂，连服 30 天，疗效佳，且无副作用。

Collect the whole plant with roots during flowering, decoct in water, take one dose twice daily for 30 consecutive days; efficacy is good and there are no side effects.

《民族医药报》

Ethnic Medicine News

12. 青龙方组成及用法

12. Composition and Usage of Qinglong Formula

喘息期服汤剂：炙麻贵、杏仁、陈皮、制半夏、甘草各 10 克，金银花 30 克，柴胡、大青叶、茯苓各 12 克，葶苈子 15 克，地龙 6 克（瓦片焙黄研末）及琥珀末 4 克，分 2 次服。

During the wheezing phase, take a decoction: 10g each of honey-fried ephedra, apricot kernels, tangerine peel, prepared pinellia, and licorice root; 30g honeysuckle flower; 12g each of bupleurum, Isatis leaf, and poria; 15g Lepidium seed; 6g earthworm (roasted on a tile until yellow and ground into powder); and 4g amber powder; divide into two doses.

每日一剂，水煎麻黄去沫，纳入诸药同煎。

One dose per day; decoct ephedra in water first, skim off the foam, then add the remaining herbs and decoct together.

西药：扑尔敏 8 毫克及维生素 K4 8 毫克，一次服，日 2 次。

Western medicine: Chlorpheniramine 8 mg and Vitamin K4 8 mg, taken together twice daily.

加减法：白色稀痰量多加白芥子 15 克，黄痰量多加川青母：10 克。

Modifications: Add 15g white mustard seed if profuse thin white phlegm is present; add 10g Fritillaria cirrhosa if profuse yellow phlegm is present.

缓解期服散剂：蛤蚧、紫河车、白术各 100 克，生黄芪 150 克，阿胶、防风各 50 克。

During the remission phase, take a powdered formula: 100g each of gecko, human placenta, and Atractylodes macrocephala; 150g raw astragalus; and 50g each of donkey-hide gelatin and fangfeng.

研末，每服 6 克，日 3 次。

Grind into powder; take 6g per dose, three times daily.

30 天为一疗程，休 10 天后可服第二疗程。

Thirty days constitute one course of treatment; after a 10-day break, a second course may begin.

《中药科技报》1991 年 11 月 26 日

Chinese Materia Medica Science and Technology News, November 26, 1991

13. 支气管炎患者不妨一试

13. Worth Trying for Bronchitis Patients

我患有支气管炎多年，先后经几家医院中西医治疗，不见好转，后求得一特效方，用药三天后除根。

I suffered from bronchitis for many years and received both TCM and Western medical treatments at several hospitals without improvement; later I obtained a specially effective formula that eradicated the condition after three days of medication.

现介绍于下，不妨一试。

It is introduced below for your trial.

方药：白茯苓 6 克，川贝 6 克，杏仁 6 克，桑皮 6 克，甘草 6 克，五味子 6 克，京半夏 6 克，当归 6 克，陈皮 6 克。

Formula: 6g each of white poria, Fritillaria cirrhosa, apricot kernels, mulberry bark, licorice root, Schisandra fruit, processed pinellia, Angelica sinensis, and tangerine peel.

熬药时间和服药时间：第 1 剂，第 1 天下午 5 时煎煮，晚上 9 时服；第 2 剂，第 2 天晚上 9 时煎煮，第 3 天早上 7 时服，第 3 剂，第 4 天早上 7 时煎煮，中午 11 时服。

Decoction and administration schedule: First dose—decoct at 5 p.m. on Day 1 and take at 9 p.m.; second dose—decoct at 9 p.m. on Day 2 and take at 7 a.m. on Day 3; third dose—decoct at 7 a.m. on Day 4 and take at 11 a.m.

最后，3 剂药渣全部合在一起，第 5 天下午 5 时煎煮，晚上 9 时服下。

Finally, combine all the dregs from the three doses, decoct at 5 p.m. on Day 5, and take at 9 p.m.

每剂只煎煮 1 次，均加适量冰糖 1 次服下。

Each dose is decocted only once, with an appropriate amount of rock sugar added, and taken all at once.

无论病情轻重，3 剂服完后可病愈。

Regardless of severity, the illness can be cured after completing the three doses.

注意事项：服药期间，宜忌烟、酒、茶、盐、葱、姜、蒜、辣椒等辛辣食物。

Precautions: During medication, avoid tobacco, alcohol, tea, salt, scallions, ginger, garlic, chili peppers, and other pungent foods.

《民族医药报》1993 年 2 月 26 日（内蒙古 孙福）

Ethnic Medicine News, February 26, 1993 (Inner Mongolia, Sun Fu)

14. 五味子鸡蛋治疗慢性气管炎

14. Schisandra Eggs for Chronic Bronchitis

据临床观察，五味子鸡蛋治疗慢性气管炎有良好的效果，特推荐如下：制作时，取五味子 250 克，红皮鸡蛋 10 个。

Clinical observation indicates that Schisandra eggs have good efficacy in treating chronic bronchitis; the preparation is recommended as follows: Take 250g Schisandra fruit and 10 red-shelled eggs.

将五味子放入瓷器内；加水煮沸 30 分钟，待药液凉透，放入红皮鸡蛋，置阴湿处，浸泡 7 天，每日早晨取鸡蛋 1 个，煮熟后服食，10 天为 1 疗程。

Place the Schisandra fruit in a porcelain vessel, add water and boil for 30 minutes; after the liquid cools completely, add the red-shelled eggs, store in a cool, damp place, and soak for 7 days; each morning, take one egg, boil it, and consume it; ten days constitute one course of treatment.

《民族医药报》1998 年 4 月 3 日（戴廷荣）

Ethnic Medicine News, April 3, 1998 (Dai Tingrong)

15. 治久咳、久喘验方

15. Proven Formula for Chronic Cough and Asthma

取甜杏仁（炒）250 克，放在铝锅内，加水适量，煮沸 30 分钟，再加核桃仁 250 克，煎至快干时加蜂蜜 500 克，拌匀至沸即可起锅。

Take 250g roasted sweet apricot kernels, place in an aluminum pot, add an appropriate amount of water, boil for 30 minutes, then add 250g walnut kernels; when nearly dry, add 500g honey, stir evenly until boiling, and remove from heat.

每次服 1-2 汤匙，每日 3 次。

Take 1–2 tablespoons per dose, three times daily.

本品有补肾益肺，止咳平喘润燥之功。

This product tonifies the kidney and lung, relieves cough and asthma, and moistens dryness.

近来，笔者用其治疗肺肾两虚型久咳、久喘症 20 余例，效果显著。

Recently, the author used it to treat over 20 cases of chronic cough and asthma due to dual deficiency of lung and kidney, with remarkable results.

《中医药报》（钟久春）

Traditional Chinese Medicine News (Zhong Jiuchun)

16. 醋蛋治喘咳：

16. Vinegar Eggs for Asthma and Cough:

青皮鸭蛋 24 只，花椒 10 克，醋 1 公斤。

24green-shelled duck eggs, 10g Sichuan peppercorns, and 1 kg vinegar.

鸭蛋洗净置砂锅内加水煮熟，倒去沸水，打破蛋壳并用竹签在每只蛋上扎 5-7 个透孔，然后再放入醋、花椒于砂锅内加盖再煮 20 分钟即成。

Wash the duck eggs, place in a clay pot with water, and boil; discard the boiling water, crack the shells, pierce each egg with a bamboo skewer to make 5–7 holes through it, then return the eggs to the pot with vinegar and Sichuan peppercorns, cover, and simmer for another 20 minutes.

每日早晚各食 1 只醋蛋，12 天为一疗程，可连续服食，一般 2-3 个疗程可愈。

Eat one vinegar egg each morning and evening; twelve days constitute one course of treatment, which can be taken continuously; generally, 2–3 courses lead to cure.

病情较重者，可加倍进食醋蛋。

Patients with more severe conditions may double the intake.

该验方适用于慢性支气管炎和哮喘患者，具有良好的脱敏作用。

This proven formula is suitable for patients with chronic bronchitis and asthma and has a good desensitization effect.

此方远期疗效好，复发率低。

It offers good long-term efficacy and a low recurrence rate.

《民族医药报》1992 年 3 月 20 日

Ethnic Medicine News, March 20, 1992

17. 主治：急性支气管炎。

17. Indication: Acute bronchitis.

方药：鲜萝卜汁 250 毫升、白糖 30 克。

Formula: 250 ml fresh radish juice and 30g white sugar.

用法：将萝卜汁与白糖炖热烊化，日服二次，每次服 20 毫升。

Usage: Stew the radish juice with white sugar until dissolved; take twice daily, 20 ml each time.

《民族医药报》1992 年 6 月 5 日

Ethnic Medicine News, June 5, 1992

18. 治气管炎方： 18. Formula for Bronchitis:

栀子 6 克、桃仁 6 克、杏仁 6 克、白胡椒 4 克、姜末 7 粒，五味共研成细末，用 2 个鸡蛋清调和后摊在纱布上，然后敷足底涌泉穴上（男左女右）。

Grind 6g gardenia fruit, 6g peach kernel, 6g apricot kernel, 4g white pepper, and 7grains of ginger powder into a fine powder; mix with the whites of two eggs, spread onto gauze, and apply to the Yongquan acupoint on the sole (left foot for males, right for females).

每日一换，治疗期间忌烟酒。

Change daily; abstain from tobacco and alcohol during treatment.

《民族医药报》（广东 林伟）

Ethnic Medicine News (Guangdong, Lin Wei)

19. 姜汁浸衣治哮喘

19. Ginger Juice-Soaked Clothing for Asthma

入冬以后，气候日渐转冷。

After entering winter, the weather grows increasingly cold.

患有哮喘的病人，由于寒气逼人而气喘吁吁，服药治疗又不见疗效或只能暂时解喘，故常为此痛苦异常。

Asthma patients often suffer greatly from panting caused by biting cold, as medication either fails or provides only temporary relief.

下面介绍的姜汁浸衣疗法，也许能令上述患者转忧为喜。

The ginger juice-soaked clothing therapy described below may bring joy to such patients.

取生姜一公斤左右捣碎滤汁，做一件合身的纱布内衣，用滤出的姜汁将内衣浸透，并在烈日下晒干。

Mash about one kilogram of fresh ginger and strain the juice; make a well-fitting gauze undershirt, soak it thoroughly in the ginger juice, and dry it in the blazing sun.

然后给患者贴身穿上，每隔九天换次姜汁浸衣。

Then have the patient wear it next to the skin, replacing the ginger-soaked garment every nine days.

一般患者穿三至四次后均可见效。

Most patients see improvement after wearing it three to four times.

病情较重，患病多年的老哮喘病人，则要穿八至九次甚或两个冬天方可收到显著疗效。

For patients with severe, long-standing asthma, eight to nine applications—or even two winters—may be required for significant results.

生姜味辛性温，具有发表散寒、化痰止咳、温卫固表的功能。

Fresh ginger is pungent and warm in nature, with functions of releasing the exterior, dispelling cold, transforming phlegm, relieving cough, warming the defensive qi, and securing the exterior.

食用或入药可治风寒感冒、痰盛咳喘。

Consumed as food or used medicinally, it treats wind-cold colds and cough/asthma with abundant phlegm.

又因生姜含有较丰富的挥发油，其主要成分是姜辣素、姜醇、姜烯等，当患者穿上姜汁衣后，衣服上的姜汁成分透过皮肤作用于人体，能兴奋运动中枢和呼吸中枢神经，使胸腔、背部及上呼吸道的血管扩张，促使血液循环加快，以达到祛寒、化痰定喘之功效。

Moreover, fresh ginger contains abundant volatile oils whose main components include gingerol, zingerone, and zingiberene; when patients wear the ginger-soaked garment, these constituents penetrate the skin, stimulate the motor and respiratory centers, dilate blood vessels in the thorax, back, and upper respiratory tract, and accelerate blood circulation, thereby achieving the effects of dispelling cold, transforming phlegm, and calming asthma.

《民族医药报》1993 年 1 月 1 日（安徽 朱晨荐）

Ethnic Medicine News, January 1, 1993 (Anhui, Recommended by Zhu Chen)

20. 治哮喘验方一则

20. A Proven Formula for Asthma

取用优质生姜 120 克，芝麻 250 克，冰糖、蜂蜜各 125 克。

Take 120g high-quality fresh ginger, 250g sesame seeds, and 125g each of rock sugar and honey.

先将生姜捣烂取汁，然后将芝麻洗净浸放入姜汁内，置于锅中用文火炒熟，出锅冷却，再将冰糖与蜂蜜一同溶化后加入姜汁、芝麻中搅拌均匀，置于容器备用。

First mash the ginger to extract its juice; wash the sesame seeds and soak them in the ginger juice, then stir-fry in a pan over gentle heat until cooked; after cooling, melt the rock sugar and honey together, mix evenly with the ginger juice and sesame seeds, and store in a container for use.

每天早起、晚睡前各服一汤匙，连续服用一周，病情便可明显减轻；病情严重者，可多服用几日，其疗效很好。

Take one tablespoon each morning upon rising and at bedtime; continuous use for one week significantly alleviates symptoms; severely affected patients may continue for additional days with excellent efficacy.

患哮喘病的读者不妨用此方一试。

Readers suffering from asthma are encouraged to try this formula.

《中医药信息报》1993 年 4 月 10 日（樊常宝）

TCM Information News, April 10, 1993 (Fan Changbao)

21. 向日葵治慢性支气管炎、哮喘、肺气肿。

21. Sunflower for Chronic Bronchitis, Asthma, and Pulmonary Emphysema.

菊科植物向日葵，我国大部分地区有分布。

The Compositae plant sunflower is distributed across most regions of China.

我们根据山西代县民间经验，用垂手可得的植物向日葵的花盘熬制成流浸膏治疗上述三大病症，结果有效率分别为：慢支 86%，哮喘 72%，肺气肿 34%；临床控制率分别为 74%，53%，15%。

Based on folk experience from Daixian, Shanxi, we prepared a fluid extract from readily available sunflower heads to treat the above three conditions; the effective rates were 86% for chronic bronchitis, 72% for asthma, and 34% for pulmonary emphysema; clinical control rates were 74%, 53%, and 15%, respectively.

《民族医药报》

Ethnic Medicine News

22. 膻中穴割治治疗咳喘有效

22. Incision Therapy at Tanzhong Acupoint Effective for Cough and Asthma

治疗方法：病人仰卧，膻中穴常规消毒后用 2% 普鲁卡因肾上腺素作局麻，用手术刀沿胸正中线方向切开皮肤及皮下组织，深及骨膜，切口长度约 1cm，然后用蚊式钳伸进切口，来回划动或作圆周样划动刺激骨膜，约 1 分钟左右，刺激强度以病人局部有胀痛感并向四周扩散为好。

Method: With the patient supine, routinely disinfect the Tanzhong acupoint and administer local anesthesia with 2% procaine-adrenaline; use a scalpel to incise the skin and subcutaneous tissue along the anterior median line down to the periosteum, with an incision length of about 1 cm; then insert mosquito forceps into the incision and move back-and-forth or in circular motions to stimulate the periosteum for approximately one minute, with optimal stimulation intensity producing local distending pain radiating outward.

刺激完后，盖以消毒纱布，胶布固定，3-5 天后伤口愈合，即可取下纱布。

After stimulation, cover with sterile gauze and secure with adhesive tape; the wound heals in 3–5 days, after which the gauze can be removed.

一周后可作第二次治疗，切口可在原切口上下或左右少许。

A second treatment may be performed one week later, with the new incision slightly above, below, left, or right of the original.

临床对 52 例观察结果，基本痊愈 14 人（其中哮喘 8 人，支气管炎 6 人）

有效 28 人（其中哮喘 15 人，支气管炎 13 人）无效 10 人（其中哮喘 6 人，支气管炎 4 人）。

Clinical observation of 52 cases showed basic recovery in 14 patients (8 asthma, 6 bronchitis), improvement in 28 (15 asthma, 13 bronchitis), and no response in 10 (6 asthma, 4 bronchitis).

同时表明，病程短者疗效较好，而病程 10 年以上治愈机会较小。

Results also indicate better efficacy in shorter disease duration, while cure is less likely when the course exceeds ten years.

实践证明，此法治疗咳喘之疗效确实较好，同手部割治，背部俞穴及定喘穴埋线等方法比较，效果更为满意。

Practice proves this method genuinely effective for cough and asthma, yielding more satisfactory results compared to hand incision therapy or catgut embedding at back-Shu and Dingchuan points.

《中医药信息报》1992 年 8 月 1 日（山西 韩万明）

TCM Information News, August 1, 1992 (Shanxi, Han Wanming)

23. 蜂蜜治小儿咳喘

23. Honey for Pediatric Cough and Asthma

小儿咳喘可取生蜂蜜 250 克，净锅烧热后先倒一点香油，油热后再倒入蜂蜜慢火熬煮。

For pediatric cough and asthma, take 250g raw honey; heat a clean pan, pour in a little sesame oil, and once hot, add the honey and simmer over low heat.

当蜂蜜热到膨胀起来时，可用扇子扇的办法降低液面温度，继续熬数分钟即可盛起咳装瓶备用。

When the honey expands from heating, fan the surface to lower its temperature, continue simmering for a few minutes, then transfer to bottles for storage.

每日服 3 至 4 次，每次 1 汤匙，温开水冲服，连续用 7 ~ 10 天就可见效。

Take 3–4 times daily, one tablespoon each time mixed with warm boiled water; effects appear after 7–10 consecutive days.

另外，柿饼 3 个，煮水 1 碗，冲蜂蜜频服也有一定效果。

Additionally, boiling three dried persimmons in one bowl of water and mixing with honey for frequent drinking also yields some benefit.

《民族医药报》1992 年 2 月 28 日（贵州 杨通福）

Ethnic Medicine News, February 28, 1992 (Guizhou, Yang Tongfu)

24. 缓解幼儿哮喘妙方

24. A Simple Remedy to Relieve Infantile Asthma

美国夏威夷大学医学院腊斯兰克博士介绍了一种简便的缓解哮喘的方法：哮喘发作时，让婴儿安静地、松弛地坐起，然后喝水，以喝热开水为宜，水温以不烫口为限，喝至身上发热后，哮喘可很快缓解，对 90% 的患者有效。

Dr. Raslanke of the University of Hawaii School of Medicine introduced a simple asthma-relief method: during an attack, seat the infant calmly and relaxedly, then give water—preferably hot boiled water at a temperature tolerable to the mouth—until the body feels warm; asthma often resolves quickly, effective in 90% of patients.

此法对成人哮喘也有一定缓解的作用。

This method also provides some relief for adult asthma.

《中医药信息报》（仰占）

TCM Information News (Yang Zhan)

25. 治喘方

25. Formula for Asthma

蛤蚧一对、半夏 30 克、杏仁 30 克、瓜蒌 60 克、白人参 15 克、青皮 9 克、干姜 30 克、阿胶 15 克。

One pair of geckos, 30g pinellia, 30g apricot kernels, 60g Trichosanthes fruit, 15g white ginseng, 9g green tangerine peel, 30g dried ginger, and 15g donkey-hide gelatin.

制成粉末，加蜜调匀，制成丸剂，每丸 6 克，每日早晚各服两丸、温开水送下。

Grind into powder, mix evenly with honey, form pills of 6g each; take two pills twice daily (morning and evening) with warm boiled water.

《中医药信息报》1997 年 1 月 3 日（陆生）

TCM Information News, January 3, 1997 (Lu Sheng)

老年人咳喘治疗

Treatment of Cough and Asthma in the Elderly

26. 冰糖 500 克、陈醋 500 毫升。

26. Combine 500g rock sugar and 500 ml aged vinegar.

将冰糖和醋置锅内，加热至沸，待糖全部溶化后取出，凉后装瓶备用。

Place in a pot, heat to boiling until the sugar fully dissolves, remove from heat, cool, and bottle for use.

一次服 10 毫升，一日 2 次。

Take 10 ml per dose, twice daily.

适用于肺热型咳嗽。

Suitable for lung-heat type cough.

27. 黑芝麻 30 克、红糖 15 克。

27. Use 30g black sesame seeds and 15g brown sugar.

先将黑芝麻炒至焦黄，捣成泥加入红糖搅拌，使红糖溶化后，倒入碗内冷后服用。

Roast the sesame seeds until scorched-yellow, mash into a paste, add brown sugar and stir until dissolved, pour into a bowl, cool, and consume.

一次服 6 克，一日 3 次。

Take 6g per dose, three times daily.

适应于肺肾气虚型咳喘。

Suitable for lung-kidney qi-deficiency type cough and asthma.

28. 嫩公鸡一只（约 500 克）、鲢鱼 500 克。

28. Use one young rooster (~500g) and 500g silver carp.

将嫩公鸡退净毛，开膛除去五脏洗净备用。

Pluck the rooster clean, gut it, wash, and set aside.

将鲢鱼开膛洗净与洗净公鸡加水清炖至烂后，吃肉喝汤，2-3 日服完。

Gut and wash the fish, then double-boil together with the rooster in water until tender; eat the meat and drink the broth, finishing within 2–3 days.

适应于寒型咳嗽。

Suitable for cold-type cough.

29. 香蕉 1-2 条，冰糖 10 克。

29. Use 1–2 bananas and 10g rock sugar.

香蕉去皮与冰糖加水 10 毫升炖煮。

Peel the bananas and stew with rock sugar and 10 ml water.

顿服，一日 1-2 次，连服数日。

Consume all at once, 1–2 times daily for several consecutive days.

适应于阴虚久咳。

Suitable for yin-deficiency chronic cough.

30. 柿饼 1 个、川贝粉 9 克。

30. Use one dried persimmon and 9g Fritillaria cirrhosa powder.

将柿饼去核与川贝粉置锅内，加水少许煮熟。

Remove the persimmon’s seeds, place with the powder in a pot, add a little water, and cook until done.

冷后药、水一同服下，一日 1 次，连服数日。

Cool and consume both the solids and liquid together once daily for several consecutive days.

用于风热咳嗽。

Used for wind-heat cough.

31. 大雪梨一个、川贝粉 9 克、冰糖或蜜 10 克。

31. Use one large snow pear, 9g Fritillaria cirrhosa powder, and 10g rock sugar or honey.

将梨挖去核，将川贝粉、冰糖和蜜装入，加水适量，加热炖 1 小时即可。

Core the pear, fill with the powder and sugar/honey, add an appropriate amount of water, and stew for one hour.

冷后顿服，一日 1 次，连服数日。

Cool and consume all at once daily for several consecutive days.

适应肺热阴虚型咳喘。

Suitable for lung-heat with yin-deficiency type cough and asthma.

32. 鸡蛋 2 个、冰糖 50 个。

32. Use 2 eggs and 50g rock sugar.

将冰糖置锅内加水 500 毫升，加热煮沸至糖溶化即可取出待冷后将鸡蛋去壳与冰糖溶液搅匀，置锅内蒸熟，加芝麻油数滴。

Boil rock sugar in 500 ml water until dissolved, remove and cool; shell the eggs, mix with the sugar solution, steam until cooked, and add a few drops of sesame oil.

顿服，一日 1 次，连服数日。

Consume all at once daily for several consecutive days.

用于干咳少痰。

Used for dry cough with scanty sputum.

33. 鸡蛋 2 个、陈醋 50 克。

33. Use 2 eggs and 50g aged vinegar.

将鸡蛋去壳加水 500 毫升，加入陈醋搅匀熬熟稍冷后顿服，一日 1 次，连服数日。

Shell the eggs, add 500 ml water and aged vinegar, stir, cook until done, cool slightly, and consume all at once daily for several consecutive days.

用于久嗽不止。

Used for persistent chronic cough.

34. 猪肺一具、萝卜 1 个、杏仁 10 克。

34. Use one pig lung, one radish, and 10g apricot kernels.

将猪肺洗净、萝卜洗净切片，加入杏仁，加水共煮烂。

Wash the pig lung, wash and slice the radish, add apricot kernels, and boil together in water until tender.

2-3 天服完，用于久咳不止。

Finish within 2–3 days; used for persistent chronic cough.

35. 猪瘦肉 100 克、玉竹 30 克。

35. Use 100g lean pork and 30g Polygonatum odoratum.

将猪瘦肉洗净切块与玉竹同入锅内加水煮烂，调味后吃肉喝汤。

Wash and cube the pork, cook with Polygonatum in water until tender, season, and consume meat and broth.

顿服，一日 1 次，连续数日。

Consume all at once daily for several consecutive days.

用于干咳。

Used for dry cough.

36. 生姜 120 克、红糖 120 克、核桃仁 120 克。

36. Use 120g fresh ginger, 120g brown sugar, and 120g walnut kernels.

将生姜洗净切片与红糖、核桃仁一同捣如泥。

Wash and slice the ginger, then mash together with brown sugar and walnuts into a paste.

一次服 10 克，1 日 2-3 次。

Take 10g per dose, 2–3 times daily.

用于寒咳，痰多稀薄。

Used for cold cough with copious thin sputum.

《中药科技报》1992 年 5 月 26 日（山东 孙寿芳）

Chinese Materia Medica Science and Technology News, May 26, 1992 (Shandong, Sun Shoufang)

37. 治肺气肿方

37. Formula for Pulmonary Emphysema

主治：慢性支气管炎所致的肺气肿，症见咳嗽，咳痰，气短乏力

Indication: Pulmonary emphysema due to chronic bronchitis presenting with cough, expectoration, shortness of breath, and fatigue.

组成：黄豆芽，猪脚

Composition: Soybean sprouts and pig trotters.

用法：共文火煎服，长期服用有显效，能温补虚寒之肺。

Usage: Simmer together over gentle heat and consume; long-term use yields marked effects by warmly tonifying a deficient-cold lung.

《民族医药报》

Ethnic Medicine News

38. 慢性肺心病气喘血淤：

38. Panting and Blood Stasis in Chronic Cor Pulmonale:

狗肺，羊肺各一具晒干，土鳖虫120克（瓦片焙黄），共研成粉末，每次服6克，日3次。

Sun-dry one dog lung and one sheep lung, roast 120g ground beetles on a tile until yellow, grind all into powder; take 6g per dose, three times daily.

39. 哮喘：地龙200克，蛤蚧一对，瓦片培黄存性，共研成细末。

39. Asthma: Roast 200g earthworms and one pair of geckos on a tile until charred externally but retaining internal properties, then grind into fine powder.

每服6克，日3次，黄酒引。

Take 6g per dose, three times daily, with yellow wine as a vehicle.

本方治肺肾热喘有显效，临床治疗12例，均有良效。

This formula is markedly effective for lung-kidney heat-type asthma; all 12 treated cases responded well.

《中药科技报》1992年3月26日

Chinese Materia Medica Science and Technology News, March 26, 1992

40. 治寒性喘咳痰多：炒苏子、妙白芥子、炒葶苈子、炙麻黄各15克，共研末，每服3克，日3次，连服3天。

40. For cold-type asthma/cough with copious sputum: Grind 15g each of roasted Perilla seed, stir-fried white mustard seed, roasted Lepidium seed, and honey-fried ephedra into powder; take 3g per dose, three times daily for three consecutive days.

本方治急性支气管炎及慢性支气管炎急性发作有良效。

This formula is effective for acute bronchitis and acute exacerbations of chronic bronchitis.

41. 冬桑叶15克，杏仁12克，水煎取汁，加蜂蜜一匙温服。

41. Decoct 15g winter mulberry leaf and 12g apricot kernels in water, strain, add one spoonful of honey, and drink warm.

每日一剂，连服三日。

One dose daily for three consecutive days.

适用于风热伤肺，咳嗽，咽部不舒者。

Suitable for wind-heat injuring the lung with cough and throat discomfort.

42. 细辛 6 克，杏仁 15 克，生姜 6 克，水煎温服。

42. Decoct 6g Asarum, 15g apricot kernels, and 6g fresh ginger in water, and drink warm.

每日一剂，连用二日。

One dose daily for two consecutive days.

用于肺寒咳嗽，效果良好。

Effective for lung-cold cough.

43. 冬桑叶，炙杷叶各 10 克，麦门冬 15 克，水煎取汁，加入冰糖 10 克，溶化服之。

43. Decoct 10g each of winter mulberry leaf and honey-fried loquat leaf plus 15g Ophiopogon tuber in water, strain, dissolve 10g rock sugar, and drink.

每日一剂，连用二、三日。

One dose daily for two to three consecutive days.

适用于燥热咳嗽。

Suitable for dry-heat cough.

44. 黄芩 10 克，瓜蒌 30 克，胆南星 6 克，水煎服，每日一剂，连用二、三日。

44. Decoct 10g Scutellaria root, 30g Trichosanthes fruit, and 6g bile arisaema in water; one dose daily for two to three consecutive days.

适用于痰热壅肺，咳嗽，咯吐黄痰不利者。

Suitable for phlegm-heat obstructing the lung with cough and difficult expectoration of yellow sputum.

45. 炙百部 100 克，水煎取汁，加入蜂蜜 50 克，熬成稀膏。

45. Decoct 100g honey-fried Stemona root in water, strain, add 50g honey,

and reduce to a thin syrup.

每次一匙，日二次，治愈为度。

Take one spoonful twice daily until cured.

适用于年久咳嗽痰少者。

Suitable for longstanding cough with scanty sputum.

46. 大梨一只，将顶端开一小洞，去核，加入川贝粉 5 克，冰糖适量。

46. Cut a small hole at the top of a large pear, core it, add 5g Fritillaria cirrhosa powder and rock sugar to taste.

放碗中蒸约一小时后，梨肉和药汁一并食之。

Steam in a bowl for about one hour, then eat both flesh and medicinal juice.

早晚各一次，连食七日。

Once in the morning and once at night for seven consecutive days.

适用于阴虚咳嗽，痰少咯吐不爽者。

Suitable for yin-deficiency cough with scanty, hard-to-expectorate sputum.

47. 将白萝卜去皮捣烂，压取汁，每用 30 毫升，加白糖 10 克化服。

47. Peel and mash white radish, press to obtain juice; take 30 ml mixed with 10g white sugar dissolved in it.

每日早晚各一次，连服三日。

Twice daily (morning and evening) for three consecutive days.

适用于咳嗽音哑，胸闷胃胀，饮食欠佳者。

Suitable for hoarse cough, chest tightness, gastric distension, and poor appetite.

48. 款冬花 10 克，用沸滚开水冲泡，代茶饮之，连用五日。

48. Steep 10g coltsfoot flower in boiling water and drink as tea for five consecutive days.

对慢性咳嗽，胸脘微闷，饮食欠佳者效佳。

Highly effective for chronic cough with mild chest/epigastric stuffiness and poor appetite.

49. 青黛 3 克，炙杏仁 6 克。

49. Use 3g indigo naturalis and 6g honey-fried apricot kernels.

二者共研细末，用白茅根 30 克煎水送服，每日二次。

Grind together into fine powder and swallow with a decoction of 30g Imperata rhizome twice daily.

对肝火犯肺，咳嗽痰中带血者，效果良好。

Effective for liver-fire invading the lung with blood-streaked sputum.

50. 罂粟壳(捣碎)3 克，用沸开水冲泡十五分钟后，调入蜂蜜一匙，代茶饮之，连用三、五日。

50. Steep 3g crushed poppy husk in boiling water for fifteen minutes, add one spoonful of honey, and drink as tea for three to five consecutive days.

适用于干咳日久不愈者。

Suitable for prolonged dry cough.

《中药科技报》1992 年 1 月 26 日（甘肃 良辰）

Chinese Materia Medica Science and Technology News, January 26, 1992 (Gansu, Liangchen)

51. 肾虚喘咳：核桃仁 500 克、五味子 100 克研成细末，每次服 6 克，日 3 次。

51. Kidney-deficiency asthma/cough: Grind 500g walnut kernels and 100g Schisandra fruit into fine powder; take 6g per dose, three times daily.

治 22 例均有显著疗效。

All 22 treated cases showed significant efficacy.

本方具有补肾益肺，平喘止咳祛痰作用，长期服用无副作用。

This formula tonifies the kidney and lung, calms asthma, relieves cough, and expels phlegm; long-term use has no side effects.

52. 治咽痒咳嗽：将 3 厘米见方的麝香止痛膏贴于天突穴位，一天见效。

52. For itchy-throat cough: Apply a 3 cm square musk analgesic plaster to the Tiantu acupoint; relief occurs within one day.

53. 肺虚久咳痰多：葶苈子、苦杏仁、白果仁各 250 克，研成粉末，加冰糖适量，每次服 6 克，日 3 次。

53. Lung-deficiency chronic cough with copious sputum: Grind 250g each of

Lepidium seed, bitter apricot kernel, and ginkgo nut into powder, add rock sugar to taste; take 6g per dose, three times daily.

54. 治小儿咳嗽方

54. Formula for Pediatric Cough

小儿感冒容易引起咳嗽，咳嗽时出现干咳无痰，或痰稀白色，有的浓稠，咽喉发痒，夜间咳嗽尤甚等症状。

Colds in children easily trigger cough, manifesting as dry cough without sputum, or thin white or thick sputum, itchy throat, and especially nocturnal worsening.

用下列小方治之，能获良效。

The following simple formula achieves good results.

红皮大蒜 1 个，去粗皮取其肉质盛在碗里，然后在蒜表面放两汤匙白砂糖，蒸熟为度，温热 1 次服下。

Take one red-skinned garlic clove, peel off the coarse skin, place the flesh in a bowl, sprinkle two tablespoons of white sugar on top, steam until cooked, and consume warm in one sitting.

接着服鱼腥陈皮汤：鲜鱼腥草 20 克，白茅根 50 克，陈皮 10 克，鲜枇杷叶 3 片（洗净去绒毛）鲜笔简草 20 克，生姜 3 片，每天 1 剂，连服 3 天，咳嗽痊愈。

Then take Houttuynia-Tangerine Peel Decoction: 20g fresh Houttuynia, 50g Imperata rhizome, 10g tangerine peel, 3 fresh loquat leaves (washed and dehaired), 20g fresh Equisetum, and 3 slices fresh ginger; one dose daily for three consecutive days leads to full recovery.

《民族医药报》1992 年 4 月 24 日（湖南 戴厚高）

Ethnic Medicine News, April 24, 1992 (Hunan, Dai Houga o)

55. 小偏方治咳嗽

55. A Small Folk Remedy for Cough

某君感冒后剧咳不止，久治不愈。

A certain person had relentless severe cough after a cold that failed to respond to prolonged treatment.

有位熟人给他介绍了一个单方，服一剂后就奇迹般好了。

An acquaintance recommended a single-herb formula, and miraculously he recovered after one dose.

这个方子是：用杏仁 100 克，化猪油 50 克、冰糖 100 克，将杏仁浸泡去皮捣细，在铁锅内加猪油炒成黄色再加入冰糖，冰糖化完拌匀即起锅。

The formula: Soak 100g apricot kernels, peel, mash finely; stir-fry in an iron pan with 50g rendered lard until yellow, add 100g rock sugar, stir until melted and well mixed, then remove from heat.

此剂日服 3 次，每次服指头大 1 颗，服完便好。

Take three times daily, one fingertip-sized piece each time; completion brings cure.

《民族医药报》（河池市白土乡 蓝芳 辑）

Ethnic Medicine News (Compiled by Lan Fang, Baitu Township, Hechi City)

56. 取捣烂后的独头生大蒜约豆瓣大一团，放于伤湿止痛膏或麝香虎骨膏的中心处，每晚洗脚后，先在双足涌泉穴周围涂上凡士林或猪油，以防起泡。

56. Mash a single-clove raw garlic into a bean-sized lump, place at the center of a dampness-relieving analgesic plaster or musk-tiger-bone plaster; after washing feet each night, first apply Vaseline or lard around the Yongquan acupoints on both soles to prevent blistering.

然后贴上放有蒜泥的膏药，第二天早晨揭去，连贴 3-5 次。

Then apply the plaster with garlic paste and remove the next morning; repeat for 3–5 consecutive nights.

此方对多种咳嗽、特别是夜间剧烈咳嗽均有良好疗效，大多数人 3-5 次即愈。

This formula is effective for various coughs, especially severe nocturnal ones; most people recover within 3–5 applications.

《民族医药报》1991 年 11 月 5 日（云南 朱明富）

Ethnic Medicine News, November 5, 1991 (Yunnan, Zhu Mingfu)

57. 干咳久治不愈，有碍工作与睡眠。

57. Persistent dry cough impairs work and sleep.

根据中医理论，此症多属肺气浮散干咳难愈。

According to TCM theory, this condition mostly stems from floating-scattering lung qi causing refractory dry cough.

可用：乌梅 9 克、百合 12 克、五味子 6 克、紫菀 9 克、诃子肉 9 克、甘草 5 克，水煎服日一剂。

Use: 9g mume fruit, 12g lily bulb, 6g Schisandra fruit, 9g aster root, 9g Terminalia chebula flesh, and 5g licorice root; decoct in water, one dose daily.

小儿用量酌减。

Reduce dosage appropriately for children.

《民族医药报》1992 年 8 月 28 日（广西百色 李树贞）

Ethnic Medicine News, August 28, 1992 (Baise, Guangxi, Li Shuzhen)

58. 取大蒜 30 克，去皮，磨碎，加入凉开水，用小麦面粉混合搅拌成泥糊状，再将这种黏稠的泥状物涂抹在纱布上，并另外拿一块纱布覆盖其表面，使其不与皮肤直接接触地敷在胸口上，一日一换。

58. Peel and grind 30g garlic, add cooled boiled water and wheat flour, mix into a thick paste; spread onto gauze, cover with another layer of gauze to avoid direct skin contact, and apply to the chest; change daily.

临床证明，蒜泥外敷对久咳不愈的咳嗽有较好的止咳效果，并具有见效快、无副作用的特点，劝君不妨试试。

Clinically proven, external application of garlic paste effectively stops persistent cough, acts quickly, and has no side effects—you are encouraged to try it.

《中医药信息报》1991 年 7 月 13 日（戴廷荣）

TCM Information News, July 13, 1991 (Dai Tingrong)

三、百日咳（18 方）

III. Pertussis (Whooping Cough) (18 Prescriptions)

1. 百日咳又称“顿咳”“疫咳”，为 5 岁以下小儿常见的急性呼吸道传染病。

1.Pertussis, also called “paroxysmal cough” or “epidemic cough,” is a common acute respiratory infectious disease in children under five.

易感于冬春之际，患者以阵发性痉挛性咳嗽、痉咳后鸡鸣样深吸气吼声为主要特征。

It is prevalent in winter and spring, characterized mainly by paroxysmal spasmodic cough followed by a crowing inspiratory whoop.

中医学认为本病系风邪疫疠之气由口鼻入肺，蕴伏肺系，肺气不宣，酿液成痰，痰阻气道，肺失宣降，肺气上逆而致“痉咳”。

TCM holds that the disease arises when wind-pathogen and pestilential qi enter the lung via mouth and nose, lodge in the lung system, impair lung diffusion, generate phlegm from fluids, obstruct airways, disrupt lung descent, and cause rebellious lung qi leading to "spasmodic cough."

笔者几年来用以下方法治疗小儿百日咳三十余例，皆获满意疗效。

Over several years, the author treated over thirty pediatric pertussis cases with the following method, all achieving satisfactory outcomes.

药物组成：活蟾蜍1只，干地龙、干蚱蜢、制半夏、川贝母各6克，制蜈蚣3克，牛黄米（牛苦胆浸泡谷米、阴干入药）12克。

Composition: One live toad; 6g each of dried earthworm, dried grasshopper, prepared pinellia, and Fritillaria cirrhosa; 3g processed centipede; and 12g Niuhuangmi (grain soaked in ox gallbladder and shade-dried).

制法：将蟾蜍开膛去内脏，然后把其余诸药填入腹内，细线缝合，焙干研极细末，高压蒸半小时，装瓶备用。

Preparation: Gut the toad, fill the cavity with the other herbs, sew closed with fine thread, roast dry, grind to ultrafine powder, steam under high pressure for half an hour, and bottle for use.

用法：1岁以下每次服0.5克，2岁以下服1克，3岁以下服1.5克，3岁以上服2克，每日3次。

Dosage: Under 1 year: 0.5g/dose; under 2 years: 1g; under 3 years: 1.5g; over 3 years: 2g; three times daily.

按：此方具祛风止痉、清肺涤痰、镇咳平喘之效。

Note: This formula dispels wind, stops spasms, clears the lung, sweeps phlegm, suppresses cough, and calms asthma.

一般服 3-5 天即可痊愈。

Recovery usually occurs within 3–5 days.

临床观察结果表明，对一些支气管哮喘患者亦可收到满意疗效。

Clinical observation also shows satisfactory efficacy in some bronchial asthma patients.

但值得注意的是：此方为祛风涤痰之峻剂，而小儿脏腑娇嫩，形气未充，故使用应中病即止，勿过剂量。

However, note that this is a potent formula for dispelling wind and sweeping phlegm; since children's viscera are delicate and their constitution immature, discontinue upon response and do not exceed the dosage.

《民族医药报》1992 年 4 月 3 日（广西 韦金星）

Ethnic Medicine News, April 3, 1992 (Guangxi, Wei Jinxing)

2. 取西瓜子 15 克，花生仁 16 克，梨 1 个切片，冰糖 30 克，水煎服。

2. Decoct 15g watermelon seeds, 16g peanut kernels, one sliced pear, and 30g rock sugar in water and drink.

每日 1 剂，连用 7-10 日为一疗程。

One dose daily; 7–10 consecutive days constitute one course.

3. 取桔饼 2 个，葱白 4 茎，冰糖 30 克，煮汤服食。

3. Boil two candied tangerine cakes, four scallion whites, and 30g rock sugar into a soup and consume.

4. 取荸荠 500 克，洗净取皮，切碎绞汁。

4. Wash 500g water chestnuts, peel, chop, and squeeze juice.

同蜂蜜 60 克混匀。

Mix evenly with 60g honey.

煮沸饮用。

Boil and drink.

每日 2 次。

Twice daily.

每次 1 小杯。

One small cup each time.

5. 取栗子仁 30 克，玉米须 6 克，冰糖 25 克，水煎服。

5. Decoct 30g chestnut kernels, 6g corn silk, and 25g rock sugar in water and drink.

每日 1 剂连用 10 日为一疗程。

One dose daily for 10 consecutive days as one course.

6. 取麻雀一只，拔去粗毛。

6. Pluck one sparrow.

在火上烤焦，去内脏，洗净炖服，治愈为止。

Char over fire, gut, wash, stew, and consume until cured.

7. 取白萝卜汁 30 毫升，白糖 1 匙，生姜汁 10 滴，冲入适量的开水搅匀，每天 3 次喝下。

7. Mix 30 ml white radish juice, one spoonful white sugar, and 10 drops ginger juice with an appropriate amount of hot water; drink three times daily.

8. 取胡萝卜 1000 克，洗净捣烂挤汁，煮开后加适量冰糖，每天 3 次，每次服 2 匙

8. Wash 1000g carrots, mash, squeeze juice, boil, add rock sugar to taste; take two spoonfuls three times daily.

9. 取鲜一箭球（水百足、三角草）100 克，糖适量，用水 2 碗煎至半碗，冲糖，分 3 次服。

9. Decoct 100g fresh Phyllanthus urinaria (Shuibaiizu/Sanjiaocao) in two bowls of water down to half a bowl, add sugar to taste, and divide into three doses.

10. 取鹅不食草 10 克，野甘草（冰糖草） 15 克，蜂窝草 20 克，天冬、百部各 25 克，水煎服，每日 2-3 次。

10. Decoct 10g Centipeda minima, 15g wild licorice (Bingtangcao), 20g Herba Lycopodii, and 25g each of Asparagus tuber and Stemona root in water; take 2–3 times daily.

《中药科技报》1990 年 12 月 26 日（刘永连）

Chinese Materia Medica Science and Technology News, December 26, 1990 (Liu Yonglian)

11. 鸡胆具有清热、祛痰、熄风、镇咳的功能，因此可用于治疗百日咳。

11. Chicken gallbladder clears heat, expels phlegm, extinguishes wind, and suppresses cough, hence useful for pertussis.

方法如下：取鲜鸡胆 5 只、蜂蜜 100 毫升，置于碗中，用文火炖 15 分钟。

Method: Place five fresh chicken gallbladders and 100 ml honey in a bowl, and stew over gentle heat for 15 minutes.

服用时，每次 5 毫升，每日 4-5 次，一般用药 5-7 天见效。

Take 5 ml per dose, 4–5 times daily; effects generally appear within 5–7 days.

《中医药信息报》1990 年 10 月 6 日（王飞马）

TCM Information News, October 6, 1990 (Wang Feima)

12. 马齿苋治疗百日咳。

12. Purslane for Pertussis.

马齿苋为民间治疗痢疾的有效草药。

Purslane is an effective folk herb for dysentery.

报道用于治疗百日咳患者，鲜品 200-300 克，水煎 2 次，浓缩至 100-150 毫升，每日 1 剂，分 3 次口服，7 日一疗程，总有效率为 93.3%。

Reported use for pertussis: Decoct 200–300g fresh purslane twice, concentrate to 100–150 ml; one dose daily divided into three oral doses; seven days per course; overall effective rate 93.3%.

13. 沙参 10 克，百部 12 克，杏仁、天冬，麦冬各 6 克，麻黄 3 克，五味子 2 克。

13. Use 10g Glehnia root, 12g Stemona root, 6g each of apricot kernel, Asparagus tuber, and Ophiopogon tuber, 3g ephedra, and 2g Schisandra fruit.

用法：上药加水 300 毫升，煎 15 分钟，待温后口服，每天 3 次。

Usage: Add 300 ml water, decoct for 15 minutes, cool to warm, and take orally three times daily.

1-3 岁每次口服 20-30 毫升，4-5 岁每次口服 40 毫升，6 岁每次口服 50 毫升。

Ages 1–3: 20–30 ml/dose; ages 4–5: 40 ml; age 6: 50 ml.

一般连服 3 剂可愈。

Generally curable after three consecutive doses.

14. 百部 30 克，白前 20 克，桔梗，法半夏各 10 克，川贝母 12 克，杏仁、沙参、炙桑皮、炙百合、葶苈子各 15 克，蜂蜜 100 克。

14. Use 30g Stemona root, 20g Cynanchum root, 10g each of Platycodon and processed pinellia, 12g Fritillaria cirrhosa, 15g each of apricot kernel, Glehnia root, honey-fried mulberry bark, honey-fried lily bulb, and Lepidium seed, plus 100g honey.

用法：初煎加水 800 毫升，浸 3 小时后，用文火煎 1 小时，取汁 250 毫升。

Usage: First decoction—add 800 ml water, soak 3 hours, simmer 1 hour, obtain 250 ml.

复煎加水 500 毫升，煎 1 小时，取汁 250 毫升，两煎共取汁 500 毫升，加入熟蜂蜜 100 克备用。

Second decoction—add 500 ml water, simmer 1 hour, obtain 250 ml; combine both decoctions to total 500 ml, add 100g prepared honey, and reserve.

每岁每次服 15 毫升，即 1 岁每次服 15 毫升，2 岁每次服 30 毫升，余类推。

Administer 15 ml per year of age per dose (e.g., 1-year-old: 15 ml; 2-year-old: 30 ml; etc.).

每隔 2-3 小时服药 1 次，日服 3-5 次。

Dose every 2–3 hours, 3–5 times daily.

取得较满意的疗效。

Satisfactory efficacy achieved.

15. 炙百部、鲜侧柏叶各 12 克，天竺黄、杏仁、前胡、葶苈子、甘草各 10 克，陈胆星、地龙各 6 克，鲜石胡荽 15 克，大枣 4 枚。

15. Use 12g each of honey-fried Stemona root and fresh Platycladus leaf; 10g each of bamboo silica, apricot kernel, Peucedanum root, Lepidium seed, and licorice root; 6g each of aged bile arisaema and earthworm; 15g fresh Centipeda

minima; and four jujubes.

咳而喘重者加炙麻黄 3 克，呕恶甚者加姜半夏 10 克，咳血者加炙紫菀 10 克，鼻衄者加白茅根 15 克，发热重者加生石膏（先煎）20 克。

If cough with severe wheezing, add 3g honey-fried ephedra; if severe nausea/vomiting, add 10g ginger-processed pinellia; if hemoptysis, add 10g honey-fried aster root; if epistaxis, add 15g Imperata rhizome; if high fever, add 20g raw gypsum (decoct first).

用法：每日 1 剂，水煎，分 3 次服。

Usage: One dose daily, decocted in water, divided into three servings.

疗效颇佳，一般连服 5-10 天可治愈。

Efficacy is excellent; cure generally occurs after 5–10 consecutive days.

16. 百部 50 克，杏仁、桔梗各 20 克。

16. Use 50g Stemona root and 20g each of apricot kernel and Platycodon.

用法：上药加水 700 毫升，煎至 350 毫升，滤出药渣，加入白糖 60 克，以文火将糖溶化，贮瓶备用。

Usage: Add 700 ml water, decoct to 350 ml, strain, add 60g white sugar, dissolve over gentle heat, and bottle.

日服 3 次，温开水冲服。

Take three times daily mixed with warm boiled water.

1 岁以下每次 2-4 毫升，1-3 岁每次 4-6 毫升，4-6 岁每次 7-9 毫升，7-9 岁每次 10-13 毫升，10 岁以上每次 15 毫升。

Under 1 year: 2–4 ml/dose; 1–3 years: 4–6 ml; 4–6 years: 7–9 ml; 7–9 years: 10–13 ml; over 10 years: 15 ml.

一般连服 5-10 天可痊愈。

Generally curable after 5–10 consecutive days.

17. 鲜茅根 15 克，大蒜 1 瓣，冰糖 1 块，川贝母、甘草各 3 克，炙百部、炙枇杷叶各 6 克。

17. Use 15g fresh Imperata rhizome, one garlic clove, one piece rock sugar, 3g each of Fritillaria cirrhosa and licorice root, and 6g each of honey-fried Stemona

root and honey-fried loquat leaf.

用法：上药水煎煮，待蒜熟后服汤食蒜。

Usage: Decoct in water; when garlic is cooked, drink the decoction and eat the garlic.

疗效显著，一般连服 3 剂可愈。

Markedly effective; generally curable after three consecutive doses.

《中药科技报》1992 年 2 月 26 日（李子云）

Chinese Materia Medica Science and Technology News, February 26, 1992 (Li Ziyun)

18. 活麻雀去毛和内脏后，将冰糖和麻雀放入碗内，放在锅中隔汤炖煮，煮开后 15 分钟，连汤水及雀肉一次吃完。

18. After plucking and gutting live sparrows, place them with rock sugar in a bowl, double-boil in a pot; after boiling for 15 minutes, consume broth and meat together in one sitting.

用量：周岁用麻雀 1 只冰糖 30 克；3-6 岁用麻雀 2-3 只，冰糖 30 克，连服 2 天，严重者可服 3 天，每天 1 次；7-12 岁用麻雀 4 只，冰糖 50 克，连服 3 天，每天一次，如常服，对慢性支气管炎也有一定的疗效。

Dosage: Age 1: one sparrow + 30g rock sugar; ages 3–6: 2–3 sparrows + 30g rock sugar, daily for 2 days (3 days if severe); ages 7–12: four sparrows + 50g rock sugar, daily for 3 days; regular use also benefits chronic bronchitis.

《民族医药报》1992 年 2 月 21 日（江苏 韦百胜）

Ethnic Medicine News, February 21, 1992 (Jiangsu, Wei Baisheng)

第二章 胃肠病
Chapter 2 Gastrointestinal Diseases

一、胃溃疡（18 方）
I. Gastric Ulcer (18 Prescriptions)

1. 海螵蛸 1000 克、大贝母 250 克、连翘 500 克、白芨 250 克、大黄 60 克、郁金 150 克、甘草 125 克。

1.Cuttlefish bone 1000g, Fritillaria thunbergii 250g, Forsythia fruit 500g, Bletilla rhizome 250g, Rhubarb 60g, Curcuma root 150g, Licorice root 125g.

共研为末、过 100 目筛、炼蜜为丸，每丸重 10 克，日服三次、每次 1 丸。

Grind all into powder, sift through a 100-mesh sieve, mix with refined honey to form pills weighing 10g each; take one pill three times daily.

7 天为一疗程。

Seven days constitute one course of treatment.

2. 一枝蒿 30 克（菜油炸酥）、何首乌（清水浸泡去涩味、再同黑豆同煮，去黑豆将何首乌晒干）100 克、炒黄豆 120 克。

2. Achillea wilsoniana 30g (deep-fried in rapeseed oil until crispy), Polygonum multiflorum 100g (soaked in water to remove astringency, boiled with black beans, then dried after removing the beans), Stir-fried soybeans 120g.

共研细末，每次服 6-10 克，日服二次，白开水送服。

Grind together into fine powder; take 6–10g per dose twice daily with plain boiled water.

3. 三七 100 克用鸡油煎炸酥、研末、蒸鸡蛋服，每次 10 克，一日二次。

3. Deep-fry 100g Panax notoginseng in chicken fat until crispy, grind into

powder, and steam with egg; take 10g per dose twice daily.

4. 三七、丹皮、天麻各等量，共为末，用煎好的菜油文火炒熟，每次服 6 克、日服二次。

4. Mix equal amounts of Panax notoginseng, Moutan bark, and Gastrodia tuber into powder; stir-fry in heated rapeseed oil over gentle heat until cooked; take 6g per dose twice daily.

以上四方经临床验证，具有消炎、止血、治酸、收敛、生肌，增进食欲之效，疗效颇佳。

Clinically verified, the above four formulas have excellent efficacy in reducing inflammation, stopping bleeding, neutralizing acid, promoting astringency, generating flesh, and improving appetite.

《民族医药报》1992 年 2 月 28 日（云南 柳克尊）

Ethnic Medicine News, February 28, 1992 (Yunnan, Liu Kezun)

5. 主治：胃溃疡所致的疼痛，呕吐泛酸，久治不愈者。

5. Indication: Pain caused by gastric ulcer, vomiting with acid regurgitation, refractory cases.

组成：蒲公英（全草）30 克。

Composition: Dandelion (whole plant) 30g.

用法：用水煎服，每日一剂，分早中晚三次服，每次加米酒一匙，连续服 8 天为一疗程。

Usage: Decoct in water, one dose daily divided into three servings (morning, noon, evening); add one spoonful of rice wine to each serving; eight consecutive days constitute one course.

6.Arora 和 Tandon 最近报道了维持胃酸缺乏的一种治医疗方案：甲氰咪胍 100mg/ h 静脉推注十持续鼻胃灌注解酸药。

6. Arora and Tandon recently reported a therapeutic regimen for maintaining gastric acid suppression: Cimetidine 100 mg/h IV bolus plus continuous nasogastric infusion of antacids.

与常规治疗相比，该方案能较快控制出血。

Compared with conventional treatment, this regimen controls bleeding more rapidly.

他们认为有越来越多的证据证明在胃酸、血凝块形成和消化性溃疡出血之间存在某种关系。

They believe increasing evidence suggests a relationship among gastric acid, clot formation, and peptic ulcer bleeding.

（苗芳 译）

(Translated by Miao Fang)

7. 蜂蜜 100-130 毫升，隔水蒸熟，于饭前 1 次服下。

7. Steam 100–130 ml honey over water until cooked; take all at once before meals.

1 日 3 次，连服 2-3 周。

Three times daily for 2–3 consecutive weeks.

8. 红茶 5 克，蜂蜜、白糖各适量。

8. Black tea 5g, honey and white sugar as appropriate.

将红茶放入保温杯中，沏泡 10 分钟后，加入蜂蜜、白糖，趁热饮之，每日 3 次。

Steep black tea in a thermos for 10 minutes, add honey and sugar, drink while hot, three times daily.

9. 粳米 60 克，砂仁细末 5 克。

9. Non-glutinous rice 60g, Amomum fruit fine powder 5g.

将粳米煮粥，调入砂仁末，再煮沸即可，早晚各饮用 1 次。

Cook rice into porridge, stir in Amomum powder, bring to a boil again; consume once in the morning and once in the evening.

10. 鲜马铃薯洗净切碎，捣烂挤汁，加适量凉开水、蜂蜜。

10. Wash fresh potatoes, chop, mash, squeeze juice, add appropriate amount of cooled boiled water and honey.

每日早晚各服 1 杯，连服 2-3 周。

Take one cup each morning and evening for 2–3 consecutive weeks.

11. 鸡蛋 1-2 个，95% 酒精 500 克。

11. Eggs 1–2, 95% alcohol 500g.

将鸡蛋、酒精放在锅内点燃，待鸡蛋水分蒸发，呈粉末即可。

Place eggs and alcohol in a pan and ignite; when egg moisture evaporates and turns to powder, it is ready.

若不成粉末，可烘干研末。

If powder does not form, dry and grind.

1日分4次服完，3日为1疗程，连服2-3个疗程。

Divide into four doses daily; three days per course; take 2–3 consecutive courses.

12. 牛奶250克煮沸，调入蜂蜜30克，白芨粉6克，顿服，每日1次。

12. Boil 250g milk, stir in 30g honey and 6g Bletilla powder; take all at once daily.

13. 鲜包心菜捣烂绞汁1杯（约200- 300毫升），略温，饭前服用。

13. Mash fresh cabbage and squeeze one cup of juice (~200–300 ml); warm slightly and take before meals.

1日2次，连服10日为1疗程。

Twice daily for 10 consecutive days as one course.

14. 饴糖1-2匙，温水化服。

14. Dissolve 1–2 spoonfuls maltose in warm water and drink.

有缓解胃痛之效。

Effective in relieving stomach pain.

（唐蔚波）(Tang Weibo)

15. 蛇舌草治胃溃疡效果好

15. Hedyotis diffusa Effective for Gastric Ulcer

蛇舌草又名蛇针草，分为硬枝和软枝两种，以软枝为佳。

Hedyotis diffusa, also called Snake Needle Grass, has hard-stem and soft-stem varieties; the soft-stem type is preferred.

属一年生草本，味甘淡，性凉。

It is an annual herb, sweet and bland in taste, cool in nature.

患有十二指肠、胃慢性溃疡，常有微痛或阵痛而引起横膈停水现象均可服用。

Suitable for chronic duodenal or gastric ulcers with mild or paroxysmal pain causing diaphragmatic fluid retention.

取青鲜蛇舌草 100 克洗净，放于陶锅，加水 500 毫升煎沸 10 分钟，去渣，用一碗加入一个鸡蛋、20 克红糖（勿用其它糖代替），充分搅匀，再把刚煎好的蛇舌草水慢慢冲入蛋液中，边冲边拌，隔水炖 20 分钟，取出候温服用，既香甜又顺口。

Wash 100g fresh Hedyotis diffusa, place in a clay pot, add 500 ml water, boil for 10 minutes, strain; mix one bowl of decoction with one egg and 20g brown sugar (do not substitute other sugars), stir thoroughly, slowly pour the hot decoction into the egg mixture while stirring, double-boil for 20 minutes, cool to warm, and consume—it is fragrant, sweet, and palatable.

每晚临睡前服用，每 10 天为一个疗程，轻则 4 个疗程，重则 5 个疗程可愈。

Take nightly before sleep; ten days per course; mild cases require 4 courses, severe cases 5 courses for cure.

《中医药信息报》1992 年 6 月 13 日（非马）

TCM Information News, June 13, 1992 (Fei Ma)

16. 地龙治疗消化性溃疡。

16. Earthworm for Peptic Ulcer.

地龙常用于息风清热，通经活络。

Earthworm is commonly used to extinguish wind, clear heat, unblock meridians, and activate collaterals.

文献报道有抗组织胺作用。

Literature reports antihistamine effects.

用于治疗经纤维胃镜检查确诊的消化性溃疡患者 40 例，每次服地龙粉 2 克，每日 3-4 次，饭后一小时内服，服 4 次者睡前加服一次，治愈率为 85.0%。

In 40 patients with endoscopically confirmed peptic ulcer, earthworm powder 2g per dose was given 3–4 times daily within one hour after meals; those taking four doses added one bedtime dose; cure rate was 85.0%.

17. 主治：胃溃疡。

17. Indication: Gastric ulcer.

方药：蚌壳粉 45 克。

Formula: Mussel shell powder 45g.

用法：取蚌壳煅灰研细末，过筛，日服 3 次，每次 15 克。

Usage: Calcine mussel shells to ash, grind to fine powder, sift; take 15g per dose three times daily.

《民族医药报》1992 年 6 月 5 日

Ethnic Medicine News, June 5, 1992

18. 胃、十二指肠溃疡：乌贼骨 60 克、元胡 30 克、鸡内金 60 克、炒五灵脂 20 克、山药 60 克、甘草 30 克，共研细末，以蜂蜜为丸，每丸重 3 克，每日服 2-3 次，每次 2-3 丸。

18. Gastric and duodenal ulcer: Cuttlefish bone 60g, Corydalis rhizome 30g, Chicken gizzard lining 60g, Stir-fried Flying squirrel feces 20g, Chinese yam 60g, Licorice root 30g; grind into fine powder, make honey pills weighing 3g each; take 2–3 pills per dose, 2–3 times daily.

散剂每次服 8-10 克，每日 2-3 次。

As powder, take 8–10g per dose, 2–3 times daily.

《中药科技报》1992 年 3 月 26 日 Chinese Materia Medica Science and Technology News, March 26, 1992

二、溃疡性结肠炎（1 方）
II. Ulcerative Colitis (1 Prescription)

河南许昌市中医院张明昌医师自拟肠炎散保留灌肠治疗 300 例慢性溃疡性结肠炎，效果良好。

Dr. Zhang Mingchang of Xuchang TCM Hospital, Henan, formulated Changyan San for retention enema in 300 cases of chronic ulcerative colitis with good results.

300 例中男 193 例，女 107 例，年龄最大 74 岁，最小 13 岁，病程最长 25 年，最短 36 天。

Among 300 cases: 193 male, 107 female; age range 13–74 years; disease duration 36 days to 25 years.

治疗方法：将治疗药物分为两组，肠炎散Ⅰ号和肠炎散Ⅱ号。

Method: Medications were divided into two groups—Changyan San No. I and No. II.

Ⅰ号由珍珠 9g、牛黄、红力参 6g、冰片、五倍子各 12g、琥珀 3g、孩儿茶 10g 共研为粉而成。

No. I consists of Pearl 9g, Bezoar, Red Ginseng 6g, Borneol, Chinese gallnut 12g each, Amber 3g, Gambir 10g, ground into powder.

具有健脾固肠、消肿生肌功用。

Functions: Strengthens spleen, secures intestines, reduces swelling, generates flesh.

本方适用于结肠黏膜溃疡糜烂、泄泻、次数频多或体重较弱者。

Indicated for colonic mucosal ulceration/erosion, frequent diarrhea, or low body weight.

Ⅱ号由珍珠、牛黄、白力参各 6g、冰片、血竭各 12g、琥珀 3g、孩儿茶 6g 共研为粉而成，具有健脾渗湿、活血化瘀、消肿止痛作用，适用于结肠黏膜充血水肿、泄泻或便秘、里急后重或大便不爽、结肠黏膜糜烂溃疡者。

No. II consists of Pearl, Bezoar, White Ginseng 6g each, Borneol, Dragon’s blood 12g each, Amber 3g, Gambir 6g, ground into powder; functions: strengthens spleen, drains dampness, activates blood, resolves stasis, reduces swelling, relieves pain; indicated for colonic mucosal congestion/edema, diarrhea or constipation, tenesmus, unsatisfactory defecation, or mucosal erosion/ulceration.

根据症状分别选用肠炎Ⅰ号或Ⅱ号，每次 2g，加温开水 50ml，调匀，温度控制在 37℃ - 38℃为宜，保留灌肠，每日 1 次，30 天为一疗程。

Select No. I or II based on symptoms; use 2g mixed with 50 ml warm boiled water at 37–38° C for retention enema once daily; thirty days per course.

结果300例中痊愈（症状消失、乙状镜检查结肠黏膜恢复正常，随访半年未复发）122例，基本痊愈（临床症状消失，肠黏膜接近正常或未完全恢复者）67例，好转（临床症状有所减轻，肠黏膜溃疡有所改善）102例，无效9例，总有效率为97 %，其中肠炎散Ⅰ号有效率为98.3%，肠炎散Ⅱ号有效率为96.2%。

Results: Of 300 cases, 122 cured (symptoms resolved, sigmoidoscopy showed normal mucosa, no relapse in 6-month follow-up), 67 basically cured (symptoms resolved, mucosa near-normal or incompletely recovered), 102 improved (symptoms alleviated, ulcers improved), 9 ineffective; total effective rate 97%; No. I effective rate 98.3%, No. II effective rate 96.2%.

《中医药信息报》1990年10月6日（朱炳麟）

TCM Information News, October 6, 1990 (Zhu Binglin)

三、痢疾（49方）

III. Dysentery (49 Prescriptions)

1. 石榴皮15克、水煎服，每天1次，连服3天。

1.Pomegranate peel 15g, decocted in water; once daily for 3 consecutive days.

2. 乌梅9克、诃子6克、肉豆蔻6克，水煎后空腹服，每天1次。

2. Mume fruit 9g, Terminalia chebula 6g, Nutmeg 6g; decoct and take on empty stomach once daily.

3. 绿茶6克，黄柏15克，水煎服，每天2-3次。

3. Green tea 6g, Phellodendron bark 15g; decoct and take 2–3 times daily.

4. 马齿苋60克，蒲公英30克水煎服，每天2-3次。

4. Purslane 60g, Dandelion 30g; decoct and take 2–3 times daily.

5. 韭菜250克，马齿苋50克，黄花菜50克，红糖100克，水煎服，每天1剂，连用了3-5天。

5. Chives 250g, Purslane 50g, Daylily flower 50g, Brown sugar 100g; decoct, one dose daily for 3–5 consecutive days.

6. 大蒜头 3-5 瓣，捣烂温开水送服，每天 2 次，连服 3 天。

6. Garlic 3–5 cloves, mashed and taken with warm boiled water twice daily for 3 consecutive days.

7. 大蒜 2 头，炒山楂 30 克，水煎服，每天 2-3 次。

7. Garlic 2 bulbs, Stir-fried Hawthorn fruit 30g; decoct and take 2–3 times daily.

8. 金银花 20 克，秦皮 10 克，西红柿叶 15 克，水煎服，每天 2 次。

8. Honeysuckle flower 20g, Ash bark 10g, Tomato leaf 15g; decoct and take twice daily.

9. 生姜、绿豆各 10 克，加水适量浓煎温服，对下痢赤白，呕吐不止者佳。

9. Fresh ginger and Mung bean 10g each; decoct concentrated in appropriate water and drink warm; excellent for red-white dysentery with persistent vomiting.

10. 地肤子 15 克，高粱叶 15 克，茶叶 6 克，水煎服，每天 2-3 次。

10. Kochia fruit 15g, Sorghum leaf 15g, Tea leaves 6g; decoct and take 2–3 times daily.

11. 生苦瓜 1 个，搗烂如泥，加糖 100 克，搅匀，2 小时滤汁去渣，一次饮服，每天 2 次。

11. One raw bitter melon, mashed to paste, add 100g sugar, mix well; after 2 hours strain juice, discard residue, drink all at once twice daily.

12. 南瓜藤 30 克，苦参 15 克，炒山楂 10 克，水煎服，每天 1-2 次。

12. Pumpkin vine 30g, Sophora flavescens root 15g, Stir-fried Hawthorn fruit 10g; decoct and take 1–2 times daily.

13. 苦参 30 克，秦皮 15 克，甘草 6 克，水煎服，每天 2 次。

13. Sophora flavescens root 30g, Ash bark 15g, Licorice root 6g; decoct and take twice daily.

14. 绿豆 15 克，干姜 6 克，栀子 12 克，水煎服，每天 2 次。

14. Mung bean 15g, Dried ginger 6g, Gardenia fruit 12g; decoct and take twice daily.

15. 桃花 12 克，干姜 10 克，秦皮 12 克，水煎服，每天 2 次。

15. Peach blossom 12g, Dried ginger 10g, Ash bark 12g; decoct and take twice daily.

16. 荷叶烧研，每服 6 克，红痢加蜜服，白痢用砂糖汤送下。

16. Char lotus leaf and grind; take 6g per dose—with honey for red dysentery, with sugar water for white dysentery.

17. 苇叶 6 克，红扁豆花 30 克，水煎服，每天 2-3 次。

17. Reed leaf 6g, Red hyacinth bean flower 30g; decoct and take 2–3 times daily.

18. 木贼 15 克，莲子 30 克，水放服，每天 2-3 次。

18. Equisetum hiemale 15g, Lotus seed 30g; decoct and take 2–3 times daily.

19. 胡萝卜子 15 克，马齿苋 30 克，水煎服，每天 3 次。

19. Carrot seed 15g, Purslane 30g; decoct and take three times daily.

20. 苹果皮 20 克，陈皮 10 克，生姜 6 克，水煎服，每日 2-3 次。

20. Apple peel 20g, Tangerine peel 10g, Fresh ginger 6g; decoct and take 2–3 times daily.

21. 山楂 30 克，茶叶 15 克，大蒜 1 头，红糖 30 克，水煎代茶饮。

21. Hawthorn fruit 30g, Tea leaves 15g, Garlic 1 bulb, Brown sugar 30g; decoct and drink as tea.

22. 冬瓜 250 克，洗净切片，马齿苋 250 克，洗净切碎，冰糖适量，共炖汤服食。

22. Winter melon 250g (washed, sliced) and Purslane 250g (washed, chopped), stewed with rock sugar to taste; consume soup and solids.

23. 乌梅 10 克，冰糖 15 克，加水煎汁，趁热饮，适用于慢性久痢，口干伤津者。

23. Mume fruit 10g, Rock sugar 15g; decoct and drink hot; suitable for chronic prolonged dysentery with dry mouth and fluid injury.

但痢疾初起，实证较著者不宜。

Not suitable for early-stage dysentery with prominent excess patterns.

24. 鳝鱼活杀，去内脏，洗净切碎，瓦上焙干，研末，每天热黄酒调 8 克，加红糖内服。

24. Slaughter live eel, gut, wash, chop, roast dry on tile, grind to powder; mix 8g daily with hot yellow wine and brown sugar for oral intake.

25. 龟肉 200 克，砂糖 50 克，共炖汤服食，适用于久痢泻血。

25. Turtle meat 200g, Sugar 50g; stew into soup and consume; suitable for chronic dysentery with bloody stools.

26. 炒山楂 10 克，野麻草 15 克，煎汤服。

26. Stir-fried Hawthorn fruit 10g, Wild hemp herb 15g; decoct and drink.

27. 鲜竹笋与米煮粥食，对久痢、久泻、脱肛者好。

27. Cook fresh bamboo shoots with rice into porridge; beneficial for chronic dysentery, chronic diarrhea, and rectal prolapse.

28. 桔饼 30 克，龙眼肉 15 克，冰糖 15 克，水 2 碗，煎至 1 碗，温服。

28. Candied tangerine cake 30g, Longan aril 15g, Rock sugar 15g; decoct two bowls of water to one bowl, drink warm.

29. 红菱角晒干研末，空腹服下 9 克，红痢老酒送下，白痢未汤送下。

29. Sun-dry red water caltrop, grind to powder; take 9g on empty stomach—with aged wine for red dysentery, with rice water for white dysentery.

30. 鹌鹑 1 只，赤小豆 30 克，生姜数片，煮熟食之。

30. Quail 1, Adzuki bean 30g, Fresh ginger several slices; cook until done and eat.

31. 黄瓜叶 60 克，黄瓜藤 30 克，水煎服，每天 1-2 次。

31. Cucumber leaf 60g, Cucumber vine 30g; decoct and take 1–2 times daily.

32. 丝瓜根、茎、叶均可，洗净后捣烂挤汁，每次服 2 匙，每天 3 次。

32. Luffa root, stem, or leaf—all usable; wash, mash, squeeze juice; take 2 spoonfuls per dose three times daily.

33. 葡萄 60 克，洗净挤汁，用沸水冲泡绿茶 1 杯，兑入挤出的葡萄汁液，趁热喝下，每天 2 次。

33. Grapes 60g, washed and juiced; brew one cup green tea with boiling water, mix in grape juice, drink hot twice daily.

34. 陈石榴焙干，研为细末，仍以酸石榴汤送服，每日 10-12 次。

34. Roast aged pomegranate dry, grind to fine powder; take with sour pomegranate decoction 10–12 times daily.

35. 香蕉花 30 克，捣烂开水冲服，或加蜂蜜调服。

35. Banana flower 30g, mashed and infused with boiling water, or mixed with honey.

36. 杨梅烧存性，研末，米汤调服，每天 2 次，每次 6 克，或以陈酒浸杨梅，每次食 1-2 枚，每天 2 次。

36. Char bayberry retaining properties, grind to powder, mix with rice water; 6g twice daily—or soak bayberries in aged wine and eat 1–2 pieces twice daily.

37. 白豆腐煎醋食之，或大麻子水研滤汁，煮绿豆食之。

37. Pan-fry white tofu in vinegar and eat; or grind hemp seeds in water, strain, and cook mung beans in the liquid to eat.

38. 沙梨皮 100 克，石榴果壳 30 克，水煎服。

38. Sand pear peel 100g, Pomegranate husk 30g; decoct and drink.

39. 用扁蓄水煎浓缩成 40% 溶液，每次服 40 毫升，每天 3 次。

39. Decoct Polygonum aviculare and concentrate to 40% solution; take 40 ml per dose three times daily.

40. 荸荠 60 克，用水煮熟，切碎后大蒜汁调食，每天 2 次。

40. Water chestnut 60g, boiled until cooked, chopped and mixed with garlic juice; twice daily.

《中药科技报》1992 年 7 月 26 日（刘永连）

Chinese Materia Medica Science and Technology News, July 26, 1992 (Liu Yonglian)

41. 急性菌痢：生姜 50-100 克，红糖 50 克，共捣为糊状，分 3 次服用，连续 1 周。

41. Acute bacillary dysentery: Fresh ginger 50–100g, Brown sugar 50g; mash into paste, divide into three doses daily for one week.

42. 痢疾腹痛里急后重：白萝卜一个切碎，焦山楂片 20 克，槐花 15 克。

42. Dysentery with abdominal pain and tenesmus: One chopped white radish, Scorched hawthorn slices 20g, Pagoda tree flower 15g.

每日一剂，水煎服，连服二剂。

One dose daily, decocted; two consecutive doses.

43. 治久痢验方：单用车前子 30 克，水煎，过滤，收集滤液。

43. Proven formula for chronic dysentery: Plantago seed 30g alone, decoct, filter, collect filtrate.

备用红（白）糖 20 克；临床应用时，若为红痢，则车前子滤液加入白糖，一次顿服，即效；若为白痢，则将红糖加至车前子滤液中一次顿服，即有效果。

Reserve 20g red or white sugar; clinically, for red dysentery add white sugar to filtrate and take all at once for immediate effect; for white dysentery add brown sugar and take all at once for prompt effect.

《中医药信息报》

TCM Information News

44. 治疗急性菌痢方 处方及用法：白头翁、金银花、山楂各 15 克，马齿苋（鲜品可用 150 克），黄连、丹皮、白芍各 10 克，黄柏、秦皮各 12 克，木香 9 克，甘草 3 克。

44. Formula for acute bacillary dysentery—Prescription and usage: Pulsatilla root, Honeysuckle flower, Hawthorn fruit 15g each; Purslane (fresh 150g if available); Coptis rhizome, Moutan bark, White peony root 10g each; Phellodendron bark, Ash bark 12g each; Aucklandia root 9g; Licorice root 3g.

日 1 剂水煎服。

One dose daily, decocted in water.

运用本法共收治 36 例，结果：痊愈 30 例，显效 5 例，无效 1 例。

Applied to 36 cases: 30 cured, 5 markedly effective, 1 ineffective.

《民族医药报》1998 年 1 月 23 日（郁金）

Ethnic Medicine News, January 23, 1998 (Yu Jin)

45. 绿茶 30 克，鲜姜 50 克，红糖 30 克，水 600 毫升。

45. Green tea 30g, Fresh ginger 50g, Brown sugar 30g, Water 600 ml.

将鲜姜洗净去皮捣碎，置入砂锅内加入水文火煮沸十五至二十分钟，然后放入茶叶，待成棕色后，再加入红糖，去渣取汤趁热服下，早晨空腹，晚上睡前各服一次，一般连服三至五天疗效显著。

Wash, peel, and mash fresh ginger; place in clay pot with water, simmer 15–20 minutes; add tea leaves until brown, then add brown sugar; strain and drink hot on empty stomach in morning and before bed at night; marked efficacy usually after 3–5 consecutive days.

茶叶主要成分是生物碱。

Main component of tea is alkaloids.

有抑菌、保护肠黏膜、肠道毛细血管收缩和收敛作用。

Has antibacterial, intestinal mucosa-protective, capillary-constricting, and astringent effects.

生姜温中散寒，其挥发性油能使血液循环增加，并有兴奋神经和止血功效。

Fresh ginger warms the middle and dispels cold; its volatile oils increase circulation, stimulate nerves, and stop bleeding.

红糖温补祛寒，有补虚冷、健脾胃、温中益气之功能。

Brown sugar warmly tonifies and dispels cold, supplementing deficiency-cold, strengthening spleen/stomach, warming the middle, and boosting qi.

《中药科技报》1992 年 5 月 6 日

Chinese Materia Medica Science and Technology News, May 6, 1992

46. 痢疾多发于夏秋季节，主要是由饮食不节，抵抗力减弱，吃了被细菌污染的食物所引起。

46. Dysentery occurs mostly in summer-autumn, mainly due to dietary indiscretion, weakened resistance, and ingestion of bacteria-contaminated food.

现介绍简便方数则，既经济又简便。

Several simple, economical formulas are introduced below.

只要对症下药，可望获得满意的疗效。

With proper pattern-based treatment, satisfactory efficacy is expected.

发病初期：①金银花 50 克焙干研末用白开水调白糖空腹服，2-4 次可愈。

Early stage: ① Roast 50g honeysuckle flower dry, grind, mix with white sugar and plain boiled water, take on empty stomach; curable in 2–4 doses.

②厚朴 20 克，水煎服，1 日 3 次，2 日即愈。

② Magnolia bark 20g, decocted three times daily; curable in two days.

里急后重：厚朴 15 克煎水冲槟榔末 10 克服，其效佳。

Tenesmus: Decoct 15g Magnolia bark and infuse 10g Areca seed powder; highly effective.

痢疾先红后白：怀牛膝 100 克，研细末用白酒 100 毫升浸泡 7 天，每次服 10 毫升，每日 3 次。

Red-then-white dysentery: Achyranthes bidentata 100g, ground fine, soaked in 100 ml liquor for 7 days; take 10 ml three times daily.

红痢不止：马齿苋（即瓜子菜）适量，洗净捣汁兑蜂蜜、酒各适量，温热空腹服，日服 3 次，2 日可愈。

Persistent red dysentery: Appropriate amount of purslane, washed, juiced, mixed with honey and wine as appropriate; take warm on empty stomach three times daily; curable in two days.

白痢不止：干饭锅巴 100 克，炒槐花 100 克，腊猪肉 15 克，共煮食，有良效。

Persistent white dysentery: Rice crust 100g, Stir-fried pagoda tree flower 100g, Cured pork 15g; cook together and eat; good effect.

红白痢：苦参 300 克，木香 60 克，甘草 20 克，研末米汤送服。

Red-white dysentery: Sophora flavescens root 300g, Aucklandia root 60g, Licorice root 20g; grind to powder, take with rice water.

赤白暴痢：龙牙草 75 克，陈茶少许，水煎服。

Acute red-white dysentery: Agrimony 75g, Aged tea a little; decoct and drink.

休息痢：白豆腐以醋煎食，有效。

Relapsing dysentery: Pan-fry white tofu in vinegar and eat; effective.

下痢脱肛：延胡索 45 克，研细末，温酒冲服。

Dysentery with rectal prolapse: Corydalis rhizome 45g, ground fine, taken with warm wine.

阿米巴痢疾：鸦胆子 10-15 粒，打碎后用龙眼肉包或装于胶囊内，开水送服。

Amebic dysentery: Brucea fruit 10–15 seeds, crushed and wrapped in longan aril or encapsulated, taken with boiled water.

日服 3 次，连服 7 天，有良效。

Three times daily for seven consecutive days; good effect.

《民族医药报》1992 年 5 月 28 日（湖南 杨玉钊）

Ethnic Medicine News, May 28, 1992 (Hunan, Yang Yuzhao)

47. 民间偏方治急性菌痢

47. Folk Remedy for Acute Bacillary Dysentery

夏季，常因饮食不当或不注意饮水卫生，易于发生急性菌痢。

In summer, acute bacillary dysentery often occurs due to improper diet or poor drinking-water hygiene.

患者表现为腹部阵痛，腹泻红白冻样大便，肛门有坠胀感等症状。

Patients present with cramping abdominal pain, red-white mucoid stools, and anal bearing-down sensation.

我们采用民间偏方酒炒山楂治疗菌痢，疗效显著，现介绍如下。

We use the folk remedy wine-stir-fried hawthorn for dysentery with remarkable efficacy, introduced below.

取山楂 100 克，红糖 100 克，白酒适量。

Take Hawthorn fruit 100g, Brown sugar 100g, Liquor as appropriate.

将山楂置文火上炒成略焦状，离火加酒搅拌，再置于锅内炒至酒干即可。

Stir-fry hawthorn over gentle heat until slightly scorched, remove from heat, add liquor and stir, return to pan and fry until liquor evaporates.

服时将焦楂加水一碗（约 200 毫升）煎 15 分钟左右，去楂加入红糖再煎到沸，趁温服下，每日一剂，一次服用。

To administer, decoct scorched hawthorn in one bowl (~200 ml) water for ~15 minutes, remove hawthorn, add brown sugar, boil again, drink warm; one dose daily taken at once.

《民族医药报》1992 年 7 月 10 日（南京 孙哲）

Ethnic Medicine News, July 10, 1992 (Nanjing, Sun Zhe)

48. 主治：菌痢。

48. Indication: Bacillary dysentery.

方药：一见喜 10 克或马齿苋 300 克。

Formula: Andrographis paniculata 10g or Purslane 300g.

用法：水煎服。

Usage: Decoct in water and drink.

《民族医药报》1992 年 6 月 5 日

Ethnic Medicine News, June 5, 1992

49. 扁蓄 治疗细菌性痢疾。

49. Polygonum aviculare for Bacillary Dysentery.

扁蓄常用于治疗泌尿系炎症。

Polygonum aviculare is commonly used for urinary tract inflammation.

用扁蓄水煎浓缩成 40% 溶液，每次 40 毫升口服，每日 3 次，总有效率为 91.9%。

Decoct and concentrate to 40% solution; take 40 ml orally three times daily; overall effective rate 91.9%.

四、胃肠炎（32 方）

IV. Gastroenteritis (32 Prescriptions)

胃寒多由过食生冷或用寒凉之药，或胃阳不足，寒从内生引起。其症常见胃脘痛，胃部发凉，得热则减，遇冷痛甚，呕吐清涎，口谈喜热饮，舌淡胖，苔白润，脉沉迟等。当温胃散寒，理气止痛。下列验方用之，均有显著效果。

Stomach cold is mostly caused by overconsumption of raw and cold foods, the use of cold and cool medicines, or insufficient stomach yang leading to internal cold generation. Common symptoms include epigastric pain, a cold sensation in the stomach, relief with heat, aggravated pain with cold, vomiting of clear saliva, a bland taste in the mouth with a preference for hot drinks, a pale and plump tongue with a white and moist coating, and a deep and slow pulse. The treatment should warm the stomach, dispel cold, regulate qi, and relieve pain. The following proven prescriptions have shown significant effects when used.

1. 毕橙茄研末，水泛为丸，每服 1 克，日服 3 次，连服 2 日即效。

1.Grind cubeb (Bi Cheng Qie) into powder, make pills with water, take 1g each time, 3 times a day; it takes effect after 2 consecutive days.

2. 白盐久腌高良姜 15 克，洗去盐，捣烂，以温开水冲服，日服 2 次。

2. Take 15g of galangal rhizome (Gao Liang Jiang) preserved in white salt for a long time, wash off the salt, mash it, and brew it with warm boiled water; take it twice a day.

3. 丁香 15 克，肉桂 9 克，共研细末，分 10 次服，日服 2 次，连服 3 日，效捷。

3. Grind 15g of clove (Ding Xiang) and 9g of cassia bark (Rou Gui) into fine powder together, divide into 10 doses, take twice a day for 3 consecutive days for rapid effect.

4. 苍术 60 克，吴萸 6 克，炒研末，每次用温开水冲服 6 克，日服 2 次。3 日即效。

4. Stir-fry 60g of atractylodes rhizome (Cang Zhu) and 6g of evodia fruit (Wu Zhu Yu), grind into powder, take 6g each time with warm boiled water, twice a day; it takes effect in 3 days.

5. 香附子 120 克，高良姜 30 克，共研细末，每服 6 克，早晚用盐姜汤送下。

5. Grind 120g of nutgrass flatsedge rhizome (Xiang Fu Zi) and 30g of galangal rhizome (Gao Liang Jiang) into fine powder, take 6g each time, washed down with salt and ginger soup in the morning and evening.

6. 老生姜、红糖各 250 克。将生姜捣汁去渣，隔水蒸 10 分钟，再将红糖溶入为膏，4 日服完，日服 2 次。

6. Take 250g each of old ginger and brown sugar. Mash the ginger to extract the juice and remove the dregs, steam it over water for 10 minutes, then dissolve the brown sugar into it to form a paste; finish it in 4 days, taking it twice a day.

7. 薏苡仁 30 克，附片 15 克，研末，每服 1.5 克，日服 2 次，连服 7-15 日。

良效。

7. Grind 30g of coix seed (Yi Yi Ren) and 15g of prepared aconite lateral root (Fu Pian) into powder, take 1.5g each time, twice a day, for 7-15 consecutive days; it has good effects.

8. 香附子 15 克，首乌 60 克，共研细末，水、醋煮，面和为丸，每服 6 克，日服 2-3 次。其效甚佳。

8. Grind 15g of nutgrass flatsedge rhizome (Xiang Fu Zi) and 60g of fleeceflower root (Shou Wu) into fine powder, boil with water and vinegar, mix with flour to make pills, take 6g each time, 2-3 times a day; its effect is excellent.

9. 白胡椒 30 粒，全蝎 1 个，共研细末，分 4 次服，日服 2 次。其效速而持久。

9. Grind 30grains of white pepper (Bai Hu Jiao) and 1 whole scorpion (Quan Xie) into fine powder, divide into 4 doses, take twice a day; its effect is rapid and lasting.

10. 干姜 15 克，砂仁 9 克，水煎分 2 次服。连服 3 日。《民族医药报》1996 年 12 月 27 日（陈国华）

10. Decoct 15g of dried ginger (Gan Jiang) and 9g of amomum fruit (Sha Ren) in water, divide into 2 doses; take for 3 consecutive days. "National Medicine News", Dec 27, 1996 (Chen Guohua).

11. 仙人掌根 30 至 60 克，配猪肚炖服，治久患胃痛。

11. Stew 30 to 60g of cactus root with pig stomach and eat it, to treat chronic stomachache.

12. 胃痛患者应合理选用中成药

12. Patients with stomachache should rationally choose Chinese patent medicines.

胃痛的常见原因有病邪犯胃、肝气郁结、脾胃虚寒、瘀血凝滞等。治疗胃痛的中成药很多，如应用合理，效如桴鼓。

Common causes of stomachache include pathogenic factors invading the stomach, stagnation of liver qi, deficiency and cold of spleen and stomach, and stagnation of blood stasis. There are many Chinese patent medicines for treating stomachache; if applied rationally, the effect is as prompt as a drumstick hitting a drum.

感受寒邪：多因寒邪侵袭和嗜食性冷所致。可见胃脘痛而感冷，喜吃热食，热敷可使疼痛减轻，舌苔白等症状。按“寒者热之”的治则宜选用散寒止痛的中成药，如良附丸，十香丸，胃气痛片或取丁桂散少许放在膏药中外贴患处。

Exposure to cold evil: Mostly caused by the invasion of cold evil and a fondness for cold foods. Symptoms include epigastric pain with a cold sensation, preference for hot food, pain relief with hot compresses, and a white tongue coating. According to the treatment principle of "treating cold with heat", one should choose Chinese patent medicines that dispel cold and relieve pain, such as Liangfu Pill, Shixiang Pill, Weiqitong Tablet, or apply a small amount of Dinggui Powder on a plaster and stick it externally to the affected area.

饮食积滞：胃痛伴嗳腐吞酸、脘腹胀闷、吐后痛减，大便溏泻不爽，苔垢腻。治以消食导滞，应选用保和丸（片）、胃痛散，食积较重者可用槟榔四消丸。

Food stagnation: Stomachache accompanied by belching with a rotten smell, acid regurgitation, epigastric and abdominal distension and fullness, pain relief after vomiting, loose and unsmooth stools, and a greasy and dirty tongue coating. Treat by promoting digestion and relieving food stagnation; Baohe Pill (Tablet) and Weitong Powder should be selected, and Binglang Sixiao Pill can be used for severe food stagnation.

肝气犯胃：胃脘胀满、攻撑作痛、连及两胁、嗳气频繁。治应疏肝理气，可用舒肝丸、拈痛丸或心腹气痛丸，若疼痛伴烧心，泛酸、口干、口苦、心烦易怒则可选用左金丸。

Liver qi invading the stomach: Epigastric distension and fullness, distending and supporting pain, extending to both flanks, and frequent belching. Treatment should soothe the liver and regulate qi; Shugan Pill, Niantong Pill, or Xinfu Qitong Pill can be used. If the pain is accompanied by heartburn, acid regurgitation, dry mouth, bitter taste, and irritability, Zuojin Pill can be selected.

脾胃虚寒：疼痛以空腹时为甚，得食则缓，喜热熨、按压痛减、伴神疲乏力，手足欠温、大便溏薄，舌淡白，宜用温中散寒的中成药，如黄芪建中丸，香砂养胃丸或香砂六君丸等。

Deficiency and cold of spleen and stomach: Pain is most severe on an empty stomach, relieved by eating, prefers hot compresses, pain reduced by pressure, accompanied by mental fatigue, lack of warmth in hands and feet, loose stools, and a pale white tongue. It is appropriate to use Chinese patent medicines that warm the middle and dispel cold, such as Huangqi Jianzhong Pill, Xiangsha Yangwei Pill, or Xiangsha Liujun Pill.

瘀血凝滞：多见于老胃痛患者，痛有定处，痛如针刺或刀割，或见吐血黑便，舌紫暗，有瘀斑等，治宜化瘀通络，可选用血府逐瘀丸、七制香附丸、失笑散、云南白药等。

Stagnation of blood stasis: More common in patients with chronic stomachache, pain has a fixed location, pain is like needle pricks or knife cuts, or accompanied by vomiting blood and black stools, dark purple tongue with ecchymosis, etc. Treatment should resolve blood stasis and unblock collaterals; Xuefu Zhuyu Pill, Qizhi Xiangfu Pill, Shixiao Powder, or Yunnan Baiyao can be selected.

胃酸过多：症见胃脘疼痛，嗳气呕恶、泛酸水、胃部嘈杂不舒等。可选用治酸止痛的中成药，如胃痛宁片、舒胃片、胃乐片、胃痛散等。《民族医药报》（王廷兆）

Excessive stomach acid: Symptoms include epigastric pain, belching, nausea and vomiting, acid regurgitation, and a noisy and uncomfortable feeling in the stomach. Chinese patent medicines that treat acid and relieve pain can be selected, such as Weitongning Tablet, Shuwei Tablet, Weile Tablet, or Weitong Powder. "National Medicine News" (Wang Tingzhao).

13. 慢性腹泻：羊骨200克，打碎炙酥，糯米、小米各100克，炒黄存性。共研末，每服10克，日3次，连服7-10天。《中药科技报》1992年3月26日13.

Chronic diarrhea: Crush 200g of sheep bone and roast it until crispy, stir-fry 100g each of glutinous rice and millet until yellow while retaining their properties. Grind them all into powder, take 10g each time, 3 times a day, for 7-10 consecutive days. "Chinese Materia Medica Science and Technology News", Mar 26, 1992.

14. 肠风下血：选用紫色细长经霜茄子 300 克，火烧存性研成粉末，早晚空腹服 10 克，连服 1 周。本方临床应用 6 例，均获治愈。

14. Intestinal wind with bloody stools: Select 300g of purple, slender, frost-bitten eggplants, burn them in fire to retain their properties, and grind into powder. Take 10g on an empty stomach in the morning and evening for 1 consecutive week. This prescription has been clinically applied to 6 cases, all of which were cured.

15. 治泄泻方：鸡蛋 2 个，醋 50 毫升，黑糖 1 汤匙（红糖也可）。将醋倒入铁锅烧热，鸡蛋去壳（蛋黄不拌碎）入锅煮熟，捞出鸡蛋拌入黑糖，趁热吃下，一次见效。

15. Prescription for diarrhea: 2 eggs, 50ml of vinegar, 1 tablespoon of dark brown sugar (brown sugar is also fine). Pour the vinegar into an iron pan and heat it, peel the eggs (do not break the yolks), put them into the pan and boil until cooked. Remove the eggs, mix in the dark brown sugar, and eat them while hot; it takes effect in one dose.

16. 急性肠胃炎，吐、泻、烦躁：取绿茶、干姜丝各 3 克，放入瓷杯中，用沸水冲泡，盖好保温 10 分钟，代茶饮。

16. Acute gastroenteritis with vomiting, diarrhea, and irritability: Take 3g each of green tea and dried ginger shreds, put them in a porcelain cup, brew with boiling water, cover and keep warm for 10 minutes, and drink it as tea.

治肠胃炎验方二则

Two Proven Prescriptions for Gastroenteritis

17. 高良姜、玄胡、吴芋、苏子、乌药、槟榔、大腹皮、广木香、藿香、猪苓、泽泻、车前仁、款冬花各 10 克。用法：水煎服，连服 5 剂。适应症：慢性胃炎。

17. 10g each of galangal rhizome (Gao Liang Jiang), corydalis tuber (Yan Hu Su), evodia fruit (Wu Zhu Yu), perilla fruit (Su Zi), lindera root (Wu Yao), areca

seed (Bing Lang), areca peel (Da Fu Pi), costus root (Guang Mu Xiang), patchouli (Huo Xiang), polyporus (Zhu Ling), alisma rhizome (Ze Xie), plantain seed (Che Qian Ren), and coltsfoot flower (Kuan Dong Hua). Usage: Decoct in water and take, for 5 consecutive doses. Indication: Chronic gastritis.

18. 野产子草、灶心土、芦根各 5 克，米炭、细茶叶各 50 克，海蚌含珠 20 克。用法：芦根用火烧成炭，同上述其余各药煮水内服。适应症：慢性肠炎。《中国医药报》1992 年 8 月 23 日（孙志海）

18. 5g each of wild Euphorbia humifusa (Ye Chan Zi Cao), stove center earth (Zao Xin Tu), and reed rhizome (Lu Gen), 50g each of rice charcoal (Mi Tan) and fine tea leaves (Xi Cha Ye), and 20g of Acalypha australis (Hai Bang Han Zhu). Usage: Burn the reed rhizome into charcoal with fire, boil it in water with the rest of the above medicines, and take it internally. Indication: Chronic enteritis. "China Medical News", Aug 23, 1992 (Sun Zhihai).

19. 治胃痛方：白胡椒 15 克、吴萸 15 克、鱼腥草 100 克、小木通 100 克，共研末加糯米 500 克入猪肚中，将口缝合入锅中，方厚朴 15 克水炖，去厚朴加白糖食之，每日一剂。

19. Prescription for stomachache: Grind 15g of white pepper (Bai Hu Jiao), 15g of evodia fruit (Wu Zhu Yu), 100g of heartleaf houttuynia herb (Yu Xing Cao), and 100g of clematis stem (Xiao Mu Tong) into powder, add 500g of glutinous rice and put them into a pig stomach. Sew the opening, put it into a pot, add 15g of magnolia bark (Hou Po) and stew in water. Remove the magnolia bark, add white sugar, and eat it; one dose per day.

20. 鸡蛋壳 1 个，洗净放入锅内炒黄，研成细末，每天 1-2 次，用开水冲服。主治过饥过饱胃痛，嗳气吐酸水。

20. Wash 1 eggshell clean, put it into a pan and stir-fry until yellow, grind it into fine powder. Take it 1-2 times a day, brewed with boiling water. It is mainly used for stomachache caused by over-hunger or over-eating, belching, and vomiting acid water.

21. 田螺壳 10 个、鸡内金 2 个，用新瓦片焙干，研成细末，每天 1-2 次，红糖水送服。主治胃痛、反胃吐酸、吐食等。

21. Take 10 river snail shells and 2 chicken gizzard linings (Ji Nei Jin), roast them dry on a new tile, and grind them into fine powder. Take it 1-2 times a day, washed down with brown sugar water. It is mainly used for stomachache, regurgitation, vomiting acid, and vomiting food.

22. 猪肚 1 个、胡椒 10 克、生姜 5 片，将猪肚洗净，纳入胡椒和姜片，隔水炖烂，加盐少许调味，每天早晚佐餐吃。主治胃部冷痛、呕吐清水、身体虚弱、饮食减少等。《中药科技报》1992 年 11 月 26 日（黄海平）

22. Wash 1 pig stomach clean, put in 10g of pepper and 5 slices of ginger, stew it over water until thoroughly cooked, add a little salt for seasoning, and eat it as a side dish in the morning and evening every day. It is mainly used for cold pain in the stomach, vomiting clear water, physical weakness, and reduced appetite. "Chinese Materia Medica Science and Technology News", Nov 26, 1992 (Huang Haiping).

23. 急性肠炎：公丁香 10 克。取马酸奶 100 毫升，将丁香倒入，浸泡 24 小时，每晚空腹服 15 毫升，连服 7-9 天疗效佳。

23. Acute enteritis: Take 10g of clove (Gong Ding Xiang). Take 100ml of mare's milk yogurt, pour the cloves into it, soak for 24 hours, take 15ml on an empty stomach every night, and take it for 7-9 consecutive days for good curative effect.

24. 霉菌性肠炎治验方

24. Proven Prescription for Mycotic Enteritis

由于抗生素的广泛应用，霉菌性肠炎有日益增多的趋势。我科应用内服基本方加减和中药保留灌肠治疗，取得了较为满意的疗效。

Due to the widespread use of antibiotics, there is an increasing trend of mycotic enteritis. Our department has applied modified basic oral prescriptions and traditional Chinese medicine retention enemas for treatment, achieving relatively satisfactory curative effects.

一、治疗方法：

I. Treatment Methods:

内服基本方组成：党参10克、白术10克、防风10克、白芍15克、陈皮10克、淮山12克、乌梅6克、槟榔10克、肉蔻6克。

Composition of the basic oral prescription: 10g of pilose asiabell root (Dang Shen), 10g of largehead atractylodes rhizome (Bai Zhu), 10g of divaricate saposhnikovia root (Fang Feng), 15g of white peony root (Bai Shao), 10g of dried tangerine peel (Chen Pi), 12g of yam rhizome (Huai Shan), 6g of dark plum fruit (Wu Mei), 10g of areca seed (Bing Lang), and 6g of nutmeg (Rou Kou).

加减法：有热象者加川连6克、葛根15克、槐花10克；气虚者加黄芪20克；阳虚有寒加肉桂3克、小茴香6克；湿重者加苡仁30克、泽泻15克；腹胀加厚朴10克；久泄不止者加罂粟壳6克、石榴皮10克。

Modifications: For those with heat signs, add 6g of coptis rhizome (Chuan Lian), 15g of kudzu root (Ge Gen), and 10g of pagoda tree flower (Huai Hua); for those with qi deficiency, add 20g of astragalus root (Huang Qi); for those with yang deficiency and cold, add 3g of cassia bark (Rou Gui) and 6g of fennel fruit (Xiao Hui Xiang); for those with heavy dampness, add 30g of coix seed (Yi Ren) and 15g of alisma rhizome (Ze Xie); for abdominal distension, add 10g of magnolia bark (Hou Po); for prolonged and unceasing diarrhea, add 6g of poppy capsule (Ying Su Ke) and 10g of pomegranate peel (Shi Liu Pi).

灌肠方组成：白头翁30克、苦参30克、地榆30克、藿香20克、加水煎取150毫升，保留灌肠，每晚一次，七天为一疗程。

Composition of the enema prescription: Decoct 30g of pulsilla root (Bai Tou Weng), 30g of lightyellow sophora root (Ku Shen), 30g of garden burnet root (Di Yu), and 20g of patchouli (Huo Xiang) in water to obtain 150ml. Perform retention enema once every night, with seven days as one course of treatment.

二、注意事项：

II. Precautions:

服药期间饮食宜清淡及营养丰富易消化之品，忌辛辣刺激性及生冷不洁之食物；适当休息，避免过劳；妇女月经期暂停用灌肠治疗。

During the medication period, the diet should be light, nutritious, and easy to digest; avoid spicy, irritating, raw, cold, and unclean foods; rest appropriately and avoid overwork; women should suspend enema treatment during menstruation.

《民族医药报》1992 年 4 月 3 日（广西民族医院 黄超坚）

National Medicine News, Apr 3, 1992 (Guangxi National Hospital, Huang Chaojian).

25. 霉菌性肠炎方

25. Prescription for Mycotic Enteritis

治方药组成：炙黄芪、苦参各 10 克，炒淮山 12 克，莲子肉 12 克，炒麦芽 12 克，大叶桉叶 12 克，补骨脂 8 克，鸡内金 6 克，银花 6 克，土茯苓 20 克，炙甘草 5 克，每日 1 剂，水煎服，每剂煎 2 次，混合 2 次药液分 3 次服。对照组全部口服制霉菌素片。结果：治疗组 110 例，全部治愈；对照组 70 例，痊愈 22 例，显效 39 例，有效 7 例，无效 2 例，两组比较有显著差异。

Composition of the treatment prescription: 10g each of honey-fried astragalus root (Zhi Huang Qi) and lightyellow sophora root (Ku Shen), 12g of stir-fried yam rhizome (Chao Huai Shan), 12g of lotus seed (Lian Zi Rou), 12g of stir-fried malt (Chao Mai Ya), 12g of eucalyptus robusta leaf (Da Ye An Ye), 8g of malaytea scurfpea fruit (Bu Gu Zhi), 6g of chicken gizzard lining (Ji Nei Jin), 6g of honeysuckle flower (Yin Hua), 20g of glabrous greenbrier rhizome (Tu Fu Ling), and 5g of honey-fried licorice root (Zhi Gan Cao). Take 1 dose daily, decoct in water, decoct each dose twice, mix the two decoctions, and take it in 3 divided doses. The control group all took nystatin tablets orally. Results: In the treatment group of 110 cases, all were cured; in the control group of 70 cases, 22 were cured, 39 showed marked effect, 7 were effective, and 2 were ineffective. There was a significant difference between the two groups.

《民族医药报》1998 年 3 月 6 日（明秀 荐）

National Medicine News, Mar 6, 1998 (Recommended by Ming Xiu).

26. 牡荆叶治肠炎

26. Vitex negundo Leaves for Treating Enteritis

据《常用中草药手册》介绍：牡荆，别名五指柑。性味功能：微辛苦平，解表化湿。主治流感、肠炎、痢疾等。

According to the "Manual of Commonly Used Chinese Herbal Medicines": Vitex negundo, also known as Wuzhigan. Properties and functions: Slightly pungent, bitter, and neutral; relieves exterior syndromes and transforms dampness. Mainly treats influenza, enteritis, dysentery, etc.

本人患慢性肠炎多年，屡治不愈，时好时坏，发作时痛苦至极。服西药不起作用。一次偶然机会得到一民间医生介绍牡荆叶可治肠炎的经验。后又查了有关资料，决定试一试，结果效果极佳。

I have suffered from chronic enteritis for many years, repeatedly treated without cure, sometimes better and sometimes worse, and extremely painful during attacks. Taking Western medicine did not work. By chance, I got the experience from a folk doctor that Vitex negundo leaves can treat enteritis. Later, I checked relevant materials and decided to give it a try, and the result was excellent.

具体用法：采嫩牡荆叶适量，放入茶杯内，倒入滚开水，加盖，闷几分钟后便可饮用。一般服后不到两小时，症状缓解，1-2 天可基本恢复。注意：牡荆叶有 3 片、5 片、7 片叶之分，采 5-7 片叶的。效果才佳，3 片叶的次之。

Specific usage: Pick an appropriate amount of tender Vitex negundo leaves, put them in a teacup, pour in boiling water, cover, and steep for a few minutes before drinking. Generally, within less than two hours after taking it, symptoms are relieved, and basic recovery can be achieved in 1-2 days. Note: Vitex negundo leaves are divided into 3-leaf, 5-leaf, and 7-leaf types; pick the 5-7 leaf ones for the best effect, while the 3-leaf ones are secondary.

《民族医药报》1992 年 6 月 5 日（广西 黄光赐）

"National Medicine News", Jun 5, 1992 (Huang Guangci, Guangxi).

27. 核桃莲子糊治腹泻

27. Walnut and Lotus Seed Paste for Treating Diarrhea

药物组成：核桃肉 30 克，莲子肉 30 克，淮山 15 克，黑大豆 15 克。

Drug composition: 30g of walnut kernel (He Tao Rou), 30g of lotus seed (Lian Zi Rou), 15g of yam rhizome (Huai Shan), and 15g of black soybean (Hei Da Dou).

制法及用法：将核桃肉、莲子肉、淮山、黑大豆混合碾磨成细粉，加入适量水置于锅中煮成糊，最后加入适量白糖，每日随意食用。

Preparation and usage: Mix and grind the walnut kernel, lotus seed, yam rhizome, and black soybean into fine powder, add an appropriate amount of water, put it in a pot and boil it into a paste, finally add an appropriate amount of white sugar, and eat it at will every day.

功效及主治：有补胃、健脾、收敛止泻之功。主治脾肾虚弱，脾虚腹泻之症。

Efficacy and indications: It has the effects of tonifying the stomach, invigorating the spleen, and astringing to stop diarrhea. It is mainly used for syndromes of spleen and kidney deficiency, and diarrhea due to spleen deficiency.

《民族医药报》1992 年 5 月 26 日（广西柳州地区人民医院 陈文贵）

"National Medicine News", May 26, 1992 (Chen Wengui, Liuzhou Prefecture People's Hospital, Guangxi).

五、胃下垂（5 方）

V. Gastroptosis (5 Prescriptions)

1. 胃下垂：麻仁 2 份，五倍子 1 份，共捣烂敷脐，外用伤湿止痛膏固定，每日换药一次，也可服用成药补中益气丸。

1.Gastroptosis: Take 2 parts of hemp seed (Ma Ren) and 1 part of Chinese gall (Wu Bei Zi), mash them together and apply to the navel, fix externally with Shangshi Zhitong Plaster, change the dressing once a day, and you can also take the patent medicine Buzhong Yiqi Pill.

2. 治胃下垂便方

2. Convenient Prescription for Treating Gastroptosis

取鸡内金 15 克、米糠 1500 克。将米糠置锅内炒至黄褐色后，再放入鸡内金，将鸡内金炒至膨胀时冷却。然后筛去米糠，将鸡内金捣研成末。成人每次服 3-5 克，黄酒送服，每日 2-3 次，一般服药半个月后即可见效。

Take 15g of chicken gizzard lining (Ji Nei Jin) and 1500g of rice bran (Mi Kang). Put the rice bran in a pan and stir-fry until yellowish-brown, then add the chicken gizzard lining, and cool it when it expands. Then sift out the rice bran, and pound and grind the chicken gizzard lining into powder. Adults take 3-5g each time, washed down with yellow wine, 2-3 times a day. Generally, it takes effect after taking the medicine for half a month.

《民族医药报》1992 年 5 月 8 日（安徽省青阳县 胡可）

"National Medicine News", May 8, 1992 (Hu Ke, Qingyang County, Anhui Province).

3. 用白胡椒 10 克、猪肚一具。将猪肚洗净，再将胡椒粉冲细，纳入锑锅中加水浸过猪肚，不放油盐，用文火炖熟。1 次或多次服完猪肚和汤。 3. Use 10g of white pepper (Bai Hu Jiao) and 1 pig stomach. Wash the pig stomach clean, grind the white pepper into fine powder, put it into an aluminum pot, add water to submerge the pig stomach, do not add oil or salt, and stew it over a slow fire until cooked. Finish the pig stomach and soup in one or multiple times.

4. 药用：党参 30 克，炙升麻 10-15 克，枳实 10 克，小茴香 10 克（系成人量）。水煎，3 次分服。两日 1 剂。连服 10- 20 剂即愈。该方能升提理气，故能获效。

4. Medication: 30g of pilose asiabell root (Dang Shen), 10-15g of honey-fried cimicifuga rhizome (Zhi Sheng Ma), 10g of immature bitter orange (Zhi Shi), and 10g of fennel fruit (Xiao Hui Xiang) (adult dose). Decoct in water, divide into 3 doses. One dose for two days. Take for 10-20 consecutive doses to cure. This prescription can raise and regulate qi, so it can achieve effects.

5. 取蓖麻籽仁、升麻粉适量。混合捣烂后做成药饼，用此饼外敷“百会穴”。并用热水袋熨烫。每日 3 次，每次半小时。每块药饼可连续使用 5 天。间隔一天后又换用新药饼，10 天为一疗程。一般 3-4 个疗程即能痊愈。此法用于饭后 2 小时为宜。但患有心脏病、高血压、呕吐、咯血及孕妇忌用。治疗期间应注意休息，不得暴饮暴食，不做剧烈运动，禁止房事。药饼不得内服，以防中毒。

（邓朝纲）

5. Take an appropriate amount of castor bean kernel (Bi Ma Zi Ren) and cimicifuga rhizome powder (Sheng Ma Fen). Mix and mash them to make a medicinal cake, and apply this cake externally to the "Baihui acupoint". Use a hot water bag for ironing. Do this 3 times a day, half an hour each time. Each medicinal cake can be used continuously for 5 days. Change to a new medicinal cake after an interval of one day, with 10 days as one course of treatment. Generally, 3-4 courses of treatment can cure it. This method is suitable to be used 2 hours after meals. However, it is contraindicated for patients with heart disease, hypertension, vomiting, hemoptysis, and pregnant women. During the treatment period, pay attention to rest, do not overeat or drink, do not do strenuous exercise, and abstain from sexual intercourse. The medicinal cake must not be taken internally to prevent poisoning. (Deng Chaogang).

六、便秘（22 方）
VI. Constipation (22 Prescriptions)

1. 热秘：证见大便干结，小便短赤，口干口臭，腹胀而痛。拟方：大黄 10 克、元参 30 克、生地 30 克、决明子 15 克、枳实 10 克、黄芩 10 克，煎服，每日 1 剂。

1.Heat constipation: Symptoms include dry and hard stools, short and dark urine, dry mouth and bad breath, abdominal distension and pain. Proposed prescription: 10g of rhubarb (Da Huang), 30g of figwort root (Yuan Shen), 30g of rehmannia root (Sheng Di), 15g of cassia seed (Jue Ming Zi), 10g of immature bitter orange (Zhi Shi), and 10g of scutellaria root (Huang Qin). Decoct and take, 1 dose per day.

2. 气秘：证见忧愁郁闷，情志不舒，欲便不出，嗳气频频，胸胁痞满。拟：木香 10 克、厚朴 10 克、槟榔 15 克、枳实 15 克、番泻叶 10 克，煎服，每日 1 剂。

2. Qi constipation: Symptoms include sorrow and depression, uncomfortable emotions, desire to defecate but unable to, frequent belching, and fullness in the

chest and flanks. Proposed prescription: 10g of costus root (Mu Xiang), 10g of magnolia bark (Hou Po), 15g of areca seed (Bing Lang), 15g of immature bitter orange (Zhi Shi), and 10g of senna leaf (Fan Xie Ye). Decoct and take, 1 dose per day.

3. 气虚秘：证见神疲气短，动则自汗，头昏乏力，虽有便意而临厕久解难出。拟方：黄芪 30 克、党参 20 克、白术 15 克、麻仁 30 克、蜂蜜 60 克（后下），煎服，每日 1 剂。

3. Qi deficiency constipation: Symptoms include mental fatigue and shortness of breath, spontaneous sweating upon movement, dizziness and weakness, although there is an urge to defecate, it is difficult to pass after a long time in the toilet. Proposed prescription: 30g of astragalus root (Huang Qi), 20g of pilose asiabell root (Dang Shen), 15g of largehead atractylodes rhizome (Bai Zhu), 30g of hemp seed (Ma Ren), and 60g of honey (Feng Mi) (added later). Decoct and take, 1 dose per day.

4. 血虚秘：证见大便秘结，面色萎黄，头晕目眩，心悸耳鸣。拟方：当归 20 克、何首乌 30 克、熟地 20 克、柏子仁 15 克、麻仁 30 克，煎服，每日 1 剂。

4. Blood deficiency constipation: Symptoms include constipation, sallow complexion, dizziness and vertigo, palpitations and tinnitus. Proposed prescription: 20g of angelica root (Dang Gui), 30g of fleeceflower root (He Shou Wu), 20g of prepared rehmannia root (Shu Di), 15g of arborvitae seed (Bai Zi Ren), and 30g of hemp seed (Ma Ren). Decoct and take, 1 dose per day.

5. 阴虚秘：证见大便干结，口燥咽干，手足心热，烦躁不安。拟方：沙参 30 克、麦冬 30 克、生地 30 克、通大海 10 克。煎服，每日 1 剂。

5. Yin deficiency constipation: Symptoms include dry and hard stools, dry mouth and throat, heat in the palms and soles, and restlessness. Proposed prescription: 30g of glehnia root (Sha Shen), 30g of dwarf lilyturf tuber (Mai Dong), 30g of rehmannia root (Sheng Di), and 10g of sterculia seed (Tong Da Hai). Decoct and take, 1 dose per day.

6. 阳虚秘：证见大便艰涩，排出困难，四肢不温，喜热畏寒，腰膝酸软。拟方：

肉苁蓉 30 克、锁阳 20 克、黑芝麻 30 克、肉桂 5 克、蜂蜜 60 克（后下），煎服，每日 1 剂。《中药科技报》1990 年 9 月 6 日（四川 谢继光）

6. Yang deficiency constipation: Symptoms include difficult and unsmooth stools, difficulty in excretion, cold limbs, preference for heat and aversion to cold, and soreness and weakness of the waist and knees. Proposed prescription: 30g of cistanche (Rou Cong Rong), 20g of cynomorium songaricum (Suo Yang), 30g of black sesame (Hei Zhi Ma), 5g of cassia bark (Rou Gui), and 60g of honey (Feng Mi) (added later). Decoct and take, 1 dose per day. “Chinese Materia Medica Science and Technology News”, Sep 6, 1990 (Xie Jiguang, Sichuan).

7. 便秘：干青果、大黄、天然碱各 25 克。研细，调匀。每日 2-3 次，每次 3 克，加水 100 毫升，煎服。《民族医药报》1992 年 10 月 16 日

7. Constipation: 25g each of dried Chinese olive (Gan Qing Guo), rhubarb (Da Huang), and natural alkali (Tian Ran Jian). Grind into fine powder and mix well. Take 2-3 times a day, 3g each time, add 100ml of water, decoct and take. “National Medicine News”, Oct 16, 1992.

8. 大黄猪肠丸治便秘。

8. Rhubarb and Pig Intestine Pill for Treating Constipation.

药物组成及制作方法：取近肛门端的猪大肠一节，酒制大黄研末填塞至猪肠饱和为度。用绳子将猪肠两端扎紧。慢火煎煮至猪肠熟透为度。然后捣烂为丸。大黄生用泻下力强，制熟以酒，性味俱减，作用缓和，仅能缓以润肠。猪大肠性味甘平，入大肠经。也取以形治形之义，功能润肠治燥，补下焦。二药制作为丸，则作用更为缓和，功慢性能润肠通便。

Drug composition and preparation method: Take a section of pig large intestine near the anus, grind wine-processed rhubarb into powder and stuff it into the pig intestine until saturated. Tie both ends of the pig intestine tightly with a string. Simmer over a slow fire until the pig intestine is thoroughly cooked. Then mash it into pills. Raw rhubarb has a strong purgative effect, but when processed with wine, its properties and flavors are reduced, its effect is mild, and it can only gently moisten the intestines. Pig large intestine is sweet and neutral in nature, and enters the large intestine meridian. It also takes the meaning of treating shape with shape, with the function of moistening the intestines, treating dryness, and tonifying the lower jiao. Making the two drugs into pills makes the effect milder, acting slowly to moisten the intestines and relieve constipation.

用法及治疗：每服五至十克，用以治疗习惯性便秘，老年性便秘等一切慢性虚性便秘。笔者用此丸治疗多例病人都取得满意效果。《中药科技报》1993年3月11日

Usage and treatment: Take 5 to 10g each time, used to treat habitual constipation, senile constipation, and all other chronic deficiency constipation. The author has used this pill to treat many patients and achieved satisfactory results. "Chinese Materia Medica Science and Technology News", Mar 11, 1993.

9. 花粉治疗便秘。花粉清热生津、消肿排脓。习惯性便秘患者171例，口服花粉胶囊0.8克/次，每日3次，7天为一疗程，总有效率为95.9%。《中药科技报》1992年7月6日

9. Pollen for treating constipation. Pollen clears heat, generates fluid, reduces swelling, and discharges pus. 171 patients with habitual constipation took pollen capsules orally, 0.8g/time, 3 times a day, with 7 days as one course of treatment, and the total effective rate was 95.9%. “Chinese Materia Medica Science and Technology News”, Jul 6, 1992.

10. 大便秘结：杏仁50克，蓖麻籽50克，大黄30克，芒硝30克，煅寒水石30克。上药共研成细粉，每日1-2次，每次3-4克，水煎服。

10. Severe constipation: 50g of apricot kernel (Xing Ren), 50g of castor bean (Bi Ma Zi), 30g of rhubarb (Da Huang), 30g of mirabilite (Mang Xiao), and 30g of calcined gypsum (Duan Han Shui Shi). Grind the above drugs into fine powder together, take 1-2 times a day, 3-4g each time, decoct in water and take.

11. 体虚便秘：黑芝麻500克，蓖麻籽500克，加炼蜜适量制成膏剂，酌量服用。

11. Constipation due to body deficiency: 500g of black sesame (Hei Zhi Ma), 500g of castor bean (Bi Ma Zi), add an appropriate amount of refined honey to

make a paste, and take it at discretion.

12. 肠燥便秘：桃仁 9 克，火麻仁 15 克，郁李仁 12 克，上药共研成粗粉，水煎服用。

12. Constipation due to intestinal dryness: 9g of peach kernel (Tao Ren), 15g of hemp seed (Huo Ma Ren), and 12g of bush cherry seed (Yu Li Ren). Grind the above drugs into coarse powder together, decoct in water and take.

13. 习惯性便秘：肉苁蓉 30 克，火麻仁 15 克，当归 15 克。共研成细粉，每日 2-3 次，每次 3-5 克，水煎服。

13. Habitual constipation: 30g of cistanche (Rou Cong Rong), 15g of hemp seed (Huo Ma Ren), and 15g of angelica root (Dang Gui). Grind into fine powder together, take 2-3 times a day, 3-5g each time, decoct in water and take.

14. 实热便秘：大黄、芒硝、白碱各 50 克，煅寒水石 60 克，上药共研成细粉，每日 1-2 次，每次 3-5 克，开水冲服。

14. Excess heat constipation: 50g each of rhubarb (Da Huang), mirabilite (Mang Xiao), and white alkali (Bai Jian), and 60g of calcined gypsum (Duan Han Shui Shi). Grind the above drugs into fine powder together, take 1-2 times a day, 3-5g each time, brew with boiling water and take.

15. 一般性便秘：大黄 50 克，蓖麻籽 100 克。上药共研成粗粉，每日 1-2 次，每次 3-5 克，开水沏服。

15. General constipation: 50g of rhubarb (Da Huang) and 100g of castor bean (Bi Ma Zi). Grind the above drugs into coarse powder together, take 1-2 times a day, 3-5g each time, brew with boiling water and take.

16. 腹痛便秘：煅寒水石 25 克，土木香 5 克，诃子 5 克，山柰 10 克，大黄 15 克，碱面（炒）10 克，上药研细粉，用茶水加适量奶油，取药粉 3-5 克煎服。

16. Abdominal pain and constipation: 25g of calcined gypsum (Duan Han Shui Shi), 5g of inula root (Tu Mu Xiang), 5g of medicine terminalia fruit (He Zi), 10g of sand ginger (Shan Nai), 15g of rhubarb (Da Huang), and 10g of fried edible alkali powder (Jian Mian). Grind the above drugs into fine powder, use tea water with an appropriate amount of cream, take 3-5g of the medicinal powder, decoct

and take.

17. 顽固性便秘：诃子 50 克，大黄 100 克，碱面 250 克，研成细粉，每日 1-2 次，一次 3-5 克，水煎服。《民族医药报》（内蒙古制药厂 包金垚）

17. Stubborn constipation: 50g of medicine terminalia fruit (He Zi), 100g of rhubarb (Da Huang), and 250g of edible alkali powder (Jian Mian). Grind into fine powder, take 1-2 times a day, 3-5g each time, decoct in water and take. "National Medicine News" (Bao Jinyao, Inner Mongolia Pharmaceutical Factory).

18. 治便秘：蜂蜜、猪板油各等量。猪板油切碎，二味调匀置于碗内隔水蒸熟，早晚空腹服一匙，1-2 天即可见效

18. Treating constipation: Equal amounts of honey (Feng Mi) and pig leaf lard (Zhu Ban You). Chop the pig leaf lard, mix the two ingredients evenly, put them in a bowl and steam over water until cooked. Take one spoonful on an empty stomach in the morning and evening, and it will take effect in 1-2 days.

19. 主治：便秘。方药：全瓜蒌 40 克，鲜首乌 50 克。用法：水煎服，日服 2 次。《民族医药报》1992 年 6 月 5 日

19. Indication: Constipation. Prescription: 40g of whole trichosanthes fruit (Quan Gua Lou) and 50g of fresh fleeceflower root (Xian Shou Wu). Usage: Decoct in water and take, twice a day. "National Medicine News", Jun 5, 1992.

20. 便秘：每顿饭前取凉开水一杯（不可用热开水），加蜂蜜两调羹，饮下。或用新鲜薯叶 500 克，加油盐适量炒熟当菜吃，每天 2 次。

20. Constipation: Take a cup of cool boiled water before each meal (do not use hot boiled water), add two tablespoons of honey, and drink it. Or use 500g of fresh sweet potato leaves, add an appropriate amount of oil and salt, stir-fry until cooked, and eat it as a vegetable, twice a day.

21. 治便秘：炒决明子 15 克，蜂蜜 30 克。先将决明子捣碎，水煎 15 分钟，冲入蜂蜜中搅拌分二次服，每日一剂。《中药科技报》

21. Treating constipation: 15g of stir-fried cassia seed (Chao Jue Ming Zi) and 30g of honey (Feng Mi). First mash the cassia seed, decoct in water for 15 minutes, pour it into the honey, stir, and take it in two divided doses, one dose per

day. “Chinese Materia Medica Science and Technology News”.

22. 中医治疗老年性便秘

22. Traditional Chinese Medicine Treatment for Senile Constipation

气虚便秘：病人虽有便意，却解便困难，便后汗出，体倦无力，舌淡苔薄，脉虚。治宜益气润肠。方用黄芪白术汤（党参、白术、黄芪、茯苓、陈皮、火麻仁、白蜜）加减。

Qi deficiency constipation: Although the patient has the urge to defecate, defecation is difficult, sweating after defecation, physical fatigue and weakness, pale tongue with thin coating, and weak pulse. Treatment should benefit qi and moisten the intestines. The prescription used is Huangqi Baizhu Decoction (pilose asiabell root, largehead atractylodes rhizome, astragalus root, poria, dried tangerine peel, hemp seed, white honey) with modifications.

血虚便秘：病人大便秘结，面色无华，头晕心悸，唇舌淡，脉细涩。治宜养血润肠，方用润肠益血汤（当归、生地、麻仁、枳壳、玄参、知母、山药、熟地、薏苡仁、甘草）等加减。

Blood deficiency constipation: The patient has constipation, lusterless complexion, dizziness and palpitations, pale lips and tongue, and a thready and choppy pulse. Treatment should nourish blood and moisten the intestines. The prescription used is Runchang Yixue Decoction (angelica root, rehmannia root, hemp seed, immature bitter orange, figwort root, anemarrhena rhizome, yam rhizome, prepared rehmannia root, coix seed, licorice root) with modifications.

上述气虚、血虚的便秘，有时单一出现，有时相兼而至，治宜两者合参。

The above qi deficiency and blood deficiency constipation sometimes appear singly and sometimes occur together, and treatment should consider both.

阳虚便秘：病人大便艰涩，小便清长，四肢不温，喜热恶寒，舌淡苦白，脉沉迟。治宜温阳通便，配方为当归、川牛膝、肉苁蓉、佛手、泽泻、升麻、枳壳、肉桂、甘草等。

Yang deficiency constipation: The patient has difficult and unsmooth stools, clear and copious urine, cold limbs, preference for heat and aversion to cold, pale tongue with white coating, and a deep and slow pulse. Treatment should warm yang and relieve constipation. The prescription includes angelica root, cyathula root, cistanche, bergamot fruit, alisma rhizome, cimicifuga rhizome, immature bitter orange, cassia bark, licorice root, etc.

老年便秘虽多以虚为主，但也有少数实证，因此，治疗上也不可一味攻下，而宜攻补兼施。此外，老年便秘除了药物治疗外还可配合食疗。如将黑芝麻、核桃仁、松子仁等研细，稍加白蜜冲服。对阴血不足的便秘，颇有功效。

Although senile constipation is mostly based on deficiency, there are also a few excess syndromes. Therefore, in treatment, one should not blindly use purgatives, but should combine attacking and tonifying. In addition, in addition to drug treatment, senile constipation can also be combined with dietary therapy. For example, grind black sesame, walnut kernel, pine nut kernel, etc., into fine powder, add a little white honey, and brew with water. It is quite effective for constipation due to insufficient yin and blood.

《民族医药报》（江苏 蔡秀芳）

"National Medicine News" (Cai Xiufang, Jiangsu).

七、肛肠科（30 方）
VII. Proctology (30 Prescriptions)

外敷：External Application:

1. 笔者用鲜无花果叶煎汤熏洗治痔疮，经临床观察有明显的治疗效果，现报告如下：

The author used a decoction of fresh fig leaves for fumigation and washing to treat hemorrhoids, and clinical observation has shown significant therapeutic effects; the report is as follows:

方药与治法：取鲜无花果树叶适量，加水煎沸 15-20 分钟，先熏后洗，每日一次，5 天为 1 疗程，未愈者，可进行第 2 疗程。一般只需 1 疗程可告愈。本法可用于内、外痔，混合痔等痔科病症。

Prescription and Method: Take an appropriate amount of fresh fig leaves, add water and boil for 15-20 minutes; first fumigate then wash, once daily, with 5 days constituting one course of treatment. If not cured, a second course may be administered. Generally, one course is sufficient for recovery. This method can be used for internal hemorrhoids, external hemorrhoids, mixed hemorrhoids, and other anal disorders.

据《救荒本草》记载，无花果为桑科植物的聚花果，性味甘、平，入肺、脾、大肠经。具有润肺止咳、清肠、消肿等功效，临床可用于治疗支气管炎、便秘、痔疮等疾病。为此应用该树叶煎汤薰洗，可促进局部血循环，改善痔静脉瘀血状态，起到清肠、消肿、止痛之效。

According to the Jiuhuang Bencao (Materia Medica for Famine Relief), the fig is a multiple fruit of the Moraceae family, sweet and neutral in nature, entering the Lung, Spleen, and Large Intestine meridians. It has the effects of moistening the lungs and relieving cough, clearing the intestines, and reducing swelling, and can be clinically used to treat bronchitis, constipation, hemorrhoids, and other diseases. Therefore, applying a decoction of its leaves for fumigation and washing can promote local blood circulation, improve venous stasis in hemorrhoidal veins, and achieve the effects of clearing the intestines, reducing swelling, and relieving pain.

《中医药信息报》1991 年 7 月 27 日（福建省连江县凤城医院 吴耀嵩 洪秀琪）

TCM Information News, July 27, 1991 (Fengcheng Hospital, Lianjiang County, Fujian Province; Wu Yaosong, Hong Xiuqi)

2. 脱肛：篦麻籽捣烂取汁涂患处，同时用鲜篦麻叶捣烂揉搽双脚涌泉穴。

2. Rectal Prolapse: Crush castor beans to extract juice and apply to the affected area; simultaneously, crush fresh castor leaves and rub them onto the Yongquan acupoints on both feet.

3. 提肛汤熏洗脱肛效果好 笔者自拟提肛汤治疗脱肛。一日量：苦参 100 克、升麻、五倍、白芷各 50 克，水煎每次加入明矾 20 克溶化，趁热先熏后洗，一日两三次。用药期间适当卧床休息，避免重力劳动和远行久蹲，保持大便通畅，避免用力排便。一般 5-7 剂可收良效。

3. Ti Gang Tang (Anal-Lifting Decoction) Shows Good Effects for Rectal Prolapse via Fumigation and Washing: The author formulated Ti Gang Tang to treat rectal prolapse. Daily dosage: Sophora flavescens 100g, Cimicifuga rhizome, Chinese gallnut, and Angelica dahurica 50g each. Decoct in water and dissolve 20g of alum in each dose; fumigate first while hot, then wash, two to three times daily. During medication, patients should rest in bed appropriately, avoid heavy labor, long-distance travel, and prolonged squatting, maintain smooth bowel movements, and avoid straining during defecation. Generally, 5-7 doses yield good results.

《中医药信息报》（卢毅）

TCM Information News (Lu Yi)

4. 中药白芨治疗肛裂 肛裂是临床上较为常见的一种肛周疾患。表现为肛周疼痛，大便时出血。因肛裂处易于合并感染，创口常不易愈合，患者不堪痛苦。我院肛肠科采用中药白芨治疗肛裂，收到良好的效果，现介绍如下，不妨一试。

4. Treatment of Anal Fissure with TCM Bletilla striata: Anal fissure is a relatively common perianal disorder in clinical practice, manifesting as perianal pain and bleeding during defecation. Because anal fissures are prone to secondary infection, the wounds often fail to heal easily, causing great suffering to patients. The Department of Proctology in our hospital has adopted the TCM herb Bletilla striata to treat anal fissures with good results; it is introduced below for your reference.

治疗方法：取中药白芨 200 克，加入适量清水（水稍稍超过药面），待药液黏稠时，去除白芨，取出药液以文火浓缩成糊状。兑入煮沸去沫的蜂蜜 50 克，充分搅匀，冷却后即可使用。用时先用温水洗浴肛周部，再以纱布蘸取白芨液外涂于肛裂患处，每日 2 次，一般涂搽 3 至 5 天创口即会结痂而愈。

Treatment Method: Take 200g of the Chinese herb Bletilla striata (Baiji), add an appropriate amount of water (just enough to slightly cover the herb), and decoct until the liquid becomes viscous. Remove the herb residue, then simmer the extracted liquid over low heat to concentrate it into a paste-like consistency. Blend in 50g of boiled and skimmed honey, stir thoroughly, and allow the mixture to cool before use. For application, first cleanse the perianal area with warm water, then apply the prepared Bletilla paste externally to the anal fissure using a piece of gauze. Apply twice daily; typically, after 3 to 5 days of treatment, the wound will scab over and heal.

《中药科技报》1993 年 3 月 11 日（南京　孙扬）

Chinese Journal of Traditional Chinese Medicine Science and Technology, March 11, 1993 (Sun Yang, Nanjing)

5. 治痔疮肛裂出血方

处方及用法：白芨 30 克，花蕊石、黄柏各 15 克，冰片 5 克，共研成细末，撒于出血溃疡之创面，或撒于油纱条上贴敷患处。每日 1-2 次，连用 3-6 次可愈。近年来，笔者在医疗实践中，用其治疗痔疮出血 20 例，肛裂出血 10 例，效果显著。

《民族医药报》1993 年 1 月 15 日（久春）

5.Prescription for Hemorrhoids and Anal Fissure with Bleeding

Prescription and Usage: Take 30g of Bletilla striata (Baiji), 15g each of Ophicalcitum (Huaruishi) and Phellodendron Bark (Huangbai), and 5g of Borneol (Bingpian). Grind all ingredients together into a fine powder. Sprinkle the powder directly onto the bleeding or ulcerated wound, or apply it to an oil-soaked gauze strip and place it over the affected area. Apply once or twice daily; healing is typically achieved after 3 to 6 consecutive applications. In recent years, the author has applied this remedy in clinical practice to treat 20 cases of hemorrhoidal bleeding and 10 cases of anal fissure bleeding, achieving remarkable results.

Ethnic Medicine News, January 15, 1993 (Jiu Chun)

6. 治外痔一法

处方：生姜汁或干姜末。

适用症：各种外痔，尤适于炎性外痔，血栓外痔以及混合痔的突出部分。

用法：生姜榨汁直接涂于局部。每日数次，睡前再涂 1 次，或以纱布浸取姜汁敷于患处。干姜末用麻油调敷，干湿适中，外用纱布及胶布固定。经用 1-2

天即可消肿止痛，内痔下垂者可自行回纳。局部有溃疡者慎用。

《民族医药报》1993 年 4 月 2 日（李志民）

6. A Remedy for External Hemorrhoids

Prescription: Ginger juice or dried ginger powder.

Indications: Various types of external hemorrhoids, especially inflammatory hemorrhoids, thrombosed hemorrhoids, and protruding parts of mixed hemorrhoids.

Usage: Apply freshly extracted ginger juice directly to the affected area several times a day, with an additional application before bedtime. Alternatively, soak gauze in ginger juice and apply it to the area. For dried ginger powder, mix it with sesame oil to form a paste (neither too dry nor too wet), apply it externally, and secure with gauze and adhesive tape. Swelling and pain typically subside within 1–2 days of use, and prolapsed internal hemorrhoids may retract spontaneously. Caution: Avoid use if there are local ulcers.

Source: "Ethnic Medicine News," April 2, 1993 (by Li Zhimin)

7. 韭菜汁外洗方：

江南民间验方，用于治疗痔疮大便出血、滴血、流血严重者。取韭菜 250 克，洗净，切碎、放入锅内，加清水 500 毫升，煎煮 10 分钟，用纱布滤出汁液，待温度降至 40℃ 左右（成温水）时，用清洁纱布蘸药液，在大便前后擦洗肛门，可取得立即止血的功效，严重者可连续应用 3-5 天，但第 2 天要重新煮汁，原汁无效。

7.Leek Juice External Wash:

A traditional folk remedy from the Jiangnan region, used to treat severe cases of hemorrhoidal bleeding during bowel movements, including dripping or profuse bleeding. Take 250grams of fresh leeks, wash them thoroughly, and chop finely. Place in a pot, add 500 ml of water, and decoct for 10 minutes. Strain the liquid through gauze, and allow it to cool to approximately 40 ° C (lukewarm). Using a clean piece of gauze soaked in the solution, gently cleanse the anal area before and after each bowel movement. This method can provide immediate hemostatic relief. For more severe cases, treatment may be continued for 3–5 consecutive days; however, a fresh batch must be prepared daily, as leftover decoction loses its efficacy.

8. 肤轻松外用法：

晚上睡觉前，用温水洗净患处，将适量肤轻松涂抹患处，最好将药膏挤入肛门内。本人临床运用时，效果是用药次日即便软血止。一般应再用 4-5 次以巩固疗效。

8.Topical Application of Fluocinolone Acetonide:

Before bedtime, gently cleanse the affected area with warm water and apply an appropriate amount of Fluocinolone Acetonide ointment to the site. For optimal results, it is advisable to squeeze the ointment directly into the anal canal. In my clinical practice, this treatment has proven highly effective, typically resulting in softened stools and cessation of bleeding by the very next day. To consolidate the therapeutic effect, it is generally recommended to continue application for an additional 4–5 doses.

9. 痔疮薰洗方：苦参 50 克、黄芩 20 克、连翘 20 克、赤芍 20 克、土茯苓 30 克、大黄 15 克、蒲公英 20 克、山栀子 20 克，水煎熏洗，每日 2 次，30 日为 1 疗程。

9.Hemorrhoid Fumigation and Wash Formula: Ingredients: Sophora Root 50g, Scutellaria Root 20g, Forsythia Fruit 20g, Red Peony Root 20g, Glabrous Greenbrier Rhizome 30g, Rhubarb 15g, Dandelion Herb 20g, and Gardenia Fruit 20g. Decoct these ingredients in water for fumigation and sitz baths twice daily. A full course of treatment consists of 30 days.

10. 肛裂薰洗方：鱼腥草 30 克、苦参 30 克、五倍子 20 克、乌梅 30 克，水煎熏洗，或趁热外敷。

10.Anal Fissure Fumigation and Wash Formula: Ingredients: Houttuynia Herb 30g, Sophora Root 30g, Chinese Gallnut 20g, and Smoked Plum 30g. Decoct these ingredients in water for fumigation and sitz baths, or apply the hot decoction topically as a warm compress while still steaming.

11. 肛门瘙痒薰洗方：苦参 20 克、蛇床子 20 克、地肤子 20 克、蝉蜕 10 克、生地 20 克，煎水熏洗。

11.Anal Pruritus Fumigation and Wash Formula: Ingredients: Sophora Root 20g, Cnidium Fruit 20g, Kochia Fruit 20g, Cicada Slough 10g, and Rehmannia Root 20g. Decoct these ingredients in water for fumigation and sitz baths.

12. 肛门湿疹薰洗方：马齿苋 30 克、苦参 30 克、白藓皮 30 克、黄芩 30 克、地肤子 30 克，青黛 20 克，水煎熏洗。

12.Anal Eczema Fumigation and Wash Formula: Ingredients: Purslane Herb 30g, Sophora Root 30g, Densefruit Pittany Root-bark 30g, Scutellaria Root 30g, Kochia Fruit 30g, and Natural Indigo 20g. Decoct these ingredients in water for fumigation and sitz baths.

13. 脱肛薰洗方：五倍子 20 克、柴胡 20 克、枳壳 30 克、升麻 20 克、明矾 30 克，水煎以熏为主。

13.Rectal Prolapse Fumigation and Wash Formula: Ingredients: Chinese Gallnut 20g, Bupleurum Root 20g, Immature Bitter Orange Fruit 30g, Cimicifuga Rhizome 20g, and Alum 30g. Decoct these ingredients in water, with the treatment focusing primarily on fumigation.

14. 肛肠手术后并发症：石榴皮 30 克，鱼腥草 30 克、野菊花 30 克、乌梅 30 克、紫花地丁 30 克，水煎熏洗，有清洁创口作用，有利于新肉生长。

《民族医药报》1992 年 9 月 11 日（江苏省盐城市郊永丰医院 吉联军）

14.Postoperative Complications of Anorectal Surgery: Ingredients: Pomegranate Peel 30g, Houttuynia Herb 30g, Wild Chrysanthemum Flower 30g, Smoked Plum 30g, and Purpleflower Violet Herb 30g. Decoct these ingredients in water for fumigation and sitz baths. This preparation serves to cleanse the surgical wound and promote granulation tissue growth. National Journal of Ethnomedicine, September 11, 1992 (Ji Lianjun, Yongfeng Hospital, Yancheng Suburbs, Jiangsu Province)

15. 一、消痔散的配制及用法：

I. Preparation and Usage of Xiaozhi Powder:

处方：明矾 20 千克，芒硝 40 千克，冰片 2 千克。如为个人使用可按比例酌情减量。

Prescription: Alum 20 kg, Mirabilite 40 kg, Borneol 2 kg. For individual use, the quantities may be reduced proportionally as appropriate.

制法：将上述三种药物研成细末（数量多者最好过 100 目筛），装瓶备用，每瓶 200 克。

Preparation Method: Grind the above three ingredients into a fine powder (for larger quantities, it is advisable to sift through a 100-mesh sieve), then store in bottles for later use, with 200g per bottle.

用法：患者排除大小便后，将消痔散半瓶倒入 2000 毫升 50℃左右的热水中，搅拌片刻，使药物充分溶解。然后暴露臀部坐入盆中浸泡，每次 15-20 分钟，边坐浴边用手指轻柔地按摩局部，毕后用干毛巾擦干患处。如有伤口，可用消毒纱布覆盖，以免污染。每日 2-3 次，3 天为一疗程。

Usage: After urination or defecation, pour half a bottle of Xiaozhi Powder into 2000 ml of hot water at approximately 50 ° C, and stir briefly until fully dissolved. Then, sit in the basin with the buttocks exposed to soak for 15–20 minutes each time; during the sitz bath, gently massage the affected area with your fingers. Afterward, pat the area dry with a clean towel. If there is an open wound, cover it with sterile gauze to prevent contamination. Use 2–3 times daily; a full course of treatment lasts 3 days.

二、适应证及禁忌证：

II. Indications and Contraindications:

适应证：凡内痔脱垂或嵌顿、血栓性外痔初期，炎性外痔，静脉曲张性外痔，结缔组织性外痔，混合痔，脱肛，各种痔疮术后水肿等发炎肿胀明显，疼痛剧烈者及老年体弱不宜手术者，均为用药适应证。

Indications: This formula is indicated for cases presenting with marked inflammatory swelling and severe pain, including prolapsed or incarcerated internal hemorrhoids, early-stage thrombosed external hemorrhoids, inflammatory external hemorrhoids, varicose external hemorrhoids, connective tissue external hemorrhoids, mixed hemorrhoids, rectal prolapse, and postoperative edema following various hemorrhoid surgeries. It is also suitable for elderly or frail patients who are not candidates for surgery.

禁忌证：妇女经期及孕妇且有习惯性流产史者禁用。

Contraindications: Contraindicated during menstruation and in pregnant women with a history of habitual abortion.

三、疗效分析：

III. Analysis of Therapeutic Efficacy:

因肛肠疾病多为湿热阻滞，气血凝滞，经络不通所致，治宜清热解毒，消肿收敛止痛。而在消痔散中，明矾解毒燥湿，收敛止血；芒硝清热泻火，解毒消肿；冰片清热止痛，芳香通络，三药合用，故可取得较好效果。此外，消痔散为白色粉末，易溶于水，溶解后呈乳白色，性质稳定，不易变质，不须煎药，携带使用方便，用药后有凉爽舒适之感，无明显刺激及副作用，药源丰富。价格低廉，易于在一般患者中推广使用。

Anorectal diseases are mostly caused by damp-heat obstruction, qi and blood stagnation, and meridian blockage; therefore, treatment should focus on clearing heat and removing toxins, reducing swelling, promoting astringency, and relieving pain. In Xiaozhi Powder, Alum removes toxins, dries dampness, promotes astringency, and stops bleeding; Mirabilite clears heat, purges fire, removes toxins, and reduces swelling; Borneol clears heat, relieves pain, and unblocks meridians through its aromatic properties. The combination of these three herbs yields favorable therapeutic results. Furthermore, Xiaozhi Powder is a white powder that dissolves easily in water to form a milky-white solution. It is chemically stable, resistant to spoilage, requires no decoction, and is convenient to carry and use. Application produces a cool and comfortable sensation without significant irritation or side effects. With abundant raw material sources and low cost, it is easy to promote among general patients.

《民族医药报》1992 年 2 月 7 日（广西中医学院二附院 黄新 李廷冠）

National Journal of Ethnomedicine, February 7, 1992 (Huang Xin & Li Tinguan, Second Affiliated Hospital of Guangxi College of Traditional Chinese

Medicine)

16. 我们在临床上，用民间验方醋韭汁治疗痔疮（内痔 31 例，外痔 20 例，混合痔 5 例），效果满意，现简单介绍如下。

16.In our clinical practice, we have applied a traditional folk remedy—vinegar and leek juice—to treat hemorrhoids (31 cases of internal hemorrhoids, 20 cases of external hemorrhoids, and 5 cases of mixed hemorrhoids), achieving satisfactory results. A brief introduction is presented as follows.

治疗方法：

Treatment Method:

外痔：韭菜 500 克，米醋 1000 毫升，将韭菜切碎用醋煎煮，待药液烧开后，改用文火慢煎，用一中间有孔（孔大直径 5-6 厘米）的木板将锅罩紧，患者肛门对准板孔坐着，令徐徐上升之药液蒸气慢熏外痔，（温度以患者能忍受为宜），持续一小时左右，继之倒出药液，待冷后慢慢外洗痔部，每天早晚各一次，慢者 10-15 天见效，快者 3-4 天治愈，平均 7- 8 天左右收效。

External Hemorrhoids: Take 500g of fresh leeks and 1000 ml of rice vinegar. Chop the leeks finely and decoct them in the vinegar. Once the liquid comes to a boil, reduce to low heat and simmer gently. Cover the pot tightly with a wooden board that has a central hole (5–6 cm in diameter). The patient should sit over the board,Allow the gently rising herbal steam to slowly fumigate the external hemorrhoids (at a temperature tolerable to the patient) for approximately one hour. Subsequently, pour out the decoction, allow it to cool, and then use it to gently wash the affected area. Perform this procedure twice daily, once in the morning and once in the evening. Therapeutic effects are typically observed within 10–15 days in slower-responding cases, while milder cases may resolve within 3–4 days, with an average response time of approximately 7–8 days.

内痔：将韭菜洗净捣烂取汁，以韭菜汁 2 份，米醋 1 份比例混匀，用脱脂棉卷成荔枝果大小，浸湿药液，外涂少量石蜡油作润滑剂，令病人解便后塞入肛内，每天一次，5 天为一疗程，每疗程间隔 2 天，连续 2-3 疗程收效。

nternal Hemorrhoids: Wash fresh leeks thoroughly, crush them into a pulp, and extract the juice. Mix the leek juice with rice vinegar in a 2:1 ratio. Roll absorbent cotton into balls approximately the size of a lychee fruit, soak them thoroughly in the prepared solution, and apply a small amount of liquid paraffin as a lubricant. Instruct the patient to insert one soaked cotton ball into the anal. Administer once daily; a course of treatment consists of 5 days, with a 2-day interval between courses. Satisfactory results are typically achieved after 2–3 consecutive courses.

混合痔：则按上述两法合为运用，即先药液熏洗外痔部分，后再用浸好药液之药棉团塞肛处理内痔部分。

Mixed Hemorrhoids: For mixed hemorrhoids, combine the two methods described above. Specifically, first fumigate and wash the external component with the herbal decoction, and then insert a cotton ball soaked in the same solution into the internal hemorrhoids.

《民族医药报》（广西天等县民族医院 张国宁 龙锦娘）

National Journal of Ethnomedicine (Zhang Guoning & Long Jinniang, Tiandeng County Ethnic Hospital, Guangxi)

17. 外用药：冰片、朱砂各等份，共为细末，装瓶备用。另取田螺 1 个，取上药末少许，共打碎调匀。洗净肛门后取液汁搽于痔疮上，每日 3 次。二方并用，一般 3-4 天有效。

17. External Application: Mix equal parts of Borneol and Cinnabar, grind into a fine powder, and store in a bottle for later use. Separately, take one river snail, add a small amount of the above powder, and crush them together until well blended. After cleansing the anal area, apply the Hemorrhoids，Three times a day. Use both prescriptions together; generally effective in three to four days.

内服：

Oral administration：

1. 槐榆煎：槐花、地榆、黄芩、桃仁、火麻仁各 10 克，陈皮、甘草各 3 克。每日 1 剂，水煎服。适用于内痔出血，有收敛止血、消炎通便。

1.Huaiyu Decoction: Sophora Flower 10g, Sanguisorba Root 10g, Scutellaria

Root 10g, Peach Kernel 10g, Hemp Seed 10g, Tangerine Peel 3g, and Licorice Root 3g. Take one dose daily as a water decoction. Indicated for bleeding from internal hemorrhoids; it has the effects of promoting astringency to stop bleeding, reducing inflammation, and relieving constipation.

2. 凉血地黄汤：生地、槐花、天花粉各 10 克，当归尾、升麻、黄连、赤芍各 5 克，枳壳、荆芥、甘草各 3 克，黄芩 6 克，每日 1 剂，水煎服。适用于便血严重者。

《民族医药报》（张英俊 荐）

2.Liangxue Dihuang Decoction: Rehmannia Root 10g, Sophora Flower 10g, Trichosanthes Root 10g, Angelica Tail 5g, Cimicifuga Rhizome 5g, Coptis Rhizome 5g, Red Peony Root 5g, Immature Bitter Orange Fruit 3g, Schizonepeta Herb 3g, Licorice Root 3g, and Scutellaria Root 6g. Take one dose daily as a water decoction. Indicated for severe cases of hematochezia. National Journal of Ethnomedicine (Recommended by Zhang Yingjun)

3. 苦参鸡蛋：乃民间验方，取苦参、 红糖各 60 克，鸡蛋 2 枚。先将苦参放适量水煎煮，取浓液去渣，再放入红糖、鸡蛋，继续煎煮。蛋熟后去壳带汤 1 次服完。每日 1 剂，连服 5 天。

3.Sophora Root and Egg Decoction: A traditional folk remedy consisting of 60g Sophora Root, 60g brown sugar, and 2 eggs. First, decoct the Sophora Root in an appropriate amount of water to obtain a concentrated liquid; strain off the dregs, then add the brown sugar and eggs, and continue to simmer until the eggs are fully cooked. Peel the eggs and consume them together with the decoction in a single serving. Take one dose daily for 5 consecutive days.

4. 乙字汤：乃日本民间验方，原方组成：大黄 1 克，柴胡 5 克，升麻 2 克，甘草 2 克，黄芩 3 克，当归 6 克，水煎服。应用时可适当加大用量 2-3 倍。经本人临床验证，2-3 剂即可取得止痛止血、痔核逐渐内收的效果。

4.Yizi Decoction: A traditional Japanese folk remedy. The original formula consists of Rhubarb 1g, Bupleurum Root 5g, Cimicifuga Rhizome 2g, Licorice Root 2g, Scutellaria Root 3g, and Angelica Root 6g, prepared as a water decoction for oral administration. In clinical application, the dosage may be appropriately increased by 2 to 3 times. My own clinical experience has verified that after just 2–3 doses, this formula can effectively relieve pain, stop bleeding, and promote gradual retraction of hemorrhoidal masses.

5. 小儿脱肛：用清洁之陈艾叶 1 把，煎水泡洗肛头后，再用竹林中之嫩气笋子烧灰，同芝麻油调敷肛头上，数次有效。可同时取生黄芪 15 克、五倍子 10 克、升麻 10 克煎水内服，一日一剂，连服七天疗效更佳。

5.Pediatric Rectal Prolapse: Take a handful of clean, aged mugwort leaves, decoct them in water, and use the liquid to wash and soak the prolapsed rectum. Next, calcine tender bamboo shoots harvested from a bamboo grove into ash, mix the ash with sesame oil to form a paste, and apply it topically to the prolapsed tissue; this treatment is effective after several applications. Concurrently, an oral decoction of 15g Raw Astragalus Root, 10g Chinese Gallnut, and 10g Cimicifuga Rhizome may be administered at one dose per day for seven consecutive days to further enhance therapeutic efficacy.

《中药科技报》1991 年 2 月 6 日（李念秋）

Journal of Traditional Chinese Medicine Science and Technology, February 6, 1991 (Li Nianqiu)

6. 治小儿脱肛一法

便后清洁肛门，将药粉（五味子、煅龙骨、煅牡蛎、诃子各等份，研末，过筛）均匀撒于脱出的肠黏膜上，厚约 1-2 毫米，将脱出肠黏膜纳入肛门内，每次大便后必用。并用补中益气丸 1/4-1/ 3 丸 / 日 2 次口服。本法共收治 78 例，结果：痊愈 63 例，好转 11 例，无效 4 例。

6.A Method for Treating Pediatric Rectal Prolapse After defecation, cleanse the anal area and evenly sprinkle a medicinal powder (prepared by grinding equal parts of Schisandra Fruit, Calcined Dragon Bone, Calcined Oyster Shell, and Chebula Fruit into a fine powder and sifting it) onto the prolapsed intestinal mucosa to a thickness of approximately 1–2 mm. Gently reduce the prolapsed mucosa back into the anal canal. This procedure must be performed after every bowel movement. Concurrently, administer Buzhong Yiqi Pills orally at a dose of 1/4 to 1/3 pill twice daily. A total of 78 cases were treated using this method. Results: 63 cases were cured, 11 cases showed improvement, and 4 cases were unresponsive to treatment.

《民族医药报》1998 年 1 月 2 日（闻文）

National Journal of Ethnomedicine, January 2, 1998 (Wen Wen)

7. 痔疮出血：木瓜 200 克，打碎炒黑。研末，每服 10 克，日 3 次，蜜糖水送服。连服 5 天。临床应用 20 例，均有效。

7.Hemorrhoidal Bleeding: Take 200g of papaya, crush it, and stir-fry until charred. Grind into a fine powder and take 10g per dose, three times daily, with honey water as a vehicle. Administer for 5 consecutive days. In clinical application involving 20 cases, the treatment was effective in all instances.

8. 预防痔疮方：取炒过的决明子 20 克置杯内，以开水冲内浸，20 分钟后水呈淡黄色，即可饮用。该药液有一种特异的芳香味，以之代茶常饮，能健胃利尿，软便通肠，用治习惯性便秘、高血压及预防痔疮有效，久用可增强视力，健壮体质。

8.Hemorrhoid Prevention Formula: Place 20g of stir-fried Cassia Seeds in a cup, pour boiling water over them, and steep for 20 minutes until the liquid turns pale yellow; it is then ready to drink. This herbal tea has a distinctive aromatic fragrance. When consumed regularly as a substitute for ordinary tea, it helps strengthen the stomach, promote diuresis, soften stools, and relieve constipation. It is effective in treating habitual constipation and hypertension, as well as in preventing hemorrhoids. Long-term use may also improve eyesight and enhance overall physical constitution.

《民族医药报》（容小翔 辑）

National Journal of Ethnomedicine (Compiled by Rong Xiaoxiang)

9. 蕹菜治痔疮 蕹菜又称空心菜，味甘性寒，有清热，解毒，止血之功。民间用其治疗痔疮出血、便秘等症效果显著。方法是：取鲜蕹菜 1 公斤，洗净，切碎，捣汁。将菜汁放在锅内，先以急火，后以文火煎煮浓缩，至煎液较稠厚时加入蜂蜜 250 克，煮沸，停火起锅，待冷装瓶。每次一汤匙，每日 2- 3 次，以开水调服之。

9.Water Spinach for Hemorrhoids: Water spinach, also known as hollow-stem vegetable, is sweet in flavor and cold in nature, possessing the properties of clearing heat, removing toxins, and stopping bleeding. Folk remedies have demonstrated remarkable efficacy in using it to treat hemorrhoidal bleeding and constipation. Preparation method: Take 1 kg of fresh water spinach, wash thoroughly, chop finely, and crush to extract the juice. Place the juice in a pot, bring to a boil over high heat, then simmer over low heat to concentrate. When the decoction becomes relatively thick, add 250g of honey, bring back to a boil, remove from heat, and allow to cool before bottling. Take one tablespoon per dose, 2–3 times daily, diluted with warm boiled water.

《中医药信息报》（章辑）

Journal of Traditional Chinese Medicine Information (Compiled by Zhang)

10. 内服方：生地 30 克，当归 15 克，地榆 15 克，赤芍 15 克，黄芩 18 克，枳壳 15 克，槐角 30 克，升麻 12 克，大黄 15 克（后下），水煎服，早晚各 1 次。

1.10.Oral Formula: Rehmannia Root 30g, Angelica Root 15g, Sanguisorba Root 15g, Red Peony Root 15g, Scutellaria Root 18g, Immature Bitter Orange Fruit 15g, Sophora Fruit 30g, Cimicifuga Rhizome 12g, and Rhubarb 15g (added near the end of decoction). Prepare as a water decoction for oral administration, taken twice daily in the morning and evening.

11. 解放军 86170 部队（四川彭山县 612760）石贤富医师采用生何首乌配伍枳壳治疗肛裂 33 例，均获临床治愈（便秘、疼痛、出血均消失，裂隙愈合，半年内不复发）。

治疗方法：生何首乌 60 克，枳壳 30 克，水煎沸后熬 15-20 分钟，待温时饭前半小时服，2 日 1 剂，连服 4 剂。在服药期间乃至愈后禁食辣椒，以防影响药效及复发。

作者认为，生何首乌配伍枳壳，能润肠通便结，理气宽肠，使胃肠蠕动规律化，大肠对水份的重吸收正常，消除了便秘的原因，有利于肛裂的愈合。何首乌含蒽昆类，主要含大黄酚，能促进肠管运动。枳壳含挥发油和黄酮甙等物质，使皮肤黏膜血管收缩而止血。这是治愈肛裂的三因素。

Dr. Shi Xianfu from PLA Unit 86170 (Pengshan County, Sichuan Province, 612760) treated 33 cases of anal fissure using a combination of Raw Polygonum Multiflorum Root and Immature Bitter Orange Fruit, achieving clinical cure in all cases (constipation, pain, and bleeding resolved; fissures healed with no recurrence within six months). Treatment Method: Decoct 60g of Raw Polygonum Multiflorum Root and 30g of Immature Bitter Orange Fruit in water; after boiling, simmer for 15–20 minutes. Administer lukewarm half an hour before meals, one dose every two days for four consecutive doses. During treatment and even after recovery, spicy chili peppers must be strictly avoided to prevent compromising efficacy or causing relapse. The author notes that the combination of Raw Polygonum Multiflorum Root and Immature Bitter Orange Fruit moistens the intestines, relieves constipation, regulates qi, expands the intestinal tract, normalizes gastrointestinal peristalsis, and restores normal water reabsorption in the large intestine, thereby eliminating the underlying cause of constipation and facilitating fissure healing. Polygonum Multiflorum contains anthraquinones, primarily chrysophanol, which promote intestinal motility. Immature Bitter Orange Fruit contains volatile oils and flavonoid glycosides, which constrict mucosal blood vessels to stop bleeding. These constitute the three key factors in curing anal fissures.

《中医药信息报》1992 年 10 月 3 日（刘永连 摘）

Journal of Traditional Chinese Medicine Information, October 3, 1992 (Excerpted by Liu Yonglian)

12. 治脱肛：炙黄芪 30 克，赤石脂 15 克，党参、白术、柴胡、当归、白芷各 10 克，陈皮、炙甘草、黄连、川芎、升麻各 6 克，黄芩 9 克，枳壳 12 克。水煎分二次服，每日一剂。Treatment for Rectal Prolapse: Honey-fried Astragalus Root 30g, Red Halloysite 15g, Codonopsis Root 10g, Atractylodes Rhizome 10g, Bupleurum Root 10g, Angelica Root 10g, Angelica Dahurica Root 10g, Tangerine

Peel 6g, Honey-fried Licorice Root 6g, Coptis Rhizome 6g, Ligusticum Rhizome 6g, Cimicifuga Rhizome 6g, Scutellaria Root 9g, and Immature Bitter Orange Fruit 12g. Prepare as a water decoction divided into two doses, taken once daily.

《中药科技报》1992 年 11 月 26 日

Journal of Traditional Chinese Medicine Science and Technology, November 26, 1992

13. 药物组成：槐米 30 克，猪直肠一具，白蜜 30 克

13.Formula Composition: Sophora Flower Bud 30g, one pig rectum, and honey 30g.

煮制方法: 把洗净的槐米和白蜜置于洗净的猪直肠内，两头扎紧，文火煮烂、食猪肠饮汤。连服五天为一疗程。

Preparation Method: Place the washed Sophora Flower Buds and honey inside the cleaned pig rectum, tie both ends tightly, and simmer over low heat until thoroughly soft. Consume the pig intestine and drink the broth. Five consecutive days constitute one course of treatment.

第三章　心脑血管病

Chapter 3　Cardiovascular and Cerebrovascular Diseases

一、心脏病（11方）

I. Heart Disease (11 Formulas)

风湿性心瓣膜病调治方

Therapeutic Formulas for Rheumatic Valvular Heart Disease

严重危害人体健康的疾病——风湿性心瓣膜病，好发于20-40岁年龄的人，女性多于男性，大部分病人起病前有风湿热病史。

Rheumatic valvular heart disease, a condition that poses a serious threat to human health, predominantly affects individuals aged 20–40, with a higher incidence in females than males; most patients have a history of rheumatic fever prior to onset.

风湿性心瓣膜炎遗留的慢性瓣膜病，主要表现为全身乏力、咳嗽、咯粉红色泡沫状痰、气喘、心悸、头晕、尿少、下肢浮肿等症状。

Chronic valvular disease resulting from rheumatic valvulitis primarily manifests as generalized fatigue, coughing with pink foamy sputum, dyspnea, palpitations, dizziness, oliguria, and lower limb edema.

对于患有风湿性心瓣膜病者可选用下列简便可行的方法治疗，效果颇好。

For patients with rheumatic valvular heart disease, the following simple and practical treatment methods can be selected, yielding favorable therapeutic outcomes.

1. 玉竹15-30克，水煎服，每日一剂，治风湿性心瓣膜病，适宜于心悸、乏力、口渴、舌红者。

1.Fragrant Solomonseal Rhizome 15–30g, prepared as a water decoction taken once daily; indicated for rheumatic valvular heart disease, particularly suitable for patients presenting with palpitations, fatigue, thirst, and a red tongue.

2. 鸭跖草 50-100 克，生玉竹、生地各 12 克，甘草 6 克，每日一帖，水煎分服，治风湿性心肌炎、风湿性心瓣膜病。

2. Common Dayflower Herb 50–100g, Raw Fragrant Solomonseal Rhizome 12g, Raw Rehmannia Root 12g, and Licorice Root 6g; take one dose daily as a water decoction divided into multiple servings for the treatment of rheumatic myocarditis and rheumatic valvular heart disease.

3. 老茶树根 30-60 克，加糯米酒适量，水煎 2 次，混合，临睡前一次服，连服一月余。

3. Old Tea Tree Root 30–60g with an appropriate amount of glutinous rice wine; decoct twice in water, combine the two decoctions, and take as a single dose before bedtime daily for over one month.

4. 万年青 20-30 克，红糖适量。将万年青加水 150 毫升，煎至 50 毫升，滤出。原药再加水 120 毫升，再煎煮 40 毫升。混合两次煎液成 90 毫升，加红糖，分 3 次服，每天一剂，7 天为一疗程。治胸闷、气喘、唇色紫绀、舌质紫暗或有瘀点。

4. Rohdea Japonica Rhizome 20–30g and an appropriate amount of brown sugar. Add 150 ml of water to the herb, decoct to 50 ml, and strain. Add another 120 ml of water to the residue, decoct again to obtain 40 ml. Combine both decoctions to yield 90 ml, add brown sugar, and divide into three doses per day; one dose daily constitutes a 7-day course of treatment. Indicated for chest tightness, dyspnea, cyanotic lips, and a dark purple tongue or petechiae.

5. 土牛膝、臭梧桐各 30 克，万年青根 15 克，灯芯草 3 克，水煎服。

5. Wild Achyranthes Root 30g, Harlequin Glorybower Twig 30g, Rohdea Japonica Root 15g, and Rush Pith 3g; prepare as a water decoction for oral administration.

6. 猪肾 1 个，党参、当归各 15 克。将猪肾臊腺剔净，切片，把党参、当归用白纱布包好，同放锅内加水适量煮汤。熟后，去药渣调味服食，隔天一剂，连服数剂。

6. One pig kidney, Codonopsis Root 15g, and Angelica Root 15g. Remove the adrenal glands from the pig kidney completely, slice it, wrap the herbs in white gauze, place all ingredients in a pot with an appropriate amount of water, and simmer into a soup. After cooking, remove the herb residue, season to taste, and consume; take one dose every other day for several consecutive doses.

7. 猪心 1 个，琥珀粉 5 克，党参 5 克。将猪心的血液洗净，放入琥珀粉、党参粉，置砂锅内加水用小火炖煮，经调味，食肉喝汤，隔天一次，连服数剂。治风湿性心瓣膜病，见心性、气短、眩晕、乏力、纳差者。

7. One pig heart, Amber Powder 5g, and Codonopsis Root Powder 5g. Wash away blood from the pig heart, fill it with amber powder and Codonopsis root powder, place in a clay pot with water, and stew over low heat. Season to taste, then consume both meat and broth once every other day for several doses. Indicated for rheumatic valvular heart disease presenting with palpitations, shortness of breath, dizziness, fatigue, and poor appetite.

《中医药信息报》1992 年 4 月 11 日（祯 恒）

Journal of Traditional Chinese Medicine Information, April 11, 1992 (Zhen Heng)

8. 淫羊藿治疗心绞痛。淫羊藿为传统的温肾壮阳药物。在研治冠心病的药物筛选动物实验中，有显著增加冠状动脉血流量，改善心肌缺血缺氧状态的作用，以淫羊藿片 0.3 克 / 片，每次 4-6 片，每日 2 次，30 天为一疗程，改善心绞痛总有效率为 77.8%，改善心电图总有效率为 74.3%。

8. Epimedium Herb for Angina Pectoris. Epimedium is a traditional herbal medicine used to warm the kidneys and tonify yang. In animal screening experiments for coronary heart disease therapeutics, it demonstrated significant effects in increasing coronary artery blood flow and improving myocardial ischemia and hypoxia. Administered as Epimedium tablets (0.3g/tablet), 4–6 tablets per dose, twice daily, with a 30-day course of treatment, the overall effective rate for relieving angina pectoris was 77.8%, and the overall effective rate for ECG improvement was 74.3%.

《中药科技报》1992年7月6日

Journal of Traditional Chinese Medicine Science and Technology, July 6, 1992

9. 山楂茶 山楂能改善冠状动脉供血，具有增进消化、降低血脂、扩张血管、调节血压等作用。故茶对高血压、高血脂及老年心脏衰弱、冠心病患者，可以长期饮用。取山楂压扁，每次30克，放茶杯中，沸水冲泡，焖20分钟，代茶饮用。以味淡为度。

9. Hawthorn Tea: Hawthorn fruit improves coronary artery blood supply and has the effects of promoting digestion, lowering blood lipids, dilating blood vessels, and regulating blood pressure. Therefore, this tea can be consumed long-term by patients with hypertension, hyperlipidemia, senile cardiac weakness, and coronary heart disease. Crush 30g of hawthorn fruit per serving, place in a teacup, infuse with boiling water, steep for 20 minutes, and drink as a tea substitute until the flavor becomes mild.

10. 三七茶 三七花具有清热平肝降压的作用，尤其能降低脉压兼有改善心肌供血功能，故经常饮用此茶，可防治高血压。配制方法是取三七花5克，开水冲泡，每日3-4次。

10. Notoginseng Flower Tea: Notoginseng flowers clear heat, calm the liver, and lower blood pressure; they are particularly effective in reducing pulse pressure while also improving myocardial blood supply. Regular consumption of this tea can help prevent and treat hypertension. Preparation: Steep 5g of notoginseng flowers in boiling water, taken 3–4 times daily.

11. 冠心病、心绞痛：白檀香、玉果各25克，广枣15克。研细，调匀，每日1-2次，每次3-6克，加50-100毫升水，用文火煮，凉服。

11. Coronary Heart Disease and Angina Pectoris: White Sandalwood 25g, Nutmeg 25g, and Guangzao Fruit 15g. Grind into a fine powder and mix thoroughly. Take 3–6g per dose, 1–2 times daily, add 50–100 ml of water, simmer over low heat, and take when cool.

《民族医药报》1992年10月16日

National Journal of Ethnomedicine, October 16, 1992

二、（一）肥胖症（6方）
II. (I) Obesity (6 Formulas)

1. 治疗肥胖症方

1.Formula for Treating Obesity

方剂组成：黄芪、防己、白术、川芎、制首乌各15克，生山楂、丹参、茵陈、水牛角各30克，生大黄9克。

Formula Composition: Astragalus Root 15g, Fangji Root 15g, Atractylodes Rhizome 15g, Ligusticum Rhizome 15g, Prepared Polygonum Multiflorum Root 15g, Raw Hawthorn Fruit 30g, Salvia Root 30g, Artemisia Scoparia Herb 30g, Buffalo Horn 30g, and Raw Rhubarb 9g.

服用方法：将以上药物加水煎成100毫升，分2次服；特别肥胖的，每天增服50毫升。服药时间一般应在4周以上。服药期间，胖病人的生活规律可以照旧，如能适当控制饮食和增加一些体力活动则效果更好些，如饭后散步半小时以上就有一定效果。

Administration Method: Decoct the above herbs in water to obtain 100 ml of liquid, divided into two doses per day; for severely obese patients, increase the daily intake by an additional 50 ml. The treatment course should generally last at least 4 weeks. During medication, patients may maintain their regular daily routines; however, better results can be achieved with appropriate dietary control and increased physical activity, such as walking for more than half an hour after meals.

《民族医药报》1998年4月3日（唐蔚波）

National Journal of Ethnomedicine, April 3, 1998 (Tang Weibo)

2. 山楂决明子茶

2. Hawthorn and Cassia Seed Tea

山楂15克，荷叶15克，决明子10克。将三味药共切细末，沸水冲泡。代茶饮，每日一剂，分3-5次饮用。功效：降脂化瘀，利水减肥。

Hawthorn Fruit 15g, Lotus Leaf 15g, and Cassia Seeds 10g. Grind all three ingredients into a fine powder and infuse with boiling water. Drink as a tea substitute, one dose daily divided into 3–5 servings. Efficacy: Lowers blood lipids, resolves blood stasis, promotes diuresis, and reduces weight.

3. 冬瓜茶

3. Wax Gourd Tea

冬瓜 500 克。将冬瓜去皮和瓤，洗净切块，绞汁，煮开后饮用。每日分早晚两次饮用，每次 200 毫升。功效：利水减肥，轻身延年。

Wax Gourd 500g. Peel and deseed the wax gourd, wash thoroughly, cut into pieces, extract the juice, bring to a boil, and drink. Consume twice daily in the morning and evening, 200 ml per serving. Efficacy: Promotes diuresis, reduces weight, lightens the body, and prolongs life.

4. 荷叶茶

4. Lotus Leaf Tea

荷叶 9 克，山楂 9 克，陈皮 9 克。洗净，混合，沸水冲泡。代茶饮，连服 3 个月为一疗程。功效：理气祛湿减肥。

Lotus Leaf 9g, Hawthorn Fruit 9g, and Tangerine Peel 9g. Wash clean, mix together, and infuse with boiling water. Drink as a tea substitute; a full course of treatment consists of 3 consecutive months. Efficacy: Regulates qi, dispels dampness, and reduces weight.

5. 枸杞菊花茶

5. Wolfberry and Chrysanthemum Tea

枸杞子 30 克，菊花 20 克。沸水冲泡。代茶饮，每日一剂，分 3 次饮用。功效：减肥降脂。

Wolfberry Fruit 30g and Chrysanthemum Flower 20g. Infuse with boiling water. Drink as a tea substitute, one dose daily divided into 3 servings. Efficacy: Reduces weight and lowers blood lipids.

6. 辨证分型治疗脂肪肝

6. Syndrome Differentiation-Based Treatment for Fatty Liver Disease

肝气郁结型：用柴胡疏肝散（含柴胡、陈皮、川芎、白芍、香橼、郁金、枳壳、香附、甘草等）。

Liver Qi Stagnation Type: Treated with Chaihu Shugan Powder (containing Bupleurum Root, Tangerine Peel, Ligusticum Rhizome, White Peony Root, Citron Fruit, Curcuma Tuber, Immature Bitter Orange Fruit, Cyperus Rhizome, Licorice Root, etc.).

痰湿困阻型：用平胃散加味（含苍术、厚朴、泽泻、茯苓、生黄芪、白术、薏苡仁、砂仁、菖蒲等）。

Phlegm-Dampness Obstruction Type: Treated with Modified Pingwei Powder (containing Atractylodes Rhizome, Magnolia Bark, Alisma Rhizome, Poria, Raw Astragalus Root, Atractylodes Rhizome, Coix Seed, Amomum Fruit, Acorus Rhizome, etc.).

湿热内蕴型：用加味柴胡汤加减（含茵陈、柴胡、黄芩、黄连、葛根、大黄、瞿麦、薏苡仁、泽泻、香橼、车前子等）。

Internal Accumulation of Damp-Heat Type: Treated with Modified Chaihu Decoction (containing Artemisia Scoparia Herb, Bupleurum Root, Scutellaria Root, Coptis Rhizome, Kudzu Root, Rhubarb, Dianthus Herb, Coix Seed, Alisma Rhizome, Citron Fruit, Plantain Seed, etc.).

瘀血阻络型：用复元活血汤加减（含柴胡、当归、郁金、丹参、天花粉、桃仁、红花、大黄、王不留行、芍药、川芎、炮甲片、地龙等）。

Blood Stasis Blocking Collaterals Type: Treated with Modified Fuyuan Huoxue Decoction (containing Bupleurum Root, Angelica Root, Curcuma Tuber, Salvia Root, Trichosanthes Root, Peach Kernel, Safflower, Rhubarb, Vaccaria Seed, Peony Root, Ligusticum Rhizome, Processed Pangolin Scale, Earthworm, etc.).

日 1 剂水煎服，3 个月为 1 疗程。运用本法共收治 76 例，结果：治愈 17 例，好转 56 例，无效 3 例。

Take one dose daily as a water decoction; a full course of treatment lasts 3 months. A total of 76 cases were treated using this method. Results: 17 cases were cured, 56 cases showed improvement, and 3 cases were unresponsive to treatment.

《民族医药报》1998 年 1 月 23 日（茵 荐）

National Journal of Ethnomedicine, January 23, 1998 (Recommended by Yin)

二、（二）高血脂症（4 方）

II. (II) Hyperlipidemia (4 Formulas)

1. 治高脂血症方

1.Formula for Treating Hyperlipidemia

方药组成：栝蒌 25 克，黄精 25 克，法半夏 10 克，海藻 15 克，泽泻 15 克，苍术 12 克，何首乌 30 克，生山楂 30 克，丹参 30 克，决明子 18 克，大黄 5 克，水煎服，每日 1 剂。治疗 92 例，总有效率 92.39%。全部病例均未发现明显毒副反应，且其合并症及并发症均有不同程度的改善。

Formula Composition: Trichosanthes Fruit 25g, Polygonatum Rhizome 25g, Processed Pinellia Rhizome 10g, Seaweed 15g, Alisma Rhizome 15g, Atractylodes Rhizome 12g, Polygonum Multiflorum Root 30g, Raw Hawthorn Fruit 30g, Salvia Root 30g, Cassia Seeds 18g, and Rhubarb 5g. Prepare as a water decoction, taken once daily. In the treatment of 92 cases, the total effective rate was 92.39%. No significant toxic or adverse reactions were observed in any case, and concomitant conditions and complications showed varying degrees of improvement.

《民族医药报》1998 年 1 月 23 日（广医 荐）

National Journal of Ethnomedicine, January 23, 1998 (Recommended by Guangyi)

2. 取决明子 10 克，制首乌 10 克，桑寄生 10 克，泽泻 10 克，生山楂 10 克。每日煎服两次，或以开水泡饮频服，一日一贴，一月为一疗程。治疗高脂血症，效果明显。经几十例临床观察，此方适用于冠心病、慢性肝炎、高血压病兼有高血脂症患者，它服用方便，无副作用，同时还具有一定的降血压作用。

2. Take Cassia Seeds 10g, Prepared Polygonum Multiflorum Root 10g, Taxillus Twig 10g, Alisma Rhizome 10g, and Raw Hawthorn Fruit 10g. Administer as a decoction twice daily, or infuse with boiling water and drink frequently

throughout the day; one dose per day constitutes a one-month course of treatment. This formula demonstrates marked efficacy in treating hyperlipidemia. Clinical observation of dozens of cases indicates that it is suitable for patients with coronary heart disease, chronic hepatitis, or hypertension accompanied by hyperlipidemia. It is convenient to take, free of side effects, and also possesses a certain degree of antihypertensive effect.

《民族医药报》1991 年 10 月 25 日（江苏 吴自强）

National Journal of Ethnomedicine, October 25, 1991 (Wu Ziqiang, Jiangsu Province)

3. 高脂血症：红花 10 克，白檀香、紫檀香各 5 克。研细，调匀。每日 2 次，每次 10 克，水煎凉服，3 周为 1 疗程。

3. Hyperlipidemia: Safflower 10g, White Sandalwood 5g, and Red Sandalwood 5g. Grind into a fine powder and mix thoroughly. Take 10g per dose, twice daily, prepared as a water decoction and taken when cool; a full course of treatment lasts 3 weeks.

4. 双耳汤治血管硬化 取白木耳、黑木耳各 15 克，以冷水泡发并洗净，放在小碗内，加水和冰糖适量，将碗置蒸锅内，蒸 1 小时。一次或分次吃木耳饮汤，每日 2-3 次，连服 2-3 个月。用其治疗老年人血管硬化、高血压和眼底出血等症，效果显著。

4. Double Fungus Soup for Arteriosclerosis: Take 15g each of white fungus and black fungus, soak in cold water until rehydrated, wash clean, place in a small bowl, add an appropriate amount of water and rock sugar, and steam in a steamer for 1 hour. Consume the fungi and broth either at once or in divided portions, 2–3 times daily, for 2–3 consecutive months. This remedy has shown remarkable efficacy in treating arteriosclerosis, hypertension, and fundus hemorrhage in elderly patients.

《中医药信息报》（吴建平）

Journal of Traditional Chinese Medicine Information (Wu Jianping)

三、脑血栓（5方）
III. Cerebral Thrombosis (5 Formulas)

1. 医学家最近研究发现，豆豉具有意外的保健作用。科学家对170多种食物的研究发现，豆豉中尿激酶的含量位居榜首，还含有大量的维生素B和抗生素，能有效地预防脑血栓的形成，改善脑血流量，防治老年性痴呆。

1.Medical researchers have recently discovered that fermented soybeans possess unexpected health benefits. A scientific study of over 170 types of food revealed that fermented soybeans rank first in urokinase content; they also contain abundant vitamin B and antibiotics, which can effectively prevent cerebral thrombosis, improve cerebral blood flow, and help prevent and treat senile dementia.

《中药科技报》1991年6月26日（仰占辑）

Journal of Traditional Chinese Medicine Science and Technology, June 26, 1991 (Compiled by Yang Zhan)

2. 治脑血栓形成后遗症方

2. Formula for Sequelae of Cerebral Thrombosis

处方：黄芪50克，丹参30克，制马钱子粉1克（冲服），土鳖虫10克，地龙20克，当归15克，乳香10克，没药10克，花粉15克，三七粉2克（冲服）。

Prescription: Astragalus Root 50g, Salvia Root 30g, Processed Strychnos Seed Powder 1g (taken with the decoction), Ground Beetle 10g, Earthworm 20g, Angelica Root 15g, Frankincense 10g, Myrrh 10g, Trichosanthes Root 15g, and Notoginseng Powder 2g (taken with the decoction).

用法：每日1剂，水煎服，10天为1个疗程，连用2-3个疗程。

Usage: Take one dose daily as a water decoction; a course of treatment consists of 10 days, with 2–3 consecutive courses recommended.

主治：脑血栓形成后遗症，半身不遂，语言謇涩，头晕，脉沉细等。

Indications: Sequelae of cerebral thrombosis, hemiplegia, slurred speech, dizziness, and deep-thready pulse.

《民族医药报》（徐文）

National Journal of Ethnomedicine (Xu Wen)

3. 适应于高血压引起的脑血栓。

3. Indicated for Cerebral Thrombosis Caused by Hypertension

处方：桂枝、川牛膝、川椒、地风、甘草、制乳香、制没药、木瓜、明天麻、自然铜（醋淬）、血竭花、威灵仙各九克，何首乌、川军、川乌、草乌、破故子、麻黄、生麻、杜仲、续断、川羌活各六克，千年见、黄芪、苍术各十二克，洋金花三克，马钱子三十克，蜂蜜一百五十克，共为细末密制为十五丸，每天晚上服一丸，开水送下。

Prescription: Cassia Twig 9g, Cyathula Root 9g, Sichuan Pepper 9g, Fangfeng Root 9g, Licorice Root 9g, Processed Frankincense 9g, Processed Myrrh 9g, Papaya Fruit 9g, Gastrodia Rhizome 9g, Natural Copper (quenched in vinegar) 9g, Dragon's Blood Flower 9g, Clematis Root 9g, Polygonum Multiflorum Root 6g, Rhubarb 6g, Sichuan Aconite Root 6g, Kusnezoff Monkshood Root 6g, Psoralea Fruit 6g, Ephedra Herb 6g, Raw Sesame 6g, Eucommia Bark 6g, Dipsacus Root 6g, Notopterygium Rhizome 6g, Homalomena Rhizome 12g, Astragalus Root 12g, Atractylodes Rhizome 12g, Datura Flower 3g, Strychnos Seed 30g, and Honey 150g. Grind all ingredients into a fine powder, mix with honey to form 15 pills. Take one pill each evening with warm boiled water.

晚上服药丸时，注射维生素 B1 和 B12，多喝蜂蜜，每日三次，以防马钱子中毒。

When taking the pill in the evening, administer injections of vitamin B1 and B12, and consume honey three times daily to prevent strychnos poisoning.

每天早晨、中午服胃酶，以防毒药伤胃。如果病情严重昏迷时，用西药抢救。输液加右旋糖酐，细胞色素丙等，注射维脑路通、清醒后用此秘方。也可用针灸，取人中、内关、三阴交，每晚强刺激，快速取穴重刺而不留针，每日一次，针灸一周，对任何致迷（如脑痉挛、脑溢血），针灸效果颇佳。

Administer pepsin every morning and at noon to protect the stomach from toxic damage. In cases of severe coma, use Western medicine for emergency resuscitation, including intravenous infusion of dextran and cytochrome C, along with injections of troxerutin; resume this secret formula once the patient regains consciousness. Acupuncture may also be applied, selecting Renzhong (GV26), Neiguan (PC6), and Sanyinjiao (SP6) points; apply strong stimulation each evening with rapid insertion and heavy manipulation without needle retention, once daily for one week. Acupuncture shows excellent efficacy for coma caused by various conditions such as cerebral vasospasm or cerebral hemorrhage.

4. 主治重型瘫痪（一至五年血压高低均可）。

4. Indicated for Severe Paralysis (Applicable Regardless of High or Low Blood Pressure Within One to Five Years of Onset)

处方: 爬山虎六十克，西洋参一百二十克，麝香一点二克，酩馏酒一千五百克，将前三味泡入酒内，半月后服用，每次二十毫升。

Prescription: Boston Ivy 60g, American Ginseng 120g, Musk 1.2g, and Distilled Liquor 1500g. Steep the first three ingredients in the liquor for half a month before consumption; take 20 ml per dose.

体会和评价：

Clinical Experience and Evaluation:

经临床对一百例患者统计分析：凡是高血压动脉硬化所致的瘫痪发病在十天之内者疗效达百分之九十六；在一年之内者，疗效百分之七十；在一百天之内者，疗效百分之九十；对高血压所致的半身不遂，显效率百分之一百，三年以上或血压稳定的患者、疗效欠佳。

Statistical analysis of 100 clinical cases showed that the effective rate reached 96% for paralysis caused by hypertensive arteriosclerosis with onset within 10 days; 70% for onset within one year; and 90% for onset within 100 days. For hemiplegia caused by hypertension, the markedly effective rate was 100%; however, efficacy was poor for patients with disease duration exceeding three years or those with stable blood pressure.

一般一周消，两周愈，重者可服二料，二料无效不可再服。服药后出现抽搐、口渴、大便干、难受等症状、为马钱子的副作用，无关大局，但心、肝、肺、肾、胃有严重并发症时慎用或少用。

Generally, symptoms resolve within one week and recovery occurs within two weeks; severe cases may take a second batch of preparation, but discontinue if no response is observed after the second batch. Symptoms such as convulsions, thirst, dry stools, and discomfort after administration are side effects of strychnos seed and are generally not clinically significant; however, use cautiously or reduce dosage in patients with severe complications involving the heart, liver, lungs, kidneys, or stomach.

《中药科技报》1991 年 11 月 26 日

Journal of Traditional Chinese Medicine Science and Technology, November 26, 1991

5. 茜草根可治疗脑梗塞

5. Madder Root for Cerebral Infarction

单味茜草根（生用）30 克，水 1200 毫升，文火煎 1 小时，滤出药液，剩余药渣再煎两次，将 3 次滤液集中浓缩至 1200 毫升，分三次服用，每日一剂。

Single herb Raw Madder Root 30g, decocted in 1200 ml of water over low heat for 1 hour; strain the liquid, decoct the residue twice more, combine all three filtrates, and concentrate to 1200 ml. Divide into three doses taken daily, one dose per day.

病案举例 Case Report

洪 XX，女，67 岁，农民，1985 年冬发生脑梗塞后，出现右侧偏瘫，生活不能自理，经中西医治疗约 1 月余，症状未见明显好转后，改用单味茜草根（生用）30 克，水煎服，每日一剂，连续服用 93 天，症状完全消失，可自行行走，生活自理，现仍存活，多次随访，无复发。

Patient Hong XX, female, 67 years old, farmer. After suffering cerebral infarction in winter 1985, she developed right-sided hemiplegia and was unable to care for herself. Following approximately one month of combined TCM and Western medical treatment with no significant improvement, she switched to single-herb Raw Madder Root 30g as a water decoction, one dose daily for 93 consecutive days. All symptoms completely resolved; she regained independent ambulation and self-care ability. She remains alive today with no recurrence confirmed through multiple follow-up visits.

体会 Clinical Insights

脑梗塞是由于脑的血液供应障碍，致脑组织缺血、缺氧而引起的脑软化，其中包括脑血栓形成和脑栓塞。脑梗塞的临床表现，可因血管闭塞的部位不同而有所差异。在治疗方面以改善脑的血液供应为治疗原则。茜草根生用能引血活血，消瘀通经。大剂量应用，其效力更大。

Cerebral infarction refers to encephalomalacia caused by impaired cerebral blood supply leading to ischemia and hypoxia of brain tissue, encompassing both cerebral thrombosis and cerebral embolism. Clinical manifestations vary depending on the site of vascular occlusion. The therapeutic principle focuses on improving cerebral blood supply. Raw madder root promotes blood circulation, activates blood flow, dissipates stasis, and unblocks meridians; its efficacy is further enhanced when used in large doses.

《中国医药报》

China Medical News

四、高血压（23 方）
IV. Hypertension (23 Formulas)

1. 田七花、野菊花各 15 克，水煎服，日一剂。

1.Notoginseng Flower 15g and Wild Chrysanthemum Flower 15g; prepare as a water decoction, taken once daily.

2. 菠菜 500 克、炒时加小麻油 25 克和盐，急火炒熟，每日食用一次。

2.Spinach 500g; stir-fry over high heat with 25g sesame oil and salt until cooked, consumed once daily.

3. 水鱼一个，洗净去内脏，加麦冬 10 克、熟地 10 克，酒盐姜葱各适量，清蒸烂熟即可食用，每日一次。

3.One soft-shelled turtle; wash clean, remove internal organs, add Ophiopogon Root 10g, Prepared Rehmannia Root 10g, and appropriate amounts of cooking wine, salt, ginger, and scallion; steam until thoroughly tender and consume once daily.

4. 白嫩萝卜（去皮）100 克、海蜇皮 100 克、洗净切成细丝，用醋、麻油、盐、味精拌匀、做凉拌菜食用，每日一次。

4.Tender white radish (peeled) 100g and jellyfish skin 100g; wash clean, shred finely, mix evenly with vinegar, sesame oil, salt, and MSG to make a cold salad, consumed once daily.

5. 里脊肉 250 克切片、枸杞子 20 克、贡菊 6 克（拍碎），里脊肉用淀粉味精盐葱酒浆好，入油锅爆炒。另起油锅将枸杞子、贡菊在油中略加翻炒，再倒入里脊肉炒匀，加适量调味品即可食用，每日一次。

5.Pork tenderloin 250g (sliced), Wolfberry Fruit 20g, and Gongju Chrysanthemum 6g (crushed); marinate the pork slices with starch, MSG, salt, scallion, and cooking wine, then deep-fry briefly in hot oil. In a separate pan, lightly stir-fry the wolfberry fruit and chrysanthemum in oil, add back the pork tenderloin, stir-fry evenly, season to taste, and consume once daily.

《民族医药报》（桂林 何建华）

National Journal of Ethnomedicine (He Jianhua, Guilin)

6. 治高血压验方

6. Empirical Formula for Hypertension

单用丹皮（15 克）一味，水煎服，每天一剂分早晚二次服。21 天为一疗程。检查有效。

Single herb Moutan Bark 15g; prepare as a water decoction, one dose daily divided into morning and evening servings. A course of treatment consists of 21 days. Clinical examinations confirmed its efficacy.

《中医药信息报》

Journal of Traditional Chinese Medicine Information

7. 醋浸花生米治高血压

7. Vinegar-Soaked Peanuts for Hypertension

（用料）：花生米、醋各适量。

Ingredients: Appropriate amounts of peanuts and vinegar.

（制法）：生花生米（带衣者 ）半碗即可，用好醋倒入满碗浸泡 7 天，每日早晚各服 10 粒。血压下降后可隔数日服用。

Preparation Method: Take half a bowl of raw peanuts (with red skins intact), fill the bowl with good-quality vinegar, and soak for 7 days. Take 10 peanuts each morning and evening. After blood pressure decreases, the dosage may be taken once every few days.

（功效）：清热活血。可治高血压，对保护血管壁，阻止血栓形成都有较好的作用。

Efficacy: Clears heat and activates blood circulation. It is effective in treating hypertension, protecting vascular walls, and preventing thrombosis.

《中医药信息报》1992 年 8 月 1 日

Journal of Traditional Chinese Medicine Information, August 1, 1992

8. 大血藤 15 克、十大功劳 15 克、杜仲 30 克、夏枯草 9 克，泡酒 500 毫升，一周后，每日服 2 次，每次 20 毫升，治疗原发性高血压。

8. Sargentodoxa Stem 15g, Mahonia Stem 15g, Eucommia Bark 30g, and Prunella Spike 9g; steep in 500 ml of liquor for one week. Thereafter, take 20 ml twice daily for the treatment of primary hypertension.

9. 红花 20 克，玉簪花 15 克，菊花 10 克。研细，每日 3 次，每次 5 克，白开水送服。7 天为 1 疗程。

9. Safflower 20g, Plantain Lily Flower 15g, and Chrysanthemum Flower 10g. Grind into a fine powder and take 5g per dose, three times daily, with plain boiled water. A course of treatment consists of 7 days.

《民族医药报》1992 年 10 月 16 日

National Journal of Ethnomedicine, October 16, 1992

10. 生绿豆磨粉治疗高血压病

10. Raw Mung Bean Powder for Hypertension

绿豆性凉味甘，有清热解毒、清暑止渴、利水消肿之功。民间用生绿豆磨粉治疗高血压有一定的疗效。

Mung beans are cool in nature and sweet in flavor, possessing the effects of clearing heat and removing toxins, relieving summer heat and quenching thirst, as well as promoting diuresis and reducing swelling. Folk use of ground raw mung bean powder has shown certain efficacy in treating hypertension.

方法是：将绿豆充分晒干，磨为极细粉末，装入瓶内密封备用。高血压病患者，每日服三次，每次服 15-20 克，饭前用温开水送下，随后再按 1 比 1 量服白糖。持续服两个月，如停药后观察一段时间血压仍高，一般再按上法服 1-2 个月，血压即会降至正常。

Method: Sun-dry the mung beans thoroughly, grind them into an extremely fine powder, and store in a sealed bottle for later use. For hypertensive patients, take 15–20g per dose, three times daily before meals with warm boiled water, followed immediately by an equal amount (1:1 ratio) of white sugar. Continue administration for two months; if blood pressure remains elevated after a period of observation following discontinuation, resume the same regimen for another 1–2 months, after which blood pressure typically returns to normal levels.

注意事项：绿豆用绿色表皮为好，黄色次之。绿豆不能炒熟和退皮，否则无效。备用之绿豆粉应防潮湿及防霉变。

Precautions: Mung beans with green skins are preferred; yellow-skinned ones are less desirable. The beans must not be roasted or dehulled, otherwise they will lose their efficacy. The prepared mung bean powder should be protected from moisture and mold.

《民族医药报》（笔 闻）

National Journal of Ethnomedicine (Bi Wen)

患高血病者采用春季饮食疗法往往对于降压有明显效果。现介绍三种春季饮食疗法如下

Hypertensive patients often achieve significant blood pressure-lowering effects through spring dietary therapy. Three spring dietary therapies are introduced as follows:

11. 用新鲜的绿茶、菊花、槐花各 5 克放入茶壶中用沸开水中泡当茶饮，每日数次。

11. Place 5g each of fresh green tea, chrysanthemum flower, and sophora flower into a teapot, infuse with boiling water, and drink as a tea substitute several times daily.

12. 山楂 15 克，荷叶 10 克，水煎当茶饮。

12. Hawthorn fruit 15g and lotus leaf 10g; prepare as a water decoction and drink as a tea substitute.

13. 高血压食疗方很多，但要注意饮食，应"三低、两多、一少"即低热量，低胆固醇、低盐饮食，多食维生素纤维素和无机盐。少吃脂肪性食物。

13. There are many dietary remedies for hypertension, but attention must be paid to diet, following the principle of "three lows, two highs, and one reduction": low-calorie, low-cholesterol, and low-salt intake; high intake of vitamins, fiber, and inorganic salts; and reduced consumption of fatty foods.

《民族医药报》1993 年 4 月 2 日（广西 黄科锦）

National Journal of Ethnomedicine, April 2, 1993 (Huang Kejin, Guangxi)

14. 菊花茶 菊花有清热解毒，平肝降压的作用，其味甘甜，可每次取菊花 3 克，沸水泡服，每日 3-4 次，对早期高血压、更年期高血压所致的眩晕、头痛、耳鸣等症尤其有效。

14. Chrysanthemum Tea: Chrysanthemum has the effects of clearing heat and removing toxins, calming the liver, and lowering blood pressure. With its sweet flavor, take 3g per serving, infuse with boiling water, and drink 3–4 times daily. It is particularly effective for dizziness, headache, and tinnitus caused by early-stage or menopausal hypertension.

15. 荷叶茶 取鲜荷叶洗净切碎，加适量水煎煮，待凉后代茶频饮。荷叶具有清热解暑、扩张血管和降脂降压作用。同时，荷叶又是减肥之良药。故此茶特别适用于肥胖合并高血压患者饮用。

15. Lotus Leaf Tea: Wash fresh lotus leaves clean, chop them, decoct in

an appropriate amount of water, and drink frequently as a tea substitute after cooling. Lotus leaf clears heat, relieves summer heat, dilates blood vessels, lowers lipids, and reduces blood pressure. It is also an excellent herb for weight loss, making this tea especially suitable for obese patients with hypertension.

16. 钩藤茶 钩藤有清热平肝和降压的作用，对高血压引起的头胀头痛，耳鸣目眩等有较好的疗效。一般以钩藤 12-15 克，加水适量煮沸 10 分钟，待放凉后加适量冰糖调饮。

16. Uncaria Tea: Uncaria clears heat, calms the liver, and lowers blood pressure, showing good efficacy for head distension, headache, tinnitus, and dizziness caused by hypertension. Generally, take 12–15g of uncaria, boil in an appropriate amount of water for 10 minutes, cool, add rock sugar to taste, and drink.

17. 玉米须茶 玉米须具有良好的利尿、消肿、止泻和健胃等功效。临床上广泛用于治疗因肾炎引起的浮肿和高血压，疗效明显且稳定，每次取 25 克玉米须，开水冲泡。代茶饮用。

17. Corn Silk Tea: Corn silk has good diuretic, anti-edema, antidiarrheal, and stomach-strengthening effects. It is widely used clinically to treat edema and hypertension caused by nephritis, with obvious and stable efficacy. Take 25g of corn silk per serving, infuse with boiling water, and drink as a tea substitute.

18. 夏枯草茶 取夏枯草的花蕾适量泡水代茶饮用，每日 3-5 次，不但有较好的平肝降压作用，而且还能治疗目赤肿病，头昏头痛等症状。

18. Prunella Spike Tea: Steep an appropriate amount of prunella flower buds in water and drink as a tea substitute 3–5 times daily. It not only calms the liver and lowers blood pressure effectively but also treats red swollen eyes, dizziness, and headache.

19. 车前子茶 车前子有明显的利尿和降压作用，故此茶适用于高血压、慢性肾炎浮肿患者长期饮用。取车前子 30 克，洗净煮汁代茶饮，也可放入杯中，沸水冲泡代茶饮用。

19. Plantain Seed Tea: Plantain seed has significant diuretic and

antihypertensive effects, making this tea suitable for long-term use by patients with hypertension or chronic nephritic edema. Take 30g of plantain seed, wash clean, decoct to obtain juice, and drink as a tea substitute; alternatively, place it in a cup, infuse with boiling water, and drink as a tea substitute.

20. 决明子茶 决明子除风散热、平肝明目、利水通便，故可治疗高血压，同时对高胆固醇血症以及便秘、目赤肿痛的人也有效。每天 15-30 克，炒黄、水煮，待凉后代茶饮。

20. Cassia Seed Tea: Cassia seed dispels wind and dissipates heat, calms the liver, brightens the eyes, promotes diuresis, and relieves constipation, thus treating hypertension. It is also effective for hypercholesterolemia, constipation, and red swollen painful eyes. Take 15–30g daily, stir-fry until yellowish, boil in water, cool, and drink as a tea substitute.

21. 西瓜翠衣茶 将新鲜西瓜外面的绿皮薄薄削下，洗净后加冷水煎煮 15 分钟，去渣，放入适量白糖，待凉后搅拌一下代茶饮。此茶既有清热解暑，利尿减肥功效，又能较好地降低血压。

21. Watermelon Rind Tea: Thinly peel the outer green skin of a fresh watermelon, wash clean, decoct in cold water for 15 minutes, strain off the residue, add white sugar to taste, stir after cooling, and drink as a tea substitute. This tea clears heat, relieves summer heat, promotes diuresis, aids weight loss, and effectively lowers blood pressure.

《中药科技报》1992 年 6 月 26 日（王玉平）

Journal of Traditional Chinese Medicine Science and Technology, June 26, 1992 (Wang Yuping)

22. 海带一尺，决明子、旱莲草各 30 克，水煎时，每日一剂，食海带喝药汤，连服 7-10 天。本方治疗原发性高血压有显效。

22. Kelp 30 cm (approx. 1 chi), Cassia Seeds 30g, and Eclipta Herb 30g; prepare as a water decoction, one dose daily. Consume both the kelp and the herbal broth for 7–10 consecutive days. This formula demonstrates marked efficacy in treating primary hypertension.

《中药科技报》1992 年 1 月 16 日

Journal of Traditional Chinese Medicine Science and Technology, January 16, 1992

23. 前些年，一位民间医生介绍，其好友李某被高血压病困扰了 20 多年，四方求医用药也无效。后来，一位亲戚推荐给李某一个治高血压病的偏方，李某坚持用药 5 个月后，血压基本恢复正常。现将此方写于下，供同病者参考。

23. Years ago, a folk doctor reported that his friend Mr. Li had suffered from hypertension for over 20 years without relief despite seeking medical treatment and medication everywhere. Later, a relative recommended a folk remedy for hypertension to Mr. Li. After adhering to this regimen for 5 months, his blood pressure essentially returned to normal. The formula is presented below for the reference of fellow sufferers.

大红枣 6 枚（小的 10-20 枚），入锅炒至有糊香味，北山楂肉 6g-10g，鬼针草（广西玉林人称虾钳草，路边、村边、屋旁常有野生）4g-6g，水煎或开水冲泡当茶饮，每日 1 剂。此方简、便、廉，经过验证疗效确切，且喝时酸甜可口，无副作用。

Take 6 large red dates (or 10–20 small ones), stir-fry them in a pan until they emit a slightly scorched aroma, then add 6–10g Northern Hawthorn Fruit Pulp and 4–6g Bidens Herb (commonly known as "Shrimp Pincer Grass" by locals in Yulin, Guangxi; often found growing wild along roadsides, village edges, and near houses). Prepare as a water decoction or infuse with boiling water to drink as a tea substitute, one dose daily. This formula is simple, convenient, and inexpensive, with verified definite efficacy. It has a pleasant sweet-and-sour taste and no side effects.

《健康报》

Health News

五、头痛（19 方）
V. Headache (19 Formulas)

1. 填精补肾法：主治肾阴阳虚。

1.Method of Replenishing Essence and Tonifying the Kidneys: Indicated for deficiency of kidney yin and yang.

“头统诸阳，而脑为髓海，不任受邪”。禀赋素亏，年老体弱：久病肾虚，元气不足则不能上营于脑，脑海空虚而见头脑空痛，重者脑鸣，眩晕耳聋，神疲善欠，腰膝无力，遗精带下，舌红少苔或舌胖淡白，脉细无力或脉沉微。宜以大补元煎加味：党参、熟地黄、当归、山药、山茱萸、枸杞子、杜仲、甘草、菊花、肉苁蓉。肾阴虚者加女贞子、旱莲草；肾阳亏者加附子、肉桂。“善补阳者，必阴中求阳，则阳得阴助而化生无穷；善补阴者，必阳中求阴，则阴得阳生而源泉不竭。”阴阳互根，滋阴助阳同用，元气充足则头痛自安。

“The head governs all yang, and the brain is the sea of marrow, which cannot tolerate pathogenic invasion.” In cases of congenital deficiency, old age, or physical weakness, prolonged illness leads to kidney deficiency; when primordial qi is insufficient, it fails to ascend and nourish the brain. Emptiness of the brain manifests as a hollow pain in the head; in severe cases, this is accompanied by tinnitus, vertigo, deafness, mental fatigue with frequent yawning, weakness of the lower back and knees, seminal emission, and leukorrhea. The tongue may be red with scant coating or pale, swollen, and white; the pulse is fine and weak or deep and faint. Treatment should employ Modified Dabu Yuan Decoction: Codonopsis Root, Prepared Rehmannia Root, Angelica Root, Chinese Yam, Dogwood Fruit, Wolfberry Fruit, Eucommia Bark, Licorice Root, Chrysanthemum Flower, and Cistanche Herb. For kidney yin deficiency, add Glossy Privet Fruit and Eclipta Herb; for kidney yang deficiency, add Prepared Aconite Root and Cinnamon Bark. As the classic saying goes, “Those skilled at tonifying yang must seek yang within yin, so that yang, assisted by yin, generates endlessly; those skilled at tonifying yin must seek yin within yang, so that yin, generated by yang, flows from an inexhaustible source." Since yin and yang are mutually rooted, simultaneous use of yin-nourishing and yang-assisting herbs ensures sufficient primordial qi, thereby resolving the headache naturally.

2. 消积导滞法：用于食积郁滞。

2. Method of Dissolving Accumulation and Guiding Stagnation: Indicated for food accumulation and stagnation.

饮食不节，食滞中院，阻碍气机，清阳不升，浊阴不降，每见头脑跳痛，肢困体重，脘腹胀满，胸膈痞塞，吞酸嗳腐，恶心呕吐，溺畅矢臭，舌苔白腻，脉濡涩或缓而滑。仿保和丸意，处方：山楂、神曲、莱服子、枳实、半夏、陈皮、茯苓、连翘、白术、黄连。胀满甚者加木香、厚朴；若便秘则加大黄、槟榔。食滞所致头痛，临床上亦不少见。治疗此类患者，须注意理气，气行则滞化，方不致有误。

Irregular diet leads to food retention in the middle jiao, obstructing the qi mechanism; clear yang fails to ascend while turbid yin fails to descend. This often presents as throbbing headache, heavy limbs with a sensation of heaviness, abdominal distension and fullness, chest and diaphragm oppression, acid regurgitation with foul belching, nausea and vomiting, smooth urination with foul-smelling stools, a white greasy tongue coating, and a soft-choppy or slow-slippery pulse. Following the principle of Baohe Pill, the prescription includes: Hawthorn Fruit, Medicated Leaven, Radish Seed, Immature Bitter Orange Fruit, Pinellia Rhizome, Tangerine Peel, Poria, Forsythia Fruit, Atractylodes Rhizome, and Coptis Rhizome. For severe distension and fullness, add Aucklandia Root and Magnolia Bark; for constipation, add Rhubarb and Betel Nut. Headaches caused by food retention are not uncommon clinically. When treating such patients, attention must be paid to regulating qi; when qi moves, stagnation resolves, ensuring accurate treatment without error.

3. 平开潜阳法：适应肝阳头痛。

3. Method of Calming and Submerging Yang: Indicated for liver-yang headache.

诸风掉眩，皆属于肝。情志不畅，肝失条达，肝滞气机；肝阴不足，肝阳上亢，气血充盈于上，故头痛晕眩，胀痛攻逆，怒后更甚；面红目涩，口苦舌干，心烦失眠，胁肋不适，舌红苔薄黄，脉弦有力。常以天麻钩藤饮加减：钩藤、天麻、桑寄生、栀子、朱茯苓、石决明，夜交藤、怀牛膝、白芍药、菊花、生龙牡。阴亏者加女贞子、枸杞子；眩晕甚者加珍珠母、刺藜蒺。肝阳头痛，犹似现代医学高血压所致头痛，故于辨证用药时，适当加入降压药如刺藜蒺、菊花、钩藤、夏枯草、石决明等，疗效更佳。

"All wind-induced tremors and dizziness belong to the liver." Emotional distress causes the liver to lose its free-coursing function, leading to qi stagnation; insufficient liver yin allows liver yang to hyperactively ascend, filling the upper body with qi and blood. This results in headache with dizziness, distending pain that surges upward, worsening after anger; red face with dry eyes, bitter taste and dry mouth, irritability with insomnia, hypochondriac discomfort, red tongue with thin yellow coating, and a wiry forceful pulse. Treatment commonly employs Modified Tianma Gouteng Decoction: Uncaria Hook, Gastrodia Rhizome, Taxillus Twig, Gardenia Fruit, Cinnabar-Processed Poria, Abalone Shell, Fleeceflower Vine, Achyranthes Root, White Peony Root, Chrysanthemum Flower, and Raw Dragon Bone & Oyster Shell. For yin deficiency, add Glossy Privet Fruit and Wolfberry Fruit; for severe vertigo, add Pearl Mother and Tribulus Fruit. Liver-yang headache resembles hypertension-induced headache in modern medicine; therefore, during syndrome differentiation-based treatment, appropriately adding antihypertensive herbs such as tribulus fruit, chrysanthemum flower, uncaria hook, prunella spike, and abalone shell yields better therapeutic outcomes.

4. 清肝降火法：适用于肝火上逆。

4. Method of Clearing the Liver and Descending Fire: Indicated for rebellious liver fire.

肝郁日久化火，肝火冲逆于上，扰乱清窍，故见头晕胀痛，甚则头痛如劈；面红目赤，口苦胁痛，烦躁易怒，便秘溲黄，舌边尖红，舌苔黄干，脉弦而数。守龙胆泻肝汤方义，选用龙胆草、柴胡、黄芩、栀子、地龙、青黛、代赭石、夏枯草，决明子，甘草。头痛重者加川牛膝；吐衄者加白茅根。本法所治为肝阳上冲，肝火宁则头痛止。注意药多苦寒，中病即止，以免伤脾碍胃。

Prolonged liver depression transforms into fire; rebellious liver fire surges upward, disturbing the clear orifices, causing dizziness with distending pain, or even splitting headache; red face and eyes, bitter taste and hypochondriac pain, irritability and easy anger, constipation with dark urine, red tongue edges and tip, yellow dry coating, and a wiry rapid pulse. Following the principle of Longdan Xiegan Decoction, select Gentian Root, Bupleurum Root, Scutellaria Root, Gardenia Fruit, Earthworm, Natural Indigo, Hematite, Prunella Spike, Cassia Seeds, and Licorice Root. For severe headache, add Cyathula Root; for vomiting or epistaxis, add Imperata Rhizome. This method treats upward-surging liver yang; when liver fire is calmed, the headache ceases. Note that most herbs are bitter and cold; discontinue once the condition improves to avoid damaging the spleen and stomach.

5. 温经散寒法：用于肝寒头痛。

5. Method of Warming Meridians and Dispelling Cold: Indicated for liver-cold headache.

厥阴之脉上于巅顶属肝，性喜条达。若因寒气中伤，肝胃虚寒，浊阴之气上乘于清阳之位，遂致头痛以巅顶为重，遇寒发作更甚，常喜裹头戴帽；面色青白，肢冷肤凉，口淡不渴，呕吐稀涎，舌苔淡白而润，脉微细或沉迟。《伤寒论》曰："干呕，吐涎沫，头痛者，吴茱萸汤主之"。故用吴茱萸汤加味：党参、吴茱萸、生姜、白豆蔻、藁本、细辛、川芎、桂枝、大枣。呕甚者加半夏、丁香；畏寒者加附子、干姜。方中吴茱萸用量宜大（15-30 克），量小则如隔靴抓痒，莫能敌邪。

The Jueyin meridian ascends to the vertex and belongs to the liver, which favors free coursing. When injured by cold, liver-stomach deficiency-cold allows turbid yin qi to ascend to the position of clear yang, causing headache centered at the vertex, worsening upon cold exposure, with a preference for wrapping the head or wearing a hat; greenish-white complexion, cold limbs and skin, bland taste without thirst, vomiting of thin saliva, pale white moist tongue coating, and a faint-fine or deep-slow pulse. The Treatise on Cold Damage states: «For dry retching, spitting of saliva, and headache, Wuzhuyu Decoction is indicated.» Therefore, use Modified Wuzhuyu Decoction: Codonopsis Root, Evodia Fruit, Fresh Ginger, White Cardamom Fruit, Ligusticum Rhizome, Asarum Herb, Ligusticum Wallichii Rhizome, Cassia Twig, and Jujube Fruit. For severe vomiting, add Pinellia Rhizome and Clove Flower; for aversion to cold, add Prepared Aconite Root and Dried Ginger. The dosage of evodia fruit should be large (15–30g); a small dose would be ineffective, like scratching an itch through boots, unable to overcome the pathogen.

6. 化痰祛淤法：本法治偏头痛。

6. Method of Resolving Phlegm and Removing Blood Stasis: Indicated for migraine.

"久病入络"。久病经久不愈，瘀阻脑络；痰湿阻滞少阳经脉，故而头痛偏于一侧，持续不止，眩晕心烦，面目虚浮紫黯，纳少呕恶，舌质淤斑或舌苔厚浊，脉濡细或细涩。笔者常用川芎、当归、苍术、半夏、枳壳、地龙、陈皮、五灵脂、生蒲黄、香附等药治疗。痰积甚者加白芥子、桔梗；淤血重者加三棱、红花。关幼波老先生云："治痰要活血，血活则痰化"。故对痰淤为犯之偏头痛，熔化痰与祛淤于一炉。临床上的脑血管意外后遗症所致偏头痛，出现上述见证，亦可按此治疗。

"Prolonged disease enters the collaterals." Chronic unresolved illness leads to blood stasis blocking cerebral collaterals; phlegm-dampness obstructs the Shaoyang meridian, resulting in unilateral persistent headache, vertigo with irritability, puffy dark-purple face, poor appetite with nausea, tongue with stasis spots or thick turbid coating, and a soft-fine or fine-choppy pulse. The author commonly uses Ligusticum Wallichii Rhizome, Angelica Root, Atractylodes Rhizome, Pinellia Rhizome, Immature Bitter Orange Fruit, Earthworm, Tangerine Peel, Flying Squirrel Feces, Raw Cattail Pollen, and Cyperus Rhizome. For severe phlegm accumulation, add White Mustard Seed and Platycodon Root; for severe blood stasis, add Sparganium Rhizome and Safflower. The late master Guan

Youbo said: "To treat phlegm, one must activate blood; when blood flows freely, phlegm resolves." Thus, for migraine caused by phlegm-stasis interplay, this method integrates phlegm resolution and stasis removal. Clinically, migraine due to cerebrovascular accident sequelae presenting with the above signs can also be treated accordingly.

7. 搜风豁痰法：此法适用于头风。

7. Method of Expelling Wind and Resolving Phlegm: Indicated for head wind syndrome.

禀赋体丰痰盛，感受外邪，久病郁滞，风痰交结上升于头，清空被扰以致头部阵发性闪电样掣痛，甚则目不能开，头不多举，时作时止，一触即发，头皮麻木或头皮肌肉抽搐；伴食欲不振，胁肋胀痛，舌苔薄白，脉象弦滑。治以自制四白汤。白附子、白芥子、白僵蚕、白芷、川芎、防风、天南星、苍术、甘草。头痛难忍者加全蝎、蜈蚣研末吞服；兼眩晕者加钩藤、地龙。头风类似现代医学慢性神经性头痛和三叉神经痛，发作短暂，以女性多见。祖国医学认为，风性主动，升发向上，挟痰上扰清空所致。治以搜风豁痰法，每收良效。

Patients with a constitutional tendency toward obesity and abundant phlegm, when invaded by external pathogens or suffering from prolonged qi stagnation, develop an intermingling of wind and phlegm that ascends to the head. This disturbs the clear orifices, causing paroxysmal lightning-like pulling pain in the head; in severe cases, the eyes cannot be opened and the head can barely be lifted. The pain is intermittent, triggered by slight contact, and accompanied by scalp numbness or muscle twitching; other symptoms include poor appetite, hypochondriac distension and pain, thin white tongue coating, and a wiry-slippery pulse. Treatment employs the self-formulated Sibai Decoction: White Aconite Rhizome, White Mustard Seed, Silkworm Batryticatus, Angelica Dahurica Root, Ligusticum Wallichii Rhizome, Fangfeng Root, Arisaema Tuber, Atractylodes Rhizome, and Licorice Root. For unbearable headache, add scorpion powder and centipede powder to be swallowed directly; for concurrent vertigo, add Uncaria Hook and Earthworm. Head wind syndrome corresponds to chronic neurogenic headache and trigeminal neuralgia in modern medicine, characterized by brief attacks and higher prevalence in females. Traditional Chinese medicine holds that wind is active and ascending in nature, carrying phlegm upward to disturb the clear orifices. The method of expelling wind and resolving phlegm consistently yields excellent results.

《中药科技报》1990 年 9 月 6 日

Journal of Traditional Chinese Medicine Science and Technology, September 6, 1990

8. 治顽固性头晕偏方

8. Folk Remedy for Refractory Dizziness

天麻、黄芪各40克，白菊花30克，川芎、蔓荆子各15克，约1公斤重鸡1只。将上述五味药加水2500毫升，以文火煎煮50分钟，滤汁备用，再将煎过的天麻(煎药时不要打碎)放进洗净的鸡腹内，另加丁香2克，玉果5克，良姜、白芷、三奈、砂仁各10克，山楂20克，食盐少许与先前煎得的药汁一道煲至全鸡熟烂，吃肉饮汤，一般服用三次均可收到理想效果。

Gastrodia Rhizome 40g, Astragalus Root 40g, White Chrysanthemum Flower 30g, Ligusticum Wallichii Rhizome 15g, Vitex Fruit 15g, and one chicken weighing approximately 1 kg. Add 2500 ml of water to the five herbs above, decoct over low heat for 50 minutes, strain and reserve the liquid. Place the used gastrodia rhizome (do not crush during decoction) into the cleaned chicken cavity, then add Clove Flower 2g, Nutmeg 5g, Galangal Rhizome 10g, Angelica Dahurica Root 10g, Sand Ginger 10g, Amomum Fruit 10g, Hawthorn Fruit 20g, and a pinch of salt. Stew together with the reserved herbal liquid until the chicken is thoroughly tender. Consume both meat and broth; satisfactory results are typically achieved after three servings.

《民族医药报》1993 年 1 月 1 日（江西上犹县寺下中心卫生院 钟久春）

National Journal of Ethnomedicine, January 1, 1993 (Zhong Jiuchun, Sixia Central Health Center, Shangyou County, Jiangxi Province)

9. 取川芎 50 克、白芷 50 克、炙远志 50 克、冰片 7 克，共研细末，用绸布包少许药末塞鼻，右侧头痛塞左鼻，左侧头塞右鼻，效果较一般止痛药迅速，且无副作用。

9. Take Ligusticum Wallichii Rhizome 50g, Angelica Dahurica Root 50g, Prepared Polygala Root 50g, and Borneol 7g; grind all into a fine powder. Wrap a small amount of the powder in silk cloth and insert into the nostril: for right-sided headache, plug the left nostril; for left-sided headache, plug the right nostril. The analgesic effect is faster than that of common painkillers, with no side effects.

《中医药信息报》1992 年 8 月 1 日（四川省温江县中医院 宁蔚夏）

Journal of Traditional Chinese Medicine Information, August 1, 1992 (Ning Weixia, Wenjiang County TCM Hospital, Sichuan Province)

10. 治头痛、头昏芎茶汤

10. Chuanxiong Tea Decoction for Headache and Dizziness

川芎 9 克，茶叶 9 克。以上两味共用冷水微火煎到适当浓度，日服三次，三日见效。笔者借用外祖父此方，治愈了自己的头痛头昏症。

Ligusticum Wallichii Rhizome 9g and Tea Leaves 9g. Decoct both ingredients in cold water over low heat to an appropriate concentration; take three times daily, with effects observed within three days. The author adopted this formula from her maternal grandfather and successfully cured her own headache and dizziness.

（湖北省中医药研究院 徐卫红）

(Hubei Provincial Academy of Traditional Chinese Medicine, Xu Weihong)

治头痛验方

Empirical Formulas for Headache

11. 治顽固性头痛：白芷 10 克、川芎 6 克、羊脑 1 付、红枣 5 枚、加水 0.5 公斤，煮沸 1 小时，去渣，吃脑饮汤。1 日 1 剂，服 3-5 剂愈，顽固性强的再多服几剂。

11. For Refractory Headache: Angelica Dahurica Root 10g, Ligusticum Wallichii Rhizome 6g, one sheep brain, and Jujube Fruit 5 pieces; add 500 ml of water, boil for 1 hour, strain off the residue, and consume both the brain and the broth. Take one dose daily; recovery typically occurs after 3–5 doses, with

additional doses recommended for highly stubborn cases.

12. 周期性头痛：适用“五花汤”：金银花 15 克、菊花 10 克、桃花 10 克、月季花 10 克，旋复花 10 克。水煎服，每日 1 剂。

12. For Periodic Headache: “Five-Flower Decoction” is indicated—Honeysuckle Flower 15g, Chrysanthemum Flower 10g, Peach Blossom 10g, Chinese Rose Flower 10g, and Inula Flower 10g. Prepare as a water decoction, taken once daily.

13. 高血压性头痛：当归、桃仁、柴胡各 10 克、红花、生地、枳壳、白芷各 15 克，牛膝、川芎，黄芩各 20 克，玄参 40 克、甘草 5 克。焙干，研成细末。每次 5 克，开水冲服，日 3 次。

13. For Hypertensive Headache: Angelica Root 10g, Peach Kernel 10g, Bupleurum Root 10g, Safflower 15g, Raw Rehmannia Root 15g, Immature Bitter Orange Fruit 15g, Angelica Dahurica Root 15g, Achyranthes Root 20g, Ligusticum Wallichii Rhizome 20g, Scutellaria Root 20g, Figwort Root 40g, and Licorice Root 5g. Roast until dry and grind into a fine powder. Take 5g per dose with boiling water, three times daily.

14. 治血虚性头痛：当归、川芎、连翘 15 克，熟地 15 克，薄荷 10 克。水煎吸其气，待药液温后服下，安睡即愈。

14. For Blood-Deficiency Headache: Angelica Root 15g, Ligusticum Wallichii Rhizome 15g, Forsythia Fruit 15g, Prepared Rehmannia Root 15g, and Mint Herb 10g. Prepare as a water decoction; first inhale the steam, then drink the liquid when lukewarm. Recovery follows after a restful sleep.

15. 治火旺上攻性头痛：内脏火盛，上逆，取金银花 10 克，菊花 7 克、花茶 5 克。水煎服。

15. For Upward-Attacking Fire Headache: Caused by excessive internal organ fire surging upward; take Honeysuckle Flower 10g, Chrysanthemum Flower 7g, and Tea Flower 5g. Prepare as a water decoction for oral administration.

《中药科技报》（河北 张金声）

Journal of Traditional Chinese Medicine Science and Technology (Zhang

Jinsheng, Hebei Province)

16. 头痛、偏头痛：川芎、白芷各 6 克，菊花 3 克，冰片 2 克，麝香 0.5 克。研细，调匀。头痛，双鼻孔吸入；右偏头痛，左鼻孔吸入；左偏头痛，右鼻孔吸入，药末刺激鼻黏膜，打喷嚏即可。每日 3 次，每次少许。本方对各种原因引起的头痛均有较好的疗效。

16. For Headache and Migraine: Ligusticum Wallichii Rhizome 6g, Angelica Dahurica Root 6g, Chrysanthemum Flower 3g, Borneol 2g, and Musk 0.5g. Grind into a fine powder and mix thoroughly. For general headache, inhale through both nostrils; for right-sided migraine, inhale through the left nostril; for left-sided migraine, inhale through the right nostril. The powder stimulates the nasal mucosa to induce sneezing. Use a small amount three times daily. This formula shows good efficacy for headaches of various etiologies.

《民族医药报》1992 年 10 月 26 日（内蒙古区蒙药厂 徐青）

National Journal of Ethnomedicine, October 26, 1992 (Xu Qing, Inner Mongolia Mongolian Medicine Factory)

17. 治神经性头痛：炒酸枣仁、熟地、石决明（先煎）各 30 克，当归、白芍、龙眼肉各 15 克，天麻、川芎、丹皮各 10 克，僵蚕、甘草各 8 克，全蝎 4 克，蜈蚣 2 条。合煎两遍。分次温服，每日一剂。

17. For Neurogenic Headache: Stir-Fried Spine Date Seed 30g, Prepared Rehmannia Root 30g, Abalone Shell 30g (decocted first), Angelica Root 15g, White Peony Root 15g, Longan Aril 15g, Gastrodia Rhizome 10g, Ligusticum Wallichii Rhizome 10g, Moutan Bark 10g, Silkworm Batryticatus 8g, Licorice Root 8g, Scorpion 4g, and Centipede 2 pieces. Decoct all ingredients together twice. Take in divided doses while warm, one dose daily.

《中药科技报》1992 年 11 月 26 日（子云）

Journal of Traditional Chinese Medicine Science and Technology, November 26, 1992 (Zi Yun)

18. 治三叉神经痛验方

18. Empirical Formula for Trigeminal Neuralgia

三叉神经痛属中医偏头痛范畴。这是一种以面部的三叉神经分布区域出现阵发性剧烈的刀割样、针刺样、火灼样疼痛为特点的病症。此病发作时疼痛难忍、苦不堪言，不发作时又如常人般。

Trigeminal neuralgia falls under the category of migraine in traditional Chinese medicine. It is characterized by paroxysmal, severe knife-like, needle-like, or burning pain in the distribution area of the trigeminal nerve on the face. During attacks, the pain is unbearable and excruciating; between episodes, patients appear completely normal.

西医治疗三叉神经痛的方法较多，但效果不太理想。有关资料介绍下述中药方治疗，效果较好。白芷 30 克、川芎 30 克、荜茇 15 克、川椒 15 克、胆南星 9 克、栀子 15 克，煎水分两次服，每日一剂，连服 10 天为一疗程，不愈可隔数天再服一个疗程，若服药期间能配合针灸治疗，收效更佳。

Although there are many Western medical treatments for trigeminal neuralgia, their efficacy is often suboptimal. Relevant literature suggests that the following herbal formula yields better results: Angelica Dahurica Root 30g, Ligusticum Wallichii Rhizome 30g, Long Pepper 15g, Sichuan Pepper 15g, Bile Arisaema Tuber 9g, and Gardenia Fruit 15g. Prepare as a water decoction divided into two doses, taken once daily. A course of treatment consists of 10 consecutive days; if not cured, another course may be administered after an interval of several days. Better therapeutic outcomes can be achieved when combined with acupuncture during medication.

《民族医药报》1991 年 7 月 5 日（陈晓录）

National Journal of Ethnomedicine, July 5, 1991 (Chen Xiaolu)

19. 头痛的中药外治法

19. External Herbal Therapies for Headache

嗡鼻法。油菜籽 1 克，川大黄 2 克研细末，取少许吹鼻中，用后有黄水流出即生效，治疗偏头痛。

Nasal Insufflation Method: Grind Rapeseed 1g and Sichuan Rhubarb 2g into a fine powder. Blow a small amount into the nostrils; efficacy is indicated when yellow fluid flows out after application. Used for treating migraine.

塞鼻法。细辛、生石膏、花粉、白芷各6克研细末，用水和成丸如绿豆粒大小，左头痛塞右鼻孔，右头痛塞左鼻孔，见汗则愈。用于风、火、痰之头痛。

Nasal Plugging Method: Grind Asarum Herb 6g, Raw Gypsum 6g, Trichosanthes Root 6g, and Angelica Dahurica Root 6g into a fine powder. Mix with water to form pills the size of mung beans. For left-sided headache, plug the right nostril; for right-sided headache, plug the left nostril. Recovery occurs upon sweating. Indicated for headaches caused by wind, fire, or phlegm.

点滴法。鲜萝卜捣汁加少许冰片溶解后仰卧，点鼻中，每日2-3次，每次2-3滴，5日为一疗程，用于风热头痛。

Nasal Drop Method: Extract juice from fresh radish, dissolve a small amount of borneol in it, then lie supine and instill into the nostrils. Apply 2–3 drops per dose, 2–3 times daily. A course of treatment lasts 5 days. Indicated for wind-heat headache.

贴敷法。

Plaster Application Method.

①胡椒、艾叶各等份共研细末，用鸡蛋清调为糊状，敷百会穴，每日换1次，5-7日为一疗程，用于风寒头痛。

① Grind equal amounts of black pepper and mugwort leaf into a fine powder, mix with egg white to form a paste, and apply to the Baihui (GV20) acupoint. Change the dressing once daily; a course of treatment lasts 5–7 days. Indicated for wind-cold headache.

②蚕砂15克，生石膏30克共为细末，用醋调为糊状敷前额，每日换药一次，3-5次一疗程，用于风热头痛。

② Grind Silkworm Feces 15g and Raw Gypsum 30g into a fine powder, mix with vinegar to form a paste, and apply to the forehead. Change the dressing once daily; a course of treatment consists of 3–5 applications. Indicated for wind-heat headache.

③吴茱萸研末醋调敷足心，每日换一次，7日为一疗程。用于肝阳头痛。

③ Grind Evodia Fruit into a fine powder, mix with vinegar, and apply to the soles of the feet. Change the dressing once daily; a course of treatment lasts 7 days. Indicated for liver-yang headache.

烟叶热渍法。黄烟叶用热水浸透，趁热敷头部及两侧太阳穴，凉则更换热的，每日 2 次，每次 30 分钟，3-5 日一疗程，适用于急性头痛。

Hot Tobacco Leaf Compress Method: Soak yellow tobacco leaves thoroughly in hot water, apply warm to the head and both temples, and replace with fresh warm leaves when cooled. Apply twice daily for 30 minutes each time; a course of treatment lasts 3–5 days. Indicated for acute headache.

药帽法。白防风、荆芥、钩藤、苍术、川芎各 20 克，藁本 6 克，细辛 4 克共研细末，将药末装帽中，每日带 2- 3 小时，7 日为一疗程，适用于老年性风寒头痛（不宜急性头痛）。

Medicated Hat Method: Grind Fangfeng Root 20g, Schizonepeta Herb 20g, Uncaria Hook 20g, Atractylodes Rhizome 20g, Ligusticum Wallichii Rhizome 20g, Ligusticum Rhizome 6g, and Asarum Herb 4g into a fine powder. Place the powder inside a hat and wear it for 2–3 hours daily; a course of treatment lasts 7 days. Indicated for senile wind-cold headache (not suitable for acute headache).

催嚏法。瓜蒂研末吹鼻取嚏，每日 3 次，5-7 日一疗程，适用于痰浊头痛。

Sneeze-Inducing Method: Grind Melon Pedicel into a fine powder and blow into the nostrils to induce sneezing. Use three times daily; a course of treatment lasts 5–7 days. Indicated for phlegm-turbidity headache.

姜热敷法。生姜 1 坨，火内煨热，切成四片，分贴前额及太阳穴，以手帕束之，凉则更换，每次 15-20 分钟，每日 2 次，3-5 日为一疗程。用于风寒头痛。

Hot Ginger Compress Method: Roast a piece of fresh ginger in fire until heated through, cut into four slices, apply to the forehead and temples, and secure with a handkerchief. Replace when cooled. Apply for 15–20 minutes per session, twice daily; a course of treatment lasts 3–5 days. Indicated for wind-cold headache.

《中药科技报》1992 年 6 月 26 日（董万法）

Journal of Traditional Chinese Medicine Science and Technology, June 26, 1992 (Dong Wanfa)

头痛：生草乌适量泡酒外揉搽痛处。

Headache: Steep an appropriate amount of Raw Kusnezoff Monkshood Root in liquor and rub externally onto the painful area.

第四章　肝胆病
Chapter 4　Hepatobiliary Diseases

一、肝炎（23 方）
I. Hepatitis (23 Formulas)

1. 苦参 20 克、胆草、郁金各 10 克，茵陈 30 克、柴胡 10 克，每日一剂。水煎服，连服一周。治急性肝炎有良效。

1.Sophora Root 20g, Gentian Root 10g, Curcuma Tuber 10g, Artemisia Scoparia Herb 30g, and Bupleurum Root 10g; take one dose daily as a water decoction for one consecutive week. This formula shows good efficacy in treating acute hepatitis.

2. 钱草、满天星、车前草各 60 克，水煎服，每日二次，治慢性肝炎。

2. Lysimachia Herb 60g, Serissa Herb 60g, and Plantain Herb 60g; prepare as a water decoction taken twice daily for the treatment of chronic hepatitis.

3. 茵陈 30 克，龙胆草 10 克，田鸡黄 15 克，鸡内金 15 克，鸡蛋二个，每次煎药时放鸡蛋二个，服药汁吃鸡蛋。每日一剂，日服 2 次。一周为一疗程。适用于慢性肝炎。

3. Artemisia Scoparia Herb 30g, Gentian Root 10g, Chicken Gallstone 15g, Chicken Gizzard Lining 15g, and two eggs. Add two eggs each time when decocting the herbs; consume both the herbal liquid and the eggs. Take one dose daily in two divided servings; a course of treatment lasts one week. Indicated for chronic hepatitis.

4. 藿香、苍术、厚朴、陈皮各 20 克，黄芩 15 克、马尾莲 30 克，赤芍 12 克，败酱草 20 克，茵陈 30 克，水煎服，每日 1 剂，服用 1- 2 周。孕妇忌用，适用于甲肝。

4. Agastache Herb 20g, Atractylodes Rhizome 20g, Magnolia Bark 20g, Tangerine Peel 20g, Scutellaria Root 15g, Coptis Rhizome 30g, Red Peony Root 12g, Patrinia Herb 20g, and Artemisia Scoparia Herb 30g; prepare as a water decoction taken once daily for 1–2 weeks. Contraindicated during pregnancy; indicated for hepatitis A.

5. 瓜蒌 15 克，黄连 6 克，半夏 16 克，水煎服，每日 1 剂，服 1-2 周，若伴有吐、泻者，加茶叶，生姜各 10 克，适用于甲肝。

5. Trichosanthes Fruit 15g, Coptis Rhizome 6g, and Pinellia Rhizome 16g; prepare as a water decoction taken once daily for 1–2 weeks. If accompanied by vomiting or diarrhea, add Tea Leaves 10g and Fresh Ginger 10g. Indicated for hepatitis A.

6. 大青叶、蒲公英各 20 克，甘草 10 克，大枣 10 克，用法同煎，服用 1- 2 周，适用于甲肝。

6. Isatis Leaf 20g, Dandelion Herb 20g, Licorice Root 10g, and Jujube Fruit 10g; decoct all ingredients together and administer for 1–2 weeks. Indicated for hepatitis A.

7. 茵陈、板蓝根各 30 克，金钱草 15 克，焦三仙各 20 克，甘草 10 克，大枣 15 克，每日一剂服用一周。适于甲肝。

7. Artemisia Scoparia Herb 30g, Isatis Root 30g, Lysimachia Herb 15g, Three Charred Digestives (Charred Hawthorn, Charred Medicated Leaven, Charred Malt) 20g each, Licorice Root 10g, and Jujube Fruit 15g; take one dose daily for one week. Suitable for hepatitis A.

8. 茵陈（或大青叶）20 克，蜂蜜 20 克，先煎茵陈取汁，再加蜂蜜调匀，约 150 毫升，分 2 次服。每日一剂，服 1-2 周。适用于甲肝。

8. Artemisia Scoparia Herb (or Isatis Leaf) 20g and Honey 20g. First decoct the herb to obtain the juice, then mix in honey evenly to yield approximately 150 ml, divided into two doses. Take one dose daily for 1–2 weeks. Indicated for hepatitis A.

9. 金银花、甘草、白术各 15 克，黄芩 10 克，每日一剂。服用 1-2 周，用于孕妇防治甲肝。

9. Honeysuckle Flower 15g, Licorice Root 15g, Atractylodes Rhizome 15g, and Scutellaria Root 10g; take one dose daily for 1–2 weeks. Used for the prevention and treatment of hepatitis A in pregnant women.

10. 党参、甘草、白术各 20 克，炒扁豆、薏苡仁、淮山药各 15 克，丹参、莲子、枣皮、桑椹各 12 克，五味子 5 克，黄芪 15 克，生姜 3 片，大枣 3 枚为引，水煎服。30 剂为一疗程。适用于乙肝。

10. Codonopsis Root 20g, Licorice Root 20g, Atractylodes Rhizome 20g, Stir-Fried Hyacinth Bean 15g, Coix Seed 15g, Chinese Yam 15g, Salvia Root 12g, Lotus Seed 12g, Dogwood Fruit 12g, Mulberry Fruit 12g, Schisandra Fruit 5g, Astragalus Root 15g, with Fresh Ginger 3 slices and Jujube Fruit 3 pieces as guiding herbs; prepare as a water decoction. A course of treatment consists of 30 doses. Indicated for hepatitis B.

《中药科技报》1991 年 10 月 16 日（欧阳军）

Journal of Traditional Chinese Medicine Science and Technology, October 16, 1991 (Ouyang Jun)

甲型肝炎食疗方

Dietary Therapy Formulas for Hepatitis A

11. 湿热型：面目周身俱黄，胸闷腹胀，纳呆，恶心，口淡，尿赤，便结。

11. Damp-Heat Type: Yellow discoloration of the face, eyes, and entire body; chest tightness and abdominal distension; poor appetite; nausea; bland taste in the mouth; dark urine; and constipation.

方一：瘦猪肉 100 克，红枣 10 枚，茵陈 60 克，板蓝根 30 克。加水适量煎煮，放盐少许，去药渣，喝汤吃肉，每天 1 剂。

Formula 1: Lean Pork 100g, Jujube Fruit 10 pieces, Artemisia Scoparia Herb 60g, and Isatis Root 30g. Decoct in an appropriate amount of water, add a pinch of salt, strain off the residue, and consume both the broth and meat. Take one dose daily.

方二：猪肝 100 克，红枣 20 枚，田基黄 30 克，猪肝切碎，用清水适量煎煮，放盐少许调味，去药渣，喝汤吃猪肝。

Formula 2: Pig Liver 100g, Jujube Fruit 20 pieces, and Hypericum Japonicum Herb 30g. Mince the pig liver, decoct with the herbs in an appropriate amount of water, season with a little salt, strain off the residue, and consume both the broth and pig liver.

12. 肝肾亏损型：胁痛隐隐，低热，口干，舌燥，手足心热。

12. Liver-Kidney Deficiency Type: Dull hypochondriac pain, low-grade fever, dry mouth, dry tongue, and heat sensation in the palms and soles.

方一：荸荠 100 克，瘦猪肉 100 克，梨 100 克。荸荠，梨去皮，猪肉切片，加水同煮熟，放盐吃肉吃梨吃荸荠。

Formula 1: Water Chestnut 100g, Lean Pork 100g, and Pear 100g. Peel the water chestnuts and pears, slice the pork, boil all ingredients together until cooked, add salt, and consume the meat, pear, and water chestnuts.

方二：西瓜汁、番茄汁适量，和匀，加白糖少许。随意饮用。

Formula 2: Mix appropriate amounts of watermelon juice and tomato juice evenly, add a little white sugar, and drink freely as desired.

《民族医药报》1993 年 4 月 2 日（湖南江华林业采育场职工医院李润）

National Journal of Ethnomedicine, April 2, 1993 (Li Run, Staff Hospital of Jianghua Forestry Cultivation Farm, Hunan Province)

13. 消疸退黄散是笔者家传秘方，对各种原因引起的黄疸均有很好的疗效。本散组方简单，成本低廉，使用方便，收效迅速，现公开介绍如下。

13. Xiaodan Tuihuang Powder is a secret family formula of the author, showing excellent efficacy for jaundice caused by various etiologies. This powder features simple composition, low cost, convenient application, and rapid onset. It is now publicly introduced as follows.

处方：甜瓜蒂，龙脑冰片，比例为 6：1。

Prescription: Melon Pedicel and Borneol, in a ratio of 6:1.

制法：将上二药分别研为极细末，和匀，密贮瓶中备用。

Preparation Method: Grind the two herbs separately into extremely fine powders, mix thoroughly, and store in a sealed bottle for later use.

用法：每取 0.2 克，摊于纸上，以鼻吸入，吸药后先出现鼻塞、继则打喷嚏、流泪等上呼吸道刺激症状，之后鼻孔会流出黏稠或淡薄不同的淡黄色液体，经几次用药后黄液流尽后黄疸即基本消失。

Usage: Take 0.2g per dose, spread on paper, and inhale through the nose. After inhalation, upper respiratory irritation symptoms such as nasal congestion, followed by sneezing and tearing, will occur first; subsequently, pale yellow fluid of varying viscosity will flow from the nostrils. After several applications, once the yellow fluid has been completely discharged, the jaundice will essentially resolve.

注意事项：

Precautions:

本散可消除黄疸，但对改变其他病症则无效，故非单纯性黄疸患者应用本法应根据具体病情酌情配合有关药物。流出的黄液体切不可吞入口中。

This powder can eliminate jaundice but is ineffective for other symptoms; therefore, patients with non-simple jaundice should combine this method with appropriate medications based on their specific condition. The discharged yellow fluid must never be swallowed.

此法解放前在河南、江苏及安徽等地江湖行医者曾有流传，但配方极为保密，有传媳不传女之规。50 年代中医界献方活动中曾有披露，但该方中只有甜瓜蒂一味，经我们对照观察，疗效远不如本方。

Before 1949, this method was circulated among itinerant folk healers in Henan, Jiangsu, and Anhui provinces, but the formula was kept strictly secret, following a tradition of passing it only to daughters-in-law and not to daughters. It was disclosed during the TCM formula contribution campaign in the 1950s, but that version contained only melon pedicel as a single ingredient. Our comparative observations show that its efficacy is far inferior to this complete formula.

《民族医药报》1992 年 4 月 17 日（江西 俞林）

National Journal of Ethnomedicine, April 17, 1992 (Yu Lin, Jiangxi Province)

14. 肝硬化：鲜骨碎补捣烂兑甜酒炒热外敷肝部，1 日 1 换，有良效。

14. Liver Cirrhosis: Mash fresh Fortune’s Drynaria Rhizome, mix with sweet rice wine, stir-fry until warm, and apply externally over the liver region. Change the dressing once daily; this method shows good efficacy.

15. 治黄疸性肝炎方：以冰糖、蜂蜜各适量调成糊状食之，每日数次不计分量，约吃 1 公斤后即可见效。

15. Formula for Icteric Hepatitis: Mix appropriate amounts of rock sugar and honey into a paste and consume several times daily without fixed dosage. Therapeutic effects are typically observed after consuming approximately 1 kg in total.

《民族医药报》1993 年 1 月 13 日（河南 王敏泽）

National Journal of Ethnomedicine, January 13, 1993 (Wang Minze, Henan Province)

16. 从刚宰杀的公猪腹腔内取出新鲜猪胆后，立即划破胆囊将胆汁倒入杯中一口喝完，随即取适量白砂糖或其它甜食放入口中改变口味。每天一次，连服 5 天为一疗程，轻症一个疗程即可治愈，重症则须服用两个疗程。此方对甲型肝炎特别有效。不妨一试。

16. Immediately after removing the fresh gallbladder from a freshly slaughtered boar, puncture it, pour the bile into a cup, and drink it all at once; then immediately place an appropriate amount of white sugar or other sweets in the mouth to mask the taste. Take once daily for 5 consecutive days as one course of treatment. Mild cases can be cured within one course, while severe cases require two courses. This formula is particularly effective for hepatitis A and is worth trying.

《民族医药报》1993 年 1 月 15 日（贵州 吴彬）

National Journal of Ethnomedicine, January 15, 1993 (Wu Bin, Guizhou Province)

17. 急性黄疸型肝炎：虎杖 20 克、茵陈 30 克、焦山楂 20 克，水煎服，每日一剂。临床应用 25 例，服 20 剂，痊愈。

17. Acute Icteric Hepatitis: Giant Knotweed Rhizome 20g, Artemisia Scoparia

Herb 30g, and Charred Hawthorn Fruit 20g; prepare as a water decoction taken once daily. In clinical application involving 25 cases, all patients achieved full recovery after taking 20 doses.

治肝硬化腹水验方

Empirical Formulas for Ascites Due to Liver Cirrhosis

18. 中药敷脐治腹水：甘遂 3 克（或商陆 6 克）、连头葱白 5 棵（畏寒者加肉桂粉 6 克），共捣糊，用时先用陈醋涂擦患处以防感染和刺激皮肤，后将药敷脐 4 小时。小便自利，腹水减少，一周后可基本消失。

18. Herbal Umbilical Application for Ascites: Kansui Root 3g (or Pokeweed Root 6g) and 5 scallion whites with roots (add Cinnamon Bark Powder 6g for patients with aversion to cold); mash all ingredients into a paste. Before application, rub the area with aged vinegar to prevent infection and skin irritation, then apply the medicated paste to the umbilicus for 4 hours. This promotes spontaneous urination and reduces ascites, which typically resolves substantially within one week.

19. 疏肝理脾丸（湖北中医学院方）：北柴胡、醋三棱、醋莪术、蒲黄、醋灵脂、茜草、地龙各 10 克、炙鳖甲、白茅根各 15 克、炒杭芍 12 克、炒枳实、青皮各 6 克、鸡内金 3 克、猪肝粉 30 克。共研细末，水泛为丸。每服 6 克。日服 3 次，饭前温开水送下。功能疏肝理脾、软坚通络、活血化瘀。用于早期肝硬化、肝硬化腹水及原因不明的脾肿大。腹水重者可加服消水丹（蝼蛄 3 个、蜣螂 1 个。研为细末）。每次 0.5 克，每日 1 次，可连服 2-3 天。

19. Shugan Lipi Pill (Formula from Hubei College of Traditional Chinese Medicine): Northern Bupleurum Root 10g, Vinegar-Processed Sparganium Rhizome 10g, Vinegar-Processed Curcuma Rhizome 10g, Cattail Pollen 10g, Vinegar-Processed Flying Squirrel Feces 10g, Madder Root 10g, Earthworm 10g, Honey-Fried Soft-Shelled Turtle Shell 15g, Imperata Rhizome 15g, Stir-Fried White Peony Root 12g, Stir-Fried Immature Bitter Orange Fruit 6g, Green Tangerine Peel 6g, Chicken Gizzard Lining 3g, and Pig Liver Powder 30g. Grind all ingredients into a fine powder and form pills with water. Take 6g per dose,

three times daily before meals with warm boiled water. Functions: Soothes the liver, regulates the spleen, softens hardness, unblocks collaterals, activates blood circulation, and resolves blood stasis. Indicated for early-stage liver cirrhosis, ascites due to liver cirrhosis, and splenomegaly of unknown origin. For severe ascites, add Xiaoshui Pellet (3 mole crickets and 1 dung beetle, ground into fine powder); take 0.5g once daily for 2–3 consecutive days.

《民族医药报》1992 年 2 月 7 日（广西 钟祖仁辑）

National Journal of Ethnomedicine, February 7, 1992 (Compiled by Zhong Zuren, Guangxi)

20. 方组："益肝茶"由黄芪、旱莲草各 300 克，茵陈、白花蛇舌草各 500 克，甘草、赤小豆、竹叶各 200 克等组成。

20. Formula Composition: "Yigan Tea" consists of Astragalus Root 300g, Eclipta Herb 300g, Artemisia Scoparia Herb 500g, Hedyotis Diffusa Herb 500g, Licorice Root 200g, Adzuki Bean 200g, and Bamboo Leaf 200g.

制法：将全药净选、混合，轧成粗末，拌匀即得。

Preparation Method: Clean and select all herbs, mix them thoroughly, crush into coarse powder, and blend evenly.

功能：增强机体组织代谢，冲刷脏器，促进其体内废物及肝炎病毒排出体外。

Functions: Enhances tissue metabolism, flushes the viscera, and promotes the excretion of metabolic waste and hepatitis viruses from the body.

用法：取益肝茶 10-15 克，沸水浸泡或煎汤均宜，日服 2-3 次，或随喝随服。

Usage: Take 10–15g of Yigan Tea, steep in boiling water or decoct as a soup; consume 2–3 times daily or drink freely as desired.

方解：黄芪、旱莲草主治五脏虚损，长于强心，护肝、健脾、益肺肾为基本功，可增强机体活力，提高细胞免疫功能，茵陈、白花蛇舌草、甘草增强肝脏解毒力，使肝功能获得改善和修复，竹叶、赤小豆除烦利尿，涤浊下行，助前药促其体内废物排出，使陈浊其去，促其新生，全药共效取"扶正祛邪"的有机结合。

Formula Analysis: Astragalus root and eclipta herb primarily treat deficiency of the five zang organs, excelling in strengthening the heart; their fundamental actions include protecting the liver, fortifying the spleen, and tonifying the lungs and kidneys, thereby enhancing vitality and improving cellular immune function. Artemisia scoparia herb, hedyotis diffusa herb, and licorice root enhance hepatic detoxification capacity, facilitating improvement and repair of liver function. Bamboo leaf and adzuki bean relieve irritability, promote diuresis, and drain turbidity downward, assisting the preceding herbs in expelling bodily waste, eliminating stale turbidity, and promoting regeneration. The combined effect of all ingredients embodies the organic integration of "supporting healthy qi and eliminating pathogenic factors."

《中医药信息报》1992 年 2 月 1 日（孟福厚）

Journal of Traditional Chinese Medicine Information, February 1, 1992 (Meng Fuhou)

21. 将泥鳅放入清水中，加生茶油数滴，放养 1-2 天后煮熟（不加油盐），捞出晒干研末，装瓶备用。每次取 2-3 克，开水冲服。日服 3 次。服至症状略有好转，可间断一段时期再服。

21. Place loaches in clean water with a few drops of raw tea oil, keep them for 1–2 days, then boil without adding oil or salt. Remove, sun-dry, grind into powder, and store in a bottle for later use. Take 2–3g per dose with boiling water, three times daily. Once symptoms show slight improvement, treatment may be paused for a period before resuming.

《民族医药报》1993 年 2 月 26 日

National Journal of Ethnomedicine, February 26, 1993

22. 乌梅治疗病毒性肝炎：乌梅为传统的收涩药。77 例病毒性肝炎患者，取乌梅 40-50 克，加水 500 毫升，浓煎至 250 毫升，顿服或分 2 次服，每日一剂，显效 66 例，有效 7 例，无效 1 例。

22. Smoked Plum for Viral Hepatitis: Smoked plum is a traditional astringent herb. In a study of 77 patients with viral hepatitis, 40–50g of smoked plum was decocted in 500 ml of water and concentrated to 250 ml. The decoction was taken as a single dose or divided into two doses daily. Results showed marked efficacy in

66 cases, improvement in 7 cases, and no response in 1 case.

《中药科技报》1992 年 7 月 6 日（江苏 刘永连）

Journal of Traditional Chinese Medicine Science and Technology, July 6, 1992 (Liu Yonglian, Jiangsu Province)

二、胆囊炎（5 方）

II. Cholecystitis (5 Formulas)

治胆道疾病以“利胆汤”为基本方，随症加减治疗胆道疾病，效果很好。

Using "Lidan Decoction" as the base formula and modifying it according to symptoms yields excellent results in treating biliary tract diseases.

“利胆汤”的药物组成是：茵陈、芒硝各 18 克，柴胡、枳壳、郁金各 10 克，赤芍 12 克，黄连、广香各 6 克。临床应用时须根据各种胆道疾病的分型对证加减：

The composition of Lidan Decoction is: Artemisia Scoparia Herb 18g, Mirabilite 18g, Bupleurum Root 10g, Immature Bitter Orange Fruit 10g, Curcuma Tuber 10g, Red Peony Root 12g, Coptis Rhizome 6g, and Aucklandia Root 6g. In clinical application, modifications should be made based on syndrome differentiation for various types of biliary tract diseases:

治胆囊炎。

Treatment of Cholecystitis:

1. 湿热型：宜清热利胆，佐以解毒。用利胆汤加银花 18 克，连翘 10 克，栀子 12 克。

1.Damp-Heat Type: Treatment principle is clearing heat and promoting gallbladder function, supplemented with detoxification. Use Lidan Decoction plus Honeysuckle Flower 18g, Forsythia Fruit 10g, and Gardenia Fruit 12g.

2. 气郁型：宜疏肝解郁，行气利胆。用利胆汤加香附、青皮各 10 克。

2. Qi Stagnation Type: Treatment principle is soothing the liver, relieving depression, moving qi, and promoting gallbladder function. Use Lidan Decoction plus Cyperus Rhizome 10g and Green Tangerine Peel 10g.

3. 血瘀型；宜活血祛瘀，通络利胆。用利胆汤加丹参、延胡、川牛膝、三棱各 10 克。

3. Blood Stasis Type: Treatment principle is activating blood circulation, removing stasis, unblocking collaterals, and promoting gallbladder function. Use Lidan Decoction plus Salvia Root 10g, Corydalis Rhizome 10g, Cyathula Root 10g, and Sparganium Rhizome 10g.

以上药物均为日一剂，水煎分两次服。

All the above formulas are taken as one dose daily, prepared as a water decoction divided into two servings.

《民族医药报》1992 年 8 月 7 日

National Journal of Ethnomedicine, August 7, 1992

4. 取新鲜猪苦胆一只，刺一小孔并将约 100 克洗净绿豆放入苦胆内，以装满和胆汁不外溢能扎上口为准，然后用细绳将口扎好，挂在阴凉通风处待风干后即可食用。每日服 2-3 次，每次服（饭前饭后均可）15-20 粒绿豆。绿豆食完，可再用新鲜猪苦胆如前法制做，一般坚持服用 2-3 个苦胆后胆囊炎即可痊愈。

4. Take one fresh pig gallbladder, make a small hole, and insert approximately 100g of washed mung beans into it, filling it without overflowing bile so that the opening can be tied securely. Tie the opening tightly with a thin string and hang it in a cool, well-ventilated place to air-dry before consumption. Take 15–20 mung beans per dose, 2–3 times daily (before or after meals). Once the mung beans are finished, prepare another fresh pig gallbladder using the same method. Generally, cholecystitis can be cured after consistently consuming 2–3 prepared gallbladders.

《民族医药报》1992 年 3 月 13 日（云南临沧 35106 部队医院 朱明富）

National Journal of Ethnomedicine, March 13, 1992 (Zhu Mingfu, Hospital of PLA Unit 35106, Lincang, Yunnan Province)

5. 消炎利胆汤治疗胆囊炎

5. Xiaoyan Lidan Decoction for Cholecystitis

笔者自拟消炎利胆汤，治疗胆囊炎，效果满意。一般服药 3-5 剂，疼痛可止，服药 15-20 剂，炎症基本消失或明显减轻。

The author formulated Xiaoyan Lidan Decoction for treating cholecystitis with satisfactory results. Generally, pain can be relieved after 3–5 doses, and inflammation essentially resolves or significantly improves after 15–20 doses.

消炎利胆方的组成：柴胡 8 克，黄芩 10 克，郁金 10 克、金钱草 30 克、炒枳实 10 克，玄胡 10 克、生军 10 克（后下），木香 10 克，炙甘草 6 克。

Composition of Xiaoyan Lidan Formula: Bupleurum Root 8g, Scutellaria Root 10g, Curcuma Tuber 10g, Lysimachia Herb 30g, Stir-Fried Immature Bitter Orange Fruit 10g, Corydalis Rhizome 10g, Raw Rhubarb 10g (added near the end of decoction), Aucklandia Root 10g, and Honey-Fried Licorice Root 6g.

用法：每日煎服一剂，每剂分二次早晚煎服，服药后大便转稀或泻下，停药则泻止。

Usage: Take one dose daily as a water decoction, divided into morning and evening servings. Stools may become loose or diarrhea may occur after administration; discontinuation of the medication will stop the diarrhea.

加减法：伴有胆囊结石者加鸡内金 15 克，海金沙 30 克（布包），芒硝 10 克（冲服）；胁胀痛者加青皮 15 克；体虚者加党参 10 克；恶心呕吐加黄连 3 克，制半夏 10 克；食欲不振加神曲、白术、炒麦芽各 15 克；有黄疸者加茵陈 20 克。

Modifications: For patients with gallstones, add Chicken Gizzard Lining 15g, Lygodium Spore 30g (wrapped in cloth), and Mirabilite 10g (taken with the decoction); for hypochondriac distension and pain, add Green Tangerine Peel 15g; for body deficiency, add Codonopsis Root 10g; for nausea and vomiting, add Coptis Rhizome 3g and Processed Pinellia Rhizome 10g; for poor appetite, add Medicated Leaven 15g, Atractylodes Rhizome 15g, and Stir-Fried Malt 15g; for jaundice, add Artemisia Scoparia Herb 20g.

本方具有疏肝利胆、消炎止痛的作用。经笔者多年临床实践，证明疗效确切，对非胆囊炎患者，用之无效。在服药前，需做 B 超检查，以明确诊断。

This formula has the effects of soothing the liver, promoting gallbladder function, reducing inflammation, and relieving pain. Years of clinical practice by the author have confirmed its definite efficacy; however, it is ineffective for patients without cholecystitis. A B-ultrasound examination is required before medication to confirm the diagnosis.

《中医药信息报》1992 年 10 月 3 日（江苏泰县中医院 谢兆丰）

Journal of Traditional Chinese Medicine Information, October 3, 1992 (Xie Zhaofeng, Taixian TCM Hospital, Jiangsu Province)

三、胆结石（2 方）
III. Cholelithiasis (2 Formulas)

1. 威灵仙治疗胆石症。威灵仙常用于祛风除湿。用来治疗胆石症患者 120 例，病程 1-10 年，威灵仙煎水内服，治愈 60 例，好转 44 例，无效 16 例，总有效率 86.7%。

1.Clematis Root for Cholelithiasis: Clematis root is commonly used to dispel wind and remove dampness. In the treatment of 120 patients with cholelithiasis (disease duration ranging from 1 to 10 years) using oral administration of clematis root decoction, 60 cases were cured, 44 cases showed improvement, and 16 cases were unresponsive, yielding a total effective rate of 86.7%.

2. 治胆石症。利胆汤的组成：柴胡 8 克，黄芩 10 克，郁金 10 克、金钱草 30 克、炒枳实 10 克，玄胡 10 克、生军 10 克（后下），木香 10 克，炙甘草 6 克。

2. Treatment of Cholelithiasis: Composition of Lidan Decoction: Bupleurum Root 8g, Scutellaria Root 10g, Curcuma Tuber 10g, Lysimachia Herb 30g, Stir-Fried Immature Bitter Orange Fruit 10g, Corydalis Rhizome 10g, Raw Rhubarb 10g (added near the end of decoction), Aucklandia Root 10g, and Honey-Fried Licorice Root 6g.

湿热型：宜清热利湿，排石利胆。用利胆汤加银花 18 克，连翘、鸡内金各 10 克，金钱草 30 克。

Damp-Heat Type: Treatment principle is clearing heat, removing dampness, expelling stones, and promoting gallbladder function. Use Lidan Decoction plus Honeysuckle Flower 18g, Forsythia Fruit 10g, Chicken Gizzard Lining 10g, and

Lysimachia Herb 30g.

气郁型：宜舒肝解郁，排石利胆。用利胆汤加香附、青皮、川牛膝各 10 克，金钱草 30 克。

Qi Stagnation Type: Treatment principle is soothing the liver, relieving depression, expelling stones, and promoting gallbladder function. Use Lidan Decoction plus Cyperus Rhizome 10g, Green Tangerine Peel 10g, Cyathula Root 10g, and Lysimachia Herb 30g.

血瘀型：宜活血祛瘀，排石利胆。用利胆汤加金钱草 30 克，丹参、延胡、川牛膝、莪术各 10 克。上述药物均为日一剂，水煎分两次服。

Blood Stasis Type: Treatment principle is activating blood circulation, removing stasis, expelling stones, and promoting gallbladder function. Use Lidan Decoction plus Lysimachia Herb 30g, Salvia Root 10g, Corydalis Rhizome 10g, Cyathula Root 10g, and Curcuma Rhizome 10g. All the above formulas are taken as one dose daily, prepared as a water decoction divided into two servings.

《民族医药报》1992 年 8 月 7 日

National Journal of Ethnomedicine, August 7, 1992

第五章　五官科

Chapter 5　Otorhinolaryngology and Ophthalmology

一、眼病

I. Eye Diseases

（一）夜盲症（8方）

(I) Night Blindness (8 Formulas)

夜盲是指在夜晚或黑暗处视物不清。

Night blindness refers to impaired vision at night or in dim light.

1. 夜明砂炒干研碎、用猪胆汁和丸如绿豆大。每次五丸，米汤送服。

1.Stir-fry bat feces until dry, grind into powder, and mix with pig bile to form pills the size of mung beans. Take 5 pills per dose with rice water.

2. 薜荔果适量，煎汁蒸猪肝吃。

2. Decoct an appropriate amount of fig fruit to obtain juice, then steam pig liver with the juice and consume.

3. 羊肝一具、不见水、以朴硝揉去血，用竹刀切开，放入谷精草一撮，于砂锅内蒸熟食服。

3. Take one sheep liver (do not wash with water), rub with mirabilite to remove blood, cut open with a bamboo knife, insert a pinch of pipewort flower, and steam in a clay pot until cooked before consuming.

4. 石决明三十克（烧灰存性），苍术（去皮）九十克。共研细末。每次九克，取猪肝适量切开，放入药末，用线扎好，用砂罐煮熟，以热气熏目，待冷后吃肝饮汁。

4. Abalone shell 30g (calcined but retaining its properties) and atractylodes

rhizome (peeled) 90g; grind together into a fine powder. Take 9g per dose, slice an appropriate amount of pig liver, place the powder inside, tie securely with thread, and boil in a clay pot until cooked. First use the steam to fumigate the eyes, then consume the liver and broth after cooling.

5. 苍术三十克，石决明、夜明砂各十五克，猪肝一百克（分两次用）。前三味药加水约五百毫升。煎成二百毫升，于早空腹、晚临睡前分两次煮猪肝服。

5. Atractylodes rhizome 30g, abalone shell 15g, bat feces 15g, and pig liver 100g (divided into two portions). Add approximately 500 ml of water to the first three herbs and decoct to 200 ml. Use this liquid to cook pig liver in two divided doses, taken on an empty stomach in the morning and before bedtime at night.

6. 百草霜适量，涂熟猪肝上服后即愈。

6. Apply an appropriate amount of soot from various grasses onto cooked pig liver and consume; recovery follows immediately.

7. 夜明砂二百克，谷精草一百克，猪肝二百克。将夜明砂、谷精草煮水去渣、炖猪肝食数次即愈。忌食燥热物，忌房事。

7. Bat feces 200g, pipewort flower 100g, and pig liver 200g. Decoct bat feces and pipewort flower in water, strain off the residue, stew the pig liver in the liquid, and consume several times until cured. Avoid dry-heat foods and sexual intercourse during treatment.

8. 谷精珠二十五克，石决明二十克，双钩藤二十五克，小茴香二十克，姜黄片（末）二十克。引用白羊肝（猪肝代亦可）二百克（不落水）。此方系成年人剂量，孩童减半或三分之一。文武火煎。

8. Pipewort seed 25g, abalone shell 20g, uncaria hook 25g, fennel fruit 20g, and turmeric slices (or powder) 20g, with 200g of white sheep liver (pig liver may be substituted) as a guiding ingredient (do not wash with water). This dosage is for adults; reduce by half or to one-third for children. Decoct over alternating high and low heat.

《中药科技报》1990 年 9 月 6 日

Journal of Traditional Chinese Medicine Science and Technology, September 6,1990

（二）弱视（1方）

(II) Amblyopia (Prescription 1)

单眼或双眼矫正视力低于正常，眼球无器质性病变者称为弱视。

Amblyopia is defined as corrected visual acuity below normal in one or both eyes without any organic lesions of the eyeball.

它是一种比近视危害更大的眼科疾病，不及时治疗会失去建立完善立体视的机会。

It is an ophthalmic disease more harmful than myopia, and failure to treat it promptly may result in the loss of the opportunity to establish well-developed stereoscopic vision.

近几年来，我国医务工作者用中药治疗弱视，取得了明显疗效。

In recent years, medical professionals in China have achieved significant therapeutic efficacy in treating amblyopia with traditional Chinese medicine.

中药疗法是：

The traditional Chinese medicine therapy is as follows:

取当归、熟地、茯苓、远志、菖蒲、党参各10克，枸杞子、充蔚子各8克，川芎、赤白芍、菟丝子、五味子、车前子各5克，桔梗3克，升麻2克（以上为3-8岁量），每日一剂，水煎服连续2-3月，可使视力得到不同程度的改善和提高。

Take 10g each of Angelica sinensis, Rehmannia glutinosa (prepared), Poria cocos, Polygala tenuifolia, Acorus tatarinowii, and Codonopsis pilosula; 8g each of Lycium barbarum and Leonurus japonicus seeds; 5g each of Ligusticum chuanxiong, red and white Paeonia lactiflora, Cuscuta chinensis, Schisandra chinensis, and Plantago asiatica seeds; 3g of Platycodon grandiflorus; and 2g of Cimicifuga heracleifolia (the above dosages are for children aged 3–8 years); decoct one dose daily in water and administer orally for 2–3 consecutive months, which can improve and enhance visual acuity to varying degrees.

中医认为，眼为脏腑先天之精所成，后天之精所养，其察五色，辨万物全赖脏腑功能协调，气血旺盛。

Traditional Chinese medicine holds that the eyes are formed by the innate essence of the zang-fu organs and nourished by the acquired essence, and their ability to perceive the five colors and distinguish all things depends entirely on the coordinated functions of the zang-fu organs and abundant qi and blood.

《黄帝内经》云:“五脏六腑之精气,皆上注于目而为之精”,“肝气通于目,肝和则能辨五色矣”,“肝肾之气充,则目精光彩明”,“肝受血而能视”。

The Yellow Emperor's Inner Canon states: "The essence and qi of the five zang and six fu organs all flow upward to the eyes to sustain vision," "Liver qi communicates with the eyes, and when the liver is harmonious, the five colors can be distinguished," "When the qi of the liver and kidneys is sufficient, the eyes are bright and lustrous," and "The eyes can see only when the liver receives adequate blood."

可见,眼要发挥正常视觉功能,全仗肝肾气血滋养。

Thus, it is evident that the normal visual function of the eyes relies entirely on the nourishment from the liver, kidneys, qi, and blood.

此方补益肝肾,养血明目,故对弱视有明显疗效,且无副作用,便于长期服食。

This prescription tonifies the liver and kidneys, nourishes the blood, and improves vision; therefore, it has marked therapeutic efficacy for amblyopia, causes no side effects, and is suitable for long-term administration.

《民族医药报》(广西 张菊生)

Ethnic Medicine News (Guangxi, Zhang Jusheng)

(三)麦粒肿(4方)

(III) Hordeolum (4 Prescriptions)

麦粒肿又称“针眼”,是发生在眼睑上的急性化脓性炎症,可采取下列简单有效的方法治疗。

Hordeolum, also known as "stye," is an acute suppurative inflammation occurring on the eyelid, which can be treated with the following simple and effective methods.

1. 耳垂放血法:将患眼同侧耳垂皮肤常规消毒,术者用食指、拇指捏紧耳垂,暴露耳垂边缘，将消毒的三棱针从耳垂边缘刺入 8 毫米左右，拨针松手，让流血 10 余滴，如流不出可挤压耳垂，然后用酒精棉签压迫针孔，第二天复诊在原伤口处消毒、挤压出血。

1.Earlobe Bloodletting Method: Routinely disinfect the skin of the earlobe on the same side as the affected eye; the practitioner pinches the earlobe tightly with the index finger and thumb to expose its edge, inserts a sterilized three-edged needle about 8 mm into the edge of the earlobe, withdraws the needle and releases the grip to allow more than 10 drops of blood to flow out (if bleeding does not occur spontaneously, the earlobe may be squeezed), and then applies pressure to the puncture site with an alcohol swab; during the follow-up visit the next day, the original wound is disinfected again and squeezed to induce bleeding.

双眼发病可两耳垂同时放血。

If both eyes are affected, bloodletting can be performed on both earlobes simultaneously.

一般 2 次见效，3-4 次治愈。

Generally, improvement is observed after 2 sessions, and cure is achieved after 3–4 sessions.

2. 中趾放血法：将足中趾常规消毒，用三棱针点刺中趾尖部，放血 5 滴，患左眼刺右中趾，患右眼刺左中趾，双眼患病同刺双中趾，每日一次，三天左右可痊愈。

2. Middle Toe Bloodletting Method: Routinely disinfect the middle toe of the foot, prick the tip of the middle toe with a three-edged needle to release 5 drops of blood; for left eye involvement, prick the right middle toe; for right eye involvement, prick the left middle toe; if both eyes are affected, prick both middle toes; perform once daily, and recovery usually occurs within approximately three days.

3. 患处点刺法：将麦粒肿患处用络合碘消毒，用三棱针刺进患处让流血，如已成脓、则刺破脓头排脓，再搽络合碘，切记络合碘不要滴进眼内，万一络合碘进入眼内，或是内麦粒肿，就要用生理盐水洗眼，一般一次告成，重者只需 2-3 次。

3. Local Pricking Method: Disinfect the affected area of the hordeolum with povidone-iodine, insert a three-edged needle into the lesion to induce bleeding; if suppuration has occurred, puncture the pustule head to drain the pus, and then apply povidone-iodine externally; care must be taken to prevent povidone-iodine from entering the eye; should it accidentally enter the eye or in cases of internal hordeolum, irrigate the eye with normal saline; generally, one session suffices, while severe cases require only 2–3 sessions.

《中医药信息报》1992 年 2 月 7 日（湖南娄底市医院眼科 罗建国）

Traditional Chinese Medicine Information News, February 7, 1992 (Department of Ophthalmology, Loudi Municipal Hospital, Hunan Province; Luo Jianguo)

4. 取细线（约 2 根车线粗）1 根，将患麦粒肿一边的中指末端第一和第二指骨连接处结扎（左眼扎左手，右眼扎右手）。

4. Take one piece of fine thread (approximately the thickness of two sewing threads) and ligate the junction between the first and second phalanges at the distal end of the middle finger on the same side as the affected eye (ligate the left hand for left eye involvement and the right hand for right eye involvement).

扎时用力要适中，有压迫感即可，过松无效。

The tying force should be moderate, producing a sensation of compression; if tied too loosely, it will be ineffective.

6-8 小时将线解开。

Untie the thread after 6–8 hours.

对早期（发病第 1、第 2 天）麦粒肿一般第 2 天可愈。

For early-stage hordeolum (onset on day 1 or day 2), recovery generally occurs by the second day.

《民族医药报》1992 年 4 月 17 日（广西宜山县 胡沛斌）

Ethnic Medicine News, April 17, 1992 (Yishan County, Guangxi; Hu Peibin)

（四）青光眼（1 方）

(IV) Glaucoma (1 Prescription)

1. 青光眼：羌活 15 克，水煎服。

1.Glaucoma: Take 15g of Notopterygium incisum, decoct in water, and administer orally.

每日 1 剂，连服 1 周为 1 疗程，一般服 3-4 疗程可愈。

One dose daily for one week constitutes one course of treatment; generally, cure is achieved after 3–4 courses.

本方对急性青光眼患者有奇效。

This prescription has remarkable efficacy for patients with acute glaucoma.

（湖南省隆回县 李禹璋）

(Longhui County, Hunan Province; Li Yuzhang)

（五）红眼病（2 方）

(V) Red Eye Disease (2 Prescriptions)

红眼病，医学上称为急性流行性出血性眼结膜炎，常于夏季气温闷热时流行，具有起病急、传播广、传染速度快的特点，开始发病多为单眼，很快累及双眼。

Red eye disease, medically termed acute epidemic hemorrhagic conjunctivitis, often prevails during hot and humid summer weather; it is characterized by acute onset, widespread transmission, and rapid contagion, usually starting in one eye and quickly involving both eyes.

症见患眼红肿疼痛、畏光、流泪、目眦（俗称"眼屎"）增多、视物不清等，少数病人伴有发烧、全身酸困不适等类似感冒症状。

Symptoms include redness, swelling, pain, photophobia, tearing, increased eye discharge (colloquially called "eye gum"), and blurred vision in the affected eyes; a minority of patients also present with fever, generalized soreness, malaise, and other flu-like symptoms.

民间采用以下方法治疗此病，效果良好。

The following folk remedies have been used to treat this condition with good results.

1. 取新鲜旱莲草约 60 克，捣烂如泥，分半后分别摊于两块干净纱布上，然后让 12 岁以下健康男孩解小便于药上，尿量以湿透药物为准，立即将药物包起，趁尿液尚热分别敷于双眼上（病人取仰卧位），每次敷 30 分钟以上，每日 3-4 次（晚上睡觉时可敷药过夜），一般 1 日见效，2-3 日痊愈，无任何毒副作用。

1.Take approximately 60g of fresh Eclipta prostrata, mash it into a paste, divide it into two equal portions, and spread each onto a piece of clean gauze; then have a healthy boy under 12 years old urinate onto the herbal paste until it is thoroughly soaked; immediately wrap up the preparation and apply it warm to both eyes while the patient lies supine; keep the compress on for more than 30 minutes each time, 3–4 times daily (it may be left on overnight during sleep); generally, improvement is seen within one day and full recovery occurs within 2–3 days, with no toxicity or side effects.

治疗期间忌食辛辣、鱼腥及酒类食品。

During treatment, avoid spicy foods, fishy or strong-smelling seafood, and alcoholic beverages.

《民族医药报》1992 年 5 月 26 日（广西龙州县民族医院 韦礼贵）

Ethnic Medicine News, May 26, 1992 (Longzhou County Ethnic Hospital, Guangxi; Wei Ligui)

2. 犁头草，别名剪刀草、地草果、拔疔草等。

2. Viola inconspicua, also known as scissor grass, ground fruit grass, or boil-pulling grass.

主要分布于云南、江西两地，有散风清热，疏肝消肿的作用。

It is mainly distributed in Yunnan and Jiangxi provinces and has the effects of dispelling wind, clearing heat, soothing the liver, and reducing swelling.

现将云南民间用此药治病验方则简介如下。

A brief introduction to a proven folk remedy using this herb from Yunnan is presented below.

治红眼病：取新鲜犁头草洗净捣烂，和鸡蛋清调匀，外敷。

For treating red eye disease: wash fresh Viola inconspicua, mash it, mix evenly with egg white, and apply externally.

《民族医药报》1992 年 9 月 4 日

Ethnic Medicine News, September 4, 1992

（六）白内障（2 方）

(VI) Cataract (2 Prescriptions)

1. 白内障，属于中医瞳神疾患，多见于老年人。

1.Cataract belongs to the category of pupil-related disorders in traditional Chinese medicine and is commonly seen in the elderly.

其表现为视物微昏、眼前常黑花缭乱，眼球干燥涩痛、伴有头昏耳鸣、足跟痛等。

Its manifestations include slightly blurred vision, frequent floaters before the eyes, dryness and aching pain in the eyeballs, accompanied by dizziness, tinnitus, heel pain, etc.

究其病因，祖国医学认为本病多由肝肾两亏、脾胃虚衰，中土失于运化、精气不能上荣或因肝经风热，上攻目系，以致神水不足，睛球混浊。

Regarding its etiology, traditional Chinese medicine holds that this disease is mostly caused by deficiency of both liver and kidneys, weakness of spleen and stomach leading to impaired transportation and transformation and failure of essence and qi to nourish upward, or by wind-heat in the liver channel attacking the ocular system, resulting in insufficient aqueous humor and turbidity of the eyeball.

中医治疗本病以健脾、补肾为主。

Traditional Chinese medicine treats this disease primarily by strengthening the spleen and tonifying the kidneys.

通明补肾方经临床证明效果较好，现奉献给广大患者。

The Tongming Bushen Formula has been clinically proven effective and is now offered to patients.

方药组成：石决明30克、人参30克、生地60克、桔梗30克、车前子30克、茺蔚子60克、白芍30克、细辛15克、大黄9克为主，视病情加减：血压偏高者加菊花、钩藤；头晕者加天麻、龟板；大便干燥者加肉苁蓉等。

The formula consists mainly of 30g Haliotis diversicolor shell, 30g Panax ginseng, 60g Rehmannia glutinosa (raw), 30g Platycodon grandiflorus, 30g Plantago asiatica seeds, 60g Leonurus japonicus seeds, 30g Paeonia lactiflora, 15g Asarum sieboldii, and 9g Rheum palmatum; modifications are made according to the condition: add Chrysanthemum morifolium and Uncaria rhynchophylla for elevated blood pressure; Gastrodia elata and turtle shell for dizziness; Cistanche deserticola for dry stools, etc.

制法: 将上药共研细末，用等量的蜂蜜制成丸药，每丸重9克，早晚各服一丸，三个月为一个疗程。

Preparation: grind all the above herbs into fine powder, make pills with an equal amount of honey, each pill weighing 9g; take one pill in the morning and one in the evening, with three months constituting one course of treatment.

注意：服药期间不服其他药物，感冒发热时停服，忌吃辛辣之食物。

Note: Do not take other medications during treatment; suspend administration during colds or fevers; avoid spicy foods.

《中医药信息报》1992年1月8日（姜兆余）

Traditional Chinese Medicine Information News, January 8, 1992 (Jiang Zhaoyu)

2. 老年性白内障是眼科常见的慢性进行性眼病。

2. Senile cataract is a common chronic progressive ophthalmic disease.

随着生活水平的提高，人们寿命的延长，老年性白内障的发病率有逐渐增长的趋势，已成为老年人致盲的病种之一。

With improved living standards and extended life expectancy, the incidence of senile cataract shows a gradually increasing trend, making it one of the leading causes of blindness in the elderly.

山东省淄博市中医院著名眼科专家任弘毅副主任医师将师传家传私方与40

年临床经验融为一体，从肝脾肾入手，以补益肝肾，育阴潜阳，健脾调中，行气散郁为治疗原则，研制成“祛障明目丸”运用于临床，治疗白内障早期（初发期、膨胀期），使其达到控制晶状体混浊，延长其寿命，而提高视力之目的。

Associate Chief Physician Ren Hongyi, a renowned ophthalmology expert at Zibo Municipal Hospital of Traditional Chinese Medicine in Shandong Province, integrated inherited family formulas with 40 years of clinical experience; approaching treatment through the liver, spleen, and kidneys, and guided by the principles of tonifying the liver and kidneys, nourishing yin and anchoring yang, strengthening the spleen and regulating the middle jiao, and moving qi to dissipate stagnation, he developed the "Quzhang Mingmu Pill" for clinical use in treating early-stage cataracts (incipient and intumescent stages), aiming to control lens opacity, prolong lens viability, and improve visual acuity.

总结在案病历计 898 例，1698 眼，治愈 1320 眼，有效 296 眼，无效 82 服，有效率 17%，治愈率 71%。

A summary of documented cases includes 898 patients and 1,698 eyes, with 1,320 eyes cured, 296 eyes showing improvement, and 82 eyes unresponsive; the effective rate was 17% and the cure rate 71%.

药物组成: 当归 6 克，白芍 15 克，女贞子 15 克，枸杞子 30 克，茺蔚子 15 克，白术 20 克，防风 12 克，菊花 12 克，决明子 20 克，香附 12 克，地龙 12 克。

Composition: 6g Angelica sinensis, 15g Paeonia lactiflora, 15g Ligustrum lucidum fruit, 30g Lycium barbarum, 15g Leonurus japonicus seeds, 20g Atractylodes macrocephala, 12g Saposhnikovia divaricata, 12g Chrysanthemum morifolium, 20g Cassia obtusifolia seeds, 12g Cyperus rotundus, and 12g Lumbricus terrestris.

用法：水煎日一剂分 2 次服，20 付为一疗程。

Usage: Decoct in water, one dose daily divided into two administrations; 20 doses constitute one course of treatment.

亦可按国家制剂要求加工为水泛丸，每次服 9 克，日 3 次。

Alternatively, it can be processed into water-binded pills according to national pharmaceutical standards, taking 9g per dose, three times daily.

《中药科技报》1992 年 5 月 26 日（山东省淄博市中医院 曹元成 任鲁平）

Chinese Materia Medica Science and Technology News, May 26, 1992 (Zibo Municipal Hospital of Traditional Chinese Medicine, Shandong Province; Cao Yuancheng, Ren Luping)

（七）视神经萎缩（7 方）

(VII) Optic Atrophy (7 Prescriptions)

1. 菊花、枸杞各 15 克，地黄 20 克，水煎服，日一剂。

1.Take 15g each of Chrysanthemum morifolium and Lycium barbarum, and 20g of Rehmannia glutinosa; decoct in water and administer orally, one dose daily.

2. 野菊花、薄荷、金银花、穿心莲、桑叶、淡竹叶、秦皮、青葙子、谷精草、木贼各 15 克，水煮蒸气薰眼，日 1-2 次。

2. Take 15g each of wild chrysanthemum, Mentha haplocalyx, Lonicera japonica, Andrographis paniculata, Morus alba leaf, Lophatherum gracile, Fraxinus chinensis bark, Celosia argentea seeds, Eriocaulon buergerianum, and Equisetum hiemale; boil in water and use the steam to fumigate the eyes, 1–2 times daily.

3. 香白芷、当归叶、牵牛钻、六花钻各 25 克，泡米酒一斤，七日后每天内服一小汤匙。

3. Take 25g each of Angelica dahurica, Angelica sinensis leaf, Qianniuzuan, and Liuhuazuan; soak in 500g of rice wine for seven days, then take one small tablespoonful orally each day thereafter.

4. 益母草子 15 克，水煎服，日一剂。

4. Take 15g of Leonurus japonicus seeds; decoct in water and administer orally, one dose daily.

5. 蜜蘑菇 50 克，水煎服，日一剂。

5. Take 50g of honey mushroom; decoct in water and administer orally, one dose daily.

6. 枸杞子、菊花、熟地黄、淮山药各 20 克，山萸肉、丹皮、泽泻各 15 克，水煎服，每日一剂。

6. Take 20g each of Lycium barbarum, Chrysanthemum morifolium, Rehmannia glutinosa (prepared), and Dioscorea opposita, and 15g each of Cornus officinalis fruit pulp, Moutan cortex, and Alisma orientale; decoct in water and administer orally, one dose daily.

7. 菟丝子、熟地黄、车前子各 15 克，研末内服，日一剂。

7. Take 15g each of Cuscuta chinensis, Rehmannia glutinosa (prepared), and Plantago asiatica seeds; grind into powder and administer orally, one dose daily.

《民族医药报》（桂林市民主路临桂县 何建华）

Ethnic Medicine News (He Jianhua, Lingui County, Minzhu Road, Guilin City)

（八）近视（4 方）

(VIII) Myopia (4 Prescriptions)

近视药膳 Medicated Diets for Myopia

1. 枸杞子 10 克、萸肉 10 克、桂圆肉 15 克、白菊花 15 克，加冷开水 300 毫升，隔水蒸 60 分钟后饮汤食渣。

1.Take 10g of Lycium barbarum, 10g of Cornus officinalis fruit pulp, 15g of longan aril, and 15g of white chrysanthemum; add 300 ml of cool boiled water, steam over water for 60 minutes, then consume both the liquid and the residue.

每日一剂，连服 5 剂。

One dose daily for 5 consecutive doses.

2. 菠菜 500 克，羊肝 90 克，谷精草 15 克，加水煎服，食肝饮汤。

2. Take 500g of spinach, 90g of sheep liver, and 15g of Eriocaulon buergerianum; decoct in water, eat the liver, and drink the soup.

每日 1 剂，连服 3-4 剂。

One dose daily for 3–4 consecutive doses.

3. 甜橙 1-2 只，去皮核、捣烂如泥加入开水和蜂蜜适量调匀食用。

3. Take 1–2 sweet oranges, peel and remove seeds, mash into a paste, mix

evenly with an appropriate amount of hot water and honey, and consume.

每日 1 剂，连服数剂。

One dose daily for several consecutive doses.

4. 赤小豆 200 克、鲤鱼 250 克，将鱼去内脏，但留肝与鳔，先将豆煮熟后加入鱼再煮至熟食用。

4. Take 200g of adzuki beans and 250g of carp; remove the fish viscera but retain the liver and swim bladder; first boil the beans until cooked, then add the fish and continue boiling until fully cooked before consumption.

（九）眼结膜炎（7 方）

(IX) Conjunctivitis (7 Prescriptions)

1. 青鱼胆草（雪里梅）10 克，水煎服。

1.Take 10g of Gentiana scabra (Xuelimei); decoct in water and administer orally.

1 日 1 剂，分 3 次服。

One dose daily, divided into three administrations.

2. 马尾黄连 10 克，薄荷 10 克，水煎服。

2. Take 10g of Coptis chinensis and 10g of Mentha haplocalyx; decoct in water and administer orally.

1 日 1 剂，分 3 次服。

One dose daily, divided into three administrations.

鲜品可用 30 克，小儿减量。

For fresh herbs, 30g may be used; reduce the dosage for children.

3. 青皮 10 克，鸡脚黄连（三棵针）根皮 50 克，水煎过滤取汁，分成 2 份。

3. Take 10g of Citrus reticulata green peel and 50g of Berberis root bark; decoct in water, filter to obtain the juice, and divide into two portions.

1 份口服，1 份乘温热先薰后洗。

Take one portion orally; use the other portion while warm to first fumigate and then wash the affected area.

1 日 3 次。

Three times daily.

4. 小山茶 10 克，金银花 10 克，水煎服。

4. Take 10g of Camellia japonica and 10g of Lonicera japonica; decoct in water and administer orally.

1 日 1 剂，分 3 次服。

One dose daily, divided into three administrations.

5. 冬开花（龙胆草）6 克，金银花 6 克，山川柳（柽柳）10 克，水煎服。

5. Take 6g of Gentiana scabra, 6g of Lonicera japonica, and 10g of Tamarix chinensis; decoct in water and administer orally.

1 日 1 剂，分 3 次服。

One dose daily, divided into three administrations.

《民族医药报》（云南会泽县 马应乖）

Ethnic Medicine News (Ma Yingguai, Huize County, Yunnan Province)

6. 治疗单纯性结膜充血：星子草、鲜桃树尖嫩叶各适量，用木棒或石头捣烂；做成蚕豆大药饼，外敷“太阳穴位”（左眼患病敷右侧；右眼患病敷左侧）并用纱布敷料敷盖。

6. For treating simple conjunctival congestion: take appropriate amounts of Aster indicus and fresh tender leaves from the tip of peach tree branches, mash them with a wooden stick or stone into a paste, form into broad-bean-sized cakes, apply externally to the Taiyang acupoint (apply to the right side for left eye involvement and to the left side for right eye involvement), and cover with gauze dressing.

一般敷后 6 至 12 小时即可治愈。

Generally, cure is achieved within 6 to 12 hours after application.

《民族医药报》1992 年 8 月 21 日（湖南 王在兴）

Ethnic Medicine News, August 21, 1992 (Wang Zaixing, Hunan Province)

7. 我院眼科专家门诊老中医，总结数十年临证经验，筛选研制的“柴芩汤（丸）”治疗眼科角膜炎、虹膜炎、睑腺炎、沙眼等外眼炎症，总有效率 99.5%，治愈率 95%。

7. Senior traditional Chinese medicine physicians at our hospital' s ophthalmology specialist clinic have summarized decades of clinical experience to develop the "Chaiqin Decoction (Pills)," which has achieved a total effective rate of 99.5% and a cure rate of 95% in treating external ocular inflammations such as keratitis, iritis, hordeolum, and trachoma.

药物由柴胡10克、黄芩12克、生地12克、元参15克、钩藤30克、桑叶10克、菊花10克、防风10克、赤芍12克、双花20克、连翘12克、甘草6克组成。

The formula consists of 10g Bupleurum chinense, 12g Scutellaria baicalensis, 12g Rehmannia glutinosa (raw), 15g Scrophularia ningpoensis, 30g Uncaria rhynchophylla, 10g Morus alba leaf, 10g Chrysanthemum morifolium, 10g Saposhnikovia divaricata, 12g Paeonia lactiflora (red), 20g Lonicera japonica, 12g Forsythia suspensa, and 6g Glycyrrhiza uralensis.

功效为祛风清热、清肝解毒。

Its functions are dispelling wind, clearing heat, clearing the liver, and relieving toxicity.

服法：水煎15分钟日一剂分二次服，3至5付为一疗程。

Administration: decoct in water for 15 minutes, one dose daily divided into two administrations; 3 to 5 doses constitute one course of treatment.

本院按国家制剂标准生产为水泛丸，广泛推广于临床，疗效显著。

Our hospital manufactures this formula as water-binded pills according to national pharmaceutical standards; it has been widely promoted in clinical practice with remarkable efficacy.

《中医药信息报》1992年5月16日（山东淄博市中医院 任鲁平）

Traditional Chinese Medicine Information News, May 16, 1992 (Ren Luping, Zibo Municipal Hospital of Traditional Chinese Medicine, Shandong Province)

（十）目涩（1方）

(X) Dry Eyes (1 Prescription)

润眼汤疗目涩

Runyan Decoction for Treating Dry Eyes

人们常常因用眼过度或用眼环境恶劣而引起眼睛干涩、目暗不明、发胀、怕风等症状。

People often experience symptoms such as dry eyes, dim vision, distension, and photophobia due to excessive eye use or poor visual environments.

笔者每遇到这种情况，常饮用润眼汤而愈。

Whenever encountering such conditions, the author often recovers by drinking Runyan Decoction.

此方简便易行，常饮无妨。

This prescription is simple and easy to prepare, and regular consumption is harmless.

现介绍如下：取枸杞子 12 克，女贞子 10 克，菟丝子 10 克，加入一碗半水，用文火煮到一碗水，即可饮用。

The preparation is as follows: take 12g of Lycium barbarum, 10g of Ligustrum lucidum fruit, and 10g of Cuscuta chinensis; add one and a half bowls of water, simmer over low heat until reduced to one bowl, and then drink.

每日一剂，连服数剂。

One dose daily for several consecutive doses.

《中医药报》（粤波）

Traditional Chinese Medicine News (Yue Bo)

（十一）眼肌型重症肌无力（1 方）

(XI) Ocular Myasthenia Gravis (1 Prescription)

眼肌型重症肌无力验方

Proven Formula for Ocular Myasthenia Gravis

重症肌无力是一种与自身免疫有关的疾病，临床以眼肌型最为多见。

Myasthenia gravis is an autoimmune-related disease, with the ocular type being the most common clinically.

治疗颇为棘手。

Treatment is quite challenging.

我院试用温肾运脾，益气升陷之法治疗该病，取得了一定的疗效。

Our hospital has tried the method of warming the kidneys, activating the spleen, tonifying qi, and raising sunken yang to treat this disease, achieving certain therapeutic efficacy.

药方及用法：黄芪 18 克，党参 12 克，柴胡、升麻各 7 克，干姜、肉桂各 6 克，防风、生甘草各 8 克，赤芍、白芍、地龙各 10 克。

Prescription and usage: 18g of Astragalus membranaceus, 12g of Codonopsis pilosula, 7g each of Bupleurum chinense and Cimicifuga heracleifolia, 6g each of dried ginger and Cinnamomum cassia bark, 8g each of Saposhnikovia divaricata and raw Glycyrrhiza uralensis, and 10g each of red Paeonia lactiflora, white Paeonia lactiflora, and Lumbricus terrestris.

水煎服，每日 1 剂，日服 3 次。

Decoct in water and administer orally, one dose daily divided into three administrations.

《民族医药报》1992 年 4 月 24 日（南京市上新河医院 孙哲）

Ethnic Medicine News, April 24, 1992 (Sun Zhe, Shangxinhe Hospital, Nanjing City)

二、鼻炎（39 方）
II. Rhinitis (39 Prescriptions)

过敏性鼻炎是一种常见病，一般有其它过敏性疾病史，如哮喘、荨麻疹等，其症状为突然发作性的鼻塞、鼻痒、喷嚏，大量流清水鼻涕，检查时可见鼻黏膜颜色比较苍白（紫红色）及水肿。

Allergic rhinitis is a common disease, generally associated with a history of other allergic conditions such as asthma and urticaria; its symptoms include sudden onset of nasal congestion, nasal itching, sneezing, and profuse watery rhinorrhea, while examination may reveal pale or purplish-red and edematous nasal mucosa.

如今，治疗过敏性鼻炎药虽不少，但效果均不堪理想。

Although there are now many medications available for treating allergic rhinitis, their efficacy remains unsatisfactory.

下边介绍几种既简易速效又无任何副作用的治疗过敏性鼻炎方法，供大家参考应用。

The following simple, rapid-acting, and reportedly side-effect-free methods for treating allergic rhinitis are presented below for reference and application.

1. 滴鼻法：把牡丹皮 1500 克浸泡于清水中半天至 1 天，然后蒸馏得 2000 毫升乳白色液体，用所得液体滴鼻，1 日 3 次，一般 2-3 天可治愈。

1.Nasal Drop Method: Soak 1,500g of Moutan cortex in clear water for half a day to one day, then distill to obtain 2,000 ml of milky white liquid; use this liquid as nasal drops three times daily, and cure is generally achieved within 2–3 days.

2. 鼻吸法: 把冰片 2 克，扑尔敏片 400 毫克，共研成极细末，采用鼻吸法给药，1 日 3-5 次，曾治疗 83 例过敏性鼻炎，痊愈 80 例，好转 3 例。

2. Nasal Insufflation Method: Grind 2g of borneol and 400 mg of chlorpheniramine tablets into an extremely fine powder together, administer via nasal insufflation 3–5 times daily; this method was used to treat 83 cases of allergic rhinitis, resulting in 80 cures and 3 improvements.

3. 中药煎制法：把土黄芪 20 克、白术、防风、当归、辛夷、五味子、石菖蒲各 10 克，细辛 3 克，蝉蜕、甘草各 6 克，水煎服，1 日 1 剂。

3. Herbal Decoction Method: Take 20g of local Astragalus, 10g each of Atractylodes macrocephala, Saposhnikovia divaricata, Angelica sinensis, Magnolia biondii flower bud, Schisandra chinensis, and Acorus tatarinowii, 3g of Asarum sieboldii, and 6g each of Cryptotympana pustulata slough and Glycyrrhiza uralensis; decoct in water and administer orally, one dose daily.

河北中医学院附属医院曾用此方治疗 34 例，治愈 26 例，好转 7 例。

The Affiliated Hospital of Hebei College of Traditional Chinese Medicine once treated 34 cases with this prescription, achieving 26 cures and 7 improvements.

4. 针剂疗法：用丹参注射液在每侧下鼻甲黏膜注射 1.5 毫克，1 周两次，6-8 次为一疗程，一般 1-2 个疗程可治愈。

4. Injection Therapy: Inject 1.5 mg of Salvia miltiorrhiza injection into the mucosa of each inferior turbinate twice weekly; 6–8 injections constitute one course of treatment, and cure is generally achieved after 1–2 courses.

5. 塞鼻疗法：把鹅不食草 50 克研为细末，将药棉浸湿拧干后，包药粉少许，卷成细条塞入鼻孔内，20-30 分钟后取出，每日 1 次。

5. Nasal Packing Method: Grind 50g of Centipeda minima into a fine powder, soak absorbent cotton in water and wring it dry, wrap a small amount of the powder inside, roll it into a thin strip, insert it into the nostril, remove it after 20–30 minutes, and apply once daily.

此法除初起有喷嚏、流泪与流鼻涕外，余无不良反应。

Apart from initial sneezing, tearing, and rhinorrhea, this method causes no other adverse reactions.

《中药科技报》（河北 刘志彬）

Chinese Materia Medica Science and Technology News (Liu Zhibin, Hebei Province)

6. 过敏性鼻炎患者近年来有所增加，由于过敏源分布较广，因此较难预防也不易治疗，一般仅能对症治疗。

6. The number of patients with allergic rhinitis has increased in recent years; due to the widespread distribution of allergens, prevention is difficult and treatment is challenging, so management is generally limited to symptomatic relief.

近年来一些研究人员发现，中药方剂桑菊饮对过敏性鼻炎有较好效果。

In recent years, some researchers have found that the traditional Chinese medicine formula Sangju Yin has good efficacy for allergic rhinitis.

桑菊饮中的桑叶、菊花除有疏风清热作用外还有清肝明目作用，因此常用于眼部疾病，由过敏性鼻炎所引起的结膜炎当然也有较好疗效；薄荷具有辛凉解毒作用，对过敏性鼻炎出现的鼻塞、目红均有效；芦根具有清热生津作用，过敏性鼻炎常久病不愈，大量鼻汁流失，体内津液减少，芦根则有预防津液不足作用。

In Sangju Yin, mulberry leaf and chrysanthemum not only dispel wind and clear heat but also clear the liver and improve vision, so they are often used for ocular diseases and naturally show good efficacy for conjunctivitis caused by allergic rhinitis; peppermint has pungent-cooling and detoxifying effects, effective against both nasal congestion and red eyes associated with allergic rhinitis; reed rhizome clears heat and generates fluids, which helps prevent fluid deficiency arising from prolonged illness, massive loss of nasal secretions, and consequent depletion of body fluids in allergic rhinitis.

另外，甘草桔梗有利于消除鼻咽部黏膜水肿，与其它药物组成复方发挥协同作用，对过敏性鼻炎有显著疗效，对久治不愈的患者不妨一试。

Additionally, licorice and platycodon help alleviate nasopharyngeal mucosal edema and exert synergistic effects when combined with other herbs in compound formulas, showing significant efficacy for allergic rhinitis; patients with long-standing refractory cases may consider trying this approach.

《中医药信息报》1992 年 2 月 15 日（吕 群）

Traditional Chinese Medicine Information News, February 15, 1992 (Lü Qun)

7. 笔者自拟“龙鱼散”治疗鼻炎，经十几年临床应用，疗效确切，现介绍如下。

7. The author formulated “Longyu Powder” for treating rhinitis, which has demonstrated definitive efficacy over more than ten years of clinical application and is introduced as follows.

方药及制备：地龙 18 克，鱼腥草 15 克，薄荷 18 克，白芷 15 克，冰片 3 克。

Composition and Preparation: 18g of Lumbricus terrestris, 15g of Houttuynia cordata, 18g of Mentha haplocalyx, 15g of Angelica dahurica, and 3g of borneol.

除冰片外，上药分别烘干研末过 100 目筛后，再与冰片共研装瓶密封备用。

Except for borneol, dry the above herbs separately, grind them into powder, pass through a 100-mesh sieve, then grind together with borneol, bottle, and seal for later use.

用法：每日用消毒棉签沾少许药末撒入患鼻腔中，每日上下午各 1 次。

Usage: Apply a small amount of the powder into the affected nasal cavity daily using a sterilized cotton swab, once in the morning and once in the afternoon.

12 天为 1 疗程。

Twelve days constitute one course of treatment.

一般 2-5 日即明显见效。

Generally, significant improvement is observed within 2–5 days.

适用范围及特点：本药散适用于过敏性鼻炎、萎缩性鼻炎、鼻窦炎。

Indications and Characteristics: This powder is indicated for allergic rhinitis, atrophic rhinitis, and sinusitis.

其具有祛风解毒，散瘀通窍之功效。

It has the effects of dispelling wind, relieving toxicity, dissipating blood stasis, and unblocking the orifices.

药价廉、疗程短，见效快易于制作及推广。

The medicine is inexpensive, the course of treatment is short, it acts quickly, and it is easy to prepare and promote.

无副作用。

It has no side effects.

病例：程某，女，54 岁，退休干部。

Case Report: Ms. Cheng, female, 54 years old, retired cadre.

1991 年 9 月 17 日初诊，自诉每逢天气变化时鼻痒、打喷嚏、流鼻涕、头晕胀，此症已有 15 年，经五官科诊为过敏性鼻炎，曾经多方治疗未效，给予“龙鱼散”治疗 5 天明显见效，经 2 个疗程治疗后，上述症状全部消失，随访至今未复发。

At her first visit on September 17, 1991, she reported nasal itching, sneezing, runny nose, and head distension whenever the weather changed; these symptoms had persisted for 15 years and were diagnosed as allergic rhinitis by the ENT department without response to multiple previous treatments; after 5 days of treatment with "Longyu Powder," significant improvement was noted, and following two courses of treatment, all aforementioned symptoms completely resolved with no recurrence during follow-up to date.

《民族医药报》（广西 何波文）

Ethnic Medicine News (He Bowen, Guangxi)

8. 处方：党参 20 克，金银花 20 克，辛夷花 20 克，黄芪 20 克，白术 15 克，防风 15 克，丹参 15 克，当归 15 克，木通 15 克，牛蒡子 15 克。

8. Prescription: 20g of Codonopsis pilosula, 20g of Lonicera japonica, 20g of Magnolia biondii flower bud, 20g of Astragalus membranaceus, 15g of Atractylodes macrocephala, 15g of Saposhnikovia divaricata, 15g of Salvia miltiorrhiza, 15g of Angelica sinensis, 15g of Akebia quinata stem, and 15g of Arctium lappa seed.

用法：水煎服，每日 1 剂，温服。

Usage: Decoct in water and take orally while warm, one dose daily.

另用棉球蘸药液塞鼻，每日 3 次。

Additionally, soak a cotton ball in the decoction and pack it into the nostril three times daily.

连用 15 剂为 1 疗程。

Fifteen consecutive doses constitute one course of treatment.

主治：过敏性鼻炎，症见反复发作性鼻痒，喷嚏频作，鼻流清涕，鼻塞，常伴头痛、汗多怕风等症状。

Indications: Allergic rhinitis presenting with recurrent nasal itching, frequent sneezing, clear watery nasal discharge, and nasal congestion, often accompanied by headache, profuse sweating, and aversion to wind.

《民族医药报》（桐文）

Ethnic Medicine News (Tong Wen)

9. 辛夷煮鸡蛋：通窍、止脓涕、祛头痛，滋养扶正。

9. Boiled Eggs with Magnolia Flower: Unblocks the orifices, stops purulent

nasal discharge, relieves headache, nourishes the body, and strengthens vital qi.

主治慢性鼻窦炎，流脓涕，体弱不胜寒凉。

It is indicated for chronic sinusitis with purulent nasal discharge and physical weakness with intolerance to cold.

用辛夷花 15 克入砂锅内，加清水 2 碗，浓缩一碗，鸡蛋 2 个，煮熟去壳，刺小孔数个，将砂锅置于火上，倒入药汁煮沸，放入鸡蛋同煮片刻，饮汤吃蛋，常服有效。

Place 15g of magnolia flower buds in a clay pot, add two bowls of water, and reduce to one bowl; boil two eggs separately, peel them, and prick several small holes on each; bring the herbal decoction to a boil over heat, add the eggs and simmer briefly together; drink the soup and eat the eggs; regular consumption yields effective results.

10. 丝瓜藤煲猪瘦肉：清热消炎、解毒通窍，主治慢性鼻炎急性发作、萎缩性鼻炎、鼻流脓涕、脑重头痛。

10. Lean Pork Soup with Loofah Vine: Clears heat, reduces inflammation, relieves toxicity, and unblocks the orifices; indicated for acute exacerbation of chronic rhinitis, atrophic rhinitis, purulent nasal discharge, and head heaviness with headache.

取近根部之丝瓜藤 3-5 尺洗净，猪瘦肉 60 克切碎，同放锅内煮汤至熟加少许盐调味，饮汤吃肉，5 次为一疗程，连用 1-3 个疗程。

Take 3–5 chi (approximately 1–1.7 meters) of loofah vine near the root, wash clean, and chop 60g of lean pork; place both in a pot, cook into soup until done, season with a little salt, then consume the soup and meat; five servings constitute one course of treatment, and 1–3 consecutive courses are recommended.

11. 柏叶猪鼻汤：消炎通窍，养阴扶正。

11. Pig Snout Soup with Platycladus Leaf: Reduces inflammation, unblocks the orifices, nourishes yin, and strengthens vital qi.

主治鼻渊、脑漏、鼻流臭涕。

It is indicated for biyuan (sinusitis), brain leakage, and foul-smelling nasal discharge.

取猪鼻肉 60 克刮洗干净，用生柏叶 30 克，金钗石斛 6 克，柴胡 10 克，同入砂锅，加清水 4 碗煎浓至一碗，滤除药渣，冲入蜜糖 60 克，30 度米酒 30 克，和匀饮之，2-4 剂为一疗程，连服 3-4 个疗程。

Scrape and wash 60g of pig snout meat clean; combine with 30g of fresh platycladus leaf, 6g of Dendrobium nobile, and 10g of Bupleurum chinense in a clay pot; add four bowls of water and decoct until reduced to one bowl; strain out the dregs, mix in 60g of honey and 30g of 30-proof rice wine, stir well, and drink; 2–4 doses constitute one course of treatment, and 3–4 consecutive courses are recommended.

12. 黄花鱼头汤：扶正祛邪，补中通窍。

12. Fish Head Soup with Daylily: Strengthens vital qi, dispels pathogenic factors, tonifies the middle jiao, and unblocks the orifices.

主治慢性萎缩性鼻炎，感冒频繁，鼻炎动辄发作。

It is indicated for chronic atrophic rhinitis, frequent colds, and easily triggered rhinitis attacks.

取镛鱼头（俗称胖头鱼）100 克，洗净后用热油两面稍煎备用。

Take 100g of silver carp head (commonly known as pangtouyu), wash clean, and lightly pan-fry both sides in hot oil; set aside.

将大枣 15 克去核洗净，用黄花 30 克，白术 15 克，苍耳子 10 克，白芷 10 克，生姜 3 片共放砂锅内与鱼头一起熬汤，待熟，吃肉饮汁。

Remove the pits from 15g of jujube dates and wash clean; combine with 30g of daylily, 15g of Atractylodes macrocephala, 10g of Xanthium sibiricum fruit, 10g of Angelica dahurica, and 3 slices of ginger in a clay pot; add the fish head and simmer into soup until cooked; eat the meat and drink the broth.

13. 芎芷炖猪脑：通窍、补脑，扶正祛邪。

13. Stewed Pig Brain with Chuanxiong and Angelica: Unblocks the orifices, tonifies the brain, strengthens vital qi, and dispels pathogenic factors.

主治慢性鼻炎，体质虚弱。

It is indicated for chronic rhinitis and weak constitution.

取猪脑 2 副（牛、羊脑也可），洗净剔除血管等备用；将川芎 10 克，白芷 10 克，辛夷花 15 克，放入砂锅内，加清水 2 碗，煎浓 1 碗。

Take 2 pairs of pig brains (beef or sheep brains may also be used), wash clean, remove blood vessels and other impurities, and set aside; place 10g of Ligusticum chuanxiong, 10g of Angelica dahurica, and 15g of magnolia flower buds in a clay pot, add two bowls of water, and decoct until reduced to one bowl.

复将药汁倾炖盅内，加入猪脑，隔水炖熟，饮汤吃猪脑，常用有效。

Pour the herbal decoction into a double-boiling jar, add the pig brains, and steam-cook over water until done; drink the soup and eat the pig brains; regular use is effective.

14. 羊粉：主治慢性鼻窦炎。

14. Sheep Testicle Powder: Indicated for chronic sinusitis.

取羊睾丸一对，洗净后，放瓦片或砂锅内焙黄（不可炒焦炒黑），研成细末，用温开水或黄酒送下。

Take one pair of sheep testicles, wash clean, roast on a tile or in a clay pot until yellowish (do not scorch or char), grind into fine powder, and take with warm boiled water or yellow rice wine.

每对睾丸一日分两次服完，连续服用 2-3 天可见效。

Consume one pair of testicles in two divided doses per day; effects are typically observed after 2–3 consecutive days of administration.

《中药科技报》1991 年 6 月 26 日（彭平建）

Chinese Materia Medica Science and Technology News, June 26, 1991 (Peng Pingjian)

15. 鹅不食草 15 克，薄荷 9 克，开水沏，代茶饮。

15. Steep 15g of Centipeda minima and 9g of peppermint in boiling water and drink as a tea substitute.

16. 用鹅不食草煎成 1% 的水溶液，滴鼻，3 次 / 日，或用凡士林制成 10% 的鹅不食草软膏，均匀涂于纱条上，剪成 2 厘米长，放于消毒缸内消毒。

16. Prepare a 1% aqueous solution by decocting Centipeda minima for use as nasal drops three times daily; alternatively, prepare a 10% Centipeda minima ointment with petrolatum, spread evenly onto gauze strips, cut into 2 cm lengths, and sterilize in a disinfection container.

用时每个鼻腔放置一条，15-20 分钟取出，每日一次，7 次为 1 疗程。

When using, place one strip in each nasal cavity, remove after 15–20 minutes, apply once daily, and seven applications constitute one course of treatment.

17. 甘草、炮干姜各 6 克，泡茶，频频饮用，疗效满意。

17. Steep 6g each of licorice and processed dried ginger in hot water to make tea; sip frequently throughout the day for satisfactory therapeutic effects.

18. 用代温灸膏贴敷双侧百劳、肺俞、膏肓六穴，效果良好。

18. Apply Daiwen Moxibustion Plaster bilaterally to the Bailao, Feishu, and Gaohuang acupoints (six points total) for good efficacy.

《中药科技报》1993 年 3 月 11 日（河南常怡勇）

Chinese Materia Medica Science and Technology News, March 11, 1993 (Chang Yiyong, Henan Province)

19. 治慢性鼻炎：取辛夷、鱼脑石各等分研细末备用。

19. For treating chronic rhinitis: Take equal amounts of magnolia flower buds and fish otoliths, grind into fine powder, and store for later use.

用时取药粉少许吹入鼻腔，一日 2-3 次，坚持用药 2-3 个月可愈。

When needed, blow a small amount of the powder into the nasal cavity 2–3 times daily; persistent use for 2–3 months can achieve cure.

也可取鱼脑石 30 克，冰片 3 克，研细末备用。

Alternatively, take 30g of fish otoliths and 3g of borneol, grind into fine powder, and store for later use.

20. 治过敏性鼻炎：取苍耳子、辛夷、白芷、丝瓜藤 100 克，绿矾 50 克，薄荷 80 克。

20. For treating allergic rhinitis: Take 100g each of Xanthium sibiricum fruit, Magnolia biondii flower bud, Angelica dahurica, and loofah vine, 50g of green

vitriol, and 80g of peppermint.

将上药研细粉过 120 目筛，装入瓷瓶备用。

Grind the above herbs into fine powder, pass through a 120-mesh sieve, and store in a porcelain bottle for later use.

每日吹鼻 3 次，10 天为一疗程，间隔 3-5 天，再进行第二疗程。

Blow the powder into the nasal cavity three times daily; ten days constitute one course of treatment, with an interval of 3–5 days before starting the second course.

本方初次使用时，鼻腔内稍有痛感，且鼻涕增多，使用几次后即可适应。

Upon initial use of this prescription, there may be slight pain in the nasal cavity and increased nasal discharge, but tolerance typically develops after several applications.

21. 治鼻窦炎：取芙蓉叶、香白芷、辛夷花各 15 克，细辛 3 克，冰片 1 克。

21. For treating sinusitis: Take 15g each of Hibiscus mutabilis leaf, fragrant Angelica dahurica, and Magnolia biondii flower bud, 3g of Asarum sieboldii, and 1g of borneol.

上药共研细末和匀贮瓶备用。

Grind all the above herbs together into a fine powder, mix evenly, and store in a bottle for later use.

使用前先将鼻腔内涕液拭干，再将药末吹入，每日 3-5 次，1-2 周可获效。

Before use, first wipe the nasal cavity dry of secretions, then blow the powder in; apply 3–5 times daily, and efficacy is generally achieved within 1–2 weeks.

《民族医药报》1992 年 9 月 4 日（江苏省南通市 吴自强）

Ethnic Medicine News, September 4, 1992 (Wu Ziqiang, Nantong City, Jiangsu Province)

22. 治慢性鼻炎一法

22. A Method for Treating Chronic Rhinitis

苍耳子 6 克，白芷 6 克，辛夷 6 克，冰片粉 0.6 克，薄荷霜 0.5 克，芝麻油 50 毫升，液体石蜡 100 毫升。

Take 6g of Xanthium sibiricum fruit, 6g of Angelica dahurica, 6g of Magnolia biondii flower bud, 0.6g of borneol powder, 0.5g of menthol crystals, 50 ml of sesame oil, and 100 ml of liquid paraffin.

将苍耳子、白芷、辛夷、油同放锅内，浸泡 24 小时，加热，待药呈黑黄色捞出，再下冰片、薄荷霜、液体石蜡，搅匀，冷却后过滤，分装入滴瓶内备用。

Place the Xanthium fruit, Angelica dahurica, Magnolia flower bud, and sesame oil together in a pot, soak for 24 hours, then heat until the herbs turn blackish-yellow and remove them; add the borneol powder, menthol crystals, and liquid paraffin, stir evenly, filter after cooling, and dispense into dropper bottles for later use.

滴鼻，每次 1-2 滴，每日 1-2 次。

Apply as nasal drops, 1–2 drops per administration, 1–2 times daily.

总有效率达 92.4%。

The total effective rate reaches 92.4%.

《民族医药报》1998 年 3 月 6 日（克 锋）

Ethnic Medicine News, March 6, 1998 (Ke Feng)

23. 鲜鸡蛋 1 个，鲜苏梗叶适量。

23. Take one fresh egg and an appropriate amount of fresh Perilla frutescens stem and leaves.

蛋、药一起煎成汤剂，吃蛋喝汤。

Decoct the egg and herbs together into a soup; eat the egg and drink the broth.

24. 辛夷花 30 克，鸡蛋 10 个。

24. Take 30g of Magnolia biondii flower buds and 10 eggs.

加水共煎煮待蛋熟后吃蛋喝汤，可经常服用。

Add water and boil together until the eggs are cooked; eat the eggs and drink the soup, which may be consumed regularly.

25. 莲子心 6 克，甘草 15 克，地丁 10 克。

25. Take 6g of lotus plumule, 15g of licorice, and 10g of Viola yedoensis.

水煮饮服，每日 1 次。

Boil in water and drink the decoction once daily.

26. 紫草 30 克，麻油 500 克，苍耳子 20 克。

26. Take 30g of Lithospermum erythrorhizon, 500g of sesame oil, and 20g of Xanthium sibiricum fruit.

先将苍耳子打碎，与紫草一起泡入麻油中 4-5 小时，然后煎炸至棕色，去渣取油备用。

First crush the Xanthium fruit, soak it together with Lithospermum in sesame oil for 4–5 hours, then fry until brownish, strain out the dregs, and reserve the oil for later use.

每日滴鼻 2 次，可治疗过敏性鼻炎。

Apply as nasal drops twice daily to treat allergic rhinitis.

27. 白芷适量，研为细末，加入少许冰片，时时搐入鼻中，可治疗单纯性和肥厚性鼻炎。

27. Take an appropriate amount of Angelica dahurica, grind into fine powder, add a small amount of borneol, and apply into the nasal cavity from time to time to treat simple and hypertrophic rhinitis.

28. 瓜蒂数个，将瓜蒂置瓦上焙干，研细末，取适量吹入鼻腔内，可治疗单纯性和肥厚性鼻炎。

28. Take several muskmelon pedicels, roast them on a tile until dry, grind into fine powder, and blow an appropriate amount into the nasal cavity to treat simple and hypertrophic rhinitis.

29. 蜂房 1 个，挤去糖汁、嚼食。

29. Take one honeycomb, squeeze out the honey, and chew to consume.

每次 30 克，每日或隔日 1 次。

Take 30g per dose, once daily or every other day.

可治单纯性和肥厚性鼻炎。

This can treat simple and hypertrophic rhinitis.

30. 辛夷 6 克，苍耳子 6 克，冰片 0.6 克。

30. Take 6g of Magnolia biondii flower buds, 6g of Xanthium sibiricum fruit, and 0.6g of borneol.

研为极细末，嗅入鼻中，可治单纯性和肥厚性鼻炎。

Grind into an extremely fine powder and inhale into the nasal cavity to treat simple and hypertrophic rhinitis.

32. 香油 30 毫升，黄连 3 克。

32. Take 30 ml of sesame oil and 3g of Coptis chinensis.

将黄连浸入香油中，一周后取油滴鼻，每日 3 次。

Soak the Coptis in sesame oil for one week, then use the infused oil as nasal drops three times daily.

可治疗萎缩性鼻炎。

This can treat atrophic rhinitis.

35. 白菊花 18 克，蜂蜜适量。

35. Take 18g of white chrysanthemum and an appropriate amount of honey.

先将菊花放在蜜上蒸 2 小时，然后去菊花同蜜滴鼻，每日 1 次。

First steam the chrysanthemum over honey for 2 hours, then remove the flowers and use the honey as nasal drops once daily.

可治疗萎缩性鼻炎。

This can treat atrophic rhinitis.

36. 大蒜数头，甘油 25 毫升。

36. Take several garlic bulbs and 25 ml of glycerin.

将蒜去皮捣烂，用纱布绞汁，加入甘油混匀，放入加盖瓶中备用。

Peel and mash the garlic, squeeze out the juice through gauze, mix evenly with glycerin, and store in a capped bottle for later use.

用时取小纱布条蘸药液，填入鼻腔中，每日 2 次，每次放置 4 小时，可治疗萎缩性鼻炎。

When using, dip a small gauze strip into the liquid, pack it into the nasal cavity twice daily, leave in place for 4 hours each time, to treat atrophic rhinitis.

《中药科技报》1993 年 12 月 9 日（江苏黄河）

Chinese Materia Medica Science and Technology News, December 9, 1993 (Huang He, Jiangsu Province)

37. 益母草适量生药用 80-160 克，（干品 50-100 克干炒焦）加水 500 毫升，煎至 200 毫升，药渣再煎取 100 毫升，将两次药液混合分 2-3 次服完。

37. Take an appropriate amount of fresh Leonurus japonicus (80–160g for fresh herb, or 50–100g of dried herb stir-fried until scorched), add 500 ml of water, decoct until reduced to 200 ml, then decoct the dregs again to obtain another 100 ml; mix the two decoctions and take in 2–3 divided doses.

一般 1-3 剂就能根治。

Generally, a radical cure can be achieved with 1–3 doses.

此药较苦，药煎好后可加一些糖调味，药效一样。

Since this medicine is quite bitter, some sugar may be added for flavoring after decoction without affecting its efficacy.

38. 甘油（如无甘油用石蜡油同样有效）100 毫升，薄荷冰 1 克，樟脑（粉）1 克，三味药物混合捣匀溶解后即可。

38. Mix 100 ml of glycerin (liquid paraffin is equally effective if glycerin is unavailable), 1g of menthol crystals, and 1g of camphor powder; pound evenly until fully dissolved.

用法：可用滴管吸药滴鼻，也可用干净的药棉沾甘油合剂填塞患侧鼻腔则效果更好。

Usage: The solution can be administered as nasal drops using a dropper, or better results can be achieved by packing the affected nasal cavity with clean absorbent cotton soaked in the glycerin mixture.

《民族医药报》1992 年 4 月 17 日（广西融水苗族自治县 韦勋荣）

Ethnic Medicine News, April 17, 1992 (Wei Xunrong, Rongshui Miao Autonomous County, Guangxi)

39. 药物组成：双花 20 克，公英 30 克，黄芩 10 克，栀子 10 克，生石膏 60 克，桔梗 15 克，丹参 12 克，辛夷 6 克，菊花 12 克，芥穗 15 克，细辛 3 克，竹叶 6 克。

39. Composition: 20g of Lonicera japonica, 30g of Taraxacum mongolicum,

10g of Scutellaria baicalensis, 10g of Gardenia jasminoides fruit, 60g of raw gypsum, 15g of Platycodon grandiflorus, 12g of Salvia miltiorrhiza, 6g of Magnolia biondii flower bud, 12g of Chrysanthemum morifolium, 15g of Schizonepeta tenuifolia spike, 3g of Asarum sieboldii, and 6g of bamboo leaf.

服法：（1）水煎15分钟日一剂分二次服，10付为一疗程。

Administration: (1) Decoct in water for 15 minutes, one dose daily divided into two administrations; 10 doses constitute one course of treatment.

（2）水泛丸，每次10克，每日三次。

(2) Alternatively, prepare as water-binded pills, taking 10g per dose three times daily.

调护：（1）忌食辛辣、发性之物（2）避免感冒。

Care instructions: (1) Avoid spicy and stimulating foods; (2) Prevent catching colds.

《中医药信息报》1992年8月1日（山东淄博市中医院 任鲁平）

Traditional Chinese Medicine Information News, August 1, 1992 (Ren Luping, Zibo Municipal Hospital of Traditional Chinese Medicine, Shandong Province)

三、中耳炎（17方）
III. Otitis Media (17 Prescriptions)

1. 新鲜桑叶数片洗净后，捣烂取汁。

1.Wash several fresh mulberry leaves clean, mash them, and extract the juice.

用时先用生理盐水清洗耳内，再用消毒干棉签擦干，然后将桑叶汁滴入耳内1-2滴，每日3次，2-3天即愈。

Before use, first clean the ear canal with normal saline, then wipe dry with a sterilized dry cotton swab; instill 1–2 drops of mulberry leaf juice into the ear three times daily, and cure is generally achieved within 2–3 days.

2. 煅龙骨、煅明矾（枯矾）各等量，分别研末，过120目细筛。

2. Take equal amounts of calcined dragon bone and calcined alum (dehydrated alum), grind each separately into powder, and pass through a 120-mesh fine sieve.

用时先用 3% 过氧化氢把耳内脓液及分泌物洗清，患耳周围用 75% 酒精常规消毒，停 2-3 分钟后用消毒棉签拭干，然后取塑料管或麦秆蘸取药粉，轻轻吹入患耳道内，每日 1 次，一般 3 次即愈。

When using, first wash away pus and secretions in the ear with 3% hydrogen peroxide, routinely disinfect the area around the affected ear with 75% alcohol, wait 2–3 minutes, wipe dry with a sterilized cotton swab, then dip a plastic tube or wheat straw into the powder and gently blow it into the affected ear canal once daily; cure is generally achieved after 3 applications.

3. 黄连 10 克，枯矾、石膏各 5 克，共研极细末后，加芝麻油适量调匀。

3. Take 10g of Coptis chinensis, 5g each of dehydrated alum and gypsum, grind together into an extremely fine powder, then mix evenly with an appropriate amount of sesame oil.

用时先按常规清除外耳道积脓，然后将药滴入耳内，每次 1-2 滴，每日 2-3 次，一般 3-5 天可愈。

Before use, remove accumulated pus from the external auditory canal as usual, then instill 1–2 drops of the preparation into the ear 2–3 times daily; cure is generally achieved within 3–5 days.

4. 人指甲焙红研末，对入等量的冰片末合匀。

4. Roast human fingernails until reddish, grind into powder, and mix evenly with an equal amount of borneol powder.

先用双氧水清洗耳道，后稳妥地将药粉少量吹入耳内。

First clean the ear canal with hydrogen peroxide, then carefully blow a small amount of the powder into the ear.

每日 1 次，一般 3 次即愈。

Apply once daily, and cure is generally achieved after 3 applications.

5. 大活田螺一只洗净外壳，放置冷水中让其吐出螺体污泥，时间越长吐纳就越清。用时先用棉签蘸生理盐水或双氧水反复拭干耳内脓液。然后侧外，使患耳朝上，请他人持田螺剪开尾部，呈漏斗状，对准患耳外耳道，用物刺激螺盖，这样活螺体收缩，令从螺尖部滴出清凉黏液，使滴入患耳，滴数不限，每日1次，轻者1次愈，重者3-5次可愈。

5.Take one large live river snail, wash its shell clean, and place it in cold water to allow it to expel mud and impurities from its body; the longer it is soaked, the cleaner the expelled contents will be. Before use, repeatedly wipe away pus from the ear canal with a cotton swab dipped in normal saline or hydrogen peroxide until dry. Then have the patient lie on their side with the affected ear facing upward; ask another person to hold the snail, cut off its tail to form a funnel shape, and align it precisely with the external auditory canal of the affected ear. Gently stimulate the snail's operculum to induce contraction of the living body, causing cool, viscous fluid to drip from the tapered end directly into the ear; there is no limit to the number of drops. Apply once daily: mild cases typically resolve after a single application, while severe cases generally require 3–5 treatments for full recovery.

6. 猪胆汁1个，明矾15克，冰片1克，从胆口将明矾装入胆内（胆汁勿倒出），悬挂阴凉通风处，风干后取出明矾，加入冰片共研细末。用时以双氧水适量滴入耳内，待起泡沫，以脱脂棉拈药，将药粉吹入少许耳内，3-5日即好转，6-7日即愈。

6.Take one pig gallbladder, 15g of alum, and 1g of borneol. Insert the alum into the gallbladder through its opening without pouring out the bile, then hang it in a cool, well-ventilated place to air-dry. Once dried, remove the alum, add the borneol, and grind them together into a fine powder. When using, instill an appropriate amount of hydrogen peroxide into the ear; once foaming occurs, use absorbent cotton to apply a small amount of the powder by gently blowing it into the ear canal. Improvement is generally seen within 3–5 days, and cure is typically achieved within 6–7 days.

7. 金丝荷叶洗净晾干，捣烂后包入细纱布挤滤出药液，然后加入适量香油备用。

7. Wash Saxifraga stolonifera clean, air-dry, mash it, wrap in fine gauze, squeeze to extract the juice, then add an appropriate amount of sesame oil and set aside for later use.

用前先将患耳用双氧水洗净，再将药液滴耳，每次 1-2 滴，每日 3-4 次。

Before use, first clean the affected ear thoroughly with hydrogen peroxide, then instill 1–2 drops of the prepared liquid into the ear 3–4 times daily.

一般 3-5 天即愈。

Generally, cure is achieved within 3–5 days.

8. 黄连、黄柏各 3 克，烤焦研极细末，枯矾 2 克，冰片 1.5 克碾碎，香油 2 两，煎开冷却 5 分钟，上药共调匀成混合油剂，一日 3 次，每次 2-3 滴，2-3 天即愈。

8. Take 3g each of Coptis chinensis and Phellodendron amurense, roast until charred, and grind into an extremely fine powder; take 2g of dehydrated alum and 1.5g of borneol, crush them; heat 100 ml of sesame oil until boiling, let it cool for 5 minutes, then mix all the above ingredients evenly into a combined oil preparation; apply 2–3 drops three times daily, and cure is generally achieved within 2–3 days.

9. 麝香 1 克，75% 酒精 10 毫升。

9. Take 1g of musk and 10 ml of 75% alcohol.

将麝香溶于酒精内，贮于瓶中，勿令泄气 7 天后用。

Dissolve the musk in the alcohol, store in a sealed bottle to prevent leakage of aroma, and use after 7 days.

先用消毒棉签将耳内脓液拭净，再用麝香酊 1-2 滴，用滴管滴入耳内，间日 1 次。

First wipe away pus from the ear canal completely with a sterilized cotton swab, then instill 1–2 drops of the musk tincture into the ear using a dropper once every other day.

一般 3-5 天即愈。

Generally, cure is achieved within 3–5 days.

10. 胡桃晒干研末，蒸熟加压取油，再将冰片 1.5 克，黄连 1 克研粉加入胡桃油内。

10. Sun-dry walnuts, grind into powder, steam until cooked, and press to extract the oil; then grind 1.5g of borneol and 1g of Coptis chinensis into powder and add them to the walnut oil.

用时先用生理盐水清洗耳内，再用消毒棉签擦干，每次滴入约 0.1 毫升，一日 1-2 次，一般 3-5 天愈。

Before use, first clean the ear canal with normal saline, then wipe dry with a sterilized cotton swab; instill approximately 0.1 ml per dose, 1–2 times daily, and cure is generally achieved within 3–5 days.

《中药科技报》1992 年 5 月 16 日（江苏 张宏俊 王道俊）

Chinese Materia Medica Science and Technology News, May 16, 1992 (Zhang Hongjun & Wang Daojun, Jiangsu Province)

11. 中耳炎：栀子 12 克，黄连 6 克，黄柏、黄芩各 10 克，水煎浓缩洁净瓶贮备用。

11. For otitis media: Take 12g of Gardenia jasminoides fruit, 6g of Coptis chinensis, and 10g each of Phellodendron amurense and Scutellaria baicalensis; decoct in water, concentrate the liquid, and store in a clean bottle for later use.

先用双氧水洗净患耳滴用，每日 3-4 次。

First wash the affected ear thoroughly with hydrogen peroxide, then apply the concentrated decoction as ear drops 3–4 times daily.

《中药科技报》1992 年 1 月 16 日

Chinese Materia Medica Science and Technology News, January 16, 1992

12. 榴花酒：石榴花（鲜）20 克（干品 10 克），捣烂，加入三花酒 50 毫升，搅拌，浸半天（干品浸 1 天），绞汁滴耳，每天 4 次，每次 3-5 滴。

12. Pomegranate Flower Wine: Take 20g of fresh pomegranate flowers (or 10g dried), mash them, add 50 ml of Sanhua liquor, stir, and soak for half a day (or one full day for dried flowers); squeeze out the juice and use as ear drops four times daily, 3–5 drops per dose.

流脓停止后，仍继续滴药 3-5 天，以防复发。

After purulent discharge ceases, continue applying the drops for another 3–5 days to prevent recurrence.

13. 银花酒：金银花（鲜）30 克（干品 15 克），捣烂，加入三花酒 50 毫升，浸半天（干品浸 1 天），绞汁，滴耳，每天 4 次，每次 3-5 滴。

13. Honeysuckle Wine: Take 30g of fresh honeysuckle flowers (or 15g dried), mash them, add 50 ml of Sanhua liquor, and soak for half a day (or one full day for dried flowers); squeeze out the juice and use as ear drops four times daily, 3–5 drops per dose.

流脓停止后，仍继续滴药 2-3 天。

After purulent discharge ceases, continue applying the drops for another 2–3 days.

如能加入冰片粉末 0.5 克配制，药效更佳。

Adding 0.5g of borneol powder during preparation can further enhance the efficacy.

14. 臭草酒：臭草（鲜）10 克，捣烂，加三花酒 10 毫升，搅拌，绞汁，滴耳，每天 4-6 次，每次 3-5 滴。

14. Rue Wine: Take 10g of fresh rue, mash it, add 10 ml of Sanhua liquor, stir, and squeeze out the juice; use as ear drops 4–6 times daily, 3–5 drops per dose.

药液以当天配制当天使用为好。

It is best to prepare and use the liquid on the same day.

流脓停止后，仍应继续滴药 3-5 天。

After purulent discharge ceases, continue app

15. 化脓性中耳炎，是耳科常见的疾病，好发于青少年及儿童，且反复发作、缠绵难愈。

15. Suppurative otitis media is a common otological disease that frequently affects adolescents and children, characterized by recurrent attacks and a protracted, refractory course.

吾采用自组方治疗中耳炎，颇具良效。

The author has employed a self-formulated prescription for treating otitis media with considerable efficacy.

药物组成：白矾 70 克、全蝎 5 克、炉甘石 20 克、冰片 5 克。

Composition: 70g of alum, 5g of whole scorpion, 20g of calamine, and 5g of borneol.

制法：白矾煅制成枯矾；炉甘石煅后水飞成极细粉（120 目）干燥过筛；全蝎焙干研粉，冰片研细；四药混匀，过 120 目筛，密封备用。

Preparation: Calcine the alum to produce dehydrated alum; calcine the calamine, levigate it in water to an extremely fine powder (120-mesh), dry, and sieve; roast the whole scorpion until dry and grind into powder; grind the borneol into fine powder; mix all four ingredients evenly, pass through a 120-mesh sieve, and store in a sealed container for later use.

用法：先用双氧水，抑或热水洗净耳内分泌物，再用干棉球拭干，然后用麦秆药粉吹入耳内，一日 2 次，一般一周内可痊愈。

Usage: First wash away secretions in the ear canal with hydrogen peroxide or warm water, then wipe dry with a dry cotton ball; subsequently, use a wheat straw to gently blow the powder into the ear twice daily, and cure is generally achieved within one week.

《民族医药报》1992 年 4 月 10 日（湖南 彭平建）

Ethnic Medicine News, April 10, 1992 (Peng Pingjian, Hunan Province)

16. 将肥大的 30 条活蚯蚓，用冷开水洗净后置消毒的杯内，加白糖 50 克，用消毒筷轻轻搅拌约半小时，待白糖溶化，蚯蚓卷曲并渗出清液，呈现黄白色粘液时，用一层消毒纱布过滤装瓶。

16. Wash 30 large live earthworms clean with cool boiled water, place them in a sterilized cup, add 50g of white sugar, and stir gently with sterilized chopsticks for about half an hour; once the sugar dissolves and the earthworms curl up and exude clear fluid, forming a yellowish-white viscous liquid, filter it through a layer of sterilized gauze and bottle the filtrate.

使用前，先用 3% 双氧水清洗耳中脓性分泌物，反复洗两次后，用消毒棉球擦干，然后将滤液滴入 3-4 滴，并在外耳道塞少许无菌干棉球，每日 2-3 次。

Before use, first wash away purulent secretions in the ear with 3% hydrogen peroxide twice, wipe dry with a sterilized cotton ball, then instill 3–4 drops of the filtrate and pack a small amount of sterile dry cotton into the external auditory canal; apply 2–3 times daily.

笔者用该法治疗 62 例患者，一般一周内即痊愈。

The author treated 62 patients with this method, and cure was generally achieved within one week.

《民族医药报》1992 年 3 月 13 日（云南西双版纳 杨健）

Ethnic Medicine News, March 13, 1992 (Yang Jian, Xishuangbanna, Yunnan Province)

17. 核桃油治中耳炎: 将核桃打碎取仁，捣成泥糊，用双层消毒纱布包成丸状。

17. Walnut Oil for Otitis Media: Crack walnuts to extract the kernels, mash them into a paste, and wrap in double-layered sterilized gauze to form a ball.

将患耳用药棉拭干脓液，然后患耳取侧卧向上位置，双手捏紧核丸，挤出油液滴耳，以不往外溢出为度，10-15 分钟患耳向下将油倒出，每日一次。

Wipe the affected ear dry of pus with absorbent cotton, then have the patient lie on their side with the affected ear facing upward; squeeze the walnut ball tightly with both hands to express oil directly into the ear, taking care not to let it overflow; after 10–15 minutes, turn the affected ear downward to drain the oil out; apply once daily.

《民族医药报》1993 年 1 月 15 日

Ethnic Medicine News, January 15, 1993

四、耳聋耳鸣（12 方）

IV. Deafness and Tinnitus (12 Prescriptions)

突发性耳聋是突然发作、在短时间内致感音性耳聋的疾病。发病原因可能与病毒感染、内耳微循环障碍或因咳嗽促使迷路内压突然增高导致蜗窗膜、前庭膜破裂等引起有关。表现特点为短时（12-48 小时内）突发耳聋（多为单侧），伴有耳鸣、耳内闷塞感或伴有眩晕呕吐等症状，治疗后听力可逐渐恢复或难恢复及反复发作等。采用中西医结合治疗 80% 以上可恢复听力，伴有眩晕、有病毒感染史、老年人、治疗不及时者治愈率较差，故应早期采用中西医结合治疗方法为：

Sudden sensorineural hearing loss is a disease characterized by abrupt onset leading to sensorineural deafness within a short period. Its etiology may be associated with viral infections, microcirculatory disturbances of the inner ear, or rupture of the round window membrane and vestibular membrane caused by sudden elevation of labyrinthine pressure due to coughing. Clinically, it presents as sudden hearing loss (mostly unilateral) occurring within a short timeframe (12–48 hours), accompanied by tinnitus, aural fullness, or symptoms such as vertigo and vomiting; after treatment, hearing may gradually recover, remain difficult to restore, or relapse repeatedly. Integrated traditional Chinese and Western medicine therapy enables hearing recovery in over 80% of cases, whereas the cure rate is lower in patients accompanied by vertigo, those with a history of viral infection, the elderly, and those receiving delayed treatment; therefore, early integrated traditional Chinese and Western medicine treatment should be adopted as follows:

1. 西医药：以扩张血管、抗凝血为主。每日用低分子右旋糖酐 500 毫升加三磷酸腺苷 40 毫克静脉滴注 1 次；兼每日用维生素 B1100 毫克、维生素 B12500 微克、654-2 针 10 毫克混合肌注 1 次；兼每次口服盐酸倍它定 8 毫克、愈风宁心片（葛根制品每片 0.1 克）3 片口服，1 日 3 次。必要时兼采用高压氧舱治疗。

1.Western Medicine: Primarily focuses on vasodilation and anticoagulation. Administer intravenous infusion once daily with 500 ml of low-molecular-weight dextran plus 40 mg of adenosine triphosphate; additionally, give one intramuscular injection daily of a mixture containing 100 mg of vitamin B1, 500 mcg of vitamin B12, and 10 mg of anisodamine (654-2); also administer orally betahistine hydrochloride 8 mg and Yufeng Ningxin tablets (Pueraria lobata preparation, 0.1g per tablet) 3 tablets per dose, three times daily. Hyperbaric oxygen therapy may be added when necessary.

2. 中医药: 以益气、活血化瘀方法为主，方用: 黄芪、葛根各30克，丹参15克，川芎、红花、薤白、黄芩各12克，甘草6克。每日1剂煎汁，上下午分服。以上中西药治疗15日为1个疗程，可连用2个疗程，以恢复听力为度。在治疗中应卧床安心休息，保持大便通畅，低盐清淡饮食，防治咳嗽、喷嚏等疾病。

2. Traditional Chinese Medicine: The treatment primarily focuses on tonifying qi and promoting blood circulation to remove blood stasis, using the following prescription: 30g each of Astragalus membranaceus and Pueraria lobata, 15g of Salvia miltiorrhiza, 12g each of Ligusticum chuanxiong, Carthamus tinctorius, Allium macrostemon bulb, and Scutellaria baicalensis, and 6g of Glycyrrhiza uralensis. Decoct one dose daily in water and administer in divided doses in the morning and afternoon. The above integrated traditional Chinese and Western medicine regimen constitutes one course of treatment lasting 15 days, and up to two consecutive courses may be administered until hearing recovery is achieved. During treatment, patients should remain on bed rest with peace of mind, maintain regular bowel movements, follow a low-salt and light diet, and prevent conditions such as coughing and sneezing.

《中医药信息报》1997年9月12日（王书鸿）

Traditional Chinese Medicine Information News, September 12, 1997 (Wang Shuhong)

链霉素中毒所致耳聋，每伴有眩晕、头痛、恶心、耳鸣、步态不稳等，发病率高，颇难治疗，并有逐年增多的趋势。近年来，中药在防治本病中，有一定的疗效，某些中药不仅能克服毒副作用，防止过敏反应，又能保证继续用药。现辑验方五则供选用。

Deafness caused by streptomycin toxicity is often accompanied by vertigo, headache, nausea, tinnitus, and unsteady gait; it has a high incidence rate, is quite difficult to treat, and shows an increasing trend year by year. In recent years, traditional Chinese medicine has demonstrated certain efficacy in the prevention and treatment of this condition; some herbal medicines can not only counteract toxic side effects and prevent allergic reactions but also enable the continuation of streptomycin therapy. Five proven prescriptions are compiled below for selection and use.

3. 取黄精 10 克，水煎服，每日两次，同时辅助服用维生素 B1 和维生素 A。

3. Take 10g of Polygonatum sibiricum, decoct in water, and administer orally twice daily, supplemented concurrently with vitamin B1 and vitamin A.

4. 取骨碎补 15 克，水煎服，每日两次，本品能使有较严重的毒性反应和立即过敏反应者可以长期不间断地使用链霉素。

4. Take 15g of Davallia mariesii rhizome, decoct in water, and administer orally twice daily; this herb enables patients who have experienced severe toxic reactions or immediate allergic responses to continue long-term uninterrupted streptomycin therapy.

5. 取响铃草 30 克，水煎服，每日两次。本品具有补肾益气功效，民间常用以治疗耳鸣、耳聋、头晕目眩肾亏等病。

5. Take 30g of Crotalaria ferruginea, decoct in water, and administer orally twice daily. This herb has the effects of tonifying the kidneys and supplementing qi, and is commonly used in folk medicine to treat tinnitus, deafness, dizziness, vertigo, and kidney deficiency.

6. 取白僵蚕炙黄研粉，每次 3 克，开水冲服，每日两次，连服 1-2 月。

6. Take Bombyx batryticatus, stir-fry until yellowish, grind into powder, and take 3g per dose mixed with boiling water twice daily for 1–2 consecutive months.

7. 取黑豆 50 克，用水煮熟吃豆喝汤，或与大米共煮粥食用，每日 1 次。

7. Take 50g of black soybeans, boil in water until cooked, then eat the beans and drink the broth; alternatively, cook them together with rice into porridge for consumption once daily.

（江苏建湖县中医院 张宏俊 王道俊）

(Jianhu County Hospital of Traditional Chinese Medicine, Jiangsu Province;

Zhang Hongjun & Wang Daojun)

8. 治耳聋、耳鸣、头晕目眩：响铃草（假花生）35克，生品加倍，猪耳朵1对，炖服，可酌加适量精盐调味。每日1次，7日为一疗程。

8. For treating deafness, tinnitus, dizziness, and vertigo: Take 35g of Crotalaria ferruginea (commonly known as false peanut), doubling the amount if using fresh material, along with one pair of pig ears; stew together and consume, optionally seasoning with an appropriate amount of refined salt. Administer once daily, with seven days constituting one course of treatment.

9. 祖国医学对耳鸣的病因常有肾虚、痰火、风热之分。据临床观察，神经性耳鸣多系精神神经方面因素引起，一般属肾阴亏虚者居多。患者除应加强身体锻炼，保证睡眠，有意转移注意力外，还可用滋阴补肾的中药治疗。下面介绍一验方：生地、熟地、麦冬、元参各30克，川芎15克，香附15克，柴胡15克，菖蒲10克，水煎服，一日一剂。

9. Traditional Chinese medicine categorizes the etiology of tinnitus into kidney deficiency, phlegm-fire, and wind-heat types. Clinical observations indicate that neurogenic tinnitus is mostly caused by psychoneurological factors and generally falls under the pattern of kidney yin deficiency. In addition to strengthening physical exercise, ensuring adequate sleep, and deliberately diverting attention, patients may also be treated with traditional Chinese medicine that nourishes yin and tonifies the kidneys. A proven prescription is introduced below: 30g each of Rehmannia glutinosa (raw), Rehmannia glutinosa (prepared), Ophiopogon japonicus tuber, and Scrophularia ningpoensis root, 15g each of Ligusticum chuanxiong, Cyperus rotundus rhizome, and Bupleurum chinense root, and 10g of Acorus tatarinowii rhizome; decoct in water and administer orally, one dose daily.

《中医药信息报》1992年5月16日（戴廷荣）

Traditional Chinese Medicine Information News, May 16, 1992 (Dai Tingrong)

10. 肾虚耳鸣：一般症状有精神疲乏，头晕耳鸣，健忘，腰瘦遗精、阳痿或阴冷、带下。每日早晚各嚼食胡桃仁 5 枚，或常食胡桃粥。

10.Tinnitus due to Kidney Deficiency: Common symptoms include mental fatigue, dizziness with tinnitus, poor memory, soreness and weakness of the lower back, seminal emission, impotence or coldness in the genital region, and leukorrhea. Chew and consume five walnut kernels each morning and evening, or regularly eat walnut porridge.

11. 老年性耳鸣：双耳同时可发生蝉鸣样、金属样高音调鸣响，时轻时重，以睡眠困难时更为明显。多半由于神经紧张、疲劳，血压变化或脑血管与神经疾患等引起。每晚可嚼食胡桃仁 5 枚，持续服用一个月。日后也可常服。能减轻症状。

11.Senile Tinnitus: Both ears may simultaneously experience high-pitched ringing resembling cicada sounds or metallic tones, which fluctuate in intensity and become more pronounced during periods of sleep difficulty. It is mostly caused by nervous tension, fatigue, blood pressure fluctuations, or cerebrovascular and neurological disorders. Chew and consume five walnut kernels every night for one consecutive month; regular consumption thereafter is also recommended to help alleviate symptoms.

12. 气血不足耳鸣：多由于脏腑虚损、重病、久病损耗元气或慢性失血所致，一般面色发白，心悸短气，倦怠无力，头昏眼花，耳鸣。在早晚空腹时细细咀嚼、慢慢吞咽胡桃仁，每次 5 克左右。若效果尚不明显，可加黑芝麻 5 克左右，一同慢慢嚼咽。

12.Tinnitus due to Qi and Blood Deficiency: This condition is mostly caused by deficiency and impairment of the zang-fu organs, severe illness, depletion of vital qi from chronic disease, or chronic blood loss. Typical manifestations include a pale complexion, palpitations, shortness of breath, lassitude and weakness, dizziness, blurred vision, and tinnitus. On an empty stomach in the morning and evening, chew the walnut kernels thoroughly and swallow them slowly, taking about 5grams each time. If the effect is not yet apparent, add approximately 5grams of black sesame seeds and chew and swallow the mixture slowly together.

《中医药信息报》（湖南 彭平建）

Traditional Chinese Medicine Information News (Peng Pingjian, Hunan)

五、口腔溃疡（13 方）

V. Oral Ulcers (13 Prescriptions)

慢性复发性口腔溃疡是一种难治性口腔疾患。其病因病机多为禀赋不足，素体蕴热、外邪乘虚而入所致。对于这种顽固性口腔溃疡，目前还没有特效疗法。笔者根据辨证论治原则治疗 10 多例，取得较满意效果。

Chronic recurrent oral ulcer is a refractory oral disease. Its etiology and pathogenesis are mostly attributed to congenital insufficiency, inherent accumulation of heat in the body, and invasion of exogenous pathogenic factors taking advantage of the deficiency. There is currently no specific therapy for this stubborn type of oral ulcer. The author has treated more than 10 cases based on the principle of syndrome differentiation and treatment, achieving satisfactory results.

1. 气阴两虚型：谢某，男，48 岁，工人，1988 年 7 月 2 日就诊。自诉口腔溃疡反复发作 6 年之久，未能根治。证见：口腔颊侧可见米粒大小不等的圆形溃疡面，边界清晰，呈暗红色，无分泌物，触之略痛。伴症：口干唇燥，神疲乏力，颧红，气短，自汗，手足心热，苔少而薄，脉虚细。治与益气滋阴。方用生脉饮加味：太子参 20 克，麦冬、沙参、生地、黄精各 15 克，鳖甲、石斛各 12 克，五味子 6 克，地骨皮 24 克。每日一剂，水煎服。大便干结加肉苁蓉、麻仁各 15 克。患者服 24 剂痊愈。随访两年未复发。外用：清热解毒散：冰片 1g，黄连、马勃、青黛各 6g，共研末，涂布患处，日 3-4 次。

1.Qi and Yin Deficiency Type: Patient Xie, male, 48 years old, worker, visited on July 2, 1988. He reported that his oral ulcers had recurred repeatedly for six years without being radically cured. Clinical manifestations included round ulcer surfaces of varying sizes, from rice-grain-sized to larger, visible on the buccal mucosa, with clear boundaries and a dark red color, no secretion, and slight pain upon touch. Accompanying symptoms were dry mouth and lips, mental fatigue and weakness, malar flushing, shortness of breath, spontaneous sweating, heat in the palms and soles, a scanty and thin tongue coating, and a deficient and thready pulse. The treatment principle was to benefit Qi and nourish Yin. The modified Shengmai Yin prescription was used: Prince ginseng 20g, Ophiopogon root, Glehnia root, Rehmannia root, and Polygonatum rhizome 15g each, soft-shelled turtle shell and Dendrobium stem 12g each, Schisandra fruit 6g, and Lycium root bark 24g. One dose daily, decocted in water for oral administration. For dry constipation, add Cistanche deserticola and hemp seed 15g each. The patient recovered completely after taking 24 doses. No recurrence was observed during a two-year follow-up. External use: Heat-Clearing and Toxin-Resolving Powder: Borneol 1g, Coptis rhizome, Lasiosphaera, and Indigo naturalis 6g each, ground together into fine powder and applied to the affected area 3–4 times daily.

2. 湿热型：马某，女，27 岁，教师，1986 年 10 月 11 日就诊。患者半年前患口腔炎继发溃疡，经注射青霉素、口服维生素治愈。近一周来，溃疡复发，随即注射青霉素无效前来求治。刻诊：两侧颊黏膜各有溃疡 3、4 个，大如指甲，小如米粒，溃疡面糜烂充血水肿及黄色分泌物，触之剧痛。伴有口苦而黏，呕恶厌食，身体困重，便溏而臭，溲赤，舌红，苔黄腻，脉滑数。证属湿热，病在中焦，邪气上填。治与清热利湿解毒。方用甘露消毒丹加减：大青叶、射干、黄芩、藿香各 10 克，银花、车前草各 20 克，白花蛇舌草、连翘各 15 克，滑石 12 克（后下），焦栀子 9 克，薏苡仁 20 克，木通 6 克。每日一剂，水煎服。外用清热解毒散。患者 12 剂，痊愈。

2. Damp-Heat Type: Patient Ma, female, 27 years old, teacher, visited on October 11, 1986. Half a year prior, she developed stomatitis complicated by ulcers, which resolved after penicillin injection and oral vitamin supplementation. Over the past week, the ulcers recurred, and subsequent penicillin injection proved ineffective, prompting her to seek treatment. On examination, there were three to four ulcers on each buccal mucosa, ranging in size from a fingernail to a rice grain; the ulcer surfaces showed erosion, congestion, edema, and yellow

discharge, with severe pain upon touch. Associated symptoms included a bitter and sticky taste in the mouth, nausea and loss of appetite, heaviness of the body, loose and foul-smelling stools, dark urine, a red tongue with a yellow and greasy coating, and a slippery and rapid pulse. The syndrome was identified as damp-heat, with the pathology located in the middle jiao and pathogenic qi rising upward. The treatment principle was to clear heat, promote diuresis to remove dampness, and resolve toxins. A modified Ganlu Xiaodu Dan was prescribed: Isatis leaf, Belamcanda rhizome, Scutellaria root, and Agastache herb 10g each; Honeysuckle flower and Plantain herb 20g each; Hedyotis diffusa and Forsythia fruit 15g each; Talcum 12g (added near the end of decoction); charred Gardenia fruit 9g; Coix seed 20g; and Akebia stem 6g. One dose daily, decocted in water for oral administration. Externally, Heat-Clearing and Toxin-Resolving Powder was applied. The patient recovered completely after taking 12 doses.

3. 毒火燔炽型；孙某，男，28岁，农民，1989年4月29日就诊。患者口腔溃疡反复发作三年余，屡经治疗无显效。这次复发起因很突然，先寒后热，继之咽喉肿痛，烦躁不安，口干大渴，两目昏瞀，经静注青霉素两天后，略有好转，口腔溃疡随而发生，烧灼性疼痛，舌质红绛，干黑无苔，脉浮大而数。治与清气凉血，泻热解毒。方用清瘟败毒饮加减：生石膏60克（先煎），生地黄30克，黄连6克，栀子、桔梗、地龙各10克，知母、元参各12克，连翘20克，淡竹叶、大黄各6克，犀角粉2克（冲服）。每日一剂水煎服。外用清热解毒散。患者服9剂，痊愈。随访一年半未见复发。《中药科技报》1992年4月7日（刘启明）

3. Blazing Toxic Fire Type: Patient Sun, male, 28 years old, farmer, visited on April 29, 1989. The patient had suffered from recurrent oral ulcers for over three years without significant improvement despite repeated treatments. This relapse occurred suddenly, beginning with chills followed by fever, then sore throat, restlessness, severe dry mouth and thirst, and blurred vision. After two days of intravenous penicillin, there was slight improvement, but oral ulcers subsequently developed with burning pain; the tongue was deep red, dry, and black without

coating, and the pulse was floating, large, and rapid. The treatment principle was to clear Qi and cool blood, purge heat, and resolve toxins. A modified Qingwen Baidu Yin was prescribed: raw gypsum 60g (decocted first), raw rehmannia root 30g, coptis rhizome 6g, gardenia fruit, platycodon root, and earthworm 10g each, anemarrhena rhizome and scrophularia root 12g each, forsythia fruit 20g, lophatherum herb and rhubarb 6g each, and rhinoceros horn powder 2g (taken mixed with water). One dose daily, decocted in water for oral administration. Heat-Clearing and Toxin-Resolving Powder was applied externally. The patient recovered completely after taking 9 doses, with no recurrence during a one-and-a-half-year follow-up. Traditional Chinese Medicine Science and Technology News, April 7, 1992 (Liu Qiming)

4. 取生萝卜数个，鲜藕一斤，洗净捣烂绞汁含漱，每日几次，连用 4 天。

4. Take several raw radishes and 500g of fresh lotus root, wash them thoroughly, crush and squeeze out the juice, use it as a mouth rinse several times daily for four consecutive days.

5. 取淡竹叶 6 克，生地黄 15 克，木通 3 克，黄连 3 克，生甘草 6 克，水煎服，每日一剂，连服三天。

5. Take lophatherum herb 6g, raw rehmannia root 15g, akebia stem 3g, coptis rhizome 3g, and raw licorice root 6g; decoct in water and take one dose daily for three consecutive days.

6. 用锡类散、冰硼散撒于溃疡面，每日数次，2-3 日见效。

6. Sprinkle Xilei San or Bingpeng San onto the ulcer surface several times daily; effects are typically seen within 2–3 days.

7. 取甲氰咪胍数片研成细末，用棉签将药粉直接均匀的涂于口腔溃疡处，每日早晚饭后及睡前各涂一次，涂药后禁止饮水 10 分钟，一般 1-2 天溃疡面开始缩小，大部分在 3 天左右可愈。

7. Grind several cimetidine tablets into fine powder and apply it evenly directly onto the oral ulcer with a cotton swab once each after breakfast, dinner, and before bedtime; avoid drinking water for 10 minutes after application.

Generally, the ulcer begins to shrink within 1–2 days, and most cases heal in about 3 days.

8. 用消毒棉签蘸云南白药粉末，涂敷患处或吹入溃疡面，一般三天见效。

8. Dip a sterile cotton swab into Yunnan Baiyao powder and apply it to the affected area or blow the powder onto the ulcer surface; effects are usually seen within three days.

9. 取维生素 E 糖衣片数片，研成细末，涂敷溃疡面上，每日 4 次，3-4 天可愈。而后，每晚睡前含服维生素 E12 片，持续一个月，以防复发。

9. Grind several vitamin E sugar-coated tablets into fine powder and apply to the ulcer surface four times daily; healing typically occurs within 3–4 days. Afterwards, take 12 vitamin E tablets sublingually every night before sleep for one month to prevent recurrence.

10. 用消毒棉签蘸 4 万单位庆大霉素注射液轻涂溃疡面，一般 3 天见效。

10. Gently apply gentamicin injection (40,000 units) to the ulcer surface using a sterile cotton swab; effects are generally observed within three days.

11. 取维生素 B2 和维生素 C 各一片，研成粉末拌匀，置少许于棉球上，撒在溃疡面上，一般 3-4 次可见效。

11. Grind one tablet each of vitamin B2 and vitamin C into powder, mix well, place a small amount on a cotton ball, and sprinkle onto the ulcer surface; effects are usually seen after 3–4 applications.

12. 取细辛 5 克，黄连 3 克，共研细末，用陈醋调成糊状敷脐，每日换药一次，3-4 次可愈。

12. Grind asarum herb 5g and coptis rhizome 3g into fine powder, mix with aged vinegar to form a paste, and apply to the umbilicus; change the dressing once daily, and healing typically occurs after 3–4 applications.

13. 取女贞鲜嫩叶 3-4 片，凉开水洗净嚼烂含漱 5 分钟咽下，每日 3 次。

13. Wash 3–4 fresh tender privet leaves with cooled boiled water, chew them thoroughly, gargle for 5 minutes, then swallow; repeat three times daily.

14. 女贞鲜嫩叶适量捣烂取汁，用药棉花蘸汁敷于溃疡面上，10 分钟后吐出，

每日3次，连用3天即可痊愈。《民族医药报》1993年4月2日（北京 马宝山荐）

14. Crush an appropriate amount of fresh tender privet leaves to extract the juice, soak medicinal cotton in the juice and apply to the ulcer surface, spit out after 10 minutes; repeat three times daily for three consecutive days to achieve complete healing. Ethnic Medicine News, April 2, 1993 (Recommended by Ma Baoshan, Beijing)

六、口疮（22方）
VI. Oral Aphthae (22 Prescriptions)

1. 方药组成：干青果250克（用柴炭火烧炭存性），熊胆3克，煅硼砂12克，煅龙骨12克，孩儿茶10克，石脂10克，煅人中白12克，僵蚕10克，上等冰片3克，雄黄3克，青黛6克，黄连3克，薄荷叶1克。制法：上药研极细末和匀，以瓶装密闭收贮备用。功效：清热解毒，消肿止痛，敛疮生肌。适应证：口舌生疮，咽喉牙龈肿痛糜烂。用法：以消毒棉签或无菌布块蘸无菌凉水揩去患处痂膜，脓汁，以净为度。随用药末少许吹患处，每日3至5次，病愈为度，一般3至5天即可告愈。《中医药信息报》1992年8月1日（四川绵竹县医院 梁开发）

1.Prescription Composition: Dried Chinese olive 250g (charred over firewood charcoal to retain its medicinal properties), bear bile 3g, calcined borax 12g, calcined dragon bone 12g, catechu 10g, red halloysite 10g, calcined human urine sediment 12g, stiff silkworm 10g, premium borneol 3g, realgar 3g, indigo naturalis 6g, coptis rhizome 3g, and mint leaf 1g. Preparation Method: Grind all the above ingredients into an extremely fine powder, mix thoroughly, and store in a sealed bottle for future use. Efficacy: Clears heat and resolves toxins, reduces swelling and relieves pain, promotes ulcer healing and tissue regeneration. Indications: Aphthous ulcers on the mouth and tongue, sore throat, and swollen, painful, or eroded gums. Usage: Use a sterile cotton swab or gauze pad dipped in sterile cool water to gently wipe away scabs and pus from the affected area until clean. Then blow a small amount of the powder onto the lesion 3 to 5 times daily until recovery, which typically occurs within 3 to 5 days. Traditional Chinese Medicine Information News, August 1, 1992 (Liang Kaifa, Mianzhu County Hospital, Sichuan)

口疮，即口腔黏膜上的圆形或椭圆形溃烂，因其有反复发作的特点，又称复发性口疮。含漱法治口疮有方法简便、收效快等特点，故选验方数则介绍如下。

Oral aphthae refer to round or oval ulcerations on the oral mucosa; due to their recurrent nature, they are also known as recurrent aphthous stomatitis. Mouth rinsing therapy for oral aphthae is characterized by its simplicity and rapid efficacy, so several proven prescriptions are selected and introduced below.

2. 心火上炎：症见口疮数目较多，溃点小，多分布在舌尖、舌边缘，灼痛明显，色鲜红。药取蔷薇根（冬取根，夏取茎叶）煎浓汁含漱，每日 6-7 次；或取野菊花或金银花 15 克，黄连 5 克，煎水漱口，每日 5-6 次；亦可以黄连 3 克，甘草 9 克，水煎，频频含漱。

2. Upward Flaring of Heart Fire: Clinical manifestations include numerous small aphthous ulcers, mostly distributed on the tip and lateral edges of the tongue, with obvious burning pain and a bright red color. For treatment, decoct multiflower rose root (use the root in winter and stems/leaves in summer) into a concentrated liquid for mouth rinsing 6–7 times daily; alternatively, decoct wild chrysanthemum or honeysuckle flower 15g and coptis rhizome 5g in water for gargling 5–6 times daily; another option is to decoct coptis rhizome 3g and licorice root 9g in water for frequent mouth rinsing.

3. 脾胃热盛：症见口疮数目多，甚或融合成片，疮周红肿，溃点表面多黄白渗出物，全身伴有脾胃热盛表现。药取银花、薄荷各等分，煎水含漱，每日 5-6 次；亦可以硼砂、薄荷泡水漱口，每日数次。

3. Exuberant Spleen-Stomach Heat: Symptoms include numerous oral ulcers that may even coalesce into patches, with redness and swelling around the lesions and yellowish-white exudate on the ulcer surfaces, accompanied by systemic signs of spleen-stomach heat. Take equal amounts of honeysuckle flower and mint, decoct in water for mouth rinsing 5–6 times daily; alternatively, steep borax and

mint in hot water for gargling several times a day.

4. 阴虚火旺：症见口疮数目少，分散，大小不等，边缘清楚，表面有灰黄色膜覆盖，全身或见阴虚火旺表现。药取地黄液（成药）5-10 毫升，加入温开水中饮漱，每日 4-5 次；也可配以生地、麦冬、玄参各等分，水煎含漱，每日 5-6 次。

4. Yin Deficiency with Hyperactive Fire: Symptoms include few scattered oral ulcers of varying sizes with distinct margins, covered by a grayish-yellow membrane, possibly accompanied by systemic signs of yin deficiency and hyperactive fire. Take 5–10 ml of Rehmannia liquid (patent medicine), add to warm boiled water for drinking and gargling 4–5 times daily; alternatively, decoct equal amounts of raw rehmannia root, ophiopogon root, and scrophularia root in water for mouth rinsing 5–6 times daily.

5. 阳虚浮火：症见口疮数疮目较少，溃点大而深，表面灰白，日久不愈，全身或有阳虚表现。药取肉桂适量水煎含漱。《民族医药报》1992 年 3 月 13 日（江苏省南通市自强）

5. Yang Deficiency with Floating Fire: Symptoms include few oral ulcers that are large and deep with a grayish-white surface, persistent and slow to heal, possibly accompanied by systemic signs of yang deficiency. Decoct an appropriate amount of cinnamon bark in water for mouth rinsing. Ethnic Medicine News, March 13, 1992 (Ziqiang, Nantong City, Jiangsu Province)

6. 柿霜（从柿饼上取），用开水冲服或加入粥中服用。

6. Persimmon frost (collected from dried persimmons): brew with boiling water for oral administration or add to porridge for consumption.

7. 采鲜芭蕉叶适量，将其用火烤热贴敷于患处，每日 2-3 次。

7. Take an appropriate amount of fresh banana leaves, roast them over fire until warm, and apply as a compress to the affected area 2–3 times daily.

8. 将维生素 C 药片 1-2 片压碎，撒于溃疡面上，闭口片刻，每日 2 次。

8. Crush 1–2 vitamin C tablets and sprinkle the powder onto the ulcer surface, keep the mouth closed for a moment, twice daily.

9. 将甲氰咪胍 1-2 片研成细末状，用棉签蘸药粉涂于溃疡面上，10 分钟内不要饮水，每日 2 次。

9. Grind 1–2 cimetidine tablets into fine powder, dip a cotton swab into the powder and apply to the ulcer surface, avoid drinking water for 10 minutes after application, twice daily.

10. 取牛奶粉适量，每日 2-3 次冲服。

10. Take an appropriate amount of milk powder and brew with water for oral administration 2–3 times daily.

11. 取西红柿汁适量含在口内，每次 3-5 分钟，一日数次。

11. Hold an appropriate amount of tomato juice in the mouth for 3–5 minutes each time, several times a day.

12. 口服六味地黄丸，每日 2-3 次，每次 6-8 克。

12. Take Liuwei Dihuang Wan orally, 6–8grams per dose, 2–3 times daily.

13. 取旋复花（中药）适量、将其焙干研成细末，用香油调敷患处，治唇口生疮。

13. Take an appropriate amount of Inula flower (a traditional Chinese herb), roast it dry and grind into fine powder, mix with sesame oil to form a paste, and apply to the affected area to treat sores on the lips and mouth.

14. 治复发口疮：每晚临睡前取山茱萸 10 克，研末，加陈醋适量调成糊状，分别置于两块干净纱布（或软棉布）中央，敷贴于足底涌泉穴，次日清晨去掉，连用 7-10 日。《民族医药报》（江西 钟久春）

14. For recurrent oral aphthae: Before going to bed every night, take 10grams of Cornus fruit, grind it into powder, add an appropriate amount of aged vinegar to make a paste, place it in the center of two pieces of clean gauze (or soft cotton cloth) respectively, and apply to the Yongquan acupoints on the soles of the feet; remove the next morning, and use continuously for 7–10 days. Ethnic Medicine News (Zhong Jiuchun, Jiangxi)

口疮是临床上常见的一种疾病，易反复发作，西药治疗效果欠佳，用中药含漱治疗不仅可使药液直接作用于病变部位，提高治疗效果，还可达到清疮去秽，消肿止痛目的，且收效迅捷。现辑验方供选用。

Oral aphthae are a common clinical disease prone to recurrence, and Western medicine often yields suboptimal results. Gargling with traditional Chinese herbal decoctions not only allows the medicinal liquid to act directly on the lesion site to enhance therapeutic efficacy but also achieves the goals of cleansing ulcers, removing foulness, reducing swelling, and relieving pain, with rapid onset of action. Several proven prescriptions are compiled here for selection.

15. 取蔷薇根 60 克，煎浓汁含漱，每日 6-7 次，一般 2-3 日即痛止肿消，口疮基本愈合，用于心火上炎之口疮，症见口疮数目多，分布舌尖者。

15. Take 60grams of multiflower rose root, decoct into a concentrated liquid for gargling 6–7 times daily; generally, pain subsides and swelling diminishes within 2–3 days, and the ulcers basically heal. This is indicated for oral aphthae due to upward flaring of heart fire, characterized by numerous ulcers distributed mainly on the tip of the tongue.

16. 取黄连 3 克，甘草 9 克，水煎后取汁频频含漱。一般 2 日即效。亦用于心火上炎之口疮。

16. Decoct 3grams of coptis rhizome and 9grams of licorice root in water, and use the resulting liquid for frequent gargling. Effects are typically seen within 2 days. This is also indicated for oral aphthae caused by upward flaring of heart fire.

17. 取野菊花或银花 15 克，黄连 5 克，煎水漱口，每日 5-6 次，一般 2 日见效，5 天即愈。用于心火上炎之口舌生疮者。

17. Decoct 15grams of wild chrysanthemum or honeysuckle flower together with 5grams of coptis rhizome in water for gargling 5–6 times daily; effects usually appear within 2 days, and complete healing occurs within 5 days. This is indicated for sores on the mouth and tongue due to upward flaring of heart fire.

18. 取银花、薄荷各 10 克，煎水后含漱，每日 5-6 次，一般 2-3 日即愈。用于脾胃积热之口疮，症见口疮数目多，甚则融合成片，疮面多黄白渗出物者。

18. Decoct 10grams each of honeysuckle flower and mint in water for gargling 5–6 times daily; recovery generally occurs within 2–3 days. This is

indicated for oral aphthae due to accumulated heat in the spleen and stomach, presenting with numerous ulcers that may even coalesce into patches and ulcer surfaces covered with yellowish-white exudate.

19. 取硼砂 2 克，薄荷 5 克，二者用沸水冲泡后漱口，每日数次。一般 2-3 日即效。亦用于脾胃积热之口疮。

19. Steep 2grams of borax and 5grams of mint in boiling water for gargling several times daily; effects are generally seen within 2–3 days. This is also indicated for oral aphthae due to accumulated heat in the spleen and stomach.

20. 杞菊地黄口服液 5-10ml，加入温开水中饮漱，每日 4-5 次，一般 3 日即效。用于阴虚火旺之口疮，症见口疮散目少，分散，边缘不清，表面有灰黄色膜覆盖者。

20. Add 5–10 ml of Qiju Dihuang Oral Liquid to warm boiled water for drinking and gargling 4–5 times daily; effects typically appear within 3 days. This is indicated for oral aphthae due to yin deficiency with hyperactive fire, presenting with few scattered ulcers, indistinct margins, and surfaces covered by a grayish-yellow membrane.

21. 取生地、麦冬、玄参各等份，煎水含漱，每日 5-6 次，一般 2-3 日即效。亦用于阴虚火旺之口疮。

21. Decoct equal amounts of raw rehmannia root, ophiopogon root, and scrophularia root in water for gargling 5–6 times daily; effects are generally observed within 2–3 days. This is also indicated for oral aphthae caused by yin deficiency with hyperactive fire.

22. 取肉桂 10 克，煎水后含漱，每日 5-6 次，一般 3 日即效。用于阳虚浮火之口疮，症见口疮数目少，溃点大而深，表面灰白，日久不愈者。《中药科技报》1992 年 4 月 7 日（张宏俊 王道俊）

22. Decoct 10grams of cinnamon bark in water for gargling 5–6 times daily; effects usually occur within 3 days. This is indicated for oral aphthae due to yang deficiency with floating fire, characterized by few ulcers that are large and deep with grayish-white surfaces and prolonged failure to heal. Traditional Chinese Medicine Science and Technology News, April 7, 1992 (Zhang Hongjun, Wang Daojun)

七、慢性咽炎（9 方）
VII. Chronic Pharyngitis (9 Prescriptions)

1. 慢性咽炎是临床上的常见疾患。该病症状迁延不愈，反复发作，临床表现为咽部微痛，发胀、发痒，有异物阻塞感、灼热感，或咽部干燥不适，吞咽不利，讲话不能持久，本院采用中药含咽法治疗，收到良好的疗效。治疗方法：取法半夏、桔梗、生甘草各 30 克，共研成细末状，放于白酒 1000 毫升内浸泡 1 日，然后兑入鸡蛋清 4 个搅匀。每日含服 3 次，每次 20-30 毫升，缓慢咽下（在口腔中含的时间越长越好），10 日为 1 疗程，间隔 3 日开始含服第 2 疗程药酒。《民族医药报》1993 年 1 月 29 日（南京市上新河医院 孙哲）

1.Chronic pharyngitis is a common clinical disorder characterized by persistent and recurrent symptoms, including mild throat pain, distension, itching, sensation of a foreign body or burning, dryness and discomfort in the throat, difficulty swallowing, and inability to speak for prolonged periods. Our hospital has achieved good therapeutic efficacy using a traditional Chinese medicine gargling-and-swallowing method. Treatment method: Take 30grams each of processed pinellia tuber, platycodon root, and raw licorice root, grind them into fine powder, soak in 1000 ml of liquor for one day, then mix in four egg whites and stir well. Gargle and slowly swallow 20–30 ml three times daily (the longer the liquid is retained in the mouth, the better); one course lasts 10 days, with a 3-day interval before starting the second course of medicated wine. Ethnic Medicine News, January 29, 1993 (Sun Zhe, Shangxinhe Hospital, Nanjing)

2. 百合 80 克、生地 50 克、大米 50 克，将生地捣碎加水煮汁，去渣，加大米、百合煮为稀粥服食。能养阴益肾、清热利咽。适用于慢性咽喉炎，肺肾阴亏、咽喉疼痛、干咳少痰、声音嘶哑者。

2. Take 80g of lily bulb, 50g of raw rehmannia root, and 50g of rice; crush the raw rehmannia root, decoct it in water to extract the juice, remove the residue, then add the rice and lily bulb to cook into a thin porridge for consumption. This

recipe nourishes yin, tonifies the kidney, clears heat, and benefits the throat, and is suitable for chronic pharyngitis with lung-kidney yin deficiency presenting with sore throat, dry cough with scanty sputum, and hoarseness.

3. 玉竹 20 克、沙参 20 克、麦冬 20 克、大米 50 克、冰糖适量，将玉竹、沙参、麦冬煎水取汁，加大米煮成稀粥，加冰糖食用，有养阴润肺、化痰止咳之功，适用于肺胃阴伤之慢性咽喉炎伴干咳少痰、咽干不适、津少口干者。

3. Take 20g each of fragrant solomonseal rhizome, glehnia root, and ophiopogon root, 50g of rice, and an appropriate amount of rock sugar; decoct the three herbs in water to obtain the juice, add the rice to cook into a thin porridge, then add rock sugar for consumption. This recipe nourishes yin, moistens the lungs, resolves phlegm, and relieves cough, and is indicated for chronic pharyngitis due to lung-stomach yin injury accompanied by dry cough with scanty sputum, throat dryness and discomfort, and dry mouth due to insufficient body fluids.

4. 天冬 30 克、麦冬 30 克、大米 50 克、蜂蜜 1 匙，将天冬、麦冬水煎取汁煮粥，待熟调入蜂蜜食用。可清热利咽、养阴润肺，适用于急性咽喉炎，后期热病伤阴及慢性咽喉炎。

4. Take 30g each of asparagus root and ophiopogon root, 50g of rice, and one spoonful of honey; decoct the two herbs in water to obtain the juice, use it to cook porridge, and stir in honey when cooked for consumption. This recipe clears heat, benefits the throat, nourishes yin, and moistens the lungs, and is suitable for acute pharyngitis, yin injury in the late stage of febrile diseases, and chronic pharyngitis.

5. 鲜藕 30 克、绿豆 30 克、大米 50 克、白糖适量，先煮绿豆至沸，加入大米煮半熟调入藕片。待熟时加入白糖稍煮一下即可。此粥甘滑可口、能清热凉血、利咽除烦、生津止渴，凡急性咽喉炎及炎症后热退伤阴者均可服食。《民族医药报》1993 年 2 月 26 日（艳 荐）

5. Take 30g of fresh lotus root, 30g of mung bean, 50g of rice, and an appropriate amount of white sugar; first boil the mung beans until the water

comes to a boil, add the rice and cook until half done, then add sliced lotus root; when fully cooked, add white sugar and simmer briefly. This sweet and smooth porridge clears heat, cools blood, benefits the throat, relieves irritability, generates body fluids, and quenches thirst, and is suitable for all cases of acute pharyngitis and yin injury after fever subsides from inflammation. Ethnic Medicine News, February 26, 1993 (Recommended by Yan)

6. 咽异感症中医称之为“梅核气”，其临床表现为，患者咽部不适，如有异物，咳之不出、咽之不下、胸肋胀满，但进食无妨。我院拟用中药“三花汤”治疗，收到较好疗效。药物组成及服用法：玫瑰花、白梅花、佛手花各 6 克，金桔叶、茯神各 10 克，桔络 3 克，每日一剂，水煎分两次服。《民族医药报》1992 年 8 月 7 日（云南 罗龙）

6. Globus pharyngeus is called “Plum Pit Qi” in traditional Chinese medicine, clinically presenting as throat discomfort with a sensation of a foreign body that can neither be coughed up nor swallowed down, accompanied by chest and hypochondriac fullness, but without affecting eating. Our hospital has formulated the traditional Chinese herbal “Sanhua Decoction” for treatment, achieving good efficacy. Composition and administration: Rose flower, white plum flower, and bergamot flower 6g each; kumquat leaf and poria with hostwood 10g each; tangerine pith 3g. One dose daily, decocted in water and taken in two divided doses. Ethnic Medicine News, August 7, 1992 (Luo Long, Yunnan)

7. 慢性咽喉炎音哑：薄荷、甘草、桔梗、乌梅、玄参、胆星、僵蚕各 20 克，研末，加冰片、硼砂各 10 克，再研细，每次取 3 克口含服，每日 4 次，连服 7-10 天。

7. For hoarseness due to chronic pharyngolaryngitis: Grind 20g each of mint, licorice root, platycodon root, smoked plum, scrophularia root, bile arisaema, and stiff silkworm into powder, add 10g each of borneol and borax, and grind again into fine powder; take 3g orally for slow dissolution in the mouth four times daily for 7–10 consecutive days.

8. 声带小结息肉肿痛音哑：沙参、百合、白芍、牛蒡子、花粉各 12 克，桔梗、

射干、诃子、凤凰衣、甘草各6克，胖大海3枚，水煎服，日1剂，30日为1疗程。《民族医药报》（吴振翔）

8. For vocal cord nodules/polyps with swelling, pain, and hoarseness: Glehnia root, lily bulb, white peony root, burdock fruit, and trichosanthes root 12g each; platycodon root, belamcanda rhizome, chebula fruit, eggshell membrane, and licorice root 6g each; sterculia seed 3 pieces. Decoct in water for oral administration, one dose daily, with 30 days constituting one course of treatment. Ethnic Medicine News (Wu Zhenxiang)

9. 单方治疗化脓性扁桃体炎：急性化脓性扁桃体炎是常见的五官科疾病。以发热、咽痛、扁桃体肿大及脓性分泌物为其临床特点。以单味大黄治疗本病有特效，笔者在临床中治疗6例，均在4天内治愈。具体方法是：将生大黄15克（小儿酌减），用开水约250毫升冲泡待温后慢慢咽下，以后每隔2小时冲泡1次，每天4次，每日1剂，停用其他药物。此法简单、疗效好，患者不妨一试。《民族医药报》1993年1月15日（广东 康忠长）

9. Single-Herb Remedy for Suppurative Tonsillitis: Acute suppurative tonsillitis is a common otorhinolaryngological disease characterized clinically by fever, sore throat, tonsillar enlargement, and purulent secretions. Using rhubarb alone has shown remarkable efficacy for this condition; the author treated 6 clinical cases, all of which were cured within 4 days. The specific method is as follows: Steep 15g of raw rhubarb (reduce the dose appropriately for children) in approximately 250 ml of boiling water, allow it to cool to a warm temperature, and then swallow slowly; thereafter, steep a fresh dose every 2 hours, 4 times daily, using one dose per day, while discontinuing all other medications. This method is simple and highly effective, and patients may wish to give it a try. Ethnic Medicine News, January 15, 1993 (Kang Zhongchang, Guangdong)

八、牙痛（24 方）
VIII. Toothache (24 Prescriptions)

1. 龟板地骨皮汤治疗虚火牙痛：笔者多年来用自拟“龟板地骨皮汤”治疗虚火牙痛，效果较为满意，一般服 2-3 剂即可减轻或消除疼痛，现简介如下，供参考。方药组成：龟板 30 克、地骨皮 20 克、骨碎补 20 克、黄柏 10 克、露蜂房 10 克，水煎服，每日一剂，服 3 次。适应症：牙齿隐隐作痛，牙龈微红略肿，咬物时痛增，有松动感，伴有头晕耳鸣。腰酸盗汗，口渴不欲饮水，舌红苔薄，脉沉细者。对身体素虚，久病失于调养，年老体弱等导致肾阴不足，虚火上炎所引起的牙痛尤为有效。功效：滋肾益阴，降火止痛。《民族医药报》1992 年 8 月 7 日（云南 李宇俊）

1.Guiban Digupi Decoction for Toothache due to Deficiency Fire: The author has used the self-formulated “Guiban Digupi Decoction” for many years to treat toothache caused by deficiency fire with satisfactory results; generally, pain can be alleviated or eliminated after taking 2–3 doses. A brief introduction is provided below for reference. Prescription Composition: Tortoise plastron 30g, lycium root bark 20g, drynaria rhizome 20g, phellodendron bark 10g, and honeycomb 10g; decoct in water for oral administration, one dose daily taken in three divided doses. Indications: Dull, lingering toothache with slightly red and swollen gums, pain aggravated by chewing, looseness of teeth, accompanied by dizziness, tinnitus, soreness of the lower back, night sweats, thirst without desire to drink, a red tongue with thin coating, and a deep and thready pulse. It is particularly effective for toothache caused by kidney yin deficiency and upward flaring of deficiency fire resulting from constitutional weakness, lack of proper care during prolonged illness, or old age and debility. Efficacy: Nourishes the kidney and tonifies yin, reduces fire and relieves pain. Ethnic Medicine News, August 7, 1992 (Li Yujun, Yunnan)

2. 治虚火牙痛：熟附子、肉桂各 3 克，生地 20 克、牛漆 3 克。水煎服。若兼表证者去肉桂加桂枝 5 克，荆芥、防风各 9 克。

2. For Toothache due to Deficiency Fire: Prepared aconite root and cinnamon bark 3g each, raw rehmannia root 20g, and achyranthes root 3g; decoct in water for oral administration. If accompanied by exterior syndrome, omit cinnamon bark and add cassia twig 5g, schizonepeta herb and fangfeng root 9g each.

3. 小山茶 6 克，挖耳草 6 克。水煎服，1 日 1 剂，分 3 次服。适用于虚火牙痛。

3. Small camellia 6g and bidens herb 6g; decoct in water for oral administration, one dose daily taken in three divided doses. Suitable for toothache due to deficiency fire.

4. 秧草根 50 克，车前草 50 克，生石膏 20 克。水煎服，1 日 1 剂，分 3 次服。药用鲜品，干品减量（各 20 克）。适用于阳明实热证牙痛。

4. Rice seedling root 50g, plantain herb 50g, and raw gypsum 20g; decoct in water for oral administration, one dose daily taken in three divided doses. Use fresh herbs; if using dried herbs, reduce the dosage to 20g each. Suitable for toothache due to excess heat in the Yangming channel.

5. 杨梅根 50 克。水煎 20 分钟后过滤，加蜂蜜 20 克、鸡蛋 1 只，再煎煮 5 分钟，待温内服。1 日 2 剂，6 日为 1 疗程。适用于龋齿牙痛。

5. Wax myrtle root 50g; decoct in water for 20 minutes, strain, add 20g of honey and one egg, then simmer for another 5 minutes, allow to cool to warm temperature, and take orally. Two doses daily, with 6 days constituting one course of treatment. Suitable for toothache caused by dental caries.

6. 水杨梅 15 克，牙齿草 15 克。水煎服，1 日 1 剂，分 3 次服。适用于风火牙痛。

6. Chinese buttonbush fruit 15g and tooth grass 15g; decoct in water for oral administration, one dose daily taken in three divided doses. Suitable for toothache due to wind-fire.

7. 锣锅底（曲莲、金刁）1.5 克。1.0 克用温开水送吞服，0.5 克含于患处。1 日 3 次，6 次为 1 疗程。忌酸冷豆类，勿空腹服药。心衰、低温、虚寒病人禁用。适用于风火牙痛、阳明实热。亦可用于口腔炎、舌炎、扁桃体炎、咽喉炎、肠炎、痢疾、胃痛等证（属实热火邪所致者）。《民族医药报》1992 年 5 月 29 日（云南 马应乖）

7. Luoguodi (Hemsleya chinensis): 1.5g per dose. Swallow 1.0g with warm boiled water and hold 0.5g at the affected site. Take three times daily, with six doses constituting one course of treatment. Avoid sour, cold foods and beans; do not take on an empty stomach. Contraindicated in patients with heart failure, hypothermia, or deficiency-cold patterns. Indicated for toothache due to wind-fire and excess heat in the Yangming channel. It can also be used for stomatitis, glossitis, tonsillitis, pharyngitis, enteritis, dysentery, and stomach pain caused by excess heat and fire pathogens. Ethnic Medicine News, May 29, 1992 (Ma Yingguai, Yunnan)

8. 治疗牙痛：取白杨树皮〈去外皮〉一小片置于牙痛处，可止痛。《民族医药报》1992 年 5 月 22 日（云南 炳）

8. For Toothache: Place a small piece of white poplar bark (with the outer bark removed) directly on the painful area to relieve pain. Ethnic Medicine News, May 22, 1992 (Bing, Yunnan)

9. 反复牙痛，牙龋红肿疼痛：取露蜂房 20 克，煎浓汁含漱口，几次即愈。

9. For Recurrent Toothache with Red, Swollen, and Painful Carious Teeth: Decoct 20g of honeycomb into a concentrated liquid for gargling; recovery typically occurs after several applications.

10. 虫牙痛：取五倍子 15 克，煎浓汁含漱口两天痛即愈。

10. For Toothache due to Dental Caries: Decoct 15g of Chinese gallnut into a concentrated liquid for gargling; pain usually resolves within two days.

11. 龋齿疼痛：先用牙签将龋齿内的内容物淘尽，然后用牙签挑入鲜松叶烧成的灰将龋齿填满，用几次即止痛。

11. For Pain from Dental Caries: First use a toothpick to thoroughly clean out debris from the carious cavity, then fill it with ash made from burnt fresh pine needles using a toothpick; pain relief is typically achieved after several applications.

12. 各种牙痛：取樟脑丸 1 粒研末，取粉少许，撒于伤湿止痛膏上，贴在痛牙一侧的腮部，注意樟脑粉尽量对准痛牙处，约五分钟即效；

12. For Various Types of Toothache: Grind one camphor ball into powder, sprinkle a small amount onto a Shangshi Zhitong plaster, and apply it to the cheek on the side of the painful tooth, ensuring the camphor powder is positioned as close as possible to the affected tooth; effects are usually felt within about five minutes.

13. 各种牙痛：取切成黄豆大小的西洋参放在痛牙上，上下牙齿咬紧，约10分钟牙痛即止。

13. For Various Types of Toothache: Place a piece of American ginseng cut to the size of a soybean on the painful tooth, clench the upper and lower teeth tightly, and the toothache generally stops within about 10 minutes.

14. 各种牙痛：取新鲜的松叶10片，放在嘴里咀嚼，约10分钟牙痛即止。《中药科技报》1992年2月26日（张宏俊 王道俊）

14. For Various Types of Toothache: Chew 10 fresh pine needles in the mouth; the toothache typically subsides within about 10 minutes. Traditional Chinese Medicine Science and Technology News, February 26, 1992 (Zhang Hongjun, Wang Daojun)

牙痛为多种牙齿疾病的常见症状之一。笔者运用中医辨证施治的理论，精选药物，自拟成药，治疗各型牙痛服一至三剂见效，五剂痊愈现介绍于下。

Toothache is one of the common symptoms of various dental diseases. Based on the theory of syndrome differentiation and treatment in traditional Chinese medicine, the author has carefully selected herbs and formulated proprietary prescriptions. These remedies are effective for all types of toothache, typically showing results after 1 to 3 doses and achieving complete recovery within 5 doses. The details are presented below.

15. 组成：生地30克、石膏30克、银花30克、大黄10克（后下）。用法：水煎服，每日一剂，连服三至五剂。小儿减量。（冷服）。功效：清热解毒，消肿止痛。主治：实热牙痛。症见牙龈肿痛，进食困难，发热口渴，舌红苔脉数。

15. Composition: Raw rehmannia root 30g, gypsum 30g, honeysuckle flower 30g, and rhubarb 10g (added near the end of decoction). Usage: Decoct in water

for oral administration, one dose daily for 3 to 5 consecutive doses; reduce the dosage for children, and take the decoction cold. Efficacy: Clears heat and resolves toxins, reduces swelling and relieves pain. Indications: Toothache due to excess heat, presenting with swollen and painful gums, difficulty eating, fever, thirst, a red tongue, and a rapid pulse.

16. 组成：生地 30 克、黄芩 15 克、僵蚕 10 克，白蒺藜 10 克。用法：水煎服，每日一剂，连服三至五剂。功效：泻火熄风，止痉定痛。主治：风火牙痛。症见牙痛肿势不显，呈掣痛，牵引患则头目作痛，舌红苔薄黄，脉弦数。

16. Composition: Raw rehmannia root 30g, scutellaria root 15g, stiff silkworm 10g, and white tribulus fruit 10g. Usage: Decoct in water for oral administration, one dose daily for 3 to 5 consecutive doses. Efficacy: Purges fire and extinguishes wind, stops spasms and alleviates pain. Indications: Wind-fire toothache, presenting with toothache without obvious swelling, drawing or pulling pain that radiates to the head and eyes, a red tongue with a thin yellow coating, and a wiry and rapid pulse.

17. 组成：防风 20 克、白芷 15 克、细辛 3 克，荜茇 10 克。用法：水煎服，每日一剂，连服三剂。功效：疏风散寒，通络止痛。主治：风寒牙痛。症见牙痛不肿，遇寒痛甚，伴有恶寒发热，头身不适，舌苔薄白，脉弦紧。

17. Composition: Fangfeng root 20g, angelica dahurica root 15g, asarum herb 3g, and long pepper 10g. Usage: Decoct in water for oral administration, one dose daily for 3 consecutive doses. Efficacy: Dispels wind and scatters cold, unblocks collaterals and relieves pain. Indications: Wind-cold toothache, presenting with toothache without swelling, pain aggravated by cold exposure, accompanied by aversion to cold, fever, general malaise, a thin white tongue coating, and a wiry and tight pulse.

18. 组成：骨碎补 30 克、枸杞子 30 克、怀牛膝 10 克、地骨皮 10 克。用法：水煎服，每日一剂，连服五剂。功效：补肾固齿，退虚火。主治：肾虚牙痛，症见牙痛反复发作，痛势不重，呈空痛，伴有牙齿松动，舌淡，苔白脉细无力。（蒋玉翠）

18. Composition: Drynaria rhizome 30g, goji berry 30g, huai achyranthes root 10g, and lycium root bark 10g. Usage: Decoct in water for oral administration, one dose daily for 5 consecutive doses. Efficacy: Tonifies the kidney and secures teeth, reduces deficiency fire. Indications: Toothache due to kidney deficiency, presenting with recurrent mild toothache characterized by a hollow, empty sensation, accompanied by loose teeth, a pale tongue with a white coating, and a thready and weak pulse. (Jiang Yucui)

19. 治风火牙痛方：金银花 12 克、连翘 9 克、菊花 9 克、甘草 3 克、露蜂房 15 克，水煎服。治风火牙痛有良效。《中医药信息报》

19. Prescription for Wind-Fire Toothache: Honeysuckle flower 12g, forsythia fruit 9g, chrysanthemum flower 9g, licorice root 3g, and honeycomb 15g; decoct in water for oral administration. This formula is highly effective for treating wind-fire toothache. Traditional Chinese Medicine Information News

20. 用鲜杉树皮（山杉皮、水杉皮均可）若干，放水适量，煮成老红色，适量含于口中，少时吐出，再含再吐，切勿咽下，反复若干次，即可达到消肿、止痛功效。不管风、火、龋牙疼痛，采用此法均能生效。《民族医药报》1992 年 2 月 21 日（浙江 何校善）

20. Take an appropriate amount of fresh fir bark (either mountain fir or metasequoia bark is acceptable), add a suitable quantity of water, and decoct until the liquid turns a deep reddish-brown color. Hold a moderate amount of the warm liquid in the mouth for a short while, then spit it out; repeat this process of holding and spitting several times without swallowing to achieve the effects of reducing swelling and relieving pain. This method is effective regardless of whether the toothache is caused by wind, fire, or dental caries. Ethnic Medicine News, February 21, 1992 (He Xiaoshan, Zhejiang)

21. 治牙周炎：取中药银花、黄芩、白芷、川芎各 10 克，生石膏 20 克（先煎）、黄连 3 克、细辛 2 克，生甘草 6 克。日 1 剂水煎服，至痊愈。《中药科技报》1993 年 3 月 11 日（南京孙扬）

21. For Periodontitis: Take honeysuckle flower, scutellaria root, angelica

dahurica root, and chuanxiong rhizome 10g each; raw gypsum 20g (decocted first); coptis rhizome 3g; asarum herb 2g; and raw licorice root 6g. Decoct in water for oral administration, one dose daily until complete recovery. Traditional Chinese Medicine Science and Technology News, March 11, 1993 (Sun Yang, Nanjing)

22. 单纯牙龈炎而致出血，可给予清热凉血止血的中药如：生地 20 克，丹皮 15 克，黄芩 10 克，元参 10 克，芍药 20 克，石膏 20 克，双花 30 克，连翘 10 克，茅根 30 克，甘草 6 克，水煎服，三七粉 1 克冲服，有一定疗效。《中药科技报》1993 年 1 月 14 日（山东省 曹元成）

22. For bleeding caused by simple gingivitis, traditional Chinese herbs that clear heat, cool blood, and stop bleeding can be administered: raw rehmannia root 20g, moutan bark 15g, scutellaria root 10g, scrophularia root 10g, peony root 20g, gypsum 20g, honeysuckle flower 30g, forsythia fruit 10g, cogongrass rhizome 30g, and licorice root 6g, decocted in water for oral administration; additionally, take 1g of notoginseng powder mixed with water. This regimen has shown certain therapeutic efficacy. Traditional Chinese Medicine Science and Technology News, January 14, 1993 (Cao Yuancheng, Shandong Province)

23. 使用葵花籽油治疗牙本质过敏症，较传统的脱敏药物取材方便，具有安全简易、牙齿不变色、气味清香等特点。并可解决多发性病例，如全口性过敏，即使全口牙都涂上葵花籽油，对口腔黏膜无腐蚀刺激等副作用。尤其对重型牙本质过敏，疗效更好。此外，在某种程度上还能预防牙本质过敏症的发生，更重要的是能避免任何药物带来的副作用。《民族医药报》1992 年 9 月 4 日（广西桂林 张菊生）

23. Using sunflower oil to treat dentin hypersensitivity offers advantages over traditional desensitizing agents, including easy accessibility, safety, simplicity, no tooth discoloration, and a pleasant fragrance. It is also effective for multiple cases, such as generalized hypersensitivity; even when applied to all teeth in the mouth, it causes no corrosive or irritating side effects on the oral mucosa. It is particularly more effective for severe dentin hypersensitivity. Moreover, it can to some extent

prevent the occurrence of dentin hypersensitivity, and more importantly, avoids any side effects associated with pharmaceutical drugs. Ethnic Medicine News, September 4, 1992 (Zhang Jusheng, Guilin, Guangxi)

24. 家传有效护齿法：我的曾祖母 105 岁时还能吃花生、嚼排骨，满口牙齿完好无缺。有人问用何护齿妙法，老人家总是笑而不答。那时，我还小，和小伙伴们把开尿仗当成趣事，说笑打闹之间，一个个乐不可支地亮出“自动水枪”互相追逐。朝人“扫射”。老太太见状，急忙制止：“屙尿讲话对牙齿有害无益，咬紧牙关，尿完再讲话。”我牢记曾祖母的话，数十年如一日，坚持每次小便时憋气息声、咬牙切齿，意想不到牙齿同样整齐无龋。待有了孩子后，在保证其口腔卫生的前提下，我如法施行此家传护齿法，果然孩子满口好牙。此法是否有科学依据，我并未考究。根据经验，笔者认为这是自我护齿的有效方法。若有兴趣，不妨一试。《民族医药报》1992 年 8 月 7 日（广西 黄汉昌）

24. An Effective Family-Inherited Tooth Protection Method: My great-grandmother could still eat peanuts and chew pork ribs at the age of 105, with a full set of intact teeth. When asked about her secret to dental care, she would always smile without answering. At that time, I was young, and my friends and I thought it was fun to have “urine battles,” laughing and playing as we gleefully pulled out our “automatic water guns” to chase and “spray” each other. Seeing this, the old lady quickly stopped us: “Talking while urinating is harmful to your teeth and offers no benefit. Clench your teeth tightly, and only speak after you finish.” I kept my great-grandmother’s words firmly in mind and, for decades without fail, held my breath and clenched my teeth every time I urinated. Unexpectedly, my teeth remained just as neat and cavity-free. After having children of my own, I applied this family-inherited tooth protection method while ensuring their oral hygiene, and indeed, they also developed a full set of healthy teeth. I have not investigated whether this method has a scientific basis. Based on personal experience, however, I believe it is an effective self-care technique for dental health. If interested, you may wish to give it a try. Ethnic Medicine News, August 7, 1992 (Huang Hanchang, Guangxi)

九、颈淋巴结核（2 个）
IX. Cervical Lymph Node Tuberculosis (2 Prescriptions)

1. 颈淋巴结结核，中医谓之“痰核”，“瘰疬”，好发于小儿及女性。家祖俞济生老中医在临床中总结出一方，经多年临床应用，疗效确佳。现介绍如下。处方：猫爪草 30 克，盘肠草 60 克（即南瓜种子在果实内萌发的幼苗），夏枯草、玄参、牡蛎各 25 克，桔梗、苏梗、郁金、香附各 9 克，麦冬、生地、丹参、丹皮各 15 克。制法：上药共研为细末，炼蜜为丸、如梧子大。用法：3-6 岁每日服 9-18 克；7-9 岁每日服 27-36 克；10-15 岁每日服 45-60 克，均分 3 次。淡黄酒送服，1 个月为 1 疗程。按：济生消瘰散疬丸系家祖所创。方中猫爪草、盘肠草、夏枯草、牡蛎清热散结，软坚消肿，现代药理研究表明猫爪草、夏枯草有明显的抗痨作用；盘肠草现代药理虽未见研究，但据家祖传训有“杀痨虫”作用，故均为本方主药。玄参、丹参、丹皮活血化瘀；苏梗、郁金、香附理气解郁；麦冬、生地养阴；桔梗引药入肺经。诸药合用，共奏清热育阴，软坚散结、理气解郁，活血化瘀，抗痨杀虫之功，故有良效。《民族医药报》1992 年 5 月 29 日（江西省）

1.Cervical lymph node tuberculosis, referred to as “phlegm nodule” or “scrofula” in traditional Chinese medicine, commonly occurs in children and women. My ancestor, the veteran TCM practitioner Yu Jisheng, formulated a prescription based on clinical experience, which has proven highly effective over many years of application. The details are as follows. Prescription: Ranunculus ternatus 30g, pumpkin sprouts (seedlings germinated from pumpkin seeds inside the fruit) 60g, Prunella spike, Scrophularia root, and Oyster shell 25g each; Platycodon root, Perilla stem, Curcuma tuber, and Cyperus rhizome 9g each; Ophiopogon root, Raw Rehmannia root, Salvia miltiorrhiza root, and Moutan bark 15g each. Preparation: Grind all ingredients into fine powder, mix with refined honey to form pills the size of parasol tree seeds. Administration: Children aged 3–6 take 9–18g daily; aged 7–9 take 27–36g daily; aged 10–15 take 45–60g daily, divided into three doses. Take with mild yellow wine; one month constitutes one course of treatment. Note: The Jisheng Scrofula-Dissolving Pill was created by my ancestor. In this formula, Ranunculus ternatus, pumpkin sprouts, Prunella spike, and Oyster shell clear heat, dissipate nodules, soften hardness, and reduce swelling. Modern pharmacological studies show that Ranunculus ternatus and Prunella spike have significant anti-tubercular effects; although no modern research exists for pumpkin sprouts, ancestral teachings attribute to them the function of "killing tubercular pathogens," making them key herbs in this formula. Scrophularia root, Salvia miltiorrhiza root, and Moutan bark promote blood circulation and remove stasis; Perilla stem, Curcuma tuber, and Cyperus rhizome regulate Qi and relieve depression; Ophiopogon root and Raw Rehmannia root nourish Yin; Platycodon root guides the medicinal effects to the Lung channel. Combined, these herbs work synergistically to clear heat, nourish Yin, soften hardness, dissipate nodules, regulate Qi, relieve depression, promote blood circulation, remove stasis, combat tuberculosis, and eliminate pathogens, thus yielding excellent therapeutic results. Ethnic Medicine News, May 29, 1992 (Jiangxi Province)

2. 治颈淋巴结核方：药物组成及用法：露蜂房一个（瓦焙存性），血竭 3 克，麝香 0.3 克，山慈菇 6 克，明矾 40 克。将上药研末加香油调敷患处。《民族医药报》（西双版纳 永兴）

2. Prescription for Cervical Lymph Node Tuberculosis: Composition and usage: One honeycomb (roasted on tiles to retain its medicinal properties), Dragon's Blood 3g, Musk 0.3g, Pseudobulbus Cremastrae seu Pleiones 6g, Alum 40g. Grind all ingredients into powder, mix with sesame oil to form a paste, and apply externally to the affected area. Ethnic Medicine News (Yongxing, Xishuangbanna)

十、面神经麻痹（3 方）
X. Facial Nerve Paralysis (3 Prescriptions)

面神经瘫痪，民间俗称为“歪嘴风”，是一种神经系统的常见病。大多数患者由于头面部吹冷风引起，寒冷和风湿是主要病因。不论男女老少，春夏秋冬都可发病。患者往往在早晨起床洗脸时，感到面部动作不灵活，急忙去照镜子，发现嘴巴歪斜、眼皮合不拢、笑时不能笑、哭时不能哭、吃饭时嘴巴不听使……得了“歪嘴风”怎么办？现给你介绍民间治疗二法：

Facial nerve paralysis, commonly known as "crooked mouth wind" in folk terms, is a common neurological disorder. In most patients, it is triggered by exposure of the head and face to cold wind, with cold and dampness being the primary etiological factors. It can affect individuals of any gender or age and may occur in any season. Patients often notice facial stiffness upon waking and washing their face in the morning; upon looking in the mirror, they discover mouth deviation, incomplete eyelid closure, inability to smile or cry properly, and loss of control over mouth movements during eating... What should be done if one develops "crooked mouth wind"? Two folk remedies are introduced below:

1. 取蓖麻籽 11-15 粒，捣烂如泥，左边嘴歪敷右边嘴侧，右边嘴歪敷左边嘴侧，纱布包扎，胶布固定，每天敷药一次，一般 2-3 天可愈。

1.Take 11–15 castor seeds, mash them into a paste, and apply to the right side of the mouth if the deviation is to the left, or to the left side if the deviation is to the right; cover with gauze and secure with adhesive tape. Apply once daily; recovery typically occurs within 2–3 days.

2. 用黄鳝鱼鲜血涂嘴侧亦可，左边歪涂右侧，右边歪涂左侧，一般数天可愈。《民族医药报》1992 年 9 月 4 日（广西玉林药材站 梁庆森）

2. Fresh blood from swamp eel may also be applied to the side of the mouth: apply to the right side for left-sided deviation and to the left side for right-sided deviation; recovery generally occurs within several days. Ethnic Medicine News, September 4, 1992 (Liang Qingsen, Yulin Medicinal Materials Station, Guangxi)

3. 处方及用法：取干鹅不食草 10 克研细末与凡士林调为膏状，均匀放在纱布上，再取新鹅不食草 20 克捣烂如泥，共摊于纱布上。患者面部向左歪斜贴右面，向右歪斜贴左面，2 天换药 1 次，一般敷药 2-3 次可愈。注意事项：在治疗时可出现轻微反应，敷药 1-2 天后，面部有虫爬感或发痒感。愈后面部出现小疹，2-3 天后会自行消失。（野 荐）

3. Prescription and Usage: Grind 10g of dried Centipeda minima into fine powder and mix with Vaseline to form an ointment; spread evenly on gauze. Then mash 20g of fresh Centipeda minima into a paste and layer it over the ointment on the gauze. For left-sided facial deviation, apply to the right side of the face; for right-sided deviation, apply to the left side. Change the dressing every 2 days; recovery usually occurs after 2–3 applications. Precautions: Mild reactions may occur during treatment; 1–2 days after application, patients may experience a crawling sensation or itching on the face. A minor rash may appear after recovery but will resolve spontaneously within 2–3 days. (Recommended by Ye)

第六章 美容科
Chapter VI: Medical Aesthetics

一、皮肤美白（17 方）
I. Skin Whitening (17 Prescriptions)

在中药里，有多种具有滋润、美白肌肤功效的药物。这些药有着共同的特征：都姓“白”。

In traditional Chinese medicine, there are numerous herbs that possess the effects of moisturizing and whitening the skin. These herbs share a common characteristic: they all have "Bai" (white) in their names.

1. 白术为菊科多年生草本植物白术的根茎，味苦，性温，其对皮肤致病真菌有一定的抑制作用。古籍《药性论》称：“用白术蘸酒（或醋），均匀涂抹脸上，可治雀斑。”

1.Baizhu (Atractylodes macrocephala) is the rhizome of a perennial herb of the Asteraceae family; it is bitter in flavor and warm in nature, and has a certain inhibitory effect on skin-pathogenic fungi. The ancient text Treatise on Medicinal Properties states: «Dipping Baizhu in wine (or vinegar) and applying it evenly to the face can treat freckles.»

2. 白芷为伞形科多年生草本植物，其味香、辛，性温，历代被视为美容佳品。无论是在千金面脂方中或是在玉容散中，白芷都是制作面脂的主药。

2. Baizhi (Angelica dahurica) is a perennial herb of the Apiaceae family; it is fragrant and pungent in flavor and warm in nature, and has been regarded as an excellent beauty ingredient throughout dynasties. Whether in the Qianjin Face Cream Formula or the Yurong Powder, Baizhi is the principal herb for making

facial creams.

3. 白芨为兰科多年生草本植物白芨的地下茎，味苦、甘，性平、涩而黏滑。外用可润滑肌肤，除面疮。

3. Baiji (Bletilla striata) is the tuber of a perennial herb of the Orchidaceae family; it is bitter and sweet in flavor, neutral, astringent, and mucilaginous in nature. When used externally, it can lubricate the skin and eliminate facial sores.

4. 白苏为人工栽培。取鲜白苏叶涂擦腋下可治狐臭。

4. Baisu (Perilla frutescens var. crispa) is artificially cultivated. Rubbing fresh Baisu leaves on the armpits can treat bromhidrosis (body odor).

5. 白蔹为多年蔓生草本植物，叶子多而细，取其根茎入药。味辛、甘，性凉。《药性论》曰："可治面上疮疱而美白肌肤。"

5. Bailian (Ampelopsis japonica) is a perennial climbing herb with numerous fine leaves; its root tuber is used medicinally. It is pungent and sweet in flavor and cool in nature. The Treatise on Medicinal Properties says: «It can treat facial sores and pimples while whitening the skin.»

6. 白附子味辛、甘，可作面脂。取其捣碎成细粉，以酒拌和，用来敷面，可治粉刺和雀斑。

6. Baifuzi (Typhonium giganteum) is pungent and sweet in flavor and can be used to make facial cream. Grind it into a fine powder, mix with wine, and apply to the face to treat acne and freckles.

7. 白蒺藜又名刺蒺藜，1 年或多年生草本植物蒺藜的果实。味苦、辛，性温。含有多种生物碱和甙类及多种丰富的过氧化物分解酶，有明显抗衰老作用，可明目轻身，去除面痕。《本草纲目》曰："洗面黑，去斑。"

7. Baijili, also known as Ciji Li (Tribulus terrestris), is the fruit of an annual or perennial herb of the Zygophyllaceae family. It is bitter and pungent in flavor and warm in nature. It contains various alkaloids, glycosides, and abundant peroxide-decomposing enzymes, exhibiting significant anti-aging effects; it can brighten the eyes, lighten the body, and remove facial blemishes. The Compendium of Materia Medica states: «It washes away darkened skin and removes spots.»

8. 白果仁为银杏的成熟种子。外用可治头面手足碍容性皮肤病，并可防止皮肤粗糙。

8. Baiguoren (Ginkgo nut) is the ripe seed of the ginkgo tree. When used externally, it can treat disfiguring skin diseases on the head, face, hands, and feet, and can also prevent rough skin.

9. 白茯苓味甘、淡，性平。《本草品汇精要》曰："取白茯苓研末，与蜜和，敷面可疗面疮。"

9. Baifuling (Poria cocos) is sweet and bland in flavor and neutral in nature. The Essential Compendium of Materia Medica states: «Grind Baifuling into powder, mix with honey, and apply to the face to treat facial sores.»

10. 白丁香味辛，性温，为雄麻雀屎。用它浸蜜可防治面疮和粉刺，能莹肌如玉。

10. Baidingxiang is pungent in flavor and warm in nature; it is the feces of male sparrows. Soaking it in honey can prevent and treat facial sores and acne, making the skin lustrous and jade-like.

11. 白僵蚕为蚕蛾科家蚕的幼虫在未吐丝前，因感染白僵菌而发病致死的僵化虫体。外用其药，味咸、辛，性平。可治面黑、碍容性疾病及口眼歪斜等症。《健康报》

11. Baijiangcan (Bombyx batryticatus) is the mummified larva of the domestic silkworm (Bombycidae) that died from Beauveria bassiana infection before spinning silk. When used externally, it is salty and pungent in flavor and neutral in nature. It can treat darkened complexion, disfiguring skin diseases, and facial paralysis. Health News

12. 柠檬汁：脸洗净，抹几下柠檬汁，保持 40-50 分钟，然后洗净，涂护肤霜。连续 20 天，增白效果明显。

12. Lemon Juice: Wash the face thoroughly, apply lemon juice several times, leave it on for 40–50 minutes, then rinse off and apply moisturizer. Continuous use for 20 days yields noticeable whitening effects.

13. 胡萝卜柠檬汁：2 匙胡萝卜汁，加 20 滴柠檬汁，每天 2-3 次抹脸，30

分钟后洗掉，再涂护肤霜。

13. Carrot-Lemon Juice: Mix 2 teaspoons of carrot juice with 20 drops of lemon juice, apply to the face 2–3 times daily, rinse off after 30 minutes, and then apply moisturizer.

14. 萝卜和西红柿汁片：把脸洗净，涂护肤霜，然后在脸上放几片萝卜片或西红柿，30 分钟后再用凉牛奶洗脸。

14. Radish and Tomato Slices: Wash the face, apply moisturizer, place a few slices of radish or tomato on the face, and after 30 minutes, wash the face with cool milk.

15. 草莓汁：先洗净脸部，然后将草莓汁擦在脸上，过 15 分钟洗去，对皮肤有洁白作用，对治疗雀斑也有一定效果。《民族医药报》1996 年 12 月 27 日（吴里平）

15. Strawberry Juice: First wash the face, then rub strawberry juice onto the skin, leave it on for 15 minutes, and rinse off. It has a whitening effect on the skin and is also somewhat effective in treating freckles. Ethnic Medicine News, December 27, 1996 (Wu Liping)

16 皮肤嫩白方：该方建议每日清晨先以 30% 浓度的盐水擦拭面部，随后用米汤或淘米水清洗，再将雪花膏与珍珠粉混合涂抹于脸部；据传统经验记载，坚持使用半个月后，可使原本粗糙黝黑的皮肤变得白皙细嫩。

16.Skin Tenderizing and Whitening Formula: This formula recommends wiping the face with a 30% saline solution every morning, followed by washing with rice soup or water from rinsed rice, and then applying a mixture of vanishing cream and pearl powder to the face; according to traditional records, consistent use for half a month can transform rough and dark skin into a fair and tender complexion.

《民族医药报》1992 年 9 月 11 日（云南 刘忠平）

As published in the Ethnic Medicine News on September 11, 1992, this formula was contributed by Liu Zhongping from Yunnan.

17. 玉肌倒膜粉：药物组成：白藓皮、白僵蚕、白芨、杏仁各 18 克，冬瓜仁、白芷各 9 克，冰片、密陀僧各 3 克。共研细末。用清水洗净面部后，将中药粉剂以冷水调成糊状，涂敷于面部，40 分钟后清水洗去，涂上润肤霜。总有效率 95.5%。

17.Jade Skin Mask Powder: This formula consists of 18g each of Cortex Dictamni, Bombyx Batryticatus, Rhizoma Bletillae, and Semen Armeniacae Amarum, 9g each of Semen Benincasae and Radix Angelicae Dahuricae, plus 3g each of Borneolum Syntheticum and Lithargyrum, all ground together into a fine powder; to use, first cleanse the face with water, then mix the herbal powder with cold water into a paste and apply evenly to the face, rinse off with water after 40 minutes and apply moisturizer, with a reported total effective rate of 95.5%.

《民族医药报》1997 年 9 月 12 日（广医）

As published in the Ethnic Medicine News on September 12, 1997, this formula was contributed by Guangyi.

二、去黄褐斑和雀斑（15 方）

Removal of Chloasma and Freckles (15 Formulas)

1.1. 西红柿汁：用 1 只西红柿挤汁，加入 1 匙甘油。每天 1 次用其洗脸，干净皮肤可涂点护肤霜。长期使用可除雀斑。

1.Tomato Juice: Squeeze the juice from one tomato and mix in one spoonful of glycerin; use this mixture to wash the face once daily, and apply a small amount of moisturizer after cleansing. Long-term use may help fade freckles.

2. 金盏花叶汁：用金盏花叶汁搽脸，既能清爽和洁白皮肤，又能除去雀斑。

2.Calendula Leaf Juice: Applying calendula leaf juice to the face can both refresh and whiten the skin, as well as remove freckles.

3. 柠檬汁加牛奶：油性或中性皮肤的人，每天用白柠檬汁加牛奶涂脸，能除雀斑。

3.Lemon Juice with Milk: For those with oily or neutral skin, applying a mixture of white lemon juice and milk to the face daily can help eliminate freckles.

4. 蒲公英花水：鲜蒲公英花适量，倒入 1 茶杯沸开水，冷却后过滤，所得液体倒入瓶中。每天早晚用蒲公英花水洗雀斑。

4.Dandelion Flower Water: Take an appropriate amount of fresh dandelion flowers, pour in one teacup of boiling water, allow to cool and strain, then store the resulting liquid in a bottle. Wash the affected areas with this dandelion flower water every morning and evening to help fade freckles.

5. 黄瓜汁：黄瓜捣汁搽脸，也可切成薄片贴在面部雀斑或黄褐斑上，1-2 分钟更换 1 次。能清洁皮肤，舒展皮肤皱纹，使肌肤变得细嫩，润滑。

5.Cucumber Juice: Mash cucumber to extract the juice and apply it to the face, or cut it into thin slices and place them over freckles or chloasma patches, replacing every 1–2 minutes; this method can cleanse the skin, smooth wrinkles, and leave the skin delicate and supple.

《民族医药报》1996 年 12 月 27 日（吴里平）

As published in the Ethnic Medicine News on December 27, 1996, this formula was contributed by Wu Liping.

6. 食盐价虽廉，但运用得法可美容。鼻头毛孔粗大，浮有黑色油脂者，可涂上橄榄油后，以手指沾精制食盐按摩鼻头。肌肤较弱者，可以用精制食盐混合营养霜来按摩。皮肤晒黑者，也可以用前面的方法，将脱皮简单而彻底去除干净。同样地，食盐按摩也可应用于手肘或膝部坚硬的死皮之去除上。另外，皮肤容易长疮的人，可在八分满的脸盆水中加入一大匙盐。以盐水洗脸，能使皮肤健美，保持正常的状态。

6.Salt Beauty Method: Although salt is inexpensive, it can be used effectively for beauty purposes when applied correctly. For enlarged pores and black sebum on the nose, apply olive oil first and then massage the area with fingers dipped in refined salt; those with delicate skin may mix refined salt with nourishing cream for massage. This method can also simply and thoroughly remove peeling skin caused by sunburn, and is equally effective for eliminating tough dead skin on elbows and knees. Additionally, individuals prone to skin sores can add a tablespoon of salt to a basin filled eight-tenths full of water; washing the face with this saline solution helps maintain healthy and normal skin condition.

《民族医药报》1992 年 8 月 28 日（成都市戴廷荣）

(Ethnic Medicine News, August 28, 1992, Dai Tingrong, Chengdu).

中医认为，人体面部黄褐斑为一种全身性气血阴阳失调的表现，主要与脾肝肾机能失调有关。情志不遂，暴怒伤肝，思虑伤脾、惊恐伤肾等皆可使气机紊乱，气血悖逆，不能上荣于面，而生褐斑。现代医学则认为本病的发生可能与机体黄体酮及雌激素的增加使酪氨酸不受谷酰甘肽的抑制。同时垂体中叶分泌的黑色素细胞雌激素增加，与妊娠时血清酮含量升高有关。

Traditional Chinese Medicine holds that facial chloasma is a manifestation of systemic imbalance of qi, blood, yin, and yang, primarily related to dysfunction of the spleen, liver, and kidney; emotional distress, excessive anger damaging the liver, overthinking impairing the spleen, and fear injuring the kidney can all disrupt qi dynamics and reverse the flow of qi and blood, preventing nourishment from reaching the face and thus forming pigmentation. Modern medicine suggests that the condition may be associated with elevated levels of progesterone and estrogen, which prevent tyrosine from being inhibited by glutathione, while increased melanocyte-stimulating hormone secreted by the intermediate lobe of the pituitary is also linked to elevated serum ketone levels during pregnancy.

据有关资料介绍，使用耳针及梅花针治疗该症，效果令人满意，具体是。

According to available data, auricular acupuncture and plum-blossom needle therapy yield satisfactory results:

7. 耳针治疗：主穴为内分泌、皮质下、肺、心、肝、肾，月经不调者加子宫、卵巢。常规消毒后，用 28 号 5 分毫针轻刺透皮肤不穿透骨膜为度，每隔 5 分钟轻捻转行针 1 次，留针 30 分钟。

Auricular Acupuncture uses Endocrine, Subcortex, Lung, Heart, Liver, and Kidney as main points, with Uterus and Ovary added for irregular menstruation; after routine disinfection, a No. 28 five-fen filiform needle is inserted lightly through the skin without penetrating the periosteum, gently twisted every five minutes, and retained for thirty minutes

8. 梅花针治疗：患处常规消毒后，均匀涂抹维生素 E，用梅花针自上至下轻轻叩打，使皮肤潮红为度。

隔日治疗 1 次，15 次为一个疗程，休息 1 周继续第 2 疗程的治疗。

资料还显示：用上述方法治疗的 42 例女性患者中，临床治愈（皮肤色素减退，肤色接近正常，伴随症状消失或基本消失）者共 6 例；显效（皮肤色素明显减退，伴随症状基本消失或明显减轻）者 21 例；好转（皮肤色素及伴随症状均较治疗前减轻）者 12 例。总有效率达 92.8%。

《民族医药报》1992 年 9 月 4 日（广西伍世轰）

Plum-Blossom Needle Therapy involves routine disinfection of the affected area, even application of vitamin E, followed by gentle tapping from top to bottom until the skin becomes flushed. Treatments are administered every other day, fifteen sessions constitute one course, and a second course begins after a one-week break. Data show that among forty-two female patients treated with these methods, six were clinically cured, twenty-one showed marked improvement, and twelve showed moderate improvement, resulting in a total effective rate of 92.8%

(Ethnic Medicine News, September 4, 1992, Wu Shihong, Guangxi).

9. 黄褐斑：蜂蜜 1 份，朱砂（水飞）4 份，混合，加入雪花膏适量调匀，每晚睡前用温水洗脸后擦药 1 次，次日起床后拭去。一般用药 10-15 天见效。

9.Chloasma Formula: Mix one part honey with four parts water-levigated cinnabar, then add an appropriate amount of vanishing cream to form a paste; apply once nightly after cleansing the face with warm water before bed, and wipe off upon waking the next morning. Effects are generally observed after 10 to 15 days of continuous use.

10. 治黄褐斑方

黄褐斑也称蝴蝶斑，系发生在面部的一种色素沉着性皮肤病。该病以女性多见，影响美容。采用下述方法治疗效果较为理想。具体是：取白芷 27 克、白附子 20 克、密陀僧 8 克，烤干研末过筛，加入雪花膏 100 克调匀，消毒后装入瓶内。每日早晨洗脸后及晚睡觉前各搽药 1 次，坚持连续用 1-2 个月。用药 4

小时内患处不接触水。搽药期间忌用化妆品，忌吃辛辣燥热食物。无论病程长短均有效。随访治愈患者一般未见复发。

《民族医药报》（潘彦清）

10.Formula for Treating Chloasma Chloasma, also known as butterfly melasma, is a pigmentary skin disorder occurring on the face. It is more common in women and affects facial aesthetics. The following treatment method has proven to be quite effective: Take 27g of Radix Angelicae Dahuricae, 20g of Rhizoma Typhonii, and 8g of Lithargyrum; roast them dry, grind into a fine powder, and sift. Mix the powder evenly with 100g of vanishing cream, sterilize the mixture, and store it in a jar. Apply the ointment once daily after morning face washing and once again before bed at night, continuing consistently for one to two months. Avoid contact with water on the affected area for four hours after application. During the treatment period, refrain from using cosmetics and consuming spicy or heat-inducing foods. This formula is effective regardless of the duration of the condition. Follow-up observations indicate that cured patients generally experience no recurrence.

Ethnic Medicine News (Pan Yanqing)

11. 将新鲜黄瓜切成两段，然后往脸上雀斑处揉擦 50-60 次，用力要均匀，不宜过大，直到黄瓜的汁液干后再用温水洗脸。此法要坚持每天两遍，大约半个月可起作用。

11.Cucumber Freckle-Removal Method: Cut a fresh cucumber into two sections and gently rub the freckled areas of the face 50–60 times with even, moderate pressure; after the cucumber juice dries completely, wash the face with warm water. This method should be performed twice daily, morning and evening, and effects are typically observed after about half a month of consistent use.

12. 新鲜的柿子树叶 30 克，浓煎待温后用手巾沾之洗脸，连续半个月。

12.Take 30grams of fresh persimmon leaves, decoct them into a concentrated solution, wait until warm, dip a towel in it to wash the face, and continue for half a month.

13 鲜芹菜根 30 克，洗净切碎，加水 250 毫升，浸泡 2 小时后，滤去药渣，以药液洗脸，每天一次，每次洗 30-40 遍，连续半个月。

13.Take 30grams of fresh celery roots, wash and chop them, soak in 250 ml of water for 2 hours, strain out the residue, use the liquid to wash the face once daily, 30 to 40 times per session, for half a month.

要注意的是，在进行上述治疗的同时，外出必须戴帽遮阳防晒。

It should be noted that during the above treatments, one must wear a hat for sun protection when going outdoors.

《民族医药报》1993 年 7 月 3 日（韦文文）

Ethnic Medicine News, July 3, 1993 (Wei Wenwen)

除雀斑的方法较多，这里介绍二则民间治雀斑的验方给患者试用

There are many methods for removing freckles; here are two folk remedies presented for patients to try.

14. 白茯苓适量，研为细末，调入优质的蜜糖呈糊膏状，每晚睡前敷于患处，连续敷 8-10 天奏效。

14.Grind an appropriate amount of white poria into fine powder, mix with high-quality honey to form a paste, apply to the affected area every night before sleep, and results can be seen after 8 to 10 consecutive days.

15. 黑丑（黑牵牛）适量，研为细末，加入打匀的鸡蛋液适量，共搅成膏状，每晚睡前敷于患处，翌晨起床用温水洗除，连续 4-6 天即可。

15.Grind an appropriate amount of black morning glory seeds into fine powder, add beaten egg white to form a paste, apply to the affected area nightly before sleep, wash off with warm water the next morning, and repeat for 4 to 6 consecutive days.

《中医药信息报》1992 年 3 月 7 日（梁庆森）

Traditional Chinese Medicine Information News, March 7, 1992 (Liang Qingsen)

三、容颜不老（1方）
Everlasting Youthful Complexion (1 Prescription):

"容颜不老方"是经过长期实践证明行之有效且在我国民间广为流传的美容良方。该方的组成：生姜500克，大枣250克，白盐50克，甘草90克，丁香、沉香各15克，茴香200克。将上述药物一起捣碎并研成粗末，调匀备用。于每天早晨取10-15克，煎服或沸水泡服均可。

The "Everlasting Youthful Complexion Prescription" is a time-tested and widely circulated folk beauty remedy in China. Its composition includes 500g of fresh ginger, 250g of Chinese dates, 50g of white salt, 90g of licorice root, 15g each of clove and agarwood, and 200g of fennel. Crush all the ingredients together into a coarse powder, mix well, and store for later use. Each morning, take 10–15g of the mixture and either decoct it in water or steep it in boiling water before consumption.

祖国医学认为，面部肌肤的润泽与否，是脾胃功能盛衰的直接反映。方中以辛温健脾的生姜与甘平益脾的大枣为主药，最能生发脾胃之气；茴香、丁香、沉香芳香理气，加强温肾助阳之力，作为辅药；食盐滋阴降火为佐药；甘草甘缓，调和营卫，能缓和药性兼调味作为调引药。诸药合用可使脾胃功能旺盛，运水谷精微灌注全身，营养肌肤，致使颜面色泽红润，从而起到养颜、美容之功效。

Traditional Chinese Medicine holds that the moisture and luster of facial skin directly reflect the functional state of the spleen and stomach. In this formula, pungent-warm ginger and sweet-neutral Chinese dates serve as principal herbs to invigorate and nourish the spleen and stomach; aromatic fennel, clove, and agarwood act as auxiliary herbs to regulate qi and enhance kidney-warming and yang-tonifying effects; salt serves as an adjuvant herb to nourish yin and reduce deficiency fire; and licorice, with its sweet and moderating nature, functions as a guiding herb to harmonize nutrient and defensive qi, moderate the properties of other herbs, and improve taste. Together, these herbs strengthen spleen-stomach function, promote the distribution of refined nutrients from food and water throughout the body, nourish the skin, and impart a rosy, radiant complexion, thereby achieving beautifying and anti-aging effects.

《民族医药报》1992 年 6 月 5 日（广西民族医院 周秋培）

Ethnic Medicine News, June 5, 1992 (Zhou Qiupei, Guangxi Ethnic Hospital)

四、斑秃及脱发（6 方）
Alopecia Areata and Hair Loss (6 Prescriptions)

1. 斑秃俗称“鬼剃头”。我们采用《山东中医杂志》上介绍的验方“生发散”予以治疗，收到了良好的疗效。

1. Alopecia areata is commonly known as “ghost shaving.” We have achieved good therapeutic results by using the proven prescription “Hair Growth Powder” introduced in the Shandong Journal of Traditional Chinese Medicine.

配制及服用法：取生地、熟地、女贞子、白芍、当归、丹参各 150 克，制首乌、侧柏叶各 225 克，羌活 75 克。将上药研末，过筛（一般以通过 6 号筛为宜），混合均匀后即得“生发散”。每次服 6 克，日服 3 次，温开水送下。为便于服用，可将药物装入空心胶囊内服用。另取侧柏叶 90 克、山奈 45 克、75% 酒精 700 毫升，将药入瓶密闭，浸泡 7-10 天，过滤即得生发水。应用时，以生姜切面蘸生发水，在脱发部位反复用力涂擦，每日 2-3 次。临床验证，一般经内服和外涂药物后，三周即可长出绒毛。

Preparation and administration: Take 150g each of raw rehmannia root, prepared rehmannia root, glossy privet fruit, white peony root, Chinese angelica root, and salvia miltiorrhiza; 225g each of prepared fleeceflower root and cacumen platycladi; and 75g of notopterygium root. Grind all ingredients into powder, sift (preferably through a No. 6 sieve), and mix thoroughly to obtain the “Hair Growth Powder.” Take 6g per dose, three times daily, with warm water. For easier administration, the powder can be filled into empty capsules. Additionally, prepare a hair growth tonic by placing 90g of cacumen platycladi and 45g of sand ginger into a sealed bottle with 700ml of 75% alcohol, soaking for 7–10 days, and then filtering. When applying, dip the cut surface of fresh ginger into the tonic and vigorously rub the bald areas repeatedly, 2–3 times daily. Clinical verification shows that new vellus hair typically begins to grow within three weeks after combined oral and topical treatment.

《民族医药报》1992 年 2 月 7 日（南京市上新河医院 孙哲）

Ethnic Medicine News, February 7, 1992 (Sun Zhe, Shangxinhe Hospital of Nanjing).

2. 外治：取鲜生姜片或鲜姜汁涂于患处，并以拇指或鱼际部位摩擦，至产生热感及痒感为止，每隔 5 分钟摩擦至热 1 次，反复 3-5 次。每日姜摩一次，直至痊愈。每次姜摩前，应用硫磺皂把头洗净。内服方药：旱莲草、何首乌、枸杞子、大熟地、黑芝麻各 15-30 克，红花 6-10 克。随证加减：头痒起屑者，加荆芥、防风、白芷 6-10 克，丹皮 10 克；头昏、失眠、心烦者，加柏子仁、炒杏仁各 15-20 克，珍珠母 30 克，远志 10 克。水煎服，每日 1 剂。据笔者观察，使用上述方法治疗斑秃，多数病人经 1-6 周治疗，可获痊愈，总有效率为 86.5%。

2. External treatment: Apply fresh ginger slices or juice to the affected area and rub with the thumb or thenar eminence until a sensation of heat and itching is produced; repeat this rubbing-to-heat cycle every 5 minutes for 3–5 cycles. Perform this ginger massage once daily until full recovery. Before each session, wash the scalp thoroughly with sulfur soap. Internal prescription: Use 15–30g each of eclipta prostrata, fleeceflower root, wolfberry fruit, prepared rehmannia root, and black sesame seeds, along with 6–10g of safflower. Modify according to symptoms: for itchy scalp with dandruff, add 6–10g each of schizonepeta, fangfeng, and angelica dahurica, plus 10g of moutan bark; for dizziness, insomnia, and irritability, add 15–20g each of arborvitae seed and stir-fried almond, 30g of pearl shell, and 10g of polygala root. Decoct in water and take one dose daily. According to the author’s observations, most patients treated with this method for alopecia areata recover within 1–6 weeks, with a total effective rate of 86.5%.

斑秃多因肝肾不足，阴血亏虚，情志所伤和气滞血瘀而致，治疗关键在于补虚养血、祛瘀生新。采取生姜摩擦助热，透入毛发孔窍，增强局部血液循环，以奏祛瘀生新之效。内服之中药，能滋补肝肾，调养阴血。这种内外合治斑秃之法，疗效确切，简便易行，值得一试。

Alopecia areata is primarily caused by liver-kidney deficiency, yin-blood depletion, emotional injury, and qi stagnation with blood stasis; thus, the key to treatment lies in tonifying deficiency, nourishing blood, removing stasis, and promoting regeneration. Ginger massage generates heat that penetrates hair follicles, enhances local blood circulation, and achieves the effect of dispelling stasis and stimulating new growth. The internal herbal formula nourishes the liver and kidneys while regulating yin and blood. This integrated internal-external approach to treating alopecia areata is clinically effective, simple, practical, and worth trying.

《民族医药报》1993 年 1 月 1 日（广西 林中）

Ethnic Medicine News, January 1, 1993 (Lin Zhong, Guangxi).

3. 治秃顶：用满天星适量（俗名见面草），花椒少许，入油锅内煎熬，用鸡毛蘸药汁涂于患处，日数次。

3.Treatment for baldness: Take an appropriate amount of Gypsophila (commonly known as Jianmiancao) and a small amount of Sichuan peppercorn, fry them in a pan with oil, dip a chicken feather into the medicated oil, and apply it to the affected area several times a day.

1.4. 透骨草具有止脱发、止痒、去头屑之功。治法是：取单味透骨草 45 克，煎汤熏洗头发，每日一剂，熏洗一次，每次 20 分钟，洗后勿用水冲洗头发。用药 4-12 日，大多数患者在用药后 3 日即见效，表现为头发脱落明显减少，头皮瘙痒减轻，终获痊愈。透骨草具有祛风除湿、活血祛瘀之功，用其煎汤熏洗，简单方便，无任何不良反应。临床实践表明，本品对各种症型的脂溢性脱发均可使用。

1.4.Garden balsam stem has the effects of stopping hair loss, relieving itching, and removing dandruff. The treatment method is as follows: take 45g of garden balsam stem alone, decoct it in water, and use the steam and liquid to fumigate and wash the hair; use one dose per day, once daily for 20 minutes each time, and do not rinse the hair with plain water after washing. After 4–12 days of medication, most patients show improvement within 3 days, manifested by significantly reduced hair shedding and alleviated scalp itching, eventually achieving full recovery. Garden balsam stem has the functions of dispelling wind-dampness and activating blood circulation to remove blood stasis; fumigating and washing with its decoction is simple, convenient, and free of adverse reactions. Clinical practice shows that this herb can be used for various types of seborrheic alopecia.

《中医药信息报》1992 年 1 月 4 日（江苏 马勇）

Traditional Chinese Medicine Information News, January 4, 1992 (Ma Yong, Jiangsu).

5. 辣椒治秃法

（用料）：辣椒 10 克，白酒 50 克

（制法）：将椒切细，用酒浸泡 10 天，过滤后去渣，用纱布浸湿，每天擦几次头皮。

（功效）：治疗秃发，促进头发的生长。

5.Chili pepper treatment for baldness

(Ingredients): 10g chili peppers, 50g liquor.

(Preparation): Chop the chili peppers finely, soak them in the liquor for 10 days, filter out the residue, soak a piece of gauze in the liquid, and rub the scalp with it several times a day.

(Efficacy): Treats baldness and promotes hair growth.

6. 许多人为掉发而发愁，而用食盐水洗头可防掉发，因为盐水对头发有杀菌消毒的作用，可减少头皮和发根的感染，同时食盐水供应了头发的某种营养需要。其具体方法是：取 100-150 克食盐，投放到半盆温水中溶解，先把头发浸在盐水中，揉搓几分钟，然后在头发中加洗发精，继续在温盐水中洗，待洗掉油污后，再用清水冲洗即可，每星期洗一至二次，一般一个月可见效。

6.Many people worry about hair loss, and washing hair with salt water can help prevent it, as salt water has antibacterial and disinfectant effects on hair, reduces infections of the scalp and hair roots, and also supplies certain nutrients needed by the hair. The specific method is: dissolve 100–150g of table salt in half a basin of warm water, first soak the hair in the salt water and massage for a few minutes, then add shampoo and continue washing in the warm salt water; after removing oil and dirt, rinse with clean water. Wash once or twice a week, and results are generally visible within one month.

《民族医药报》1991 年 10 月 25 日（浙江 何校善辑）

thnic Medicine News, October 25, 1991 (Compiled by He Xiaoshan, Zhejiang).

五、痤疮（5 方）

Acne (5 Prescriptions):

痤疮俗称“米疮”。中医称本病为肺风粉刺。为青年男女较为常见的一种慢性皮肤病。这是因为青春发育期、性腺成熟、内分泌增加，刺激皮脂腺分泌过多，使毛囊上皮增生，而将毛囊皮脂腺管口阻塞，再经继发细菌感染而引起的慢性化脓性毛囊炎。皮脂溢出症，过多地吃脂肪和糖类，消化不良等，常为本病的诱发原因。现将治疗方法介绍如下：

Acne is commonly known as “rice sore” and referred to as “lung wind acne” in Traditional Chinese Medicine. It is a common chronic skin disease among young men and women, caused by increased endocrine secretion during puberty and gonadal maturation, which stimulates excessive sebum production, leads to hyperplasia of hair follicle epithelium, blocks the opening of the pilosebaceous duct, and subsequently triggers chronic suppurative folliculitis due to secondary bacterial infection. Seborrhea, excessive intake of fats and sugars, and indigestion are often predisposing factors for this condition. The treatment methods are introduced as follows:

1. 常用温热水、消毒香皂洗脸以除去油脂，勿用手挤抓痤疮。少吃脂肪和糖类，避免饮酒和刺激性食物。

1. Wash the face regularly with warm water and antiseptic soap to remove excess oil, and avoid squeezing or scratching acne lesions with hands; reduce the intake of fats and sugars, and avoid alcohol and irritating foods.

2. 内服维生素 B6 维生素 B2 或多吃蔬菜。

2. Take vitamin B6 and vitamin B2 orally, or increase vegetable consumption.

3. 中医药治疗：以清肺热，利肺气为主。枇杷叶 15 克、桑白皮 15 克、银花 20 克、黄柏 10 克、黄连 10 克、百部 10 克、连翘 20 克、甘草 10 克，加水煎服，每日一剂，如化脓性炎症较重而顽面者，可加服抗菌素治疗。

3. TCM treatment focuses on clearing lung heat and regulating lung qi: decoct 15g loquat leaf, 15g mulberry bark, 20g honeysuckle flower, 10g phellodendron bark, 10g coptis rhizome, 10g stemona root, 20g forsythia fruit, and 10g licorice root in water for oral administration, one dose per day; for severe and stubborn suppurative inflammation, antibiotics may be added.

4. 可外擦 1.2% 硫酸锌、红霉素锌（EZ 液）。

4. Topical application of 1.2% zinc sulfate or erythromycin-zinc (EZ solution) can be used.

《中药科技报》1992 年 4 月 17 日（空军沈阳医院药剂科研制）

Journal of Traditional Chinese Medicine Science and Technology, April 17, 1992 (Developed by the Pharmacy Research Department of Shenyang Air Force Hospital).

5. 治疗痤疮验方

处方及用法：枇杷叶、桑白皮、连翘各 15 克，黄柏、白花蛇舌草、黄连各 10 克，生地 20 克，甘草 5 克。脾胃积热黄连易黄芩，加生薏苡仁、生山楂、茵陈、生栀子；热毒内盛加知母、赤芍、白芷、金银花、野菊花；便秘加大黄；瘙痒难忍加蝉蜕；疹色深加紫草；有结节加皂刺、夏枯草；继发感染加板蓝根。日 1 剂水煎服，用 4-6 周。服药期间忌食辛辣、糖类及油腻之品。经治疗多例，均治愈。

5. Proven prescription for acne treatment:

Prescription and usage include 15g each of loquat leaf, mulberry bark, and forsythia fruit; 10g each of phellodendron bark, spreading hedyotis herb, and coptis rhizome; 20g raw rehmannia root; and 5g licorice root. For spleen-stomach accumulated heat, replace coptis rhizome with scutellaria root and add raw coix seed, raw hawthorn fruit, capillary wormwood, and raw gardenia fruit; for internal accumulation of heat toxin, add anemarrhena rhizome, red peony root, angelica dahurica, honeysuckle flower, and wild chrysanthemum flower; for constipation, add rhubarb; for unbearable itching, add cicada slough; for dark-colored rashes, add arnebia root; for nodules, add gleditsia spine and selfheal spike; for secondary infection, add isatis root. Take one dose daily as a water decoction for 4–6 weeks, and avoid spicy, sugary, and greasy foods during medication. Multiple cases treated with this method have all been cured.

《民族医药报》1998 年 1 月 23 日（新）

Ethnic Medicine News, January 23, 1998 (Xin).

六、白癜风（9 方）
Vitiligo (9 Prescriptions)

1. 生姜一块，用刀切开，用切面擦摩患处，汁液干后，用刀切开生姜再擦，一日数次。

1. Take a piece of fresh ginger, cut it open, and rub the affected area with the cut surface; once the juice dries, make a fresh cut and rub again, repeating several times a day.

2. 用鲜芝麻花涂抹患处，一日 5-10 次。

2. Apply fresh sesame flowers to the affected area 5–10 times daily.

3. 秋天露重时节，清晨去菜地收取韭叶上的露水，封在瓶内，用来涂抹患处。

3. During heavy dew periods in autumn, collect morning dew from chive leaves in vegetable fields, seal it in a bottle, and apply it to the affected area.

4. 用热的鳗鱼油涂擦患处，每次 3 分钟，一日两次。

4. Rub warm eel oil onto the affected area for 3 minutes each time, twice daily.

5. 把无花菜叶子切成细条，用烧酒浸泡后涂抹患处，一日 2-3 次。

5. Cut cauliflower leaves into thin strips, soak them in strong liquor, and apply the liquid to the affected area 2–3 times daily.

6. 用白酒 10-15 毫升，送服生香油 10-15 毫升，一日三次，连服两个月，忌食生冷、猪肉、鸡肉、酒、蒜。

6. Take 10–15 ml of raw sesame oil with 10–15 ml of white liquor as a vehicle, three times daily for two consecutive months; avoid raw/cold foods, pork, chicken, alcohol, and garlic during treatment.

《民族医药报》1992 年 4 月 17 日（马宝山 荐）

Ethnic Medicine News, April 17, 1992 (Recommended by Ma Baoshan).

7. 脱发及白癜风：黑豆 500 克，水 1000 毫升，文火熬煮，以水浸豆粒饱胀为度。取出，放器皿中阴干，然后撒细盐少许，贮于瓷瓶内备用。每服 6 克，饭后温开水送下，每日 2 次。.

For hair loss and vitiligo: Simmer 500g black beans in 1000 ml water over low heat until the beans are fully swollen and have absorbed the water; remove them, shade-dry in a container, sprinkle with a small amount of fine salt, and store in a porcelain jar for later use. Take 6g per dose with warm water after meals, twice daily.

（李明）白癜风，常见于头皮、颈、手指、胸、腰及四肢等部位。有的连头面、头发、眉毛及眼睫毛都同时变白。白癜风虽然不痛不痒，对健康没有多大影响，但是影响外观，给患者带来苦恼，所以急于求治。笔者在临床上常用中草药治疗此病。疗效颇佳，现简介如下。

(Li Ming). Vitiligo commonly occurs on the scalp, neck, fingers, chest, waist, and limbs; in some cases, the face, hair, eyebrows, and eyelashes may also turn white simultaneously. Although vitiligo is neither painful nor itchy and has little impact on general health, its cosmetic effects cause significant distress, prompting patients to seek urgent treatment. The author frequently uses Chinese herbal medicine for this condition in clinical practice with satisfactory results, briefly introduced as follows.

8. 取乌梅 50 克，浸泡于 95% 酒精 100 毫升中，2 周后过滤取药液备用。使用时，蘸药液用力搽患处，每次 5 分钟，每日 3 次。可同时内服下列方剂：黑豆、制首乌、地榆、石决明（打碎）各 15 克。紫草、红花、郁金、丹皮、白蒺藜各 10 克。水煎，每日 1 剂分 3 次服。

8. Soak 50g dark plum in 100 ml of 95% alcohol for two weeks, filter to obtain the medicinal liquid for external use; vigorously rub the affected area with the liquid for 5 minutes each time, three times daily. Concurrently, take the following internal formula: 15g each of black beans, prepared fleeceflower root, garden burnet root, and crushed abalone shell; 10g each of arnebia root, safflower, curcuma tuber, moutan bark, and white tribulus fruit; decoct in water and divide one daily dose into three servings.

9. 取补骨脂 30 克，白蒺藜 20 克，浸泡于 95% 酒精 100 毫升中，2 周后取用其浸出液，涂搽患处，每日 2 次。可同时用地榆、石决明（打碎）各 15 克，紫草、白蒺藜各 10 克，水煎分 2 次服；若毛发也变白的，宜用制首乌、当归、黑芝麻各 15 克，生地、熟地、桃仁、红花各 12 克，水煎分 3 次服。

在进行上述治疗时，还应注意以下四点：

精神要乐观，而且要有信心和耐心。一般以 3 个月为 1 个疗程，坚持治疗 2 个疗程。

食用丝瓜、茄子、芹菜、胡萝卜、苹果、核桃、黑芝麻、猪肝等，对病情有利。

应少吃或忌食酒、蒜、葱、鱼虾及羊肉等。

应避免日光照射和热天不要在阳光下暴晒，还要注意室内通风。

9. Soak 30g psoralea fruit and 20g white tribulus fruit in 100 ml of 95% alcohol for two weeks, then apply the extract to the affected area twice daily. At the same time, decoct 15g each of garden burnet root and crushed abalone shell together with 10g each of arnebia root and white tribulus fruit in water, and take in two divided doses; if body hair has also turned white, instead decoct 15g each of prepared fleeceflower root, Chinese angelica root, and black sesame

seeds along with 12g each of raw rehmannia root, prepared rehmannia root, peach kernel, and safflower in water, and take in three divided doses. During the above treatments, the following four points should also be observed: maintain an optimistic mindset with confidence and patience; one course of treatment generally lasts three months, and two consecutive courses should be completed. Consuming loofah, eggplant, celery, carrots, apples, walnuts, black sesame seeds, and pig liver is beneficial to the condition. Alcohol, garlic, scallions, fish, shrimp, and mutton should be reduced or avoided entirely. Avoid direct sunlight exposure, especially intense sunbathing in hot weather, and ensure good indoor ventilation.

《民族医药报》1992 年 5 月 22 日（广西 李子云）

Ethnic Medicine News, May 22, 1992 (Li Ziyun, Guangxi).

七、扁平疣（17 方）
Flat Warts (17 Prescriptions)

1. 冰醋酸药糊治良性疣：纯冰醋酸 2-3 毫升，面粉适量。取清洁干燥青霉素瓶 1 只，倒入冰醋酸，然后慢慢加入面粉，并用竹签调匀成糊状。使用时，用竹签挑糊状物涂疣，以完全盖住疣体为宜（切莫沾染好皮肤），厚度如钱币，约 10-20 分钟后药糊干燥，待 3-5 天后连同蚀死的疣组织一起自行脱落。疣的直径小于 0.5 厘米一次即可除去，大于 0. 5 厘米 2-3 次即除去。疣脱落后不留疤痕。

如涂药糊后感到轻度灼热，为正常现象。若疼痛难忍，应马上去除，并将患处浸于水中，待愈后再重新施治。

1. Glacial acetic acid paste for benign warts: Use 2–3 ml of pure glacial acetic acid and an appropriate amount of flour. Take a clean, dry penicillin vial, pour in the glacial acetic acid, then gradually add flour while stirring with a bamboo stick to form a paste. When applying, use the bamboo stick to pick up the paste and apply it to the wart, ensuring complete coverage of the lesion (avoid contact with healthy skin); the thickness should be coin-like. The paste will dry in about 10–20 minutes, and after 3–5 days, it will fall off naturally along with the necrotic

wart tissue. Warts less than 0.5 cm in diameter can be removed in one application, while those larger than 0.5 cm require 2–3 applications. No scarring remains after the wart falls off. Mild burning sensation after application is normal; if pain becomes unbearable, remove the paste immediately, soak the affected area in water, and resume treatment only after healing.

《民族医药报》（施秋林）

Ethnic Medicine News (Shi Qiulin).

2. 疣类是一种好发于手、足、面部有碍于美容的皮肤病，目前对该疾尚无特效疗法。广西融安县皮防站韦湘自 1986 年以来，采用三氯化铁酊治疗这类皮肤病患者取得较好疗效。具体是：用棉签蘸适量三氯化铁酊（三氯化铁 14. 0 克，蒸馏水 21.0 毫升，95% 酒精加至 100 毫升），涂于疣体表面，再用蘸有三氯化铁酊的棉签用力推擦疣体，一般 1 个疣体推擦 3-5 次即可脱落。后用三氯化铁酊涂布或压迫止血；扁平疣和线状疣的治疗则是先用棉签蘸三氯化铁酊涂布于疣体表面，再用刮匙将疣体刮掉，后用蘸有三氯化铁酊的棉签涂于疣的基底部。术后须预防感染，7-10 天痂皮脱落而痊愈。

2. Warts are a cosmetically disfiguring skin disease commonly occurring on the hands, feet, and face, for which there is currently no specific cure. Since 1986, Wei Xiang from the Skin Disease Prevention Station of Rong’an County, Guangxi, has achieved good therapeutic results using ferric chloride tincture. The specific method is as follows: Dip a cotton swab into an appropriate amount of ferric chloride tincture (14.0g ferric chloride, 21.0 ml distilled water, and 95% alcohol added to make 100 ml), apply it to the surface of the wart, and then vigorously rub the wart with the soaked swab; generally, rubbing 3–5 times per wart is sufficient for it to detach. Afterwards, apply ferric chloride tincture or apply pressure to stop bleeding. For flat warts and linear warts, first apply ferric chloride tincture to the wart surface with a cotton swab, scrape off the wart with a curette, and then apply the tincture to the base of the wart with another soaked swab. Postoperative infection prevention is necessary, and the scab typically falls off within 7–10 days, resulting in complete healing.

三氯化铁酊治疗疣类皮肤病每毫升可治疗几十个疣体，造价低，药液易配。只要棉签和刮匙，不论在城市、农村、家庭均可开展，不受医疗条件限制。此疗法曾在第四届全国皮肤美容学术研讨会上交流，得到专家学者的肯定。

Ferric chloride tincture is cost-effective and easy to prepare, with each milliliter capable of treating dozens of warts. Requiring only cotton swabs and a curette, this treatment can be performed in urban clinics, rural areas, or at home without being limited by medical facilities. This therapy was presented at the Fourth National Symposium on Dermatological Aesthetics and received positive recognition from experts and scholars.

《民族医药报》（广西 韦万春）

Ethnic Medicine News (Wei Wanchun, Guangxi).

扁平疣多见于青少年，好发于面、前臂与手背等部位。皮疹为米粒至黄豆大，呈肤色或淡褐色，扁平坚实的小丘疹，表面光滑发亮，有时皮疹数目众多如撒粟，或成群出现。因搔抓可自身接种，亦可沿抓痕而呈线形排列，愈后无疤痕。无自觉症状，有时微痒，日晒后常加重，病程缓慢，半数能自愈，常有新损害发生。如患有此症，可选用下述方药治疗。

Flat warts are most common in adolescents and frequently occur on the face, forearms, and dorsum of the hands. Lesions range from rice-grain to soybean size, appearing as flesh-colored or light brown, flat, firm papules with smooth, shiny surfaces; they may be numerous like scattered millet seeds or appear in clusters. Scratching can cause autoinoculation, leading to linear arrangement along scratch marks, and healing occurs without scarring. There are usually no subjective symptoms, though mild itching may occur, often exacerbated by sun exposure; the course is chronic, with spontaneous resolution in half of cases, but new lesions frequently develop. Patients with this condition may choose from the following herbal prescriptions.

3. 板蓝根 30 克，山豆根 10 克，香附 18 克，木贼草 10 克。水煎服，复渣外洗患处。

3. Decoct 30g isatis root, 10g tonkin sophora root, 18g cyperus rhizome, and

10g horsetail herb in water for oral administration; reuse the dregs for external washing of the affected area.

4. 生薏苡仁 30 克，大青叶 30 克，板蓝根 30 克，夏枯草 30 克。水煎服。

4. Decoct 30g raw coix seed, 30g folium isatidis, 30g isatis root, and 30g selfheal spike in water for oral administration.

5. 马齿苋 30 克，紫草 10 克，败酱草 15 克，大青叶 30 克煎水代茶饮。

5. Decoct 30g purslane, 10g arnebia root, 15g patrinia herb, and 30g folium isatidis in water to be drunk as tea.

6. 板蓝根 30 克，大青叶 30 克，香附 12 克，连翘 15 克，生薏苡仁 30 克水煎服。

6. Decoct 30g isatis root, 30g folium isatidis, 12g cyperus rhizome, 15g forsythia fruit, and 30g raw coix seed in water for oral administration.

7. 磁石 30 克，珍珠母 30 克，代赭石 15 克，生牡蛎 30 克，桃仁 9 克，红花 9 克，穿山甲 15 克，皂角刺 9 克，金银花 15 克，黄柏 12 克。水煎服。

7. Decoct 30g magnetite, 30g pearl shell, 15g hematite, 30g raw oyster shell, 9g peach kernel, 9g safflower, 15g pangolin scale, 9g gleditsia spine, 15g honeysuckle flower, and 12g phellodendron bark in water for oral administration.

8. 马齿苋 30 克，苍术 9 克，露蜂房 9 克，白芷 9 克，细辛 6 克，蛇床子 12 克，苦参 15 克，陈皮 6 克。煎水热洗，每天 2-3 次，至皮损处略变红色为度。

8. Decoct 30g purslane, 9g atractylodes rhizome, 9g honeycomb, 9g angelica dahurica, 6g asarum herb, 12g cnidium fruit, 15g sophora flavescens root, and 6g dried tangerine peel in water; wash the affected area with the warm decoction 2–3 times daily until the skin lesions turn slightly red.

9. 治寻常疣：以鲜田七叶、食盐各适量捣烂涂搽患处，每日搽 3-5 次，3-5 天有效。或用生田七粉每次 1 克，每日 3 次，以开水送服，5 天可愈。

《民族医药报》

Treatment for common warts: Mash an appropriate amount of fresh Panax notoginseng leaves and salt together, apply to the affected area 3–5 times daily; effective within 3–5 days. Alternatively, take 1g of raw Panax notoginseng powder three times daily with boiling water; curable within 5 days.

Ethnic Medicine News.

单位中药治扁平疣集锦

Collection of Single-Herb TCM Remedies for Flat Warts

10. 取生青苦瓜，剖开去籽，放入酸菜水中复泡一周后取出切碎，在油锅中爆炒 1 分钟，盛入盘中作菜食用，一日 3 次，每次 100 克，连续食用半月左右，可获痊愈。

10.Take fresh green bitter melon, cut open and remove seeds, soak in pickled vegetable brine for one week, then remove, chop, stir-fry in a hot pan for 1 minute, and serve as a dish; consume 100g per serving, three times daily for about half a month to achieve full recovery.

11. 鸦胆子适量，取 10 毫升左右的干净小瓶，将捣烂的鸦胆子连仁带皮倒入，加等体积 75% 乙醇，浸泡一夜，用棉签蘸取乙醇液外搽患处，每天 2-3 次，一周左右局部结痂并逐渐脱萎，不留瘢痕。

11.Take an appropriate amount of Brucea javanica fruit, place the mashed fruit (with seed and skin) into a clean 10ml vial, add an equal volume of 75% ethanol, soak overnight, dip a cotton swab into the ethanol solution and apply externally to the affected area 2–3 times daily; local scabbing occurs within about one week and gradually falls off without leaving scars.

12. 红花 10 克泡开水饮，至无色则丢去，每日一剂，局部红、热、痒感为有效反应，妇女经期停服，治疗 6 列均痊愈。

12.Steep 10g safflower in boiling water and drink until the liquid turns colorless, then discard; take one dose daily. Local redness, warmth, and itching indicate an effective response; discontinue during menstruation. All 6 treated cases were cured.

13. 鸡内金 20 克，加水 200 毫升，浸泡 2-3 天外搽患处，每日 5 至 6 次，一般外搽 10 天，扁平疣即干涸缩小而脱落，治疗 10 例皆获良效。

13.Soak 20g chicken gizzard lining in 200ml water for 2–3 days, apply externally to the affected area 5–6 times daily; after approximately 10 days of external application, flat warts dry up, shrink, and fall off. All 10 treated cases achieved good results.

14. 生香附 20 粒洗净，碾碎加鸡蛋或鸭蛋一个熟炒，隔日或 2-4 日吃，5-8 次为一疗程，儿童用 10-15 粒。孕妇忌用。

14.Wash 20 raw cyperus rhizomes, crush them, stir-fry with one chicken or duck egg until cooked, and consume every other day or every 2–4 days; 5–8 doses constitute one course of treatment. Use 10–15grains for children. Contraindicated for pregnant women.

15. 用鲜蒺藜 250 克，加水两碗水煎滤过后待用，先用 10% 的洗必泰消毒患部，然后用药液洗患处，每日 2 次，2- 3 天即愈。

《中药科技报》1997 年 9 月 26 日（王东萍）

15.Decoct 250g fresh tribulus fruit in two bowls of water, filter, and set aside; first disinfect the affected area with 10% chlorhexidine, then wash with the herbal decoction twice daily; curable within 2–3 days. Journal of Traditional

Chinese Medicine Science and Technology, September 26, 1997 (Wang Dongping).

16. 碘酒治扁平疣特效

扁平疣属慢性病毒感染引起的一种皮肤疾患，多发生在暴露部位，如发生在面部则不同程度地影响容貌。

笔者因自己孩子患扁平疣 3 年有余，用多种中药外洗，并肌注聚肌胞、干扰素均无显效，而用碘酒外涂一个月后竟痊愈；继续用此方治疗患者 40 例全部治愈。

具体方法为：用 2% 碘酒外涂患处，每日 2 次。对发生在面部的扁平疣患儿，为了不影响其容貌美观，可每晚一次，晨起洗掉，连用 1 个月即可痊愈。

碘酒对表皮组织的穿透力特强，对多种病原体均有杀灭作用，故长期涂抹患处，可将表皮组织中的病毒杀灭，继而痊愈。

16.Iodine tincture is highly effective for flat warts: Flat warts are a chronic viral skin infection that commonly occurs on exposed areas; facial involvement can affect appearance to varying degrees. The author’s child had flat warts for over three years with no significant improvement from various external TCM washes or intramuscular injections of polyinosinic-polycytidylic acid and interferon, but was unexpectedly cured after one month of topical iodine tincture application; subsequently, all 40 patients treated with this method were fully cured. Specific method: Apply 2% iodine tincture topically to the affected area twice daily. For pediatric patients with facial flat warts, to preserve cosmetic appearance, apply once nightly and wash off in the morning; continuous use for one month leads to complete healing. Iodine tincture has strong penetration into epidermal tissue and broad-spectrum pathogen-killing activity; prolonged topical application eliminates viruses within the epidermis, resulting in cure.

17. 治疗扁平疣中药（苡仁、炙黄芪、大青叶、马齿苋、红花、紫草）水煎服；西药聚肌胞肌肉注射，治疗扁平疣效果好，优于单用中药。两者合用有协同作用。

（陕西省西乡县中医院 吴照平）

17.Oral administration of a TCM decoction (coix seed, honey-fried astragalus root, folium isatidis, purslane, safflower, arnebia root) combined with intramuscular injection of polyinosinic-polycytidylic acid yields superior therapeutic effects for flat warts compared to TCM alone; the combination demonstrates synergistic action.

(Wu Zhaoping, Xixiang County TCM Hospital, Shaanxi Province)

八、白发（6方）

remature Graying of Hair (6 Prescriptions):

1. 桑椹蜜汁。到果品店买鲜桑椹二斤或到中药店买干桑椹一斤，用清水洗净，加适量的水煎煮，半小时后滤出煎好的液汁，然后再加适量的水煎煮半小时滤出液汁。将两次煎好的液汁掺和在一起后，用小火煎煮使其浓缩，待其稠粘时加入蜂蜜六两，一起煮沸后任其自然冷却，倒入玻璃瓶内密封备用。每次取一汤匙桑椹蜜汁，用开水冲化饮用；每日两次，常饮可使头发保持乌亮的光泽。

1. Mulberry Honey Syrup: Purchase two jin of fresh mulberries from a fruit

store or one jin of dried mulberries from a TCM pharmacy, wash them thoroughly with clean water, add an appropriate amount of water and decoct for half an hour, then filter out the liquid; repeat the process by adding water again, decocting for another half hour, and filtering. Combine the two batches of decocted liquid, simmer over low heat to concentrate until viscous, add six liang of honey when thickened, bring to a boil together, allow to cool naturally, and store in a sealed glass jar for later use. Take one tablespoon of mulberry honey syrup each time, dissolve in boiling water and drink twice daily; regular consumption helps maintain dark, lustrous hair.

2. 芝麻桑葚蜜。将黑芝麻、鲜桑椹各半斤，一起捣烂成糊状，再加入适量的蜂蜜调匀，置于密封瓶内。每日三次，每次取一汤匙用开水冲服，如连服两个疗程效果更佳。

2. Sesame-Mulberry Honey Paste: Mash half a jin each of black sesame seeds and fresh mulberries into a paste, mix evenly with an appropriate amount of honey, and store in a sealed jar. Take one tablespoon three times daily, dissolved in boiling water; better results can be achieved if taken continuously for two courses of treatment.

3. 黑芝麻粥。每天用黑芝麻半两与适量的大米煮成粥，佐餐食用，可起乌发护发作用。

3. Black Sesame Porridge: Cook half a liang of black sesame seeds with an appropriate amount of rice into porridge daily, and consume as a side dish with meals; this helps darken and nourish the hair.

4. 桃仁蜜饯。到中药房或药店买二斤桃仁，放在干净的冷水中浸泡三天，漂去苦味后取出，剥掉桃仁皮。然后将适量的白糖放入锅中，待其融化后即倒入桃仁中拌匀。每天二次，每次吃十粒蜜饯桃仁，不仅可护发乌发，而且对“少白头”也有一定的疗效。《民族医药报》1992 年 2 月 14 日（江苏 纪国安）。

4. Candied Peach Kernels: Purchase two jin of peach kernels from a TCM pharmacy or drugstore, soak them in clean cold water for three days, rinse to remove bitterness, remove, and peel off the skin. Place an appropriate amount of

white sugar in a pan, melt it, pour over the peeled peach kernels, and mix evenly. Consume ten candied peach kernels twice daily; this not only nourishes and darkens hair but also has certain therapeutic effects on premature graying. Ethnic Medicine News, February 14, 1992 (Ji Guoan, Jiangsu).

5. 青年白发：黑豆适量，九蒸九晒后，每次取 6 克，口嚼后用淡盐水送下，每日 2 次。

5. Premature Graying in Youth: Take an appropriate amount of black beans, steam and sun-dry them nine times alternately, then take 6g per dose, chew thoroughly, and swallow with light salt water twice daily.

6. 各种白发病：黑豆 120 克，米醋 500 克，以醋煮豆成稀糊状，过滤后，以牙刷蘸药醋外刷毛发，每日 2 次。

6. Various Types of Hair Whitening: Simmer 120g black beans in 500g rice vinegar until a thin paste forms, filter the mixture, dip a toothbrush into the medicated vinegar, and brush the hair externally twice daily.

九、头皮屑（3 方）：

IX. Dandruff (3 Prescriptions):

1. 内服四物汤加味：生地 10 克，当归 10 克，白芍 10 克，红花 10 克，桃仁 10 克，秦艽 10 克，蝉蜕 10 克，荆芥穗 10 克，防风 10 克，僵蚕 10 克，川芎 6 克，水煎 2 次，分 2 次早晚服，日 1 剂。外治方：苦杏仁、猪油各 30 克，共捣如膏状，布包，火上烤热后擦患处，日 2-3 次。去头皮屑结果：治疗 18 例，3 例在 13 天内治愈，13 例在 15-20 天内治愈，2 例在 25 天内治愈。《民族医药报》

1. Oral administration of modified Siwu Decoction: 10g each of raw rehmannia root, Chinese angelica root, white peony root, safflower, peach kernel, gentiana macrophylla root, cicada slough, schizonepeta spike, fangfeng, and stiff silkworm, plus 6g ligusticum wallichii rhizome; decoct twice in water, divide into two doses taken morning and evening, one dose per day. External prescription: Mash 30g each of bitter apricot kernel and lard into a paste, wrap in cloth, roast

over fire until warm, and rub onto the affected area 2–3 times daily. Results for dandruff removal: Of 18 treated cases, 3 were cured within 13 days, 13 within 15–20 days, and 2 within 25 days. Ethnic Medicine News.

2. 自述：很多人都知道用硫磺软膏能抑制头皮屑的产生，可没过多久，头皮屑又出现了，关键是他们不会洗头。我教赵女士一个正确的方法，保管有用。当你用硫磺软膏洗头时，在最后一遍用水清洗时，要捏点盐、倒些醋进去，少许即可。用这样的水洗后，头发不但光滑，而且消毒止痒。通常 3 天洗一次头，一个月就差不多了，同时最好吃点鱼肝油等富含维生素 A 和维生素 C 的食物。十几年前，我按此坚持洗了半个月头，头皮屑就无影无踪了，至今未犯。（王先生）

2. Personal account: Many people know that sulfur ointment can inhibit dandruff, but it often returns shortly after because they do not wash their hair correctly. I taught Ms. Zhao a proper method that is guaranteed to work. When washing your hair with sulfur ointment, during the final rinse, add a pinch of salt and a splash of vinegar—just a small amount is sufficient. Washing with this water not only makes hair smooth but also disinfects and relieves itching. Typically, washing once every three days for about a month is adequate, and it is best to simultaneously consume foods rich in vitamins A and C, such as cod liver oil. Over ten years ago, I persisted with this washing method for half a month, and my dandruff disappeared completely without recurrence to this day. (Mr. Wang)

3. 白屑病，现代医学称为“干性皮脂溢出”症，多顽固久治难愈。表现为头部瘙痒，头皮遍布白色，大量干燥白屑，瘙痒时脱屑纷纷落下。笔者用下述方治疗该症效果显著。大黄、硫磺各 15 克，共研成细末，以冷开水调成糊状，涂搽头部（先剃净头发）。过 4 小时后，再以温开水冲泡狗头骨灰将头部洗净。隔日 1 次，一般连用 3-5 次可获良效。此外，用该方治疗脂溢性皮炎、酒糟鼻及痤疮等症，疗效亦颇佳。《民族医药报》1992 年 5 月 1 日（江西 钟久春）

3. Pityriasis simplex capitis, termed “dry seborrhea” in modern medicine, is often stubborn and difficult to cure despite prolonged treatment. It manifests as scalp itching, widespread white scaling, abundant dry flakes, and shedding of scales upon scratching. The author has achieved remarkable results treating

this condition with the following prescription: Grind 15g each of rhubarb and sulfur into fine powder, mix with cool boiled water to form a paste, and apply to the scalp (after shaving the head completely). After 4 hours, wash the head clean using warm water infused with dog skull ash. Apply once every other day; generally, 3–5 consecutive applications yield excellent results. Additionally, this formula shows good efficacy in treating seborrheic dermatitis, rosacea, and acne. Ethnic Medicine News, May 1, 1992 (Zhong Jiuchun, Jiangxi).

十、口干唇裂（3 方）：

X.Dry Mouth and Chapped Lips (3 Prescriptions):

1. 药物组成：太子参 20 克，沙参 15 克，玄参 15 克，黄芪 30 克，麦冬 15 克，乌梅 15 克，玉竹 15 克，五味子 10 克，茯苓 20 克，山药 30 克。用法：每日一剂，文火水煎两次兑匀，早晚分服。方中太子参、黄芪、山药、茯苓补气健脾益胃；沙参、玄参、麦冬、玉竹养阴增液润燥；乌梅、五味子生津止渴。诸药合之，乃健脾益胃，养阴润燥，生津增液之良方。故对老年人脾胃阴虚而致口干症，颇有效验。

1. Composition: 20g Prince ginseng, 15g glehnia root, 15g scrophularia root, 30g astragalus root, 15g ophiopogon tuber, 15g dark plum, 15g fragrant solomonseal rhizome, 10g schisandra fruit, 20g poria, and 30g Chinese yam. Usage: Take one dose daily, decoct twice in water over low heat, mix the two decoctions evenly, and take in divided doses morning and evening. In this formula, Prince ginseng, astragalus root, Chinese yam, and poria tonify qi, strengthen the spleen, and benefit the stomach; glehnia root, scrophularia root, ophiopogon tuber, and fragrant solomonseal rhizome nourish yin, increase body fluids, and moisten dryness; dark plum and schisandra fruit generate fluid and quench thirst. The combination of these herbs forms an excellent prescription for strengthening the spleen and stomach, nourishing yin, moistening dryness, and generating body fluids. Therefore, it is quite effective for dry mouth caused by

spleen-stomach yin deficiency in the elderly.

2. 每晚临睡前取枸杞子（宁夏杞子最佳）30 克，用冷开水轻轻洗净后，徐徐嚼服。枸杞子 30-50 克，麦冬 10 克，甘草 3 克。水煎每日分二次服。一般连服 3-4 剂可愈。《健康报》1998 年 2 月 20 日（梁庆森）

2. Every night before bedtime, take 30g of wolfberry fruit (Ningxia wolfberry is preferred), gently wash it with cool boiled water, and chew slowly before swallowing. Alternatively, decoct 30–50g wolfberry fruit, 10g ophiopogon tuber, and 3g licorice root in water, and take in two divided doses daily. Generally, recovery can be achieved after taking 3–4 consecutive doses. Health News, February 20, 1998 (Liang Qingsen).

3. 治疗嘴唇干裂可用滋阴汤: 生地 20 克, 元参 20 克, 麦冬 15 克, 天冬 15 克，花粉 15 克，沙参 15 克，桔梗 15 克，射干 10 克，百合 30 克，玉竹 15 克，金银花 20 克，连翘 20 克，甘草 6 克，水煎服。还可以配合唇裂散等一些中成药口服。

3. For chapped lips, Nourishing Yin Decoction can be used: Decoct 20g raw rehmannia root, 20g scrophularia root, 15g ophiopogon tuber, 15g asparagus tuber, 15g trichosanthes root, 15g glehnia root, 15g platycodon root, 10g belamcanda rhizome, 30g lily bulb, 15g fragrant solomonseal rhizome, 20g honeysuckle flower, 20g forsythia fruit, and 6g licorice root in water for oral administration. It can also be combined with oral intake of patent medicines such as Chapped Lip Powder.

十一、酒糟鼻（2 方）:

XI. Rosacea (2 Prescriptions):

1. 酒糟鼻是一种常见的鼻部疾患，以鼻尖红赤灼痛为其特征。其病因系脾经湿热，肝肺火郁，熏蒸鼻窍所致。据临床报道，以如下验方治疗多例，均取得满意疗效，具体方法为：处方：绿豆 750 克，荷花瓣 100 克（晒干），滑石 25 克，白芷 25 克，白附子 25 克，冰片 10 克，密陀僧 10 克。制法及用法：以上药物共研为细末，为一料。用时将患处洗净，白天则以药末擦之，晚上则以温水将药调成糊状，封涂于患部，晨起则洗去，如此用药，至愈为度。《民族医药报》1993 年 2 月 26 日（桂 荐）。

1. Rosacea is a common nasal disorder characterized by redness and burning pain at the tip of the nose. Its etiology is attributed to damp-heat in the spleen channel and stagnated fire in the liver and lungs, which steam upward to affect the nasal orifices. Clinical reports indicate that multiple cases treated with the following proven prescription have achieved satisfactory results. Prescription: 750g mung beans, 100g dried lotus petals, 25g talcum powder, 25g angelica dahurica, 25g typhonium rhizome, 10g borneol, and 10g litharge. Preparation and usage: Grind all the above ingredients into a fine powder to make one batch. Wash the affected area thoroughly before application; during the day, rub the powder directly onto the lesion, and at night, mix the powder with warm water into a paste, apply it as a sealed coating to the affected area, and wash it off the next morning. Continue this regimen until full recovery. Ethnic Medicine News, February 26, 1993 (Recommended by Gui).

2. 治疗酒渣鼻：内服大黄、黄连、生地、葛根、红花 、赤芍、栀子、甘草，外用 10% 硫磺霜涂搽局部，治疗酒渣鼻效果好。

2. Treatment for rosacea: Oral administration of rhubarb, coptis rhizome, raw rehmannia root, kudzu root, safflower, red peony root, gardenia fruit, and licorice root, combined with topical application of 10% sulfur cream to the affected area, yields good therapeutic effects for rosacea.

十二、瘢痕疙瘩（1 方）：
XII. Keloid (1 Prescription):

1. 瘢痕疙瘩：蜂蜜 18 毫升，食醋 250 毫升，五倍子 78 克，蜈蚣 1 条，用砂锅作煎器，炭火熬成稠膏装入陶瓷器皿备用。先用浓茶水洗净患处再用药膏少许外敷患部，每日换药 1 次。连用两周，病变组织逐渐软化、萎缩。

1. For keloid: Combine 18 ml honey, 250 ml vinegar, 78g Chinese gallnut, and

one centipede in an earthenware pot, simmer over charcoal fire into a thick paste, and store in a ceramic container for later use. First wash the affected area with strong tea water, then apply a small amount of the ointment externally; change the dressing once daily. After two weeks of continuous application, the diseased tissue gradually softens and atrophies.

第七章　骨病科
Chapter VII Orthopedics

一、关节炎（13 方）
I. Arthritis (13 Prescriptions)

1. 肩周炎是以肩关节周围疼痛和关节功能活动受限为主要表现的一种常见疾病，主要好发于中老年人而尤以女性多见。下面介绍一种用中药外敷治疗肩周炎的方法。取中药川乌、草乌各 90 克，樟脑 90 克，白芷 50 克，共研细末装瓶备用。使用时根据疼痛部位大小，取药末适量，用食醋与蜂蜜调成糊状外敷于肩部疼痛点，药厚约 0.5 毫米左右，外用绷带或纱布固定，并以热水袋外敷 30 分钟，每日一次，连用一周至半月，可消除疼痛，恢复关节功能。《民族医药报》（陕西安康地委党校 绪林）。

1. Periarthritis of the shoulder is a common condition primarily characterized by pain around the shoulder joint and restricted joint mobility, predominantly affecting middle-aged and elderly individuals, especially women. The following introduces a method of external application of Chinese herbal medicine for treating periarthritis of the shoulder. Take 90g each of Sichuan aconite root and Kusnezoff monkshood root, 90g camphor, and 50g angelica dahurica; grind them together into a fine powder and store in a bottle for later use. When applying, take an appropriate amount of the powder according to the size of the painful area, mix it with vinegar and honey to form a paste, and apply externally to the painful point on the shoulder with a thickness of approximately 0.5 mm; secure it with a bandage or gauze, and apply a hot water bottle externally for 30 minutes. Use once daily for one week to half a month to eliminate pain and restore joint function.

Ethnic Medicine News (Xu Lin, Party School of Ankang Prefectural Committee, Shaanxi).

2. 肩周炎，又称漏肩风，是一种常见病，多发生于中老年人，冬天尤甚。现把民间治疗肩周炎的一则验方介绍于下，供患者试用。取生川乌、生草乌各100克，晒干或微火烘干研为细末，加入樟脑120克和适量米酒糟（或米醋）调匀，稍蒸热后敷于患处，绷带包扎固定；或把药末与米醋调匀后，装入纱布袋内，睡前放患处，药袋上放一个热水袋即可。每天晚上敷药，一般连敷4-5晚即可收到理想的疗效。《民族医药报》1992年2月14日（广西 梁庆森）。

2. Periarthritis of the shoulder, also known as "leaked shoulder wind," is a common disease that mostly occurs in middle-aged and elderly people, particularly in winter. A folk proven prescription for treating periarthritis of the shoulder is introduced below for patients to try. Take 100g each of raw Sichuan aconite root and raw Kusnezoff monkshood root, sun-dry or dry over low heat, and grind into fine powder; add 120g camphor and an appropriate amount of rice wine lees (or rice vinegar), mix evenly, steam slightly until warm, apply to the affected area, and secure with a bandage. Alternatively, mix the powder evenly with rice vinegar, place it in a gauze bag, put it on the affected area before sleep, and place a hot water bottle on top of the bag. Apply the medication every night; generally, ideal therapeutic effects can be achieved after 4–5 consecutive nights of application. Ethnic Medicine News, February 14, 1992 (Liang Qingsen, Guangxi).

土家医治关节痛偏方：3. 螃蟹泥治肩关节周围炎。方法：捉活螃蟹一个，小的则捉二个，先让螃蟹在清水中泡半天，待其把腹中的泥排完，后取出捣成肉泥，将捣好的螃蟹泥，摊在纱布上，直径不宜超过8厘米，贴敷在肩胛最疼的区域。晚上8点贴上，第二天早晨8点取掉。1-2次即有效。

Tujia Folk Remedies for Joint Pain: 3. Crab paste for periarthritis of the shoulder. Method: Catch one live crab (or two if small), soak it in clean water for half a day to allow it to expel mud from its abdomen, then remove and mash it into a meat paste. Spread the mashed crab paste on gauze with a diameter not exceeding 8 cm, and apply it to the most painful area of the scapula. Apply at 8 p.m.

and remove at 8 a.m. the next morning. Effective within 1–2 applications.

4. 近年来，笔者在医疗实践中，应用下述外治方治疗风湿性关节炎多例，效果显著。外洗：取桃树节、杉树节、桑树节、松树节各 100 克（鲜品加倍），加水煎汤去渣，趁热熏洗患处，每日 2 次，连洗 7-10 日即可。外敷：棉花籽 250 克，炒热敷患关节，每日 2 次，连用 7-10 日。《民族医药报》1992 年 4 月 24 日（钟久春）。

4. In recent years, the author has applied the following external treatment prescriptions to treat multiple cases of rheumatoid arthritis in clinical practice with remarkable results. External wash: Take 100g each of peach tree nodes, fir tree nodes, mulberry tree nodes, and pine tree nodes (double the amount for fresh herbs), decoct in water, remove the dregs, and fumigate and wash the affected area while hot twice daily for 7–10 consecutive days. External application: Stir-fry 250g cotton seeds until hot, apply to the affected joint twice daily, and continue for 7–10 consecutive days. Ethnic Medicine News, April 24, 1992 (Zhong Jiuchun).

5. 内服方：生川乌、生草乌、川木瓜、川牛膝、当归、川芎、银花、麻黄、乌梅、防风、秦艽、全虫各 9 克，白术、杜仲、仙灵脾各 12 克，蜈蚣 3 条（去头足），高粱酒或米酒 250 克，红糖 250 克。

Internal Prescription: Raw Chuanwu (Aconitum carmichaelii), Raw Caowu (Aconitum kusnezoffii), Sichuan Papaya (Chaenomeles speciosa), Sichuan Achyranthes (Cyathula officinalis), Angelica sinensis, Ligusticum chuanxiong, Honeysuckle, Ephedra, Dark Plum (Mume Fructus), Saposhnikovia divaricata, Gentiana macrophylla, and Scorpion each 9g; Atractylodes macrocephala, Eucommia bark, and Epimedium each 12g; Centipede 3 pieces (heads and feet removed); Sorghum liquor or rice wine 250g; Brown sugar 250g.

制法及用法：将上药和糖、酒一起放入一个能容纳 3 公斤水的陶罐内，用干净棉布封口，黄泥糊紧。置文火上炖 2 小时后，取出埋于潮湿之地以除火毒，24 小时后取出滤渣即成。每次服 35 毫升，于饭后服，每日 3 次。10 天为一疗程。

Preparation and Administration: Place the above herbs, sugar, and wine together in a ceramic jar capable of holding 3 liters of water. Seal the mouth with clean cotton cloth and tighten with yellow mud. Simmer over a gentle fire for 2 hours. Remove the jar and bury it in damp ground to eliminate «fire toxicity.» After 24 hours, remove it, filter out the dregs, and the liquid is ready for use. Take 35 ml each time, after meals, three times daily. Ten days constitute one course of treatment.

6. 外用方：生川乌一枚，用粗底瓷碗底盛上白酒 3 毫升，磨汁外涂于痛处。每日涂擦 2-3 次，10 天为一疗程。

External Prescription: One piece of raw Chuanwu (Aconitum carmichaelii). Grind it into juice using 3 ml of white liquor on the bottom of a coarse porcelain bowl. Apply the juice externally to the painful area. Rub 2–3 times daily. Ten days constitute one course of treatment.

《民族医药报》1992 年 5 月 15 日（江西 俞瑜 俞琳）

Source: "Ethnic Medicine News," May 15, 1992 (Jiangxi Province; Authors: Yu Yu, Yu Lin)

7. 黑木耳 150-200 克，用水浸透后，用米酒煎熟（不加油盐），日内分 2-3 次把酒和木耳吃完。

7.Soak 150–200g of black wood ear mushrooms in water until fully hydrated. Then, decoct them in rice wine (without adding oil or salt) until cooked. Consume both the wine and the mushrooms within the day, divided into 2–3 doses.

8. 枫荷桂 500 克，大活血（槟榔钻） 500 克，走马胎 500 克，川牛七 200 克，通城虎 30 克，桂枝 30 克，同 45 度米酒 4-5 公斤浸泡 30 天，每天早晚各饮 15-30 毫升（晚上睡前饮至微醉更佳）。不饮酒者，取上药各一半煎水加白酒一小杯内服，日 2 次。

8.Soak the following ingredients in 4–5 kg of 45-proof rice wine for 30 days: Fenghegui (likely Illicium verum or a local variant) 500g, Da Huoxue (Binlangzuan/Rhizoma Arisaematis or similar local herb) 500g, Zoumatai (Ardisia gigantifolia) 500g, Sichuan Niuxi (Cyathula officinalis) 200g, Tongchenghu (Stephania tetrandra or similar) 30g, and Cinnamon Twig (Guizhi) 30g. Drink 15–30 ml every morning and evening (drinking until slightly tipsy before bedtime is considered more effective). For those who do not consume alcohol, take half the amount of the above herbs, decoct them in water, add a small cup of white liquor, and take internally twice daily.

9. 走马胎 500 克，红枣 50 克，同猪脊龙骨适量煎食（可加盐），日服 2 次。

9.Decoct 500g of Zoumatai (Ardisia gigantifolia) and 50g of red dates with an appropriate amount of pork spine bones (salt may be added). Consume as food twice daily.

10. 陈茶子麸（收藏 5 年以上的）榨出油后之油茶籽饼、陈薯藤（贮藏 2-3 年以上的老红薯藤）、陈墙石灰（几十年以上的旧居壁上石灰）各 500 克，同煎水趁热洗患部，日 2 次，连洗 7 天。

10.Use 500g each of the following: Oil-extracted tea seed cake from old tea seeds (stored for more than 5 years), old sweet potato vines (stored for 2–3 years), and old wall lime (from walls of residences decades old). Decoct these ingredients in water and wash the affected area while the liquid is still hot. Do this twice daily for 7 consecutive days.

11. 樟树皮（取面向东方的二层皮）、山栀、五加皮各 12 克，共研末，加米酒糟捣匀，患部不发热者蒸热敷之；皮肤烫热者冷敷。早晚解下一小时后，另用此三味药煎水洗患部，再敷上原药，连敷 2 天。又可用此方药物浸白酒，每天酌量分服。

11.Take 12g each of Camphor tree bark (the second layer of bark facing east), Gardenia fruit, and Acanthopanax bark. Grind them into powder and mix uniformly with rice wine lees. If the affected area is not hot to the touch, apply the mixture as a hot compress (steamed); if the skin feels hot, apply it as a cold compress. Remove the compress after one hour in the morning and evening. Then, wash the affected area with a decoction made from these same three ingredients, and reapply the original medicinal paste. Continue this for 2 days. Alternatively, these herbs can be soaked in white liquor and consumed orally in moderate amounts daily.

12. 蚕砂 150 克，食盐 150 克，同炒热入布袋熨患部，立即止痛。

12.Stir-fry 150g of silkworm excrement (Can Sha) and 150g of salt until hot. Place them in a cloth bag and apply as a hot compress to the affected area to provide immediate pain relief.

关节炎患者在服药治疗期间应忌食酸、辣、生冷食品及猪肝猪血、羊肝羊血、鹅肉、草鱼等品。

Dietary Restrictions: During the course of treatment for arthritis, patients should avoid acidic, spicy, and raw/cold foods, as well as pork liver, pork blood, sheep liver, sheep blood, goose meat, and grass carp.

《民族医药报》1992 年 7 月 3 日（广西 梁庆森）

Source: "Ethnic Medicine News," July 3, 1992 (Guangxi Province; Author: Liang Qingsen)

13. 五枝煎治膝关节炎

Five-Twig Decoction for Knee Osteoarthritis:

处方：桃枝 30 克，桑枝 30 克，柳枝 30 克，竹枝 30 克，酸枣枝 30 克。

用法：上药均以鲜枝入药，粗细似筷子，切成一寸长短，放入 3000 毫升水中煎煮。煎成的五枝液，趁热放入盆中；让病人睡下，盖上棉被，不得漏气，双膝屈曲，将药盆放在双膝之下，让蒸气熏蒸膝关节，待下肢发汗为宜，约一小时左右，每天一次，连续 10 天为一疗程。

The prescription consists of 30g peach twig, 30g mulberry twig, 30g willow twig, 30g bamboo twig, and 30g sour jujube twig. For usage, all the above medicinal materials should be used as fresh twigs; select twigs with a thickness similar to chopsticks, cut them into one-cun lengths, and decoct them in 3000ml of water. Pour the prepared five-twig liquid into a basin while hot; have the patient lie down and cover with a quilt to prevent heat from escaping, bend both knees, place the medicinal basin beneath the knees, and use the steam to fumigate the knee joints until the lower limbs sweat slightly. Each session lasts about one hour, administered once daily, with 10 consecutive days constituting one course of treatment.

《民族医药报》1991 年 11 月 5 日（湖南 侯启年）

This formula was provided by Hou Qinian from Hunan and published in the Ethnic Medicine News on November 5, 1991.

二、坐骨神经痛（6 方）
Sciatica (6 Formulas):

坐骨神经痛属中医痹证（筋痹）范畴。本病虽非危急重症，然病情缠绵，给患者造成诸多不便。现介绍效方数则，供患者选用。

Sciatica falls under the category of Bi syndrome (tendon Bi) in Traditional Chinese Medicine. Although this condition is not a critical or life-threatening disease, its prolonged and lingering nature causes significant inconvenience to patients. Several effective formulas are hereby introduced for patients’ reference and selection.

1. 生鸡蛋一个，蜈蚣一条。将蜈蚣研成末，将鸡蛋敲一小孔后放入蜈蚣粉，用面粉调湿密封其孔，蒸熟或烧熟后食用，每日一次，每次一个，连服 10 日有效。

1.Take one raw egg and one centipede; grind the centipede into a fine powder, make a small hole in the egg, insert the centipede powder through the hole, seal it with moistened dough, and then steam or bake until cooked. Consume one egg daily, and effects can be observed after 10 consecutive days of administration.

2. 用八角枫根 30 克研细末，用白开水（稍冷）送服，每日服三次。

Grind 30g of Alangium chinense root into a fine powder and take it with slightly cool boiled water, three times daily.

3. 皂刺 20 克、生地 20 克、玄参 20 克、石斛 10 克、知母 10 克、桑寄生 20 克。每日一剂，水煎服。服 10 剂为一疗程。

3.The prescription includes 20g Chinese honeylocust spine, 20g raw rehmannia root, 20g figwort root, 10g dendrobium stem, 10g anemarrhena rhizome, and 20g Chinese taxillus herb; decoct one dose in water daily for oral administration, with 10 doses constituting one course of treatment.

4. 生黄芪 30 克，木瓜、玄胡各 20 克，赤白芍、当归、怀膝各 15 克，海风藤、苍术、防风各12克，土鳖10克，桂枝、甘草各6克。水煎内服，每日一剂，10剂为一疗程。

《民族医药报》1992年7月3日（四川 陶昔安）

The prescription comprises 30g raw astragalus root, 20g each of papaya fruit and corydalis tuber, 15g each of red peony root, white peony root, Chinese angelica root, and Huai achyranthes root, 12g each of kadsura pepper stem, atractylodes rhizome, and fangfeng root, 10g ground beetle, and 6g each of cassia twig and licorice root; decoct in water for oral administration, one dose daily, with 10 doses forming one course of treatment. Formulas 2 through 4 in this section were provided by Tao Xi' an from Sichuan and published in the Ethnic Medicine News on July 3, 1992.

5. 坐骨神经痛是临床上常见的综合病症，以腰腿掣痛、酸楚、着重、麻木为主要表现，重则出现功能障碍，多因风寒湿邪气阻滞经络、经脉气滞血淤所致。据此，笔者拟用"坐骨散"治疗坐骨神经痛45例。经过2-3年的详细观察，症状体征完全消失38例，症状体征明显改善减轻5例，无效2例。

Sciatica is a common clinical syndrome characterized primarily by pulling pain, soreness, heaviness, and numbness in the lower back and legs; severe cases may present with functional impairment, mostly caused by wind-cold-damp pathogens obstructing the meridians and resulting in qi stagnation and blood stasis. Based on this understanding, the author formulated "Zuogu San" (Sciatica Powder) to treat 45 cases of sciatica. After 2–3 years of detailed observation, symptoms and signs completely disappeared in 38 cases, significantly improved in 5 cases, and showed no response in 2 cases.

本方由乌蛇、全蝎、蜈蚣、土元、制乳香、制没药、当归、三七各等分组成。先将乌蛇、全蝎、蜈蚣、土元用瓦片培黄，与余药研成细末，每服6克。轻症日服2次，重症日服3次，黄酒冲服，以10天为一疗程，两个疗程间停药3-5天。一般用药1-3个疗程有显效或治愈，若服3个疗程后无效时改用他法治疗。

The formula consists of equal parts of Zaocys snake, scorpion, centipede, ground beetle, processed frankincense, processed myrrh, Chinese angelica root, and notoginseng. First, roast the Zaocys snake, scorpion, centipede, and ground beetle on a tile until yellowish, then grind them together with the remaining herbs into a fine powder. Take 6g per dose: twice daily for mild cases and three times daily for severe cases, mixed with yellow rice wine. Ten days constitute one course of treatment, with a 3–5 day break between courses. Significant improvement or cure is generally achieved within 1–3 courses; if no effect is observed after 3 courses, alternative treatments should be adopted.

《中医药信息报》1992 年 8 月 1 日（青海 刘启明）

This formula was provided by Liu Qiming from Qinghai and published in the Traditional Chinese Medicine Information News on August 1, 1992.

6. 简方治坐骨神经痛

乌梢蛇 10 克、蜈蚣 10 克、全蝎 10 克，焙干研成粉末，等分成八包，首日上下午各服 1 包，温开水送服，继之每日上午服 1 包，7 日为 1 疗程。

两个疗程间隔 3 至 5 天，一般 1 至 2 个疗程可显效至痊愈。

Simple Formula for Sciatica:

Take 10g of Zaocys snake, 10g of centipede, and 10g of scorpion; roast until dry, grind into powder, and divide equally into eight packets. On the first day, take one packet in the morning and one in the afternoon with warm boiled water; thereafter, take one packet every morning. Seven days constitute one course of treatment, with a 3–5 day interval between courses. Significant improvement to complete recovery is generally achieved within 1–2 courses.

《民族医药报》1992 年 4 月 24 日（贵州 杨通福）

This formula was provided by Yang Tongfu from Guizhou and published in the Ethnic Medicine News on April 24, 1992.

三、足跟痛（7 方）

III.Heel Pain (7 Formulas)

1. 处方及用法：威灵仙 40 克，石见穿 30 克，骨碎补 20 克，生草乌、山奈、急性子、椒目、马钱子、川乌各 10 克，蜈蚣 1 条。装纱布袋，浸入 1 公斤醋内，取液浸泡患足 30 分钟，天冷时可加热，浸泡后清水洗净。1 周换药 1 次，3 个月为 1 疗程。应用本法曾收治 500 例，结果：显效（症状消失，1 年内无复发）310 例，有效 130 例，无效 60 例，总有效率 88%。个别患者见皮肤痛，未见其它毒副反应。

Prescription and Usage: 40g Clematis root, 30g Chinese sage herb, 20g Drynaria rhizome, 10g each of raw kusnezoff monkshood root, sand ginger, impatient balsam seed, Sichuan pepper seed, strychnos seed, and Sichuan aconite root, plus 1 centipede. Place all ingredients in a gauze bag, soak in 1kg of vinegar, and use the liquid to soak the affected foot for 30 minutes; heat the liquid if the weather is cold, and rinse the foot with clean water after soaking. Replace the medicinal bag once a week, with 3 months constituting one course of treatment. This method was applied to 500 cases: 310 cases showed marked effectiveness (symptoms disappeared with no recurrence within 1 year), 130 cases were effective, and 60 cases were ineffective, yielding a total effective rate of 88%. A few patients experienced skin tingling, but no other toxic or adverse reactions were observed.

《民族医药报》

This formula was published in the Ethnic Medicine News.

2. 处方：生南星、生半夏、生草乌各 10 克。

用法：将上述三味中药共碾成细粉，充分混匀。取凡士林适量（无凡士林可用鸡蛋清）把药粉调配成糊状，均匀抹在足跟疼痛处，用胶布固定，每 3-4 天换药一次。一般用药一个月可控制足跟痛。

注意：治疗期间尽量少走路，勿过久站立。

Prescription: 10g each of raw jack-in-the-pulpit tuber, raw pinellia tuber, and raw kusnezoff monkshood root.

Usage: Grind the above three herbs into a fine powder and mix thoroughly. Add an appropriate amount of Vaseline (egg white can be used as a substitute if Vaseline is unavailable) to form a paste, apply evenly to the painful area of the heel, secure with adhesive tape, and replace the dressing every 3–4 days. Heel pain can generally be controlled after one month of treatment. Note: During treatment, minimize walking and avoid prolonged standing.

《民族医药报》1992 年 2 月 14 日（广东省　陈烈辉）

This formula was provided by Chen Liehui from Guangdong Province and published in the Ethnic Medicine News on February 14, 1992.

3. 用白芷 10 克，白术 10 克、防风 10 克，将其研末，装入一个布袋里。在使用前，将药袋放入清水中浸泡 15 分钟。另找一大半块砖头，在其中凿一个能放下药袋的凹坑，然后将砖放在炉火中，待烧热后，把砖取出放在平稳的地上，迅速往砖心凹坑里倒入食醋，把药袋放在凹坑中，再把脚跟慢慢地踏在布袋上面，熏 20 分钟，一般的病人熏二三次就见明显效果，五六次可巩固疗效。每次 1 剂。

Take 10g each of Angelica dahurica root, atractylodes rhizome, and fangfeng root; grind into powder and place in a cloth bag. Before use, soak the bag in clean water for 15 minutes. Take a large half-brick, carve a cavity in it to hold the medicinal bag, heat the brick over a stove, remove and place it steadily on the ground, quickly pour edible vinegar into the cavity, insert the medicinal bag, and then slowly step the heel onto the bag to fumigate for 20 minutes. Most patients show significant improvement after 2–3 sessions, and 5–6 sessions can consolidate the therapeutic effect; use one dose per session.

《民族医药报》1998 年 1 月 23 日（里　平）

This formula was provided by Li Ping and published in the Ethnic Medicine News on January 23, 1998.

4. 陈醋浸足法：用陈醋 2 斤，加热至足可浸入的温度，每日浸一小时。醋温下降后再次加热，一般浸 10-15 天，足跟痛开始逐渐减轻，连续浸 1-2 个月，可望恢复。

4.Aged Vinegar Foot Soak Method: Use 1kg of aged vinegar, heat to a temperature tolerable by the foot, and soak for one hour daily; reheat when the vinegar cools down. Heel pain generally begins to gradually alleviate after 10–15 days of soaking, and recovery can be expected after 1–2 consecutive months of treatment.

5. 薰洗砖烙法：先将祁艾 6 克、乌梅 15 克放入水中煎出药汁，装入盆内，使热气上蒸，患足放于气上熏冲，并用衣物遮盖。等药液稍冷后，将患足跟底部放于砖上，趁热下压数分钟，每日 1-2 次，连续 7 天为一疗程。药液可用多次。

Fumigation-Washing and Brick Pressing Method: First, decoct 6g mugwort leaf and 15g dark plum in water to obtain medicinal juice, pour into a basin to allow steam to rise, place the affected foot over the steam for fumigation, and cover with clothing. When the liquid cools slightly, press the bottom of the affected heel against a warm brick for several minutes; perform 1–2 times daily, with 7 consecutive days constituting one course of treatment. The medicinal liquid can be reused multiple times.

《中药科技报》1992 年 1 月 26 日

This formula was published in the Chinese Herbal Medicine Science and Technology News on January 26, 1992.

6. 炮山甲 30 克，炙鳖甲 40 克，威灵仙 50 克，陈米醋 1000 毫升。煎熬 30 分钟后离火，熏洗患足，每日 1-2 次，一剂可用 7 天。临床治疗 30 余例，一般患者 1 剂即可痊愈，重症患者连用 2 剂，明显见效。

Prescription: 30g processed pangolin scale, 40g honey-fried soft-shelled turtle shell, 50g Clematis root, and 1000ml aged rice vinegar. Decoct for 30 minutes, remove from heat, and use to fumigate and wash the affected foot 1–2 times daily; one dose can be used for 7 days. In clinical treatment of over 30 cases, most patients recovered with one dose, while severe cases showed significant improvement after two consecutive doses.

《民族医药报》1998 年 3 月 6 日（明秀荐）

This formula was recommended by Ming Xiu and published in the Ethnic Medicine News on March 6, 1998.

7. 川芎治足跟痛 igusticum Wallichii for Heel Pain

处方及用法：取川芎 500 克，研成细粉，分成两份，各用白布包好，置于袜内接触足跟痛处，两包轮流使用，一个月后，疼痛即止，不再复发。屡用屡验。

Take 500g Ligusticum wallichii rhizome, grind into fine powder, divide into two portions, wrap each in white cloth, place inside socks against the painful area of the heel, and alternate between the two packs. Pain stops after one month with no recurrence; this method has been repeatedly verified through clinical use.

《民族医药报》1993 年 1 月 15 日（郑州 李平）

This formula was provided by Li Ping from Zhengzhou and published in the Ethnic Medicine News on January 15, 1993.

四、骨质增生（7 方）
IV. Bone Hyperplasia (7 Formulas)

1. 随着透视诊断在临床上的普遍应用，一些不明原因的腰痛疾病结论为骨质增生者，屡见不鲜。若施以一般常规疗法，很难收到理想的效果，故在治疗上颇感棘手。笔者拟“抑骨增生汤”治愈两例，将验案介绍于下。

With the widespread clinical application of fluoroscopic diagnosis, cases of unexplained low back pain diagnosed as bone hyperplasia have become increasingly common. Conventional therapies often fail to achieve satisfactory results, making treatment quite challenging. The author formulated “Yigu Zengsheng Tang” (Bone Hyperplasia Inhibition Decoction) and successfully cured two cases, which are presented below.

病例一：患者，刘某，男，45 岁，干部。于 1958 年患腰痛，逐年加剧。1961 年经县医院和重庆市三家医院拍片结论为“四、五腰椎上角唇样性增生”。曾用封闭、针灸、埋线、注射骨宁、红茴香针等治疗及服用抗风湿、激素、镇痛等药物、疗效不佳。1964 年秋，腰痛加剧，前来求治。余参考了拍片结论及治疗情况后，用“抑骨增生汤”治之。药用：芍药 50 克，当归 15 克，鹿衔草 15 克，木瓜 30 克，续断 15 克，川牛膝 15 克，威灵仙 15 克，鸡血藤 15 克，甘草 6 克，水煎服，1 日 1 剂。1 月后，改为间日 1 剂。服至翌年 5 月，自觉症状完全消失，追访至今，未见复发。多年痼疾，终获治愈。

Case 1: Patient Liu, male, 45 years old, a cadre, suffered from progressively worsening low back pain since 1958. In 1961, X-rays taken at the county hospital and three hospitals in Chongqing confirmed "lip-like hyperplasia at the superior angles of the 4th and 5th lumbar vertebrae." Previous treatments including nerve blocks, acupuncture, catgut embedding, injections of Guning and red star anise, as well as oral antirheumatic drugs, hormones, and analgesics, were ineffective. In autumn 1964, the patient sought treatment due to aggravated pain. Based on the X-ray findings and treatment history, the author prescribed "Yigu Zengsheng Tang": 50g white peony root, 15g Chinese angelica root, 15g pyrola herb, 30g papaya fruit, 15g teasel root, 15g cyathula root, 15g clematis root, 15g spatholobus stem, and 6g licorice root, decocted in water for oral administration, one dose daily. After one month, the dosage was adjusted to one dose every other day. By May of the following year, all subjective symptoms had completely disappeared, and follow-up to date shows no recurrence; this chronic condition was ultimately cured.

病例二：患者，彭某，男，32岁，粮站保管员。1983年夏正入库时，初感左侧腰部胀痛，并放射至左腿外侧。7天后，痛如锥刺，起卧需搀扶。在XX区医院诊断为坐骨神经痛。以封闭针灸兼服中西药半月，无效。由单位介绍外出治疗。某县医院拍片（拍片号：10092）结论为1-2腰椎增生。仍用封闭、兼服抗风湿、激素、骨质增生丸等药物治疗，效果不明显。返单位后，特来请余用中药治疗。

Case 2: Patient Peng, male, 32 years old, a grain depot storekeeper, experienced distending pain in the left waist radiating to the lateral aspect of the left leg while storing grain in summer 1983. Seven days later, the pain became stabbing, requiring assistance for getting up or lying down. He was diagnosed with sciatica at a district hospital, but half a month of nerve blocks, acupuncture, and combined Chinese-Western medication proved ineffective. Referred by his workplace for external treatment, an X-ray (No. 10092) at a county hospital revealed hyperplasia of the 1st and 2nd lumbar vertebrae. Treatments including nerve blocks, antirheumatic drugs, hormones, and bone hyperplasia pills remained ineffective. Upon returning to work, he specifically requested TCM treatment from the author. Physical examination showed no redness, swelling, or heat in the affected area, only mild tenderness on palpation and difficulty moving.

观拍片结论后，细查患部、无红、肿、热等症状。局部触之微痛。行动艰难。苔白腻，边有齿痕，舌下有瘀点，脉见沉弦。余以“抑骨增生汤”随证施治。药用：赤芍、白芍各 30 克，归尾 15 克，威灵仙 20 克，川牛藤 15 克，木瓜 30 克，续断 15 克，海风藤 15 克，鸡血藤 15 克，红花 10 克，桃仁 10 克，甘草 6 克。因久病入络，加蜈蚣 2 条，炮山甲 6 克（研末兑服），1 日 1 剂。10 天后，改作间一剂减红花、桃仁量为 6 克，加黄芪 30 克。服药 80 余剂，历时半载而告愈，追访 1 年未发。

The tongue coating was white and greasy with teeth marks on the edges, sublingual stasis spots were present, and the pulse was deep and wiry. The author modified “Yigu Zengsheng Tang” according to the syndrome: 30g each of red peony root and white peony root, 15g angelica tail, 20g clematis root, 15g cyathula root, 30g papaya fruit, 15g teasel root, 15g kadsura pepper stem, 15g spatholobus stem, 10g safflower, 10g peach kernel, and 6g licorice root. Due to prolonged illness affecting the collaterals, 2 centipedes and 6g processed pangolin scale (ground into powder and mixed with the decoction) were added, one dose daily. After 10 days, the regimen was changed to one dose every other day, safflower and peach kernel were reduced to 6g each, and 30g astragalus root was added. After taking over 80 doses across six months, the patient recovered fully, with no recurrence during one-year follow-up.

按：“抑骨增生汤”用归芍以养血柔肝；川牛膝、木瓜舒筋活血；灵仙、续断、鸡血藤、海风藤祛湿活血，通络止痛；鹿衔草养肝强筋、祛风除湿；并以甘草调和诸药，共奏养血柔肝、活血通络、祛湿止痛之效。因久痛入络，用蜈蚣、山甲舒通经络；久病多虚、加黄芪以扶正，久痛必瘀，投红花、桃仁以活血祛瘀，随证化裁，故能收到满意的疗效。

（邓朝纲）

Commentary: “Yigu Zengsheng Tang” uses angelica and peony to nourish blood and soften the liver; cyathula root and papaya to relax tendons and activate blood; clematis, teasel, spatholobus, and kadsura pepper stem to dispel dampness, activate blood, unblock collaterals, and relieve pain; pyrola herb to nourish the liver, strengthen tendons, and dispel wind-dampness; and licorice to harmonize all herbs, collectively achieving the effects of nourishing blood, softening the liver, activating blood, unblocking collaterals, dispelling dampness, and relieving pain. For prolonged pain entering the collaterals, centipede and pangolin scale are added to unblock meridians; for deficiency due to chronic illness, astragalus is added to support upright qi; and for inevitable blood stasis from chronic pain, safflower and peach kernel are used to activate blood and resolve stasis. Flexible modification according to the syndrome ensures satisfactory therapeutic outcomes.

(Deng Chaogang)

2. 骨质增生是一种较为常见的疾病，治疗较为棘手，下面介绍其治疗验方一则。熟地 40 克、鹿角胶 40 克、龟板 40 克、当归 30 克、川芎 30 克、红花 30 克、麻黄 30 克、桂枝 30 克、防风 30 克、制马钱子 10 克、蜈蚣 10 克、地鳖虫 10 克、制川乌 5 克、制草乌 5 克。上药炮制后共研成细末，加蜜糖适量炼制成丸，每丸重 9 克。每日早晚各服 1 丸，1 月为 1 疗程。服药期间忌食猪肉、鱼肉，禁止房事，减少重体力劳动，避免精神刺激，纠正不良姿势；体质虚弱及伴有其它疾病者用量酌减。

Bone hyperplasia is a relatively common disease that is often difficult to treat. A proven formula is introduced below. Prescription: 40g prepared rehmannia root, 40g deer antler glue, 40g tortoise shell, 30g Chinese angelica root, 30g ligusticum rhizome, 30g safflower, 30g ephedra herb, 30g cassia twig, 30g fangfeng root, 10g processed strychnos seed, 10g centipede, 10g ground beetle, 5g processed Sichuan aconite root, and 5g processed kusnezoff monkshood root. After proper processing, grind all herbs into a fine powder, add an appropriate amount of honey to refine into pills, each weighing 9g. Take one pill twice daily (morning and evening), with one month constituting one course of treatment.

During medication, avoid pork and fish, abstain from sexual activity, reduce heavy physical labor, avoid mental stimulation, and correct poor posture; reduce the dosage for patients with weak constitutions or concurrent diseases.

此方用于治疗颈椎、腰椎、膝关节及跟骨骨质增生，疗效满意。方中马钱子有剧毒，要注意炮制和用量。

This formula has shown satisfactory efficacy in treating bone hyperplasia of the cervical vertebrae, lumbar vertebrae, knee joints, and calcaneus. Note: Strychnos seed in this formula is highly toxic; strict control over its processing method and dosage is essential.

《民族医药报》1992 年 4 月 3 日（广西 韦礼贵）

This formula was provided by Wei Ligui from Guangxi and published in the Ethnic Medicine News on April 3, 1992.

3. 治疗骨质增生方

Formula for Bone Hyperplasia

续断、骨碎补、山甲珠、桃仁、红花、土鳖虫、川楝子、甘草各 30 克，蜈蚣 30 条。颈椎增生加葛根；腰椎增生加杜仲；增生关节炎及跟骨刺加川牛膝。共研细末，每日 5 克，分 2-3 次以白开水冲服。本法共收治 148 例，结果：显效（症状、体征消失）94 例，有效 48 例，无效 6 例。

The prescription consists of 30g each of teasel root, drynaria rhizome, processed pangolin scale, peach kernel, safflower, ground beetle, toosendan fruit, and licorice root, plus 30 centipedes. Add kudzu root for cervical hyperplasia, eucommia bark for lumbar hyperplasia, and cyathula root for hyperplastic arthritis and heel spurs. Grind all ingredients into a fine powder; take 5g daily in 2–3 divided doses with plain boiled water. This method was applied to 148 cases: 94 cases showed marked effectiveness (symptoms and signs disappeared), 48 cases were effective, and 6 cases were ineffective.

《民族医药报》1998 年 1 月 23 日（洪 水）

This formula was provided by Hong Shui and published in the Ethnic Medicine News on January 23, 1998.

4. 骨质增生方

Bone Hyperplasia Formula

白芍 30 克，木瓜 12 克，甘草 12 克，鸡血藤 15 克，威灵仙 15 克。用水煎，早晚服一次。颈椎骨质增生可增加葛根 12 克；胸椎者，增加狗脊 12 克；腰椎者，增加怀牛膝、杜仲各 12 克，效果更明显。

The prescription includes 30g white peony root, 12g papaya fruit, 12g licorice root, 15g spatholobus stem, and 15g clematis root; decoct in water and take once in the morning and once in the evening. For cervical bone hyperplasia, add 12g kudzu root; for thoracic hyperplasia, add 12g cibotium rhizome; for lumbar hyperplasia, add 12g each of Huai achyranthes root and eucommia bark to enhance efficacy.

《民族医药报》

This formula was published in the Ethnic Medicine News.

5. 壁虎六十克、地龙六十克、草乌七十五克、广木香一百二十克、乳香九十克、大活六十克、梅片三克、元寸四点五克（即麝香）。用法：将壁虎用火焙干，与诸药共研为细末，加水为丸，如绿豆大，成人服三至六克，每日三次。

此方对轻型骨型骨质增生一剂即愈。

60g gecko, 60g earthworm, 75g kusnezoff monkshood root, 120g Aucklandia root, 90g frankincense, 60g Angelica pubescens root, 3g borneol, and 4.5g musk. Usage: Roast the gecko over fire until dry, grind it together with all other herbs into a fine powder, and form pills with water to the size of mung beans. Adults take 3–6g per dose, three times daily. This formula can cure mild bone hyperplasia with a single course of treatment.

6. 元寸零点一克、藤黄一点五克、朱砂一点五克、梅片一点五克、壁虎一条焙干取一半，以上诸药共为细末，用胶布将药棉贴于患处，三至四次即愈。

注意：藤黄剧毒药品：“抬头喝藤黄，低头见阎王”，患者要严加保管，胶布四周要贴严，贴后要将药面妥善处理，以免引起中毒死亡事件的发生。

此方治较重病例。我用此秘方治愈达两千五百例，治愈率百分之九十八，有效率百分之百。

0.1g musk, 1.5g gamboge, 1.5g cinnabar, 1.5g borneol, and half of one roasted-dry gecko; grind all ingredients into a fine powder, apply the medicated cotton to the affected area with adhesive tape, and cure is typically achieved after 3–4 applications. Caution: Gamboge is a highly toxic substance; as the folk saying goes, "Take gamboge with head up, meet the King of Hell with head down." Patients must store it securely, ensure the adhesive tape is sealed tightly on all sides, and properly dispose of the used medication to prevent fatal poisoning. This formula is suitable for severe cases; the author has cured 2,500 cases with this secret formula, achieving a 98% cure rate and 100% effective rate.

按：壁虎，异名守宫、天龙。为壁虎科动物的全体，多分布于我国中部和东南一带。其功能：祛风定惊、活血化瘀、散结止痛。经鉴定，具有抑制癌细胞生长的作用，经过特殊喂养的壁虎（即是人造麝香）有通窍止痛作用，可以治骨质增生、骨瘤等。

Note: Gecko, also known as Shougong or Tianlong, is the whole body of Gekkonidae animals, mainly distributed in central and southeastern China. Its functions include dispelling wind, calming convulsions, activating blood, resolving stasis, dissipating nodules, and relieving pain. It has been identified to have anti-cancer cell growth effects, and specially fed geckos (acting as artificial musk) have the effect of unblocking orifices and relieving pain, applicable to bone hyperplasia and bone tumors.

《中药科技报》1991 年 11 月 26 日（青兰 国营）

This formula was provided by Qinglan Guoying and published in the Chinese Herbal Medicine Science and Technology News on November 26, 1991.

7. 治骨质增生验方

Proven Formula for Bone Hyperplasia

方药组成：皂刺 50 克，当归 10 克，红花 10 克，山茱萸 10 克，川芎 15 克，鸡血藤 30 克，威灵仙 12 克，可随症加减。每日 1 剂，水煎 2 次，早晚分 2 次服。治疗骨质增生 41 例，总有效率为 92.7%。

The prescription comprises 50g Chinese honeylocust spine, 10g Chinese angelica root, 10g safflower, 10g dogwood fruit, 15g ligusticum rhizome, 30g spatholobus stem, and 12g clematis root; modifications can be made according to symptoms. Take one dose daily, decoct twice in water, and administer in two divided doses (morning and evening). In the treatment of 41 cases of bone hyperplasia, the total effective rate was 92.7%.

《民族医药报》1998 年 1 月 23 日（桂峰）

This formula was provided by Gui Feng and published in the Ethnic Medicine News on January 23, 1998.

五、跌打损伤（11 方）
V. Traumatic Injuries (11 Formulas)

1. 处方：全当归、桃仁泥、滴乳香、没药各 20g、京赤芍 15g、川草乌 10g、北细辛 10g、真血竭 20g、粉甘草 10g、泽兰 30g、白酒 50g

加减：局部血肿症状重者加：生大黄 15g，蒲公英 30g，黄柏 30g，玄胡索 20g；上肢重者加：八方麻 20g，上桂枝 20g；下肢重者加川牛膝 20g，五加皮 20g；腰部重者加：红杜仲 30g，骨碎补 30g；头部重者加：正川芎 30g，天麻 20g；

功能主治：活血化瘀，消肿止痛，疏通经脉，舒筋活络。适用于跌打损伤造成瘀血肿胀及一切软组织损伤疼痛者。初期用效果好。

用法：每剂加水 2000 至 3000 毫升，煎至一半，趁热熏洗。也可用毛巾浸湿敷于患处。每日三次，每次 20 至 40 分钟。每剂熏六次。每次熏洗时，可先以热气熏蒸，待药汤降至 50℃左右，可浸洗。为使热量持久，可先用两条毛巾在药盆内浸湿，交替温敷患处。直至药液凉时为止。完毕，用毛巾擦干患处。收捡用物，以备再用。轻者 1 剂，重者 2 至 3 剂即愈。

禁症：局部有皮损者禁用。对患者体质虚弱，孕妇及心脑血管病均慎用或禁用。

Prescription: 20g each of whole Chinese angelica root, peach kernel paste, frankincense, and myrrh; 15g red peony root; 10g each of Sichuan aconite root and kusnezoff monkshood root; 10g Manchurian wild ginger; 20g genuine dragon's blood; 10g licorice root powder; 30g bugleweed herb; and 50g white liquor. Modifications: For severe local hematoma, add 15g raw rhubarb, 30g dandelion, 30g amur cork-tree bark, and 20g corydalis tuber; for severe upper limb symptoms, add 20g octagonal hemp and 20g cassia twig; for severe lower limb symptoms, add 20g cyathula root and 20g acanthopanax bark; for severe lumbar symptoms, add 30g eucommia bark and 30g drynaria rhizome; for severe head symptoms, add 30g ligusticum rhizome and 20g gastrodia tuber. Functions and Indications: Activates blood and resolves stasis, reduces swelling and relieves pain, unblocks meridians, and relaxes tendons; indicated for traumatic bruising, swelling, and all soft tissue injury pain, with best results in the early stage. Usage: Add 2000–3000ml water to each dose, decoct to half volume, and fumigate/wash while hot; alternatively, soak a towel in the liquid and apply to the affected area. Use three times daily, 20–40 minutes per session, with each dose reusable for six sessions. First fumigate with steam, then wash when the liquid cools to ~50° C; to retain heat, alternate two towels soaked in the liquid as warm compresses until the liquid cools. Dry the area with a towel afterward and save materials for reuse. Mild cases resolve with one dose; severe cases require 2–3 doses. Contraindications: Do not use on broken skin; use with caution or avoid in weak patients, pregnant women, and those with cardiovascular/cerebrovascular diseases.

《中药科技报》1993 年 1 月 14 日（安徽　汪耕郭）

This formula was provided by Wang Gengguo from Anhui and published in the Chinese Herbal Medicine Science and Technology News on January 14, 1993.

2. 处方及用法：栀子 50 克，大黄 30 克，乳香 100 克，没药 100 克，姜黄 50 克。以上药味共研细末，共置于铁锅内炒热时撒上适量米酒，以药末湿润为度，取出置于一块方形干净的布料摊平外敷患处，再用一块塑料薄膜外包，以绷带固定，24 小时后取下复炒如上法再敷。此法曾治疗多例跌打损伤、关节扭伤闭合性瘀血肿痛患者，一般用药 3-5 天即取良效。个别病例外敷后出现皮肤瘙痒等反应，此为正常现象，可隔日外敷一次。

2.Prescription and Usage: 50g gardenia fruit, 30g rhubarb, 100g frankincense, 100g myrrh, and 50g turmeric rhizome. Grind all ingredients into a fine powder, stir-fry in an iron pan until hot, sprinkle with an appropriate amount of rice wine to moisten the powder, spread onto a clean square cloth, and apply externally to the affected area. Cover with plastic film and secure with a bandage; remove after 24 hours, re-stir-fry as above, and reapply. This method has treated multiple cases of traumatic injuries and closed joint sprains with bruising and swelling, generally achieving good results within 3–5 days. Occasional skin itching after application is normal; in such cases, apply every other day.

3. 处方及用法：小榕叶、七叶莲、木贼、黑心姜块根各适量（以上四味均为鲜品），洗净共捣烂，以适量男童小便拌匀，置于锅上炒热，取出摊于一块小手帕大小的纱布上，外敷跌打扭伤肿痛处，外用绷带固定，一日一换，一般用药 3-5 天有效。

Prescription and Usage: Appropriate amounts of fresh small fig leaves, schefflera arboricola leaves, horsetail herb, and black-heart ginger rhizome. Wash, pound together, mix evenly with an appropriate amount of young boy’s urine, stir-fry in a pan until hot, spread onto a handkerchief-sized gauze pad, and apply externally to the swollen/painful area from trauma/sprains. Secure with a bandage and replace daily; effective within 3–5 days.

《民族医药报》1992 年 9 月 4 日（广西 钟以林）

This formula was provided by Zhong Yilin from Guangxi and published in the Ethnic Medicine News on September 4, 1992.

4. 祖传活血消肿膏

组成：大黄、白芥子、血竭、儿茶、生半夏、骨碎补、地鳖虫、生南星、刘寄奴、生栀子、白芷、乳香、没药、广三七各 10g。

制法：以上共研细粉末，备用。

用法：用凡士林或麻油调成糊状，铺在纱布上，敷于患处。

主治：活血化瘀、消肿止痛，用于一切跌打损伤肢体肿胀。

注：笔者临床上曾治疗近 300 例，疗效显著。2 天至 7 天内损伤症状基本痊愈。

Ancestral Blood-Activating Swelling-Reducing Ointment: Composition: 10g each of rhubarb, white mustard seed, dragon’s blood, catechu, raw pinellia tuber, drynaria rhizome, ground beetle, raw jack-in-the-pulpit tuber, artemisia anomala herb, raw gardenia fruit, angelica dahurica root, frankincense, myrrh, and Panax notoginseng. Preparation: Grind all ingredients into a fine powder for later use. Usage: Mix with Vaseline or sesame oil to form a paste, spread on gauze, and apply to the affected area. Indications: Activates blood, resolves stasis, reduces swelling, and relieves pain for all traumatic limb swelling. Note: The author treated nearly 300 cases with significant efficacy; symptoms mostly resolved within 2–7 days.

（安徽省　汪耕郭）

(Wang Gengguo, Anhui Province)

5. 治急性扭伤一法

A Method for Acute Sprains

在日常生活和工作中，经常会发生扭伤，如手腕、脚踝、腰部、脖颈等处，老年人尤易发生。下面向读者介绍一种治扭伤的简易方法: 用适量生姜捣烂去汁，加食盐少许拌匀外敷患处，可用绷带固定，每日 1 次，一般 2-3 次即可痊愈。

5.Sprains of the wrist, ankle, waist, and neck are common in daily life and work, especially among the elderly. Simple treatment: Pound an appropriate amount of fresh ginger, squeeze out the juice, mix the pulp with a pinch of salt, apply externally to the affected area, and secure with a bandage. Apply once daily; cure is typically achieved in 2–3 applications.

《民族医药报》1992 年 4 月 10 日（江苏　樊常宝）

This formula was provided by Fan Changbao from Jiangsu and published in the Ethnic Medicine News on April 10, 1992.

6. 药用：大黄 15 克、生栀子 8 克，干姜 2 克、生川乌 9 克、生草乌 9 克、红花 9 克、川芎 12 克、公丁香 5 克。上药晒干，研细末，瓶装备用。

适应症：各种挫伤、扭伤。用法：根据损伤范围的大小，取上述药末适量，加白酒或陈醋调成稀糊状，涂敷患处，外用塑料纸覆盖，一日换药一次。（附：药粉干燥后，可用白酒调湿再敷）一般敷药 3- 5 天即可痊愈。

6.Medicinal Formula: 15g rhubarb, 8g raw gardenia fruit, 2g dried ginger, 9g raw Sichuan aconite root, 9g raw kusnezoff monkshood root, 9g safflower, 12g ligusticum rhizome, and 5g clove. Sun-dry all herbs, grind into fine powder, and store in a bottle. Indications: Various contusions and sprains. Usage: Take an appropriate amount of powder based on the injury size, mix with white liquor or aged vinegar to form a thin paste, apply to the affected area, cover with plastic wrap, and change dressing daily (Note: If the powder dries, remoisten with white liquor before reapplying). Cure is generally achieved in 3–5 days.

《中药科技报》（郭 一）

This formula was provided by Guo Yi and published in the Chinese Herbal Medicine Science and Technology News.

7. 祖传接骨活血汤：

Ancestral Bone-Knitting Blood-Activating Decoction

组成：当归、威灵仙、赤芍、生地、红花、地鳖虫、骨碎补、广三七、广木香、乳香、没药、五加皮各 10 克。

功用：祛瘀活血、续骨接筋。

主治：骨折筋伤及软组织损伤。

用法：水煎服，一日剂，每日服 2 次。

Composition: 10g each of Chinese angelica root, clematis root, red peony root, raw rehmannia root, safflower, ground beetle, drynaria rhizome, Panax notoginseng, Aucklandia root, frankincense, myrrh, and acanthopanax bark. Functions: Resolves stasis, activates blood, knits bones, and reconnects tendons. Indications: Fractures, tendon injuries, and soft tissue damage. Usage: Decoct in water for oral administration, one dose daily, taken twice daily.

8. 祖传续骨金丹

Ancestral Bone-Knitting Golden Elixir

组成：当归 16 克，熟地黄、骨碎补、续断、广木香各 10 克，赤芍、血竭、地鳖虫各 15 克，川红花、乳香、明没药、桃仁、煅自然铜各 6 克、北细辛 1 克。

加减：上部加桂枝、八方麻、五加皮各10克，中部加杜仲、破故纸、炒枳壳、春柴胡各10克，下部加川牛膝、木瓜、五加皮各10克。

功用：续筋接骨、消肿止痛、活血散瘀。

主治：一切骨折所致瘀血停滞、肿胀疼痛。

用法：水煎服，每日1剂，4剂为一疗程。

Composition: 16g Chinese angelica root; 10g each of prepared rehmannia root, drynaria rhizome, teasel root, and Aucklandia root; 15g each of red peony root, dragon’s blood, and ground beetle; 6g each of Sichuan safflower, frankincense, refined myrrh, peach kernel, and calcined native copper; and 1g Manchurian wild ginger. Modifications: For upper body injuries, add 10g each of cassia twig, octagonal hemp, and acanthopanax bark; for middle body, add 10g each of eucommia bark, psoralea fruit, stir-fried immature bitter orange, and spring bupleurum root; for lower body, add 10g each of cyathula root, papaya fruit, and acanthopanax bark. Functions: Reconnects tendons and knits bones, reduces swelling and relieves pain, activates blood and disperses stasis. Indications: Stasis, swelling, and pain caused by all types of fractures. Usage: Decoct in water for oral administration, one dose daily, with 4 doses constituting one course of treatment.

9. 祖传接骨散：

Ancestral Bone-Knitting Powder

组成：黄柏、大黄、白芥子、乳香、没药、田七、地鳖虫、刘寄奴、生半夏各20克。

功用：活血消肿、镇痛续骨。

主治：骨折及软组织损伤。

用法：共研细末，用凡士林或麻油调包、敷患部。

Composition: 20g each of amur cork-tree bark, rhubarb, white mustard seed, frankincense, myrrh, Panax notoginseng, ground beetle, artemisia anomala herb, and raw pinellia tuber. Functions: Activates blood, reduces swelling, relieves pain, and promotes bone healing. Indications: Fractures and soft tissue injuries. Usage: Grind all ingredients into a fine powder, mix with Vaseline or sesame oil to form a poultice, and apply to the affected area.

10. 祖传损伤活血丸：

Ancestral Trauma Blood-Activating Pills

组成：当归、赤芍、生地、红花、乳香、没药、酒大黄、刘寄奴、广三七、血竭、牛膝、木瓜、炒枳壳、威灵仙、五加皮、续断、桂枝、地鳖虫、透骨草、柴胡、丹皮各 20 克。

功用：活血消肿，散瘀止痛、续骨。

主治：全身跌打损伤，骨折后伤处疼痛，瘀血肿胀。

用法：共研细末。每次服 3 至 6 克，一日二次，用温开水或少量米酒送服。

10.Composition: 20g each of Chinese angelica root, red peony root, raw rehmannia root, safflower, frankincense, myrrh, wine-processed rhubarb, artemisia anomala herb, Panax notoginseng, dragon' s blood, achyranthes root, papaya fruit, stir-fried immature bitter orange, clematis root, acanthopanax bark, teasel root, cassia twig, ground beetle, garden balsam stem, bupleurum root, and moutan bark. Functions: Activates blood, reduces swelling, disperses stasis, relieves pain, and promotes bone healing. Indications: Systemic traumatic injuries, post-fracture pain, and bruising/swelling. Usage: Grind all ingredients into a fine powder; take 3–6g per dose, twice daily, with warm boiled water or a small amount of rice wine.

11. 接骨膏（经验方）

Bone-Knitting Ointment (Empirical Formula):

组成：鲜五加皮 50 克、鲜骨碎补 30 克、活地鳖虫 30 个。功用：续筋接骨。主治：一切骨折、筋伤。用法；将药捣烂成泥状，敷患部。24 小时敷一次。

11.Composition: 50g fresh acanthopanax bark, 30g fresh drynaria rhizome, and 30 live ground beetles. Functions: Reconnects tendons and knits bones. Indications: All fractures and tendon injuries. Usage: Pound the ingredients into a paste and apply to the affected area once every 24 hours.

《中医药信息报》（安徽省 汪耕郭）

This formula was provided by Wang Gengguo from Anhui Province and published in the Traditional Chinese Medicine Information News.

六、肾虚腰腿痛（3 方）
Kidney Deficiency-Induced Low Back and Leg Pain (3 Formulas)

1. 吾插队时收集到治疗慢性腰痛的验方三花汤。十余年来曾介绍给不少患者使用，每获良效。三花汤由红花地桃花根、黄花仔根、五色花根、千斤拨、鹿衔草各 50 克组成，另加猪尾巴一条用水同煎，食肉饮汤。红花地：桃花系锦葵科植物肖梵天花，别名小朝阳、八卦草、野桃花。黄花仔是锦葵科植物粘毛黄花稔。五色花为马鞭科植物马樱丹，又名五色梅、如意草、穿墙风。千斤拔系豆科植物千斤拔。鹿衔草为鹿蹄草科植物鹿蹄草。这些民间草药具有祛风湿，活血行血，舒筋活络，补虚益肾的作用，常用来治疗风湿筋骨痛，四肢麻木，腰膝无力等病症。猪尾巴补肾引药入病所。

1.During my years as an educated youth in the countryside, I collected a proven formula for chronic low back pain called Sanhua Tang (Three-Flower Decoction), which has been recommended to many patients over more than ten years with consistently good results. Sanhua Tang consists of 50g each of Honghuadi Taohua root, Huanghuazai root, Wusehua root, Qianjinba root, and Luxiancao herb, plus one pig’s tail; decoct all ingredients in water together, then consume both the meat and the broth. Honghuadi Taohua refers to Urena lobata (Malvaceae), also known as Xiao Chaoyang, Bagua Cao, or Ye Taohua; Huanghuazai is Sida rhombifolia (Malvaceae); Wusehua is Lantana camara (Verbenaceae), also called Wuse Mei, Ruyi Cao, or Chuanqiang Feng; Qianjinba is Flemingia prostrata (Fabaceae); and Luxiancao is Pyrola calliantha (Pyrolaceae). These folk herbs have the effects of dispelling wind-dampness, activating blood circulation, relaxing tendons and unblocking collaterals, and tonifying deficiency and reinforcing the kidney; they are commonly used to treat rheumatic bone and muscle pain, numbness of the limbs, and weakness of the waist and knees. The pig’s tail serves to tonify the kidney and guide the medicinal effects to the affected site.

《民族医药报》1992 年 2 月 7 日（广西　黄育文）

This formula was provided by Huang Yuwen from Guangxi and published in the Ethnic Medicine News on February 7, 1992.

2. 药方及用法：猪肾（猪腰）1 个，楠竹蔸 1 个（砍掉竹竿一年以后的）、杜仲 15 克，补骨脂 10 克。把杜仲、补骨脂研成细末。再把猪肾表皮薄膜剥掉，剖开，把药末放入猪肾中，用纱布包住猪肾。然后把竹蔸节锉空，放入猪肾。在竹蔸周围涂上一层黄泥土（浆），竹蔸放在柴火中烧烤，猪肾煨熟为宜，去掉猪肾中的药末。吃猪肾，同时适量米酒送服。 此方治肾虚引起的腰痛为宜。每天吃 1 次，连吃 3 次见效。

2.Prescription and Usage: One pig kidney, one nan bamboo stump (harvested one year after cutting down the culm), 15g eucommia bark, and 10g psoralea fruit. Grind the eucommia bark and psoralea fruit into a fine powder; peel off the outer membrane of the pig kidney, split it open, place the medicinal powder inside, and wrap the kidney with gauze. Hollow out the bamboo stump node, insert the wrapped pig kidney, coat the outside of the stump with a layer of yellow clay slurry, and roast it over firewood until the pig kidney is fully cooked. Remove the kidney, discard the medicinal powder inside, eat the kidney, and take it with an appropriate amount of rice wine. This formula is suitable for low back pain caused by kidney deficiency; consume once daily, and effects can be observed after three consecutive doses.

《民族医药报》1992 年 2 月 26 日（湖南　戴厚高）

This formula was provided by Dai Hougao from Hunan and published in the Ethnic Medicine News on February 26, 1992.

3. 慢性腰腿痛：乌梅、川乌、当归、甘草各 9 克，将上药加白酒 500 克，泡三天，每天一次，每次口服 15 毫升（1 汤匙）。

3.ormula for Chronic Low Back and Leg Pain: 9g each of dark plum, Sichuan aconite root, Chinese angelica root, and licorice root. Soak the above herbs in 500g white liquor for three days; take orally once daily, 15ml (one tablespoon) per dose.

《中药科技报》

This formula was published in the Chinese Herbal Medicine Science and Technology News.

七、骨髓炎（2方）
VII. Osteomyelitis (2 Prescriptions)

1. 中医治疗慢性化脓性骨髓炎
Traditional Chinese Medicine (TCM) Treatment for Chronic Suppurative Osteomyelitis

根据临床证候分为湿热病型：初有寒战，继发高热，口渴烦躁，小溲黄赤，患肢疼痛彻骨，肿胀红热，舌苔白厚或黄腻，脉洪数弦滑。破溃流脓，初多稠厚，渐转稀薄，不易收口，形成慢性窦道。患者形体消瘦，面色苍白，精神不振，食欲减退，舌淡胖、苔白、脉细弱。X线摄片可见骨质破坏，有死骨。

Based on clinical syndromes, it is divided into the Damp-Heat type: initially presenting with chills, followed by high fever, thirst, restlessness, dark yellow urine, bone-deep pain in the affected limb, swelling, redness, and heat. The tongue coating is thick white or yellow and greasy, with a surging, rapid, string-taut, and slippery pulse. Upon ulceration and pus discharge, the pus is initially thick but gradually becomes thin, making it difficult to heal and forming chronic sinus tracts. Patients appear emaciated with a pale complexion, poor spirits, and reduced appetite; the tongue is pale and swollen with a white coating, and the pulse is thin and weak. X-rays reveal bone destruction and sequestra (dead bone).

风寒湿毒：初起恶寒发热或无寒热，患处隐隐酸痛，肿胀不明显，继则局部疼痛加重，皮色隐红，脓水稀薄淋漓，疮口经久不愈，形成一个或多个窦道。

Wind-Cold-Damp-Toxin type: initially presenting with aversion to cold and fever, or no fever/chills, accompanied by dull aching pain and unobvious swelling. Subsequently, local pain worsens, the skin becomes faintly red, and thin pus oozes continuously. The sores fail to heal over a long period, forming one or more sinus tracts.

其治疗运用中医治则的消、托、补治之。

Treatment follows the TCM principles of Elimination (Xiao), Supporting (Tuo), and Tonification (Bu).

消法：湿热病型初起，内服仙方活命饮合黄连解毒汤加减（穿山甲、皂刺、金银花、归尾、赤芍、乳香、没药、白芷、黄连、黄芩、黄柏、山栀、甘草），外敷如意金黄散。风寒湿毒型初起，有寒热者，内服万灵丹合荆防败毒散加减（苍术、何首乌、羌活、荆芥、川乌、乌药、川芎、甘草、川石斛、全蝎、防风、细辛、当归、麻黄、雄黄），外敷如意金黄散。无寒热者内服阳和汤，外用熨风散（羌活、防风、白芷、当归、细辛、芫花、白芍、肉桂）醋炒热慰患处。

Elimination Method: For the initial stage of the Damp-Heat type, administer a modified Xianfang Huoming Yin combined with Huanglian Jiedu Tang internally (including pangolin scales, saponin spines, honeysuckle, angelica tail, red peony, frankincense, myrrh, angelica dahurica, coptis, scutellaria, phellodendron, gardenia, and licorice), and apply Ruyi Jinhuang San externally. For the initial stage of the Wind-Cold-Damp-Toxin type with fever/chills, administer a modified Wanling Dan combined with Jingfang Baidu San internally (including atractylodes, fleece-flower root, notopterygium, schizonepeta, Sichuan aconite, lindera, ligusticum, licorice, dendrobium, scorpion, saposhnikovia, asarum, angelica sinensis, ephedra, and realgar), and apply Ruyi Jinhuang San externally. For cases without fever/chills, administer Yanghe Tang internally, and apply Yunfeng San (including notopterygium, saposhnikovia, angelica dahurica, angelica sinensis, asarum, yuanhua, white peony, and cinnamon bark) stir-fried hot with vinegar to the affected area.

托法：脓成而未溃者，需切开排脓；已溃而余毒未尽，脓稀肿硬不消者，内服托里消毒散加减（党参、黄芪、白术、茯苓、甘草、当归、川芎、白芍、金银花、白芷、穿山甲、皂角刺），外用红升丹药线；若有较大死骨不能排出或空腔形成，则需医生手术彻底清除，作一期缝合。

Supporting Method: For abscesses that have formed but not ruptured, surgical incision and drainage are required. For ruptured abscesses with residual toxins, thin pus, and unresolved hard swelling, administer a modified Tuoli Xiaodu San internally (including codonopsis, astragalus, atractylodes, poria, licorice, angelica sinensis, ligusticum, white peony, honeysuckle, angelica dahurica, pangolin scales, and saponin spines), and use Hongsheng Dan medicinal threads externally. If large sequestra cannot be discharged or cavities form, a physician must surgically remove them thoroughly and perform primary suturing.

补法：溃后而致气血两虚，面色苍白，少气乏力者，内服八珍汤，若脾虚气滞者，治用参苓白术散加减，肝肾虚亏者，六味地黄汤加减。（永久）

Tonification Method: For patients with dual deficiency of qi and blood, pale complexion, and fatigue after ulceration, administer Bazhen Tang internally. For spleen deficiency with qi stagnation, use a modified Shenling Baizhu San. For liver and kidney deficiency, use a modified Liuwei Dihuang Tang. (Yong Jiu)

2. 民间方治慢性骨髓炎

2. Folk Prescription for Chronic Osteomyelitis

慢性骨髓炎属中医“附骨疽”“附骨流注”范围，多由外感毒邪，乘虚入里、留于筋骨，致经络受损，气血失调所致。下述民间方治疗该病，经过十余年的临床验证，治愈率高。

Chronic osteomyelitis falls under the TCM categories of “Fugu Ju” (bone-attached abscess) and “Fugu Liuzhu” (bone-attached wandering abscess). It is mostly caused by external toxic pathogens taking advantage of deficiency to enter the interior and lodge in the bones and muscles, leading to meridian damage and qi-blood imbalance. The following folk prescription has been clinically verified for over ten years with a high cure rate.

药物组成及用法：取白背叶 10 克、五加皮 15 克、抱石莲 10 克、茜草 6 克、中华常青藤 10 克、闹阳花根（岬根）6 克、淫羊藿 6 克，每日一剂，水煎服。

Composition and Usage: Take 10g of white back leaf (Bai Bei Ye), 15g of eleutherococcus bark (Wu Jia Pi), 10g of rock lotus (Bao Shi Lian), 6g of madder root (Qian Cao), 10g of Chinese evergreen vine (Zhonghua Chang Qing Teng), 6g of rhododendron root (female root) (Nao Yang Hua Gen), and 6g of epimedium (Yin Yang Huo). Boil one dose daily in water for oral administration.

药理探讨：方中白背叶微涩微苦性平具有清热利湿消瘀之功；五加皮、中华常青藤，茜草具有活血祛风、补肾、壮筋骨之神效；抱石莲、淫羊藿其性味苦凉、具有清热解毒、利湿消瘀之功能；闹阳花根性味辛温，有毒。具有驱风、除湿、消肿、止痛之奇效。诸药合用具有补肝肾、祛风湿、清热解毒、活血止痛之功，故治慢性骨髓炎有效。

Pharmacological Discussion: In this formula, Bai Bei Ye is slightly astringent, slightly bitter, and neutral in nature, with the effects of clearing heat, promoting diuresis, and resolving stasis. Wu Jia Pi, Zhonghua Chang Qing Teng, and Qian Cao have the remarkable effects of promoting blood circulation, dispelling wind, tonifying the kidneys, and strengthening bones and tendons. Bao Shi Lian and Yin Yang Huo are bitter and cool in nature and flavor, functioning to clear heat, detoxify, promote diuresis, and resolve stasis. Nao Yang Hua Gen is pungent, warm, and toxic, possessing miraculous effects in dispelling wind, removing dampness, reducing swelling, and relieving pain. Combined, these herbs tonify the liver and kidneys, dispel wind-dampness, clear heat and detoxify, and promote blood circulation to relieve pain, making them effective for treating chronic osteomyelitis.

注意事项：方中闹阳花根有毒，宜选用雌根，同时应选用次根而不应选用主根，连服本药一般不要超过七天。体虚者应加生芪、党参，白术、茯苓，熟地等补气血之药品。笔者在治疗体虚弱者时，改闹阳花根为皂角刺，取得类似疗效。

Precautions: Nao Yang Hua Gen in this formula is toxic; the female root should be selected, specifically the secondary root rather than the main root. Continuous use should generally not exceed seven days. For patients with physical deficiency, add raw astragalus, codonopsis, atractylodes, poria, and rehmannia to tonify qi and blood. When treating weak patients, the author substituted Nao

Yang Hua Gen with saponin spines (Zao Jiao Ci) and achieved similar efficacy.

《民族医药报》1992 年 5 月（浙江省东阳市中医院 卢樟文 周荣岳）

Ethnic Medicine News, May 1992 (Lu Zhangwen, Zhou Rongyue, Dongyang City TCM Hospital, Zhejiang Province)

八、骨结核（1 方）
VIII. Bone Tuberculosis (1 Prescription)

家传有治骨结核

A Family Prescription for Treating Bone Tuberculosis

笔者采用家传方治疗骨结核，经 20 多年的临床实践，收效理想。兹介绍于下。

The author has used this family prescription to treat bone tuberculosis. After more than 20 years of clinical practice, it has achieved ideal therapeutic effects. It is introduced as follows.

方药组成（一剂量）：僵蚕 25 克、龙衣 12 克、雄黄 15 克、皂刺 18 克、血余炭 10 克、蜂蜡 70 克。

Ingredients (for one dose): 25g of stiff silkworm (Jiang Can), 12g of snake slough (Long Yi), 15g of realgar (Xiong Huang), 18g of saponin spines (Zao Ci), 10g of human hair charcoal (Xue Yu Tan), and 70g of beeswax (Feng La).

加工及用法：将僵蚕、龙衣、皂刺分别在微火上炒黄，加入雄黄及血余炭共研细末，过筛，再将蜂蜡熔化后上诸药加入并搅拌，使之均匀，做成绿豆大小的小丸。每次服 15 克（小儿酌情减量），以黄酒冲服，每日二次。孕妇及产后忌服。

Preparation and Usage: Stir-fry the stiff silkworm, snake slough, and saponin spines separately over a low fire until yellowish. Add the realgar and human hair charcoal, then grind them together into a fine powder and sift. Melt the beeswax, add the powdered herbs, and stir until evenly mixed. Form the mixture into small pills the size of mung beans. The dosage is 15g each time (reduce appropriately for children), taken with yellow rice wine, twice daily. Contraindicated for pregnant women and postpartum women.

按：一般服上药数剂即显效，服药十剂以下常可痊愈。

Note: Generally, significant effects are seen after taking a few doses of this medicine. Patients can often be completely cured after taking fewer than ten doses.

《民族医药报》1992 年 4 月 3 日（江苏省泰州市中医院 王靖 国庆）

Ethnic Medicine News, April 3, 1992 (Wang Jing, Guo Qing, Taizhou City TCM Hospital, Jiangsu Province)

九、脉管炎（1 方）
IX. Vasculitis (1 Prescription)

治脉管炎方

Prescription for Treating Vasculitis

方药：全虫 30 克、蜈蚣 10 条、土鳖 30 克、地龙 60 克、川牛膝 30 克、玄胡 30 克、赤芍 30 克、制附子 15 克、干姜 10 克、肉桂 10 克、麝香 0.05 克（另包）

Ingredients: 30g of scorpion (Quan Chong), 10 centipedes (Wu Gong), 30g of ground beetle (Tu Bie), 60g of earthworm (Di Long), 30g of cyathula root (Chuan Niu Xi), 30g of corydalis tuber (Xuan Hu), 30g of red peony root (Chi Shao), 15g of processed aconite root (Zhi Fu Zi), 10g of dried ginger (Gan Jiang), 10g of cinnamon bark (Rou Gui), and 0.05g of musk (She Xiang, packed separately).

制法及服法：将上药烘燥（麝香除外）共研细末，然后加入麝香和匀，装入瓶内密封备用。用时每日服 2 次，每次服 5-10 克，早晚吃饭前半小时用温开水冲服。15 天为一疗程，服完一个疗程后，停药 5 天，再服一个疗程。

Preparation and Usage: Bake the above herbs dry (except for the musk), then grind them together into a fine powder. Add the musk and mix well, then store in a sealed bottle for future use. Take twice daily, 5-10g each time, dissolved in warm water half an hour before breakfast and dinner. A treatment course lasts for 15 days. After completing one course, stop the medication for 5 days before starting the next course.

功效：疏通经络、活血止痛。

Effects: Unblocks meridians and collaterals, promotes blood circulation, and relieves pain.

主治：寒性血栓阻塞性脉管炎。

Indications: Cold-type thromboangiitis obliterans.

禁忌：牛肉、羊肉、虾米等。

Contraindications: Beef, mutton, dried shrimp, etc.

《民族医药报》1992 年 7 月 3 日（湖南 戴厚高）

Ethnic Medicine News, July 3, 1992 (Dai Hougao, Hunan)

第八章　泌尿科

Chapter 8　Urology Department

一、肾炎（15 方）

I. Nephritis (15 Prescriptions)

1. 肾炎验方

Verified Prescription for Nephritis

急性肾炎以浮肿、尿少，尿液检查出现蛋白尿、管型尿或血尿为其主要特征。祖国医学认为本病与水湿和风邪侵袭有关。治疗以宣肺、祛风、利湿为主。下面介绍验方两则，以供参考。

Acute nephritis is mainly characterized by edema, oliguria, and the presence of proteinuria, casts, or hematuria in urine tests. Traditional Chinese Medicine (TCM) believes that this disease is related to the invasion of water-dampness and wind pathogens. Treatment mainly focuses on diffusing the lungs, dispelling wind, and promoting diuresis. The following two verified prescriptions are introduced for reference.

急性期治疗方

Prescription for the Acute Stage

炙麻黄 7 克，桔梗 5 克，银花 5 克、防风 6 克，鱼腥草 5 克，车前草 5 克、茯苓皮 5 克，生姜皮 4 克，淡竹叶 4 克，炙甘草 5 克。本方功效宣肺祛风、清热利湿。适用于急性肾炎初期，症见面目或全身浮肿，发热恶风，咳嗽、尿少，镜检见蛋白尿，管型尿或血尿者。

7g of honey-fried ephedra, 5g of platycodon, 5g of honeysuckle, 6g of saposhnikovia, 5g of houttuynia, 5g of plantain, 5g of poria peel, 4g of fresh ginger peel, 4g of light bamboo leaf, and 5g of honey-fried licorice. This formula has the effects of diffusing the lungs, dispelling wind, clearing heat, and promoting diuresis. It is suitable for the early stage of acute nephritis, presenting with edema of the face or whole body, fever and aversion to wind, cough, oliguria, and microscopic proteinuria, casts, or hematuria.

恢复期治疗方

Prescription for the Recovery Stage

急性期后，浮肿渐退，蛋白尿、管型尿减少或微量，或有少量红细胞，伴有全身疲乏，形体消瘦，食欲不振者，以益肾健脾、补益气血为主。

After the acute stage, as edema gradually subsides, proteinuria and casts decrease or become trace, or there are a few red blood cells, accompanied by systemic fatigue, emaciation, and poor appetite, the treatment should mainly focus on tonifying the kidneys and strengthening the spleen, as well as supplementing qi and blood.

药用：枸杞 8 克，女贞子 6 克，白术 5 克，淮山 6 克，陈皮 4 克，炙黄芪 10 克，党参 8 克，生地 5 克，当归 4 克，炙甘草 6 克。以上方药均以每日一剂水煎服。

Ingredients: 8g of wolfberry, 6g of glossy privet fruit, 5g of atractylodes, 6g of Chinese yam, 4g of tangerine peel, 10g of honey-fried astragalus, 8g of codonopsis, 5g of rehmannia, 4g of angelica sinensis, and 6g of honey-fried licorice. The above prescriptions are taken as one dose daily, decocted in water.

《民族医药报》1991 年 11 月 5 日（广西龙胜各族自治县中医院 陆强益）

Ethnic Medicine News, November 5, 1991 (Lu Qiangyi, Longsheng Various Nationalities Autonomous County TCM Hospital, Guangxi)

急性肾炎：

Acute Nephritis:

2. 冬瓜皮 30 克，鲜茅根 30 克。配制及用法：水煎服，每日 1 次，连服 15 日。适用于急性肾炎水肿。

2. 30g of winter melon peel and 30g of fresh cogongrass rhizome. Preparation and Usage: Decoct in water and take once daily for 15 consecutive days. Suitable

for edema in acute nephritis.

3. 陈葫芦壳 30 克。配制及用法：水煎服，每日 1 剂。亦可用陈葫芦 1 个，焙黄研末，每次 9 克，开水调服。适用于急性肾炎浮肿。

3. 30g of dried gourd shell. Preparation and Usage: Decoct in water, one dose daily. Alternatively, take one dried gourd, bake it until yellow, grind it into powder, and take 9g each time mixed with boiling water. Suitable for edema in acute nephritis.

4. 鳢鱼 1 条，赤小豆 15 克，苡仁 10 克，茯苓皮 10 克。配制及用法：取约重 500 克鳢鱼 1 条，去鳞及内脏，洗净余药加水适量，煮 1 小时，服用。

4. One snakehead fish, 15g of adzuki beans, 10g of coix seeds, and 10g of poria peel. Preparation and Usage: Take one snakehead fish weighing about 500g, remove the scales and internal organs, wash it, add the remaining herbs and an appropriate amount of water, boil for 1 hour, and consume.

说明：鳢鱼又名和鱼、乌鱼，如果没有可用鲤鱼代用。也可取鳢鱼 1 条约重 500 克，去鳞及内脏，洗净，冬瓜 1500 克，大葱 5 茎，红小豆 30 克，加水 5 碗煎至 3 碗，吃鱼喝汤后盖被取微汗。

Note: Snakehead fish is also known as He fish or Wu fish; if unavailable, it can be substituted with carp. Alternatively, take one snakehead fish weighing about 500g, remove the scales and internal organs, wash it, add 1500g of winter melon, 5green onion stalks, and 30g of adzuki beans, add 5 bowls of water and decoct to 3 bowls. After eating the fish and drinking the soup, cover up to induce mild sweating.

5. 黄母鸡 1 只，龙葵豆 7 粒，大麻仁 7 粒，黑豆 200 克，红糖 1000 克。

5. One yellow hen, 7 black nightshade seeds, 7 hemp seeds, 200g of black beans, and 1000g of brown sugar.

配制及用法：取大母鸡 1 只，去毛及内脏，洗净，将药入鸡腹内，置锅中加水及红糖煮汤，一日内服完。

Preparation and Usage: Take one large hen, remove the feathers and internal organs, wash it, put the herbs into the chicken’ s belly, place it in a pot with water and brown sugar to boil into soup, and finish it within one day.

说明：服药后盖被取汗，不要吹风，并忌盐 3 日。此方急慢性肾炎皆可服用。

Note: After taking the medicine, cover up to induce sweating, avoid wind exposure, and abstain from salt for 3 days. This prescription can be used for both acute and chronic nephritis.

慢性肾炎：

Chronic Nephritis:

6. 赤小豆 90 克，花生仁 90 克，红糖 60 克，红枣 10 个。

6. 90g of adzuki beans, 90g of peanut kernels, 60g of brown sugar, and 10 red dates.

配制及用法：共煮熟服用。每日 1 次，早饭前服，可连用 3-5 个月。

Preparation and Usage: Boil all ingredients together until cooked and consume. Take once daily before breakfast, and can be used continuously for 3-5 months.

7. 黄芪 30 克，糯米 90 克。配制及用法：糯米淘净，与黄芪共煮粥食用。

7. 30g of astragalus and 90g of glutinous rice. Preparation and Usage: Wash the glutinous rice clean, boil it together with astragalus into porridge, and consume.

8. 大西瓜 1 个，红皮蒜 13 头。用法：在西瓜上挖 1 个洞，塞入去皮的大蒜，再用瓜皮塞住洞口，将洞口向上置锅中炖至蒜熟，吃蒜和西瓜，分两天服完。

8. One large watermelon and 13 heads of red-skinned garlic. Usage: Dig a hole in the watermelon, stuff in the peeled garlic, plug the hole with the removed watermelon rind, place it in a pot with the hole facing up, and stew until the garlic is cooked. Eat the garlic and watermelon, and finish it over two days.

说明：一般 2 年以内的肾炎，服 14 次可明显好转。

Note: Generally, for nephritis within 2 years, significant improvement can be seen after taking it 14 times.

9. 大西瓜 1 个，大蒜适量。配制及用法：切开西瓜蒂部，挖去瓤及子，装满去皮的大蒜，仍以蒂盖好，以纸筋泥封固，于火中煨 1 天，取出研成细末备用。

用时每取 3 克，吞服，一日 2 次。

9. One large watermelon and an appropriate amount of garlic. Preparation and Usage: Cut off the stem of the watermelon, scoop out the pulp and seeds, fill it with peeled garlic, cover it with the stem, seal it tightly with paper-pulp mud, bake it in the fire for 1 day, take it out, and grind it into a fine powder for later use. When using, take 3g each time, swallow it, twice a day.

10. 玉米须 60 克。配制及用法：煎汤代茶饮，每日 1 剂，口渴时饮，连用 3 个月。此方适用于小儿慢性肾炎。

10. 60g of corn silk. Preparation and Usage: Decoct into soup to drink as tea, one dose daily, drink when thirsty, and use continuously for 3 months. This prescription is suitable for chronic nephritis in children.

11. 药物组成：新鲜猪胃一个，紫皮独头生大蒜 7 只。制法及服法：首先将猪胃洗净，把剥皮后的紫皮大蒜放入其中，然后将猪胃放锅里煮至烂熟，吃肉、蒜、喝汤。一次或多次服完均可。该法无副作用，一般服用 3-4 次可取效。

11. Ingredients: One fresh pig stomach and 7 raw purple-skinned single-clove garlic bulbs. Preparation and Usage: First, wash the pig stomach clean, put the peeled purple garlic into it, then boil the pig stomach in a pot until thoroughly cooked. Eat the meat and garlic, and drink the soup. It can be consumed in one or multiple sittings. This method has no side effects, and effects can generally be achieved after 3-4 servings.

《民族医药报》1992 年 8 月 2 日（贵州省绥阳县科协 吴彬）

Ethnic Medicine News, August 2, 1992 (Wu Bin, Suiyang County Association for Science and Technology, Guizhou Province)

12. 胡椒蛋治肾炎

12. Pepper Egg for Treating Nephritis

取白胡椒 7 粒，新鲜鸡蛋 1 枚。先将鸡蛋磕一小口，然后将白胡椒装入鸡蛋内，用面粉封口，外用湿纸包裹，放入蒸笼内蒸熟。服时剥去蛋壳，将鸡蛋胡椒一起吃下。成人：每日服 2 枚，儿童 1 枚。10 天为一疗程，隔 3 天再服第二疗程，此方安全可靠，无任何副作用。（本方适用于急慢性肾炎病史不长者）。

Take 7 white peppercorns and 1 fresh egg. First, crack a small hole in the egg, put the white peppercorns inside, seal the hole with flour, wrap it with wet paper, and steam it in a steamer until cooked. When taking it, peel off the shell and eat the egg and pepper together. For adults: take 2 eggs daily; for children: 1 egg. A treatment course is 10 days, with a 3-day break before the second course. This prescription is safe, reliable, and has no side effects. (This prescription is suitable for those with a short history of acute or chronic nephritis.)

《中医药信息报》1992 年 5 月 30 日（仰占）

TCM Information News, May 30, 1992 (Yang Zhan)

13. 肾炎（水肿）：铁扫帚根 30 克、珍珠菜根 24 克、六月雪根 15 克、半边莲 30 克、积雪草 30 克、一枝黄花 15 克、厚朴 12 克、白芝麻 60 克、白糖 50 克，水煎服，每日 1 剂。忌盐及动物油。

13. Nephritis (Edema): 30g of iron broom root, 24g of pearl herb root, 15g of patrinia root, 30g of Chinese lobelia, 30g of centella, 15g of goldenrod, 12g of magnolia bark, 60g of white sesame, and 50g of white sugar. Decoct in water and take one dose daily. Abstain from salt and animal fats.

《中药科技报》1992 年 3 月 26 日

Chinese Herbal Medicine Science and Technology News, March 26, 1992

14. 蛋白尿是急慢性肾炎的一个常见症状。祖国医学认为，肾炎蛋白尿的病机，属本虚标实。本虚表现在脾肾虚损，标实为湿热、痰瘀互结。蛋白尿的产生，是脾气下陷，肾精不足，导致肾失封藏，不能摄纳肾中精微，加上痰瘀湿热、胶结不化，使精微物质从溺窍泄出。笔者采用祖传药物二草汤治疗本病，疗效较为满意。

14. Proteinuria is a common symptom of acute and chronic nephritis. TCM believes that the pathogenesis of nephritis proteinuria is characterized by root deficiency and branch excess. Root deficiency manifests as spleen and kidney deficiency, while branch excess is the mutual binding of damp-heat, phlegm, and blood stasis. The production of proteinuria is due to spleen qi sinking and kidney essence deficiency, leading to the kidney’s failure to store and retain the refined

essence. Combined with the unresolved binding of phlegm, stasis, and damp-heat, the refined substances leak out through the urinary tract. The author uses the ancestral prescription Ercao Tang (Two-Herb Decoction) to treat this disease with satisfactory efficacy.

二草汤药物组成是：细种日本草 50 克，白术、山药各 30 克，益母草 20 克。每日一剂水煎 2 次，分早、晚温服，半个月为 1 疗程，一般用药 1 至 2 个疗程尿蛋白消失。此方具有补脾益肾，升清降浊，清化湿热，活血化瘀之功效，疗效可靠，无副作用。

The composition of Ercao Tang is: 50g of fine Japanese herb, 30g each of atractylodes and Chinese yam, and 20g of motherwort. Take one dose daily, decocted twice in water, and taken warm in the morning and evening. Half a month is one treatment course. Generally, proteinuria disappears after 1 to 2 courses. This formula has the effects of tonifying the spleen and kidneys, raising the clear and descending the turbid, clearing and transforming damp-heat, and promoting blood circulation to remove blood stasis. It has reliable efficacy and no side effects.

《民族医药报》1992 年 5 月 1 日

Ethnic Medicine News, May 1, 1992

15. 处方及用法：黄芪、玉米须、糯米根各 30 克，炒糯米一撮，煲水代茶，分数次服。每日 1 剂，切勿间断，连服 3 个月。

15. Prescription and Usage: 30g each of astragalus, corn silk, and glutinous rice root, and a pinch of stir-fried glutinous rice. Boil in water to drink as tea, divided into several doses. Take one dose daily, do not interrupt, and take continuously for 3 months.

注意事项：服药期间定期尿检查，若见尿蛋白消失，第 4 个月开始可隔 1-2 天服一剂。轻者服半年，较重者则服 1 年。服药期间注意休息，避免受凉，以防感冒。少食盐，要适当给予谷、肉、水果、蔬菜等食物，以助扶正治病，忌食煎炒油炸、热毒及刺激性的食物。还可结合辨证适当配服其他中药。此方对肾病蛋白尿的改善有一定的疗效，大部分患者随着尿蛋白的消失而浮肿、血尿、高血压等症状也相应得到改善。

Precautions: Undergo regular urine tests during medication. If proteinuria disappears, starting from the 4th month, take one dose every 1-2 days. Mild cases should take it for half a year, while more severe cases should take it for 1 year. Rest well during medication, avoid catching a cold to prevent colds. Consume less salt, and appropriately provide grains, meat, fruits, and vegetables to support the body' s resistance and aid treatment. Avoid fried, hot-toxic, and irritating foods. Other TCM herbs can also be appropriately combined based on syndrome differentiation. This prescription has a certain effect on improving nephrotic proteinuria. For most patients, as proteinuria disappears, symptoms such as edema, hematuria, and hypertension are also correspondingly improved.

《民族医药报》1992 年 1 月 3 日（晴野）

Ethnic Medicine News, January 3, 1992 (Qing Ye)

二、膀胱炎（6 方）

II. Cystitis (6 Prescriptions)

1. 处方及用法: 金钱草、车前草各 30 克，金银花 15 克，滑石 18 克，甘草 3 克。将药共置砂锅内，加水适量煎煮，水沸 20 分钟后去药渣，分 2 次温服，每次半小碗。

Prescription and Usage: 30g each of lysimachia and plantain, 15g of honeysuckle, 18g of talcum, and 3g of licorice. Place all the herbs in a clay pot, add an appropriate amount of water, and boil. After boiling for 20 minutes, remove the dregs. Divide the decoction into two doses and take warm, half a small bowl each time.

本方具有清热解毒、利尿通淋之功效，治疗急性膀胱炎所致的尿频、尿急、尿痛，服药 1-3 剂，即可收到显著疗效。

This formula has the effects of clearing heat and detoxifying, promoting diuresis, and relieving stranguria. For treating urinary frequency, urgency, and dysuria caused by acute cystitis, significant effects can be achieved after taking 1-3 doses.

《民族医药报》（李子云）

Ethnic Medicine News (Li Ziyun)

2. 膀胱湿热：半边莲 30 克，尿泡草 20 克，每日一次，每日 2 次，服 3 剂而愈。

2. Bladder Damp-Heat: 30g of Chinese lobelia and 20g of bladder herb. Take once daily, twice a day. It can be cured after taking 3 doses.

3. 银金花、连翘各 9 克，茅根 15 克，地龙 10 克，车前草 10 克，茜草 15 克，海金沙 10 克。水煎服，每日 1 剂。

3. 9g each of honeysuckle and forsythia, 15g of cogongrass rhizome, 10g of earthworm, 10g of plantain, 15g of madder root, and 10g of Japanese climbing fern spores. Decoct in water and take one dose daily.

4. 川木通、车前子各 12 克，生蒲黄、扁蓄各 10 克，夜关门、铁马鞭各 5 克，水煎服。

4. 12g each of Sichuan clematis and plantain seeds, 10g each of raw cattail pollen and knotweed, and 5g each of night-closing gate and iron whip. Decoct in water and take.

5. 车前草、虎杖、马鞭草各 12 克，茅根、蒲公英、海金沙 9 克，忍冬藤、紫花地丁、十大功劳各 6 克，加水煎成 300 毫升。每日 1 剂，水煎服。

5. 12g each of plantain, giant knotweed, and verbena, 9g each of cogongrass rhizome, dandelion, and Japanese climbing fern spores, and 6g each of honeysuckle stem, violet, and mahonia. Add water and decoct to 300ml. Take one dose daily, decocted in water.

6. 天胡荽、连钱草各 9 克，车前草、金银花各 10 克，十大功劳、海金沙、茅根各 12 克，水煎服。

6. 9g each of hydrocotyle and golden coin grass, 10g each of plantain and honeysuckle, and 12g each of mahonia, Japanese climbing fern spores, and cogongrass rhizome. Decoct in water and take.

《民族医药报》Ethnic Medicine News

三、泌尿系感染（3 方）
III. Urinary Tract Infection (3 Prescriptions)

1. 广金钱草 10 克，车前草、海金沙各 8 克，金银花 9 克，水煎服，每日 1 剂。

10g of desmodium, 8g each of plantain and Japanese climbing fern spores, and 9g of honeysuckle. Decoct in water and take one dose daily.

2. 茜草 12 克，夜关门 10 克，马鞭草 5 克，车前草 10 克，金钱草 12 克，水煎服，每日 1 剂。

2. 12g of madder root, 10g of night-closing gate, 5g of verbena, 10g of plantain, and 12g of lysimachia. Decoct in water and take one dose daily.

《民族医药报》

Ethnic Medicine News

3. 尿路感染

3. Urinary Tract Infection

中老年妇女患尿路感染者比较常见，现荐民间方三则选用。

Urinary tract infections are relatively common in middle-aged and elderly women. Three folk prescriptions are now recommended for selection.

车前草 30 克、萹蓄 60 克、金银花 15 克、甘草 3 克，每日一剂，水煎分二次服。

30g of plantain, 60g of knotweed, 15g of honeysuckle, and 3g of licorice. Take one dose daily, decocted in water and divided into two doses.

绿豆芽 500 克，白糖适量，将绿豆芽洗净，以纱布压挤取汁，加白糖，代茶饮服。

500g of mung bean sprouts and an appropriate amount of white sugar. Wash the mung bean sprouts, squeeze out the juice with gauze, add white sugar, and drink as tea.

鸡内金 2 个、金钱草 30 克、玉米心 3 个、车前子 15 克、地龙 1.5 克、蛇蜕 1.5 克、板蓝根 30 克、地丁 1.5 克，水煎服。本方适用于尿路感染急性发作期。

2 chicken gizzard linings, 30g of lysimachia, 3 corn cobs, 15g of plantain seeds, 1.5g of earthworm, 1.5g of snake slough, 30g of isatis root, and 1.5g of violet. Decoct in water and take. This prescription is suitable for the acute attack stage of urinary tract infections.

《民族医药报》1992 年 4 月 3 日（四川 敬海东）

Ethnic Medicine News, April 3, 1992 (Jing Haidong, Sichuan)

四、老年人尿频、尿毒症、腰痛（4 方）

IV. Frequent Urination in the Elderly, Uremia, and Lumbago (4 Prescriptions)

1. 治老年人尿频验方

Verified Prescription for Treating Frequent Urination in the Elderly

老年人有尿频（小便次数多），甚至遗尿的病症，可服以下中药组合的方剂治疗：

For elderly people suffering from frequent urination (increased frequency of urination) or even enuresis, the following combination of Chinese herbs can be taken for treatment:

太子参、山药、黄芪各 15 克，桑螵蛸、山萸肉、茯苓各 12 克，覆盆子 9 克，益智仁、乌药各 6 克，炮附子、甘草各 3 克，肉桂 2 克。水煎分两次服，每日一剂，一般连服 3-5 剂，疗效满意。

15g each of pseudostellaria root, Chinese yam, and astragalus, 12g each of mantis egg-case, dogwood fruit, and poria, 9g of raspberry, 6g each of alpinia fruit and lindera, 3g each of processed aconite and licorice, and 2g of cinnamon bark. Decoct in water and take in two divided doses, one dose daily. Generally, taking 3-5 consecutive doses yields satisfactory results.

《中药科技报》1992 年 12 月 16 日（子云）

Chinese Herbal Medicine Science and Technology News, December 16, 1992 (Zi Yun)

2. 治老人尿频

2. Treating Frequent Urination in the Elderly

处方及用法：白果 30 克，芡实 20 克，益智仁 10 克，桑螵蛸 10 克，大枣 10 枚，每日一剂，连用 3 天有良效。

Prescription and Usage: 30g of ginkgo nut, 20g of euryale seed, 10g of alpinia fruit, 10g of mantis egg-case, and 10 red dates. Take one dose daily. Good effects can be achieved after 3 consecutive days of use.

《民族医药报》（成都 戴廷荣）

Ethnic Medicine News (Dai Tingrong, Chengdu)

3. 尿毒症三方

3. Three Prescriptions for Uremia

方一：茵陈嵩的种子 20 克，水煎服。一天量，分 3-4 次服用。

Prescription 1: 20g of capillary wormwood seeds. Decoct in water and take. This is a one-day dosage, divided into 3-4 doses.

方二：糯米 100 克、生芪 5 个、淡竹叶 50 克，水煎服。约十剂后即可见效。

Prescription 2: 100g of glutinous rice, 5 raw astragalus roots, and 50g of light bamboo leaves. Decoct in water and take. Effects can be seen after about ten doses.

方三：采沼泽生长之芦根 20 克，水煎服。一天量。分 3-4 次服用。

Prescription 3: 20g of reed rhizome harvested from marshes. Decoct in water and take. This is a one-day dosage, divided into 3-4 doses.

4. 治老年腰痛

4. Treating Lumbago in the Elderly

白术 30 克、焦杜仲 15 克，水煎。早晚各一次，每日一剂，2-3 日即效。

30g of atractylodes and 15g of charred eucommia. Decoct in water. Take once in the morning and once in the evening, one dose daily. Effects can be achieved within 2-3 days.

五、蛋白尿（4方）
V. Proteinuria (4 Prescriptions)

1. 笔者在临床实践中应用经验方“茴苓汤”治疗乳糜尿，效果卓著，现介绍给大家一试。

In clinical practice, the author applied the empirical prescription “Hui Ling Tang” to treat chyluria with remarkable results, and it is now introduced for everyone to try.

小茴12克，茯苓20克，制川乌12克，桂枝10克，白术12克，芡实12克，党参12克，白花蜂10克，露蜂房10克，水煎服，每日一剂。

12g of fennel, 20g of poria, 12g of processed Sichuan aconite, 10g of cinnamon twig, 12g of atractylodes, 12g of euryale seed, 12g of codonopsis, 10g of white bee, and 10g of wasp nest. Decoct in water and take one dose daily.

《中医药信息报》1992年9月5日（山东 李祥农）

TCM Information News, September 5, 1992 (Li Xiangnong, Shandong)

2. 方法：取双侧阴陵泉、关元俞、肾俞，用75%酒精棉球常规消毒，在其附近寻找暴涨的血络，用消毒过的三棱针快速刺破，任其流血。待血止时拔火罐，视出血量多少而决定取罐时间，一般10-15分钟。取罐后碘酒棉球消毒针眼，新洁尔灭棉球擦洗血迹。

2. Method: Select bilateral Yinlingquan, Guanyanshu, and Shenshu acupoints. Routinely disinfect with 75% alcohol swabs, find the engorged blood vessels nearby, quickly puncture them with a sterilized three-edged needle, and let the blood flow freely. Apply cupping when the bleeding stops, and determine the cupping time based on the amount of bleeding, generally 10-15 minutes. After removing the cups, disinfect the puncture sites with iodine swabs and wipe away the blood traces with benzalkonium bromide swabs.

据郑策医师报道，用此法治疗60例，病程最短2月，最长20年。经刺1-2次，48例痊愈（乳科糜尿消失，能胜任重体力劳动，1年后追访无复发），10例好转（乳糜尿消失，但劳累后偶有发作，不经治疗、休息后自愈，可作轻体力劳动），2

例无效。

According to Dr. Zheng Ce, 60 cases were treated with this method, with disease durations ranging from 2 months to 20 years. After 1-2 punctures, 48 cases were cured (chyluria disappeared, able to perform heavy physical labor, and no recurrence was found during follow-up 1 year later), 10 cases improved (chyluria disappeared, but occasional attacks occurred after fatigue, which resolved spontaneously after rest without treatment, able to perform light physical labor), and 2 cases were ineffective.

《中医药信息报》1992 年 5 月 9 日（江苏 张宏俊 王道俊）

TCM Information News, May 9, 1992 (Zhang Hongjun, Wang Daojun, Jiangsu)

3. 尿浊：车前草 50 克，苦参 20 克，挣死牛（夜关门）15 克，秧草根 15 克。水煎加红糖 10 克为引。每日 1 剂，分 3 次服。6 日为 1 疗程。

3. Turbid Urine: 50g of plantain, 20g of sophora flavescens, 15g of Zheng Si Niu (night-closing gate), and 15g of rice seedling root. Decoct in water and add 10g of brown sugar as a guiding drug. Take one dose daily, divided into three servings. A treatment course lasts for 6 days.

（云南 马应乖）

(Ma Yingguai, Yunnan)

4. 治疗尿浊验方 鲜芥菜去叶留(带)根须和茎120克，入煎剂，收液一碗服用。每天 2 剂。一般连服 2-3 天即可痊愈。

4. Verified Prescription for Treating Turbid Urine: Take 120g of fresh mustard greens, remove the leaves but keep the roots and stems, decoct in water to yield one bowl of liquid, and consume. Take 2 doses a day. Generally, continuous use for 2-3 days can achieve a cure.

六、尿潴留（8方）

VI. Urinary Retention (8 Prescriptions)

1. 独头大蒜1个，栀子3枚，食盐适量，共混捣烂，做成饼状敷脐上，4小时后小便流畅。

One single-clove garlic, 3gardenia fruits, and an appropriate amount of salt. Mix and mash them together, form into a cake-like shape, and apply to the navel. Urination will become smooth 4 hours later.

2. 葱白500克，麝香适量，共捣烂分成2包加温热，交替贴敷于脐上，冷却后再用第2包替上，轮流使用，直到小便排出为止。

2. 500g of green onion white and an appropriate amount of musk. Mash them together, divide into 2 packs, warm them up, and apply them alternately to the navel. When the first pack cools down, replace it with the second pack. Use them in rotation until urination occurs.

3. 取芒硝粉30克，甘遂粉15克，2药混匀敷贴于脐上，每天换药1次，若贴敷处皮肤有发热感，马上会有小便排出。

3. Take 30g of mirabilite powder and 15g of kansui root powder, mix the two herbs evenly, and apply to the navel. Change the medication once a day. If the skin at the application site feels warm, urination will occur immediately.

4. 大田螺5个，麝香9克，食盐9克，混合捣烂后加香粉拌匀，敷肚脐或气海穴处。（注意：寒性小便不利者禁用此方）。

4. Five large field snails, 9g of musk, and 9g of salt. Mash them together after mixing, add some fragrant powder and mix well, then apply to the navel or the Qihai acupoint. (Note: This prescription is contraindicated for patients with cold-type dysuria.)

5. 蓖麻籽（去壳）10粒，田螺5个，食盐9克。混合捣烂药贴脐部，用纱布盖好固定，1小时后，小便顺畅。

5. Ten castor seeds (shelled), five field snails, and 9g of salt. Mix and mash the herbs, apply to the navel, cover with gauze, and secure it. Urination will

become smooth 1 hour later.

《民族医药报》1997 年 11 月 7 日（申高林）

Ethnic Medicine News, November 7, 1997 (Shen Gaolin)

6. 非阻塞性尿潴留是临床常见症状，多见于老人和产妇，往往令家中束手无策，现介绍一简易方法。

6. Non-obstructive urinary retention is a common clinical symptom, frequently seen in the elderly and postpartum women, which often leaves families helpless. A simple method is now introduced.

令患者仰卧，术者侧立，以两手拇指重叠压于脐眼至耻骨联合上缘中线二分之一处（相当于关元穴靠近石门穴处），其他手指卡住两侧髂骨上缘的腰部，两食指紧靠髂骨上缘，压力先轻后重，以利尿为度，待排尿终止才放手，切勿中途停止用力。

Have the patient lie supine. The operator stands on the side, overlaps both thumbs, and presses on the midpoint between the navel and the upper border of the pubic symphysis (equivalent to the area between the Guanyuan and Shimen acupoints). The other fingers grasp the waist at the upper border of the iliac bones on both sides, with the index fingers placed closely against the upper border of the iliac bones. Apply pressure starting light and gradually increasing, to the extent of promoting diuresis. Do not release the pressure until urination ceases; never stop applying force midway.

《民族医药报》（江苏 自强）

Ethnic Medicine News (Zi Qiang, Jiangsu)

7. 葱白一根（10 厘米长），白胡椒 7 粒，共捣烂如泥，填敷肚脐上，用塑料薄膜盖好后用胶布固定。本方对 12 例病人应用均获良效。对老年人因前列腺肥大所致小便不通也有较好效果。

7. One green onion white (10 cm long) and 7 white peppercorns. Mash them together into a paste, fill and apply it to the navel, cover with plastic wrap, and secure with adhesive tape. This prescription has achieved good results in 12 patients. It also has a good effect on urinary obstruction caused by prostate

hypertrophy in the elderly.

《民族医药报》1992 年 2 月 21 日（贵州 杨通福）

Ethnic Medicine News, February 21, 1992 (Yang Tongfu, Guizhou)

8. 急性尿潴留，是老年人的一种多发病。一旦患此病，痛苦难忍。下述中药方对治疗该疾有良好效果：黄芪 30 克、甘草 10 克、肉桂 6 克、知母 6 克、黄柏 6 克、王不留行 5 克、茯苓 15 克、金银花 15 克、肉苁蓉 12 克，每日一剂，每剂用水煎三次，当茶饮，一般用药一至二剂，尿潴留症即可缓解，等症状消除后服知柏地黄丸巩固疗效。

8. Acute urinary retention is a frequently occurring disease in the elderly. Once afflicted, the suffering is unbearable. The following TCM prescription has good effects on treating this disease: 30g of astragalus, 10g of licorice, 6g of cinnamon bark, 6g of anemarrhena, 6g of phellodendron, 5g of vaccaria seeds, 15g of poria, 15g of honeysuckle, and 12g of cistanche. Take one dose daily, decocted three times in water, and drink as tea. Generally, after taking 1-2 doses, the symptoms of urinary retention can be relieved. After the symptoms disappear, take Zhibai Dihuang Wan to consolidate the efficacy.

此方对於中医辨证属气阴两虚之症效果尤佳。

This prescription is particularly effective for TCM syndromes diagnosed as dual deficiency of qi and yin.

《民族医药报》（浙江 周新民）

Ethnic Medicine News (Zhou Xinmin, Zhejiang)

七、泌尿系结石（8 方）

VII. Urinary System Stones (8 Prescriptions)

1. 笔者结合临床实践自拟三金琥膝汤治疗泌尿系结石 240 例，取得良好效果，兹介绍如下。

Combining clinical practice, the author formulated Sanjin Huxi Tang to treat 240 cases of urinary system stones with good results, which are introduced as follows.

一般资料：240例中，男性170例，女性70例。年龄最小为3岁，最大为58岁。单发性结石216例，多发性结石24例；肾结石54例（单侧47例，双侧1例，单侧肾、输尿管结石4例，单侧肾多发性结石2例）；输尿管结石174例（单侧161例，双侧7例，单例多发6例）；膀胱结石11例，尿道结石1例。结石横径0.3-1.2厘米，竖径0.3-1.7厘米。肾功能一般良好，不论结石单发或多发，坚持治疗3个疗程以上为统计对象。

General Data: Among the 240 cases, 170 were male and 70 were female. The youngest patient was 3 years old, and the oldest was 58. There were 216 cases of single stones and 24 cases of multiple stones; 54 cases of kidney stones (47 unilateral, 1 bilateral, 4 unilateral kidney and ureteral stones, and 2 unilateral multiple kidney stones); 174 cases of ureteral stones (161 unilateral, 7 bilateral, and 6 single-case multiple); 11 cases of bladder stones, and 1 case of urethral stones. The transverse diameter of the stones was 0.3-1.2 cm, and the vertical diameter was 0.3-1.7 cm. Renal function was generally good. Regardless of whether the stones were single or multiple, patients who persisted in treatment for more than 3 courses were included in the statistics.

本组病例除典型病史，症状及体检外，均经X线、B型超声波探查或造影确诊。

In addition to typical medical history, symptoms, and physical examinations, all cases in this group were confirmed by X-ray, B-ultrasound, or contrast imaging.

治疗方法：本组病例均用三金琥膝汤加减治疗。处方：金钱草30克，海金砂10克，鸡内金5克（冲服），琥珀粉3克（冲服）山木通10克，滑石粉30克，牡丹皮10克，川牛膝10克，台乌药10克，甘草梢5克。加减：疼痛较剧者，加元胡索9克，赤芍12克，或针刺足三里，中等度刺激，不留针；血尿明显者加炒蒲黄9克，小蓟15克；气虚者加黄芪15克，党参20克；血虚者加熟地15克，白芍12克；脾虚者加白术12克，淮山12克；肾阳虚者加附片6克，肉桂4克；肾阴虚者加生地12克，女贞子12克。

Treatment Method: All cases in this group were treated with modified Sanjin

Huxi Tang. Prescription: 30g of lysimachia, 10g of Japanese climbing fern spores, 5g of chicken gizzard lining (taken by mixing with the decoction), 3g of amber powder (taken by mixing with the decoction), 10g of Sichuan clematis, 30g of talcum powder, 10g of moutan bark, 10g of cyathula root, 10g of lindera, and 5g of licorice tip. Modifications: For severe pain, add 9g of corydalis and 12g of red peony, or perform acupuncture at Zusanli with moderate stimulation without retaining the needles; for obvious hematuria, add 9g of stir-fried cattail pollen and 15g of small thistle; for qi deficiency, add 15g of astragalus and 20g of codonopsis; for blood deficiency, add 15g of prepared rehmannia and 12g of white peony; for spleen deficiency, add 12g of atractylodes and 12g of Chinese yam; for kidney yang deficiency, add 6g of aconite slices and 4g of cinnamon bark; for kidney yin deficiency, add 12g of rehmannia and 12g of glossy privet fruit.

诸药（冲服药除外）加水浸泡 10-15 分钟，水面高出药面 0.5-1 厘米，煎开 20 分钟，过滤取汁温服，一日 2 次，连服 10 天为 1 疗程。

Soak all the herbs (except those taken by mixing) in water for 10-15 minutes, with the water level 0.5-1 cm above the herbs. Boil for 20 minutes, filter to obtain the liquid, and take it warm, twice a day. 10 consecutive days constitute one treatment course.

疗效标准：①痊愈：排出结石，经 X 线腹部平片或 B 型超声波复查，结石阴影消失，尿常规和肾图恢复正常，临床症状消失；②显效：排出部分砂石样结石或结石位置下降 3 厘米以上，临床症状基本消失；③无效：经治疗 3 个疗程，与治疗前相比较，结石未排出或位置下移小于 3 厘米。

Efficacy Criteria: ① Cured: Stones discharged; upon re-examination with abdominal X-ray or B-ultrasound, the stone shadow disappeared, urinalysis and renogram returned to normal, and clinical symptoms disappeared; ② Markedly effective: Partial sand-like stones discharged or stone position dropped by more than 3 cm, with clinical symptoms basically disappeared; ③ Ineffective: After 3 courses of treatment, compared with before treatment, the stones were not discharged or dropped less than 3 cm.

治疗效果：痊愈 124 例，占 51.67%；有效 92 例，占 38.33%，无效 24 例，占 10%。总有效率 90%。

Treatment Results: 124 cases were cured, accounting for 51.67%; 92 cases were effective, accounting for 38.33%; and 24 cases were ineffective, accounting for 10%. The total effective rate was 90%.

体会：泌尿系结石属祖国医学的石淋、砂淋、血淋等范畴，多因脾不健运，湿邪内停，蕴久化热，结于下焦，尿液受湿热煎熬而成；或因七情所伤，肝郁气滞，升降失常，引起三焦气化失司，水液通利失常，影响肾的功能，脾、肝、肾三脏病变又相互影响，砂石渐成。笔者自拟三金琥膝汤扶助正气，祛除邪气。方中以金钱草、海金砂清热、利尿、速石；山木通、滑石粉利水通淋；牡丹皮、琥珀粉活血散瘀止痛；鸡内金化坚磨石；川牛膝活血祛瘀，引石下行；台乌药行气止痛，引石下行；引甘草梢泻火解毒，缓急止痛。诸药配合，共奏行气止痛，清热利湿，排石通淋之功。

Experience: Urinary system stones belong to the TCM categories of Shi Lin (stone stranguria), Sha Lin (sand stranguria), and Xue Lin (blood stranguria). They are mostly caused by impaired spleen transport, internal retention of dampness, prolonged accumulation transforming into heat, and binding in the lower jiao, where urine is 煎熬 (decocted) by damp-heat; or caused by emotional injuries leading to liver qi stagnation, abnormal ascending and descending, resulting in impaired Sanjiao qi transformation, abnormal water fluid passage, and affected kidney function. The pathological changes in the spleen, liver, and kidney mutually influence each other, gradually forming stones. The author formulated Sanjin Huxi Tang to support healthy qi and eliminate pathogenic factors. In this formula, lysimachia and Japanese climbing fern spores clear heat, promote diuresis, and expedite stone discharge; Sichuan clematis and talcum powder promote diuresis and relieve stranguria; moutan bark and amber powder promote blood circulation, dissipate stasis, and relieve pain; chicken gizzard lining dissolves hardness and grinds stones; cyathula root promotes blood circulation, removes stasis, and guides stones downward; lindera promotes qi circulation, relieves pain, and guides stones downward; licorice tip purges fire, detoxifies, and relieves spasms and pain. Combined, these herbs work together to promote qi circulation, relieve pain, clear heat and promote diuresis, and discharge stones to relieve stranguria.

《民族医药报》1992 年 4 月 17 日（湖南 王艳）

Ethnic Medicine News, April 17, 1992 (Wang Yan, Hunan)

2. 主治：膀胱结石。方药：鹅不食草 200 克（鲜），白糖 10 克，白酒 15 克。

2. Indications: Bladder stones. Ingredients: 200g of fresh centipeda, 10g of white sugar, and 15g of white liquor (baijiu).

用法：水煎服，每日一剂，连服 5-10 剂。

Usage: Decoct in water and take, one dose daily, continuously for 5-10 doses.

《民族医药报》1992 年 6 月 5 日（苏州 俞敏）

Ethnic Medicine News, June 5, 1992 (Yu Min, Suzhou)

3. 肾输尿管结石 23 例

3. 23 Cases of Kidney and Ureteral Stones

肾输尿管结石常表现为腰部突然发作阵发性剧烈绞痛，并沿该侧输尿管向膀胱、会阴大腿两侧放射，常伴有面色苍白，恶心，呕吐，冷汗，绞痛后可出现血尿。笔者自 1984 年以来运用自拟海金砂汤治疗肾输尿管结石 23 例，均获治愈。

Kidney and ureteral stones often present as sudden paroxysmal severe colic in the lower back, radiating along the ureter on the affected side to the bladder, perineum, and both thighs. It is often accompanied by pale complexion, nausea, vomiting, and cold sweat. Hematuria may occur after the colic. Since 1984, the author has used the self-formulated Haijinsha Tang to treat 23 cases of kidney and ureteral stones, all of which were cured.

一般资料：23 例中，男 16 例，女 7 例，年龄，20 至 30 岁 19 例，40 至 55 岁 4 例，病程 10 天以内的 20 例，30 天以上的 3 例。B 超检查肾输尿管可见大小不等的砂石。

General Data: Among the 23 cases, 16 were male and 7 were female. In terms of age, 19 cases were 20-30 years old, and 4 cases were 40-55 years old. In terms of disease duration, 20 cases were within 10 days, and 3 cases were over 30 days. B-ultrasound showed sand and stones of varying sizes in the kidneys and ureters.

治疗方法：海金砂30克（包煎），金钱草60克，冬葵子15克，广地龙10克，生鸡内金12克，车前子30克（包煎），滑石粉60克，王不留行15克，尿血：加白茅根30克，瞿麦12克。腰酸：加桑寄生18克，淮牛膝12克。便秘：加制川军9克、玄明粉12克（冲服）。气虚：加胡桃肉12克（打），菟丝子12克。肾绞痛：加生白芍30克，炒元胡12克，生甘草3克。肾阴虚：加生地15克。肾阳虚：加肉桂3克（后下）。肾盂积水：加炒白芥子10克，炒莱菔子12克。每日一剂。水煎服。服药期间，禁忌辛辣刺激性食物。

Treatment Method: 30g of Japanese climbing fern spores (decocted in a cloth bag), 60g of lysimachia, 15g of mallow seeds, 10g of earthworm, 12g of raw chicken gizzard lining, 30g of plantain seeds (decocted in a cloth bag), 60g of talcum powder, and 15g of vaccaria seeds. For hematuria: add 30g of cogongrass rhizome and 12g of dianthus. For lumbago: add 18g of mistletoe and 12g of cyathula root. For constipation: add 9g of processed rhubarb and 12g of mirabilite (taken by mixing with the decoction). For qi deficiency: add 12g of crushed walnut kernel and 12g of dodder seeds. For renal colic: add 30g of raw white peony, 12g of stir-fried corydalis, and 3g of raw licorice. For kidney yin deficiency: add 15g of rehmannia. For kidney yang deficiency: add 3g of cinnamon bark (added towards the end of decoction). For hydronephrosis: add 10g of stir-fried white mustard seeds and 12g of stir-fried radish seeds. Take one dose daily, decocted in water. During medication, spicy and stimulating foods are strictly prohibited.

疗效统计：23例全部治愈，服药3至5剂15例，6至10剂6例，10剂以上2例。

Efficacy Statistics: All 23 cases were cured. 15 cases recovered after taking 3-5 doses, 6 cases after 6-10 doses, and 2 cases after more than 10 doses.

《中医药信息报》1992年5月30日（张银慧 张达）

TCM Information News, May 30, 1992 (Zhang Yinhui, Zhang Da)

4. 笔者在临床实践中应用补气清热利水通淋法治疗尿路结石30余例（所有

病例均经 B 型超声波检查所见结石分别存在于尿路的某个部位。所有病例均在当地服用中药清热利湿剂 10 至 20 剂，以及西药抗菌素、解痉药治疗病情未见改善，后来我院经服用补气清热利水通淋法治疗。经服药后排出大小不等、形态各异、硬度不同的结石）均获得显著疗效，现报告如下：

4. In clinical practice, the author applied the method of tonifying qi, clearing heat, promoting diuresis, and relieving stranguria to treat over 30 cases of urinary tract stones (all cases were confirmed by B-ultrasound to have stones located in various parts of the urinary tract. All patients had previously taken 10-20 doses of heat-clearing and dampness-resolving TCM agents locally, as well as Western antibiotics and antispasmodics, without improvement. After coming to our hospital and receiving the above-mentioned treatment, they discharged stones of varying sizes, shapes, and hardness). All achieved significant effects, which are now reported as follows:

方剂组成、用法、主证及疗效：元芪 30 克、党参 20 克、莪术 10 克、当归 10 克、陈皮 10 克、柴胡 6 克、升麻 6 克、泽夕 10 克、车前 10 克、木通 10 克、金钱草 30 克、白茅根 30 克、甘草 10 克。水煎服。日一剂。早晚各服一次。10 至 20 剂为一疗程。病人按结石的所在部位，可有小腹稳痛，腰背剧痛，或痛不可忍，小便难，尿中夹有砂石，或溺中有血，血色红紫，脉数有力或沉弦舌红，苔白或黄等症状。病人在服药过程中排尿通畅，疼痛日渐减轻，结石随尿中排出。凡结石能从尿路通过，服用本方剂均能将结石排出。经 B 超复查结石不再存留。

Prescription Composition, Usage, Main Symptoms, and Efficacy: 30g of astragalus, 20g of codonopsis, 10g of zedoary, 10g of angelica, 10g of tangerine peel, 6g of bupleurum, 6g of cimicifuga, 10g of alisma, 10g of plantain, 10g of clematis, 30g of lysimachia, 30g of cogongrass rhizome, and 10g of licorice. Decoct in water and take. One dose daily, taken once in the morning and once in the evening. 10-20 doses constitute one treatment course. Depending on the location of the stones, patients may present with dull lower abdominal pain, severe lumbago and back pain, or unbearable pain, difficult urination, sand and stones in the urine, or blood in the urine with a red-purple color, a rapid and forceful or deep and string-taut pulse, a red tongue, and a white or yellow coating. During medication, patients experienced smooth urination, gradually alleviated pain, and discharged stones with their urine. As long as the stones could pass through the urinary tract, this prescription could successfully discharge them. Follow-up B-ultrasound confirmed that no stones remained.

中医认为结石的形成是由于湿热注于下焦，肾虚膀胱气化不利所致。小便结石淋沥涩痛是因尿路中有结石阻塞，下焦气化功能失常所造成。而本方剂是由补中益气汤加味而成，能推动三焦气化之运行。下焦气化功能正常，再配伍清热利水通淋之药品，小便通利，而使尿路结石得以顺利排出。

TCM believes that the formation of stones is caused by damp-heat pouring into the lower jiao, and kidney deficiency leading to impaired qi transformation of the bladder. The painful and difficult urination with stones is caused by the blockage of stones in the urinary tract and the dysfunction of qi transformation in the lower jiao. This prescription is a modified version of Buzhong Yiqi Tang (Tonify the Middle and Augment the Qi Decoction), which can promote the qi transformation of the Sanjiao. When the qi transformation function of the lower jiao returns to normal, combined with herbs that clear heat, promote diuresis, and relieve stranguria, urination becomes smooth, allowing the urinary tract stones to be discharged smoothly.

《中医药信息报》1992 年 8 月 1 日（河北 于洪章）

TCM Information News, August 1, 1992 (Yu Hongzhang, Hebei)

5. 治尿石症方

5. Prescription for Treating Urolithiasis

主治，泌尿系结石引起的疼痛，血尿。

Indications: Pain and hematuria caused by urinary system stones.

组成：生车前草 10 克，绿豆粉 10 克，桃仁 50 只。

Composition: 10g of raw plantain, 10g of mung bean powder, and 50 peach kernels.

用法：捣烂，开水冲服，二次服下。

Usage: Mash them into a paste, brew with boiling water, and take in two divided doses.

《民族医药报》

Ethnic Medicine News

6. 尿路结石

6. Urinary Tract Stones

石苇、半边莲、天胡荽、海金沙各 30 克，木通、茅根各 10 克，水煎服，每日 1 剂。

30g each of pyrrosia, Chinese lobelia, hydrocotyle, and Japanese climbing fern spores, and 10g each of clematis and cogongrass rhizome. Decoct in water and take one dose daily.

7. 车前草、木通、无根藤各 15 克，海金沙、石苇各 20 克，十大功劳、茅根各 25 克，水煎服，每日 1 剂。

7. 15g each of plantain, clematis, and dodder, 20g each of Japanese climbing fern spores and pyrrosia, and 25g each of mahonia and cogongrass rhizome. Decoct in water and take one dose daily.

8. 金钱草、石苇、海金沙、鸡内金各 20 克，车前草、木通、茅根、无根藤各 10 克，水煎服，每日 1 剂。

8. 20g each of lysimachia, pyrrosia, Japanese climbing fern spores, and chicken gizzard lining, and 10g each of plantain, clematis, cogongrass rhizome, and dodder. Decoct in water and take one dose daily.

《民族医药报》（广西 盘祖良）

Ethnic Medicine News (Pan Zugen, Guangxi)

第九章　男科
Chapter 9　Andrology

一、前列腺炎（5方）
I. Prostatitis (5 Prescriptions)

1. 治慢性前列腺炎验方

Verified Prescription for Treating Chronic Prostatitis

前列腺炎是青壮年男性常见疾病，往往与尿道炎、精囊炎及附睾炎等并存，有急性与慢性两种，尤以慢性多见。

Prostatitis is a common disease in young and middle-aged men, often coexisting with urethritis, seminal vesiculitis, and epididymitis. It can be acute or chronic, with the chronic form being more common.

慢性前列腺炎以会阴部不适，尿道异物感，腰骶部酸痛，小腹坠胀，尿排不尽，尿前段或后段有白浊，失眠多梦，遗精、乏力健忘为主要症状。

The main symptoms of chronic prostatitis include perineal discomfort, a foreign body sensation in the urethra, lumbosacral soreness and pain, lower abdominal distension and heaviness, incomplete urination, white turbid urine at the beginning or end of urination, insomnia with excessive dreaming, seminal emission, fatigue, and poor memory.

已婚者可有性欲减退、早泄、阳痿或不育等；

Married patients may experience decreased libido, premature ejaculation, impotence, or infertility.

直肠指检多见前列腺硬度增加，或有硬结及触痛；

Digital rectal examination often reveals increased prostate hardness, or the presence of hard nodules and tenderness upon palpation.

前列腺液镜检，每高倍视野白细胞超过10个或成堆，卵磷脂小体显著减少。

Microscopic examination of prostatic fluid shows that white blood cells exceed 10 per high-power field or appear in clusters, and lecithin bodies are significantly reduced.

方药组成及用法：大黄、半夏各10-15克，琥珀10-20克。

Prescription Composition and Usage: 10-15g each of rhubarb and pinellia, and 10-20g of amber.

先取大黄、半夏，加水适量，煎汁200毫升，用100毫升冲琥珀5-10克，一次服完，每日早晚各服一次。

First, take the rhubarb and pinellia, add an appropriate amount of water, and decoct to yield 200ml of liquid. Use 100ml of this decoction to mix with 5-10g of amber powder, and take it all at once, once in the morning and once in the evening.

初用本方，药量从轻到重，因人而异，服用前三剂时大黄、半夏用量各10克，琥珀用量5克；

When initially using this prescription, the dosage should be adjusted from light to heavy depending on the individual. For the first three doses, use 10g each of rhubarb and pinellia, and 5g of amber.

病人服药后，大便每日不超过2次，大黄、半夏可用到15克，琥珀用到10克。

If the patient has no more than two bowel movements per day after taking the medication, the dosage of rhubarb and pinellia can be increased to 15g, and amber to 10g.

个别患者服药后有轻度腹痛，不用停药，两日后腹痛可自行缓解。

A few patients may experience mild abdominal pain after taking the medication; there is no need to stop the medication, as the pain will subside on its own after two days.

多数病人服药1-2周，可望治愈。

Most patients can expect to be cured after taking the medication for 1-2 weeks.

《民族医药报》1991 年 7 月 5 日（广西 林中）

Ethnic Medicine News, July 5, 1991 (Lin Zhong, Guangxi)

2. 治疗慢性前列腺炎。

2. Treating Chronic Prostatitis

鸭跖草 30-50 克（鲜品为 100-300 克），蒲公英 50 克，以淘米水煎煮 10-20 分钟后服用。

30-50g of dayflower (100-300g if fresh) and 50g of dandelion. Decoct in rice-washing water for 10-20 minutes and take.

每日一剂，分二次服；然后再用清水煎药渣，取液水温坐浴，15 天为一疗程。

Take one dose daily, divided into two servings. Then, decoct the remaining herbal dregs in clean water, and use the warm liquid for a sitz bath. A treatment course lasts for 15 days.

适用于耻骨上阴茎根部轻度疼痛，两腹股沟部或阴部呈交替性刺痛或下腹痛，下腰部胀痛或伴有尿意不尽之感，甚至阳痿、早泄等。

This is suitable for mild pain at the base of the penis above the pubis, alternating stabbing pain in both groin areas or the genital region, or lower abdominal pain, lower back distension and pain accompanied by a feeling of incomplete urination, or even impotence and premature ejaculation.

3. 前列腺肥大的外治疗法

3. External Therapies for Prostatic Hypertrophy

①刺嚏法或探吐法。

① Sneezing or Emetic Method.

取消毒棉签探入鼻部刺激鼻中，使之引发嚏涕。

Use a sterilized cotton swab to gently stimulate the inside of the nasal cavity to induce sneezing.

或用羽毛探入口中刺激喉部，使之作呕而微吐。

Alternatively, use a feather to stimulate the throat to induce mild vomiting.

即可使小便自利。

This can promote spontaneous urination.

②熨脐法。

② Navel Ironing Method.

系用艾叶 60 克、石菖蒲 30 克，炒热以布包之，热熨于脐部（神阙穴），冷则易之即可见效。

Use 60g of mugwort leaves and 30g of sweetflag rhizome. Stir-fry them until hot, wrap them in a cloth, and apply the hot pack to the navel (Shenque acupoint). Replace it when it cools down, and it will take effect.

③暖小腹法。

③ Lower Abdomen Warming Method.

系用食盐 500 克，切碎生葱 250 克与食盐同放锅内炒热后，用布包之待温度适宜时，熨暖小腹部，冷则易之，热熨数次，小便即可自利。

Use 500g of salt and 250g of chopped raw green onions. Stir-fry them together in a pan until hot, wrap them in a cloth, and when the temperature is appropriate, apply it to warm the lower abdomen. Replace it when it cools down. After several hot applications, spontaneous urination will occur.

④中极穴贴药法。

④ Zhongji Acupoint Plaster Method.

系用甘遂细末 9 克，面粉适量及冰片少许，加温水调成糊状，贴于中极穴（脐下 4 寸）方圆两寸的位置上，一般 30 分钟就能利尿。

Use 9g of finely ground kansui root powder, an appropriate amount of flour, and a small amount of borneol. Mix them with warm water into a paste, and apply it to an area of about two cun around the Zhongji acupoint (4 cun below the navel). Diuresis can generally be achieved within 30 minutes.

⑤穴位指压法。

⑤ Acupoint Acupressure Method.

取中根（脐下 4 寸）、关元（脐下 2 寸）、阴陵泉（胫骨内侧髁宜下陷窝中）、三阴交（内髁直上 3 寸）各穴，用拇指按压几分钟或用艾炷加灸海穴气（脐下 1.5），十几分钟小便即可自利。

Select the following acupoints: Zhonggen (4 cun below the navel), Guanyuan (2 cun below the navel), Yinlingquan (in the depression below the medial condyle of the tibia), and Sanyinjiao (3 cun directly above the medial malleolus). Press each acupoint with the thumb for a few minutes, or apply moxibustion with moxa cones to the Qihai acupoint (1.5 cun below the navel). Spontaneous urination can be achieved in about ten minutes.

《中药科技报》1992 年 4 月（宋永照 宋艳敏）

TCM Science and Technology News, April 1992 (Song Yongzhao, Song Yanmin)

4. 老年男性前列腺增生多因肾气衰弱、膀胱不利、湿热内蕴所致，中医治疗重在益气补肾、升清降浊、软坚散结。

4. Prostatic hyperplasia in elderly men is mostly caused by weakened kidney qi, impaired bladder function, and internal accumulation of damp-heat. TCM treatment focuses on tonifying qi and nourishing the kidneys, raising the clear and descending the turbid, and softening hardness and dissipating nodules.

方用：黄芪 15 克，党参 15 克，淮山药 15 克，菟丝子 12 克，覆盆子 12 克，升麻 10 克，当归 10 克，山甲片 10 克，莪术 10 克，海藻 10 克，黄柏 10 克，滑石 10 克。水煎服。

Prescription: 15g of astragalus, 15g of codonopsis, 15g of Chinese yam, 12g of dodder seeds, 12g of raspberry, 10g of cimicifuga, 10g of angelica, 10g of pangolin scales, 10g of zedoary, 10g of seaweed, 10g of phellodendron, and 10g of talcum. Decoct in water and take.

10 剂为 1 疗程，可连服 3-5 个疗程。

10 doses constitute one treatment course, and 3-5 consecutive courses can be taken.

《民族医药报》1992 年 5 月 22 日（杭州 张亦华）

Ethnic Medicine News, May 22, 1992 (Zhang Yihua, Hangzhou)

5. 黄芪 60 克，地龙 10 克，当归 10 克，川芎 10 克，王不留行子 10 克，红花 10 克，桃仁 10 克，牛膝 10 克，琥珀末（冲服）3 克，皂角刺 6 克，夏枯草

15克，生牡蛎30克，每日1剂，水煎服。

5. 60g of astragalus, 10g of earthworm, 10g of angelica, 10g of ligusticum, 10g of vaccaria seeds, 10g of safflower, 10g of peach kernel, 10g of cyathula root, 3g of amber powder (taken by mixing with the decoction), 6g of honeylocust spine, 15g of prunella, and 30g of raw oyster shell. Take one dose daily, decocted in water.

《民族医药报》1998年4月3日（宁在兰）

Ethnic Medicine News, April 3, 1998 (Ning Zailan)

二、疝气（7方）

I. Hernia (7 Prescriptions)

1. 生龙眼核500克，洗净，瓦上焙干为末，每日10克，用黄酒送服。

Take 500g of raw longan seeds, wash them, roast them dry on a tile, and grind them into powder. Take 10g daily with yellow rice wine.

2. 延胡索、荔枝核、青皮各50克，桔梗10克，共研末，分9次服，1日服3次。

2. Take 50g each of corydalis, litchi seeds, and green tangerine peel, and 10g of platycodon. Grind them together into powder. Divide the powder into 9 doses, and take 3 doses a day.

3. 净地龙、透骨草各10克，白糖150克，大葱白连须去叶8克，用黄酒500克，同药装入壶内，隔水炖开，分2次服，见汗。

3. Take 10g each of cleaned earthworm and transuic grass, 150g of white sugar, and 8g of green onion white (with roots, without leaves). Put them together with the herbs into a pot, add 500g of yellow rice wine, and stew over a water bath until boiling. Divide into 2 doses. Take until sweating occurs.

4. 川楝子50克，茴香15克，木香10克，故纸6克，共为细末，每服8克，姜汤送下。

4. Take 50g of Sichuan chinaberry, 15g of fennel, 10g of costus root, and 6g of psoralea fruit. Grind them together into fine powder. Take 8g each time, swallowed with ginger soup.

5. 生枳壳 15 克，生黄芪 15 克，升麻 6 克，水煎服。

5. Take 15g of raw bitter orange, 15g of raw astragalus, and 6g of cimicifuga. Decoct in water and take.

6. 小茴香 12 克，川楝子 10 克，石菖蒲、葫芦巴各 9 克，水煎温服。

6. Take 12g of fennel, 10g of Sichuan chinaberry, and 9g each of sweetflag rhizome and fenugreek. Decoct in water and take warm.

7. 花椒 40 克，葱须 8 个，瓜蒌 1 个，陈醋 250 克，用白布包药，砂锅醋煎，洗患处。

7. Take 40g of Sichuan peppercorns, 8green onion roots, 1 Chinese cucumber, and 250g of aged vinegar. Wrap the herbs in a white cloth, decoct in a clay pot with the vinegar, and wash the affected area with the liquid.

《中国科技报》1992 年 4 月 16 日（徐国庆）

China Science and Technology News, April 16, 1992 (Xu Guoqing)

三、阴囊湿疹（5 方）

III. Scrotal Eczema (5 Prescriptions)

1. 阴囊湿疹又叫绣球风，为临床常见皮肤病。该病特点是皮疹呈多型性，局部红肿奇痒，常因过度搔抓而流黄水，若不及时治疗，易反复发作，迁延不愈。

Scrotal eczema, also known as “Xiuqiu Feng”, is a common clinical skin disease. The characteristics of this disease include polymorphic skin rashes, local redness, swelling, and severe itching. It often oozes yellow fluid due to excessive scratching. If not treated promptly, it is prone to repeated attacks and prolonged healing.

临床实践证明，“苦参荆艾汤”治阴囊湿疹，效果良好，请患者不妨试一试。

Clinical practice has proven that “Kushen Jing’ai Tang” has good effects in treating scrotal eczema. Patients are welcome to give it a try.

药物组成：苦参、荆芥、艾叶、防风、杏仁、蛇床子、猪胆汁各 16 克，细辛 10 克。

Prescription Composition: 16g each of sophora flavescens, schizonepeta, mugwort leaf, saposhnikovia, almond, cnidium fruit, and pig bile, and 10g of asarum.

配制方法：将上述药物放入药锅内，加入清水 2000 毫升，文火煮沸 30-40 分钟。

Preparation Method: Put the above herbs into a pot, add 2000ml of clean water, and boil over low heat for 30-40 minutes.

使用方法：将上述药液倒入盆中，趁热熏洗局部，每日 2 次，每次 30-40 分钟。

Usage: Pour the herbal liquid into a basin, and while it is hot, fumigate and wash the local area. Do this twice a day, 30-40 minutes each time.

《民族医药报》（徐宝庆）

Ethnic Medicine News (Xu Baoqing)

阴囊癣为一种常见的癣症，以湿热型多见。重者瘙痒、起泡、流黄水。笔者现将几年的治疗体会报道如下：

Scrotal tinea is a common type of tinea, mostly seen as the damp-heat type. Severe cases present with itching, blistering, and oozing of yellow fluid. The author now reports on several years of treatment experience as follows:

2. 鲜龙葵全草 30g、地骨皮 15g、羌活 9g、石菖蒲 9g、白藓皮 12g、龙胆草 10g、地肤子 10g、蛇床子 12g、陈艾叶 15g、川黄柏 18g、枯黄芩 15g。内服七剂。

2. 30g of fresh whole black nightshade plant, 15g of Chinese wolfberry root bark, 9g each of notopterygium and sweetflag rhizome, 12g each of dictamnus bark and cnidium fruit, 10g each of gentian and kochia fruit, 15g of aged mugwort leaf, 18g of Sichuan phellodendron, and 15g of dried scutellaria. Take 7 doses orally.

3. 鲜龙葵全草 50g、地骨皮 30g、防风 15g、白芷 15g、地肤子 25g、蒲公英 30g、蛇床子 25g、苦参 20g、土花椒 10g、陈艾叶 30g。洗浴，一日两次，连用七剂。

3. 50g of fresh whole black nightshade plant, 30g of Chinese wolfberry

root bark, 15g each of saposhnikovia and angelica dahurica, 25g each of kochia fruit and cnidium fruit, 30g of dandelion, 20g of sophora flavescens, 10g of wild Sichuan peppercorn, and 30g of aged mugwort leaf. Use for bathing, twice a day, for 7 consecutive doses.

按：本方根据《纲目》载："龙葵治天疱湿疮，苗叶捣敷之，苗消热散血。"

Note: According to the Compendium of Materia Medica (Bencao Gangmu), "Black nightshade treats pemphigus and damp sores; its stems and leaves can be mashed and applied topically to reduce heat and dissipate blood stasis."

配黄柏、黄芩、地骨皮除湿、清热，起到满意的治疗效果，一般病程二年以上的患者 15 日即愈，二年以内的患者 1 周内即愈，有效率 95%，无不适反应及副作用。

Combined with phellodendron, scutellaria, and Chinese wolfberry root bark to remove dampness and clear heat, it achieves satisfactory therapeutic effects. Generally, patients with a disease course of over two years are cured in 15 days, and those with a course of less than two years are cured within one week. The effective rate is 95%, with no adverse reactions or side effects.

《中药科技报》1991 年 11 月 26 日

TCM Science and Technology News, November 26, 1991

4. 药物和用法：龙骨（煅）牡蛎（煅）各等量研末调匀为散，装瓶备用。

4. Herbs and Usage: Take equal amounts of calcined dragon bone and calcined oyster shell. Grind them into powder and mix evenly. Store in a bottle for later use.

用法：有渗液的将龙牡散直接擦于患处，无渗液的可将龙牡散用冷开水湿润后擦于患处即可，一般 10 分钟后即可止痒，每日 2-3 次，3-5 天可愈。

Usage: If there is exudate, apply the Longmu powder directly to the affected area. If there is no exudate, moisten the powder with cooled boiled water before applying. It generally stops itching in 10 minutes. Apply 2-3 times a day, and it can be cured in 3-5 days.

对手脚趾湿疹疗效也很好，一擦即痒止痛减。

It also has very good effects on hand and toe eczema; itching and pain are relieved immediately upon application.

《民族医药报》（广西 王济仁）

Ethnic Medicine News (Wang Jiren, Guangxi)

5. 治阴囊顽癣，阴唇、会阴、臀部湿疹、奇痒难忍者。

5. For treating stubborn scrotal tinea, and eczema of the labia, perineum, and buttocks with unbearable severe itching.

可用五倍子 100 克，乌贼骨 80 克，冰片 3.5 克。共研细末，以麻油调成糊状涂搽患处，消毒纱布包裹，每日 3 次。既止痒又止痛，连续用 3-5 日即愈。

Use 100g of Chinese gallnut, 80g of cuttlebone, and 3.5g of borneol. Grind them together into fine powder, mix into a paste with sesame oil, and apply to the affected area. Wrap with sterilized gauze. Apply 3 times a day. It relieves both itching and pain, and continuous use for 3-5 days can achieve a cure.

四、阳痿（5 方）
IV. Impotence (5 Prescriptions)

1. 冬虫夏草 30 克，凹舌兰 30 克，黄精 30 克，天冬 30 克，唐古特马尿泡根 15 克，牛、羊、黄羊、石羊等之睾丸（不拘多少）。

30g of cordyceps, 30g of orchid, 30g of polygonatum, 30g of asparagus, 15g of Tangut prickly ash root, and testicles of cattle, sheep, goitered gazelle, or blue sheep (in any amount).

以上诸药共为细末，放入牦牛奶中共煮，尔后即以纸遮蔽，晒干，研为细末；

Grind the above herbs into fine powder, boil them together in yak milk, then cover with paper, sun-dry, and grind into fine powder again.

加水獭阴茎 1 条和睾丸 2 个，鹿肾 1 个，鹿睾丸 2 个，麻雀肉数只（去内脏和嘴爪，油炸），共为细末，炼密为丸如鸽蛋大。

Add 1 otter penis and 2 testicles, 1 deer kidney, 2 deer testicles, and several sparrows (eviscerated, with beaks and claws removed, then deep-fried). Grind them all into fine powder, refine with honey, and make pills the size of pigeon eggs.

早晚服 1 丸，以酒为引。服药期间，忌房事。

Take 1 pill in the morning and 1 in the evening, taken with wine as a guide. Abstain from sexual intercourse during medication.

2. 玉竹 60 克，天冬 30 克，建果芹 30 克，阴郁马先蒿 15 克，蒺藜 30 克，无患子 150 克，凹舌兰 150 克，冬虫夏草 150 克，石龙子一个，共研为细末，炼密为丸如蚕豆大，早饭前，晚饭后各服 1 丸。

2. 60g of Solomon’s seal, 30g of asparagus, 30g of Jian fruit celery, 15g of yin-yu pedicularis, 30g of tribulus, 150g of soapberry, 150g of orchid, 150g of cordyceps, and 1 skink. Grind them together into fine powder, refine with honey, and make pills the size of broad beans. Take 1 pill before breakfast and 1 pill after dinner.

《民族医药报》1992 年 4 月 17 日（青藏 王绍兴）

Ethnic Medicine News, April 17, 1992 (Wang Shaoxing, Qinghai-Tibet)

3. 治疗阳痿。

3. Treating Impotence.

党参 30 克，黑胡椒 10 克（布包），白鸽一只（去毛除内脏）加水适量，食盐少许，小火慢慢炖熟，饮汤吃鸽肉。连服 5-7 次。

30g of codonopsis, 10g of black pepper (wrapped in cloth), and 1 white pigeon (plucked and eviscerated). Add an appropriate amount of water and a little salt, and simmer slowly over low heat until cooked. Drink the soup and eat the pigeon meat. Take continuously for 5-7 times.

适用于房事不举或举而不坚，头昏耳鸣，腰膝酸软，畏寒肢冷等症候。

This is suitable for symptoms such as inability to achieve or maintain an erection during sexual intercourse, dizziness and tinnitus, soreness and weakness in the lower back and knees, and aversion to cold with cold extremities.

4. 阳萎：龙抱柱（盘龙参）100 克，小红参 100 克，一朵云（阴地蕨）20 克，枸杞 100 克，淫羊藿 20 克。白酒 2 公斤，浸泡 7 日后服。日服 3 次，每次 50-

100 毫升，30 日为 1 疗程。

4. Impotence: 100g of long-bao-zhu (spiral orchid), 100g of small red ginseng, 20g of yi-duo-yun (Botrychium ternatum), 100g of wolfberry, and 20g of epimedium. Steep in 2kg of liquor for 7 days before taking. Take 3 times a day, 50-100ml each time. 30 days constitute one treatment course.

5. 阳痿：淫羊藿 50 克，杜仲 50 克，骚羊古 50 克，梦花根 30 克，以上药味一起泡于 750 毫升酒内，7 天后早晚服用。

5. Impotence: 50g of epimedium, 50g of eucommia, 50g of sao-yang-gu, and 30g of meng-hua root. Steep the above herbs together in 750ml of liquor, and take in the morning and evening after 7 days.

五、睾丸肿痛（2 方）

V. Testicular Swelling and Pain (2 Prescriptions)

1. 香茶菜方治睾丸肿痛

Xiangchacai Prescription for Treating Testicular Swelling and Pain

香茶菜，又名棱角三七，铁棱角，铁秤锤等，是多年生草本植物。

Xiangchacai, also known as Lengjiao Sanqi, Tielengjiao, Tiechengchui, etc., is a perennial herb.

生长在山坡路边，溪沟边阴湿的草丛中或杂木林中，夏季及秋季采集。

It grows in the moist grass on roadsides of mountain slopes, along streams and ditches, or in mixed forests, and is collected in summer and autumn.

本品有活血消肿，清热解毒之功。

This herb has the effects of promoting blood circulation and reducing swelling, as well as clearing heat and detoxifying.

以此药为主治疗睾丸肿痛，疗效极佳，吾屡试屡验，现介绍如下。

Using this herb as the main ingredient to treat testicular swelling and pain has excellent efficacy. I have tested it repeatedly with consistent results, and it is now introduced as follows.

药物组成：香茶菜 15-20 克，荔枝核 12 克。

Prescription Composition: 15-20g of Xiangchacai and 12g of litchi seeds.

用法：上两味药加鸡蛋（一侧睾丸肿痛加鸡蛋 1 只，二侧加 2 只），水煎饮汁、食蛋，每日 2 次。

Usage: Add eggs to the above two herbs (add 1 egg if one testicle is swollen and painful, add 2 eggs if both are affected). Decoct in water, drink the liquid, and eat the eggs. Take twice daily.

加减法：睾丸重坠，属气虚不能升提者，加黄芪 30 克，升麻 5 克。

Modifications: For severe testicular heaviness and bearing-down sensation due to qi deficiency and inability to raise, add 30g of astragalus and 5g of cimicifuga.

疗效分析：睾丸肿痛（附睾炎或睾丸炎）。

Efficacy Analysis: Testicular swelling and pain (epididymitis or orchitis).

中医均称“子痈”。

In TCM, this condition is collectively referred to as “Ziyong” (testicular abscess).

中医认为该病症由肝气郁结，气滞血瘀所致。

TCM believes that this condition is caused by liver qi stagnation, leading to qi stagnation and blood stasis.

方中香茶菜清热解毒，活血消肿；

In this prescription, Xiangchacai clears heat and detoxifies, promotes blood circulation, and reduces swelling.

荔枝核疏肝理气，止痛散结；

Litchi seeds soothe the liver, regulate qi, relieve pain, and dissipate nodules.

加血肉有情之品的鸡蛋滋阴柔肝。

Adding eggs, which are “flesh and blood” nourishing substances, helps nourish yin and soften the liver.

且荔枝核，鸡蛋形同睾丸，中医认为同类相从，可亲和直达病所。

Moreover, litchi seeds and eggs resemble testicles in shape. TCM believes in the principle of "like attracts like," allowing them to target and reach the diseased site directly.

如是肝体得养，肝气调畅，气行瘀血散，故肿痛除。

Thus, the liver is nourished, liver qi flows smoothly, qi moves and blood stasis dissipates, thereby eliminating the swelling and pain.

《民族医药报》1992 年 4 月 3 日（浙江 程法森）

Ethnic Medicine News, April 3, 1992 (Cheng Fasen, Zhejiang)

2. 睾丸炎：王不留行果 120 克，骨碎补 30 克，煮猪脚服。

2. Orchitis: 120g of vaccaria seeds and 30g of drynaria. Boil them together with pig's trotters and consume.

六、输精管结扎术后结节痛（1 方）

VI. Nodule Pain after Vasectomy (1 Prescription)

治疗输精管结扎术后的痛性结节。

For treating painful nodules after vasectomy.

橘核 15 克，丝瓜络 15 克加水 3000 毫升煎至 1000 毫升左右，加入适量食盐，再煎煮 15-20 分钟，去渣取汁当茶饮用，每日一剂，10 天为一疗程。

Take 15g of tangerine seeds and 15g of loofah loofah sponge. Add 3000ml of water and decoct until about 1000ml remains. Add an appropriate amount of salt, and continue to decoct for 15-20 minutes. Discard the dregs and drink the liquid as tea. Take one dose daily, with 10 days constituting one treatment course.

适用于输精管结扎术后阴囊坠胀疼痛，有结节，按之固定不移，触之痛甚，尤以房事过后疼痛加剧。

This is suitable for scrotal bearing-down pain and swelling after vasectomy, with nodules that are fixed in place upon palpation, severe pain upon touch, and especially aggravated pain after sexual intercourse.

（广西民族医院 周秋培）

(Guangxi Ethnic Hospital, Zhou Qiupai)

七、性淡漠症（1 方）

VII. Sexual Apathy (1 Prescription)

性淡漠症：仙第参 20 克，枸杞子 20 克，淫羊藿 20 克，鹿胶 10 克，熟地 20 克，羊肾 2 个同煎，每日 1 剂，分 2 次服，10 日为 1 疗程。

Sexual apathy: 20g of Xian-di-shen (a type of ginseng), 20g of wolfberry, 20g of epimedium, 10g of deer-hide gelatin, 20g of prepared rehmannia, and 2 sheep kidneys. Decoct them together. Take one dose daily, divided into two servings. 10 days constitute one treatment course.

本方亦可用于女性性淡漠症及男女早衰。

This prescription can also be used for female sexual apathy and premature aging in both men and women.

八、睾丸鞘膜积液（1 方）

VIII. Hydrocele of the Tunica Vaginalis (1 Prescription)

治疗睾丸鞘膜积液验方

Verified Prescription for Treating Hydrocele of the Tunica Vaginalis

单用紫苏叶 50 克，加净水 350ml，煮沸后 15 分钟，趁热过滤，将滤液装入一容器内，趁药液之温产生的蒸气熏患部，待药液冷却到皮肤温度时，则可将有鞘膜积液之睾丸放入盛药的容器内浸泡 10-20 分钟。

Use 50g of perilla leaves alone, add 350ml of clean water, boil for 15 minutes, and filter while hot. Pour the filtrate into a container. While the hot liquid generates steam, fumigate the affected area. When the liquid cools to skin temperature, immerse the testicle with hydrocele in the container for 10-20 minutes.

每天一次，用药至积液消失。一般使用此药如法炮制 3-10 天可痊愈。

Do this once a day, and continue the medication until the effusion disappears.

Generally, preparing and using this herb as instructed for 3-10 days can achieve a cure.

《中医药信息报》

TCM Information News

九、男性龟头水肿（1方）

IX. Male Glans Penis Edema (1 Prescription)

本病以阴茎龟头包皮水肿通明为特征。

This disease is characterized by transparent edema of the glans penis and prepuce.

不痛不痒，甚者波及阴囊，常见于小儿，农村俗称“蚯蚓风”。

It is painless and non-itchy, and in severe cases, it can spread to the scrotum. It is common in children and is commonly known as “Earthworm Wind” in rural areas.

据资料报道取蝉蜕 15 克或威灵仙根 30 克任选一种，水煎取药液趁温外洗患处 10-15 分钟，一般用药后即可见效，1 次未愈者可煎第二次药液再洗。

According to reported data, choose either 15g of cicada slough or 30g of clematis root. Decoct in water and wash the affected area with the warm liquid for 10-15 minutes. It generally takes effect immediately after medication. If it is not cured after one application, decoct a second batch of liquid for another wash.

《民族医药报》1993 年 4 月 2 日（野集）

Ethnic Medicine News, April 2, 1993 (Ye Ji)

十、男子精液不化（1方）

X. Male Semen Non-liquefaction (1 Prescription)

对中、西医常规治疗后，疗效不显著的精液不液化的患者，可采用华佗再造丸（中成药店有售）治疗。

For patients with semen non-liquefaction who have not shown significant efficacy after conventional TCM and Western medicine treatments, Huatuo Zaizao Pills (available at Chinese patent medicine stores) can be used.

用法：口服，2 次 / 日，8 克 / 次，蜜糖水送服，连服 10 天，停药 1 天，再继续下一疗程，可连服 3 个疗程。

Usage: Take orally, twice a day, 8g each time, swallowed with honey water. Take continuously for 10 days, stop for 1 day, and then continue to the next course. This can be taken for 3 consecutive courses.

复查精液常规，若未愈，再继续用药 3 个疗程。

Re-examine the routine semen analysis. If not cured, continue the medication for another 3 courses.

治疗 65 例，痊愈 54 例，其中妊娠 25 例，无效 11 例。

Out of 65 treated cases, 54 were cured, including 25 cases of subsequent pregnancy, and 11 cases were ineffective.

《民族医药报》1998 年 1 月 23 日（明秀）

Ethnic Medicine News, January 23, 1998 (Ming Xiu)

十一、遗精（2 方）

XI. Spermatorrhea (2 Prescriptions)

1. 工作经验中总结出一个专治遗精的药方，他说："此方十分有效，一般患者，三剂药可愈。"

A prescription specifically for treating spermatorrhea was summarized from clinical experience. The author stated, "This prescription is highly effective; generally, patients can be cured after taking three doses."

方药：熟地 30 克，枣仁 15 克，玉米须 15 克，芋肉 12 克，云苓 15 克，白芍 15 克，当归 15 克，茯神 6 克，五味子 3 克，白芥子 3 克，肉桂 1 克，黄连 1 克。水煎服。一日一剂。

Prescription: 30g of prepared rehmannia, 15g of sour jujube seeds, 15g of corn silk, 12g of dogwood fruit, 15g of poria, 15g of white peony, 15g of angelica, 6g of poria with hostwood, 3g of schisandra, 3g of white mustard seeds, 1g of cinnamon bark, and 1g of coptis. Decoct in water and take. Take one dose daily.

《中药科技报》1992 年 2 月 16 日（河南 孙云清）

TCM Science and Technology News, February 16, 1992 (Sun Yunqing, Henan)

3. 梦遗（精）：锁阳、绵羊肉各 30 克。同煎，吃肉喝汤，每晚 1 剂。1 周为 1 疗程。

3. Nocturnal emission: 30g each of cistanche and mutton. Decoct them together, eat the meat and drink the soup. Take one dose every night. One week constitutes one treatment course.

十二、男子不育症（1 方）
XII. Male Infertility (1 Prescription)

精子减少导致的不育症。

Infertility caused by oligospermia (reduced sperm count).

菟丝子 30 克，淫羊藿 30 克（布包），猪脊肉 100 克（洗净切成小块），粳米 150 克，一同入锅煮粥，加少许食盐调味服食。

30g of dodder seeds, 30g of epimedium (wrapped in cloth), 100g of pork loin (washed and cut into small pieces), and 150g of japonica rice. Cook them together into porridge, add a little salt for flavoring, and consume.

7-10 天为一疗程。

7-10 days constitute one treatment course.

适用于婚后多年不育，阳痿、早泄及不能射精等。

This is suitable for infertility after years of marriage, impotence, premature ejaculation, and inability to ejaculate.

检查精液发现：精液量少于 2 毫升，精子总数每毫升精液中少于 2 千万，精子活动率为 50% 以下，或死精、无精子等。

Semen analysis reveals: semen volume of less than 2ml, total sperm count of less than 20 million per ml, sperm motility rate below 50%, or the presence of dead sperm or azoospermia (no sperm).

一般服用 2-3 个疗程后显效。

Generally, significant effects can be achieved after taking 2-3 treatment courses.

第十章　妇科

Chapter 10　gynecology

一、乳腺增生（6 方）

I. Mammary Gland Hyperplasia (6 Prescriptions)

1. 乳腺增生是内分泌紊乱引起乳腺小叶及乳腺管异常增殖的妇女常见慢性病，属于祖国医学“乳癖”范畴。

Mammary gland hyperplasia is a common chronic disease in women caused by endocrine disorders leading to abnormal proliferation of mammary lobules and ducts. It belongs to the category of “Rubing” (breast lumps) in traditional Chinese medicine. 临床表现为乳房胀痛及肿块，肿块表面光滑，能推动，常于情绪不佳和月经前增大。

Clinical manifestations include breast distension and pain, as well as masses. The masses have a smooth surface, are movable, and often enlarge when the patient is in a bad mood or before menstruation.

中药治疗本病的效果甚佳。

Traditional Chinese medicine has excellent effects in treating this disease.

用药方法：茯苓 30 克，夏枯草、土贝母各 20 克，炮山甲、醋玄胡、川楝子、昆布、海藻各 15 克，柴胡 12 克，甘草 6 克，水蛭、三棱、莪术各 5 克，每日 1 剂，煎成 400 毫升，分早晚 2 次服。

Medication Method: 30g of poria, 20g each of prunella and Bolbostematis Rhizoma, 15g each of pangolin scales (processed), vinegar-processed corydalis, Sichuan chinaberry, kelp, and seaweed, 12g of bupleurum, 6g of licorice, and 5g each of leech, sparganium, and zedoary. Take one dose daily, decoct into 400ml, and divide into two servings in the morning and evening.

10 天为 1 疗程，月经期不必停药。每疗程间隔 2-3 天。

10 days constitute one treatment course, and there is no need to stop the medication during menstruation. Leave an interval of 2-3 days between each course.

病程短者用药 1 疗程，乳房疼痛及肿块即消失。

For patients with a short disease course, one treatment course can make the breast pain and masses disappear.

（广西 钱方庆）

(Qian Fangqing, Guangxi)

2. 乳腺增生病是妇女常见疾病之一，患者以 40 岁以上妇女最为多见。

2. Mammary gland hyperplasia is one of the common diseases in women, most frequently seen in women over the age of 40.

近年来，许多专家认为，乳腺增生与乳腺癌有着相似的流行病学特点。

In recent years, many experts believe that mammary gland hyperplasia and breast cancer share similar epidemiological characteristics.

基于这种原因，我们读者验方交流协会专门搜集了一些有关防治乳腺增生的验方。现选一则介绍给大家。

For this reason, our Readers' Verified Prescription Exchange Association has specifically collected some verified prescriptions for the prevention and treatment of mammary gland hyperplasia. We have selected one to introduce to everyone.

处方：丹参、橘叶各 15 克，王不留行、川楝子、土鳖虫、皂角刺各 10 克，每日一剂，水煎分三次服。

Prescription: 15g each of salvia and tangerine leaves, and 10g each of vaccaria seeds, Sichuan chinaberry, ground beetle, and honeylocust spine. Take one dose daily, decocted in water and divided into three servings.

外敷生白附子或鲜蟾蜍皮。十五日为一疗程。

Apply raw aconitum or fresh toad skin topically. 15 days constitute one treatment course.

此方能疏通乳腺淤滞、消炎、止痛，疗效可靠，无副作用。

This prescription can relieve mammary gland stagnation, reduce inflammation, and relieve pain. It has reliable efficacy and no side effects.

《民族医药报》1992 年 2 月 14 日（云南 刘丽）

Ethnic Medicine News, February 14, 1992 (Liu Li, Yunnan)

3. 治急性乳腺炎：蒲公英、橘核、野菊花各 30 克，当归、柴胡、陈皮各 10 克，通草 6 克，甘草 3 克。水煎分二次服，每日一剂。

3. Treating Acute Mastitis: 30g each of dandelion, tangerine seeds, and wild chrysanthemum, 10g each of angelica, bupleurum, and tangerine peel, 6g of tetrapanax, and 3g of licorice. Decoct in water and divide into two servings. Take one dose daily.

《中药科技报》1992 年 11 月 26 日

TCM Science and Technology News, November 26, 1992

4. 乳腺小叶增生症是指中年以后妇女乳腺小叶增生，乳房内有大小不等的硬结并伴有不同程度的乳房部胀痛不适为主的病症。

4. Lobular hyperplasia of the breast refers to a condition in middle-aged and older women characterized by hyperplasia of mammary lobules, hard nodules of varying sizes in the breast, and varying degrees of breast distension, pain, and discomfort.

民间用敷脐法治疗本病有一定的疗效，兹将方药与用法简介如下。

The folk method of applying herbal plasters to the navel has a certain effect in treating this disease. The prescription and usage are briefly introduced as follows.

药物：穿山甲（炒成甲珠）20 克、蒲公英 16 克、木香 10 克、当归 8 克、白芷 12 克、薄荷 15 克、山栀子 10 克、地丁 10 克、瓜蒌仁 15 克、生黄芪 30 克、郁金 18 克、麝香 2 克。研末备用。

Herbs: 20g of pangolin scales (stir-fried into beads), 16g of dandelion, 10g of costus root, 8g of angelica, 12g of angelica dahurica, 15g of mint, 10g of gardenia,

10g of violet, 15g of trichosanthes seeds, 30g of raw astragalus, 18g of turmeric, and 2g of musk. Grind into powder and set aside.

用法：将脐部用75%酒精清洗消毒干净，取上药末适量（2-3克）填于脐眼处，外用干棉球轻压并做局部按柔三分钟，然后以一小块胶布紧贴脐部将药物固定，一周内换药两次，8次为一疗程。

Usage: Clean and disinfect the navel with 75% alcohol. Take an appropriate amount of the above herbal powder (2-3g) and fill it into the navel. Gently press with a dry cotton ball and massage the local area for three minutes. Then, use a small piece of adhesive tape to firmly fix the medicine over the navel. Change the medicine twice a week, with 8 changes constituting one treatment course.

一般用药3个疗程可使肿块缩小，疼痛缓解。

Generally, 3 treatment courses can shrink the masses and relieve pain.

《民族医药报》1991年7月5日（广西 陆强益）

Ethnic Medicine News, July 5, 1991 (Lu Qiangyi, Guangxi)

5. 急性乳腺炎，多见于初产妇哺乳期，中医称之为“乳痈”，认为该疾病系因乳汁积滞不得外泄所致。

5. Acute mastitis is common during the lactation period of primiparas. In TCM, it is called “Ruyong” (breast abscess), and is believed to be caused by the retention of breast milk that cannot be discharged.

其主要表现为乳房红肿疼痛、触之灼热、按之痛甚，可伴有恶寒发热、烦渴尿黄等症状。

Its main manifestations include redness, swelling, and pain in the breast, a burning sensation upon touch, and severe pain upon pressure, which may be accompanied by symptoms such as chills, fever, restlessness, thirst, and yellow urine.

笔者在临床上每遇此症，均取仙人掌外敷治之，屡获良效。

In clinical practice, whenever the author encounters this condition, topical application of cactus is used for treatment, which has repeatedly achieved good results.

其方法是：取3个手指大小的生仙人掌2-3瓣，去毛刺，每瓣用利刀从侧面剖成两块薄片。

The method is as follows: Take 2-3 segments of fresh cactus about the size of three fingers, remove the spines, and use a sharp knife to cut each segment laterally into two thin slices.

用火烤热后将每片的剖面贴敷于患乳上，冷后再烤再敷，连敷30-60分钟，每日3次，一般1次显效，3-6次痊愈。

Heat them over a fire, then apply the cut surface of each slice to the affected breast. When it cools, reheat and reapply. Continue applying for 30-60 minutes, 3 times a day. Generally, significant effects are seen after 1 application, and a cure is achieved after 3-6 applications.

治疗期间忌食辛辣及鱼腥食品。

During treatment, avoid spicy and fishy foods.

《民族医药报》1991年8月25日（广西 韦礼贵 郑翠萍）

Ethnic Medicine News, August 25, 1991 (Wei Ligui, Zheng Cuiping, Guangxi)

6. 治乳腺炎。取白花丹，过山香全草各100克，嘱患者自带身上；或放在睡床的床单下。一般连用数天可痊愈。

6. Treating Mastitis. Take 100g each of leadwort and Guoshanxiang whole plant. Instruct the patient to carry them on their person, or place them under the bedsheet. Generally, continuous use for several days can achieve a cure.

《民族医药报》1992年8月28日（广西）

Ethnic Medicine News, August 28, 1992 (Guangxi)

二、乳腺炎（25方）
II. Mastitis (25 Prescriptions)

1. 用鲜蒲公英全草捣烂外敷患处，同时取全草60-90克水煎服，每日2次；也可用根去皮，捣烂后塞患侧鼻孔，每日2次。

Mash fresh whole dandelion plants and apply them topically to the affected area. At the same time, take 60-90g of the whole plant, decoct in water, and take twice a day. Alternatively, peel the root, mash it, and plug it into the nostril on the affected side twice a day.

2. 鲜芫花根适量，去表皮，用白色内层，捣烂塞鼻，每日一次；或用鲜毛茛叶适量，揉烂塞患侧鼻孔，每日 2 次，每次 5 分钟；也可用天名精叶适量揉烂塞患侧鼻孔，每日两次，每次 20 分钟。

2. Take an appropriate amount of fresh yuanhua (Daphne genkwa) root, peel off the outer skin, and use the white inner layer. Mash it and plug it into the nostril once a day. Alternatively, take an appropriate amount of fresh buttercup leaves, mash them, and plug them into the nostril on the affected side twice a day for 5 minutes each time. You can also mash an appropriate amount of Tianmingjing leaves and plug them into the nostril on the affected side twice a day for 20 minutes each time.

3. 取仙人掌一块（巴掌大小）刮去外皮后捣烂，再加白酒适量搅拌贴敷患处。

3. Take a piece of cactus (about the size of a palm), scrape off the outer skin, and mash it. Add an appropriate amount of liquor, stir, and apply it to the affected area.

4. 菖蒲根 30 克研细，早晚各取 6 克，用白酒送服；或用菖蒲根 30 克水煎服。

4. Grind 30g of sweetflag rhizome into fine powder. Take 6g in the morning and evening, swallowed with liquor. Alternatively, decoct 30g of sweetflag rhizome in water and take.

5. 华山矾根 60 克，蛇葡萄根 30 克，水煎，趁热熏洗患处，日一剂，连用五日。

5. Take 60g of Huashan fan root and 30g of Ampelopsis root. Decoct in water and use the hot steam to fumigate and wash the affected area while it is hot. Take one dose a day for 5 consecutive days.

6. 半边莲、地丁草（犁头草）各 50 克（均为鲜品），加酒糟、食盐少许。共捣烂，厚敷患处，每日一换，连用 3-5 日。

6. Take 50g each of lobed cardinal flower and violet (both fresh). Add a little distillers’ grains and salt. Mash them together, apply a thick layer to the affected area, change the dressing daily, and use continuously for 3-5 days.

7. 小连翘（全草）30 克，水煎服，每日一剂，连服 3-5 日。

7. Take 30g of St. John' s wort (whole plant). Decoct in water and take. Take one dose daily for 3-5 consecutive days.

《民族医药报》1992 年 5 月 1 日（江苏 纪国安）

Ethnic Medicine News, May 1, 1992 (Ji Guo' an, Jiangsu)

8. 蒲公英 50 克，环留 25 克。每日一剂，水煎两次服。

8. 50g of dandelion and 25g of Huanliu. Take one dose daily, decocted in water and taken twice.

9. 当归 60 克，水煎头、二两汁取液 200 毫升。每隔 6 小时服药 1 次，每次 50 毫升。日服 4 次。一般早期治疗一昼夜即愈。

9. Take 60g of angelica. Decoct in water and collect 200ml of liquid from the first and second decoctions. Take 50ml every 6 hours, 4 times a day. Generally, early treatment can achieve a cure within 24 hours.

10. 鹿角霜 13 克，蒲公英 120 克，水煎，兑入黄酒二两。分 2 次口服，每日一剂。

10. 13g of deer antler frost and 120g of dandelion. Decoct in water, add 2 liang (about 100g) of yellow rice wine. Divide into 2 oral doses. Take one dose daily.

11. 银花 15 克，蒲公英 30 克，野菊花 20 克，柴胡 9 克，瓜蒌 30 克，穿山甲 6 克，甘草 3 克。水煎服，每日一剂。一般服用 2-3 剂即可痊愈。

11. 15g of honeysuckle, 30g of dandelion, 20g of wild chrysanthemum, 9g of bupleurum, 30g of trichosanthes, 6g of pangolin scales, and 3g of licorice. Decoct in water and take. Take one dose daily. Generally, taking 2-3 doses can achieve a cure.

12. 蒲公英 30 克，全瓜蒌 20 克，金银花 20 克，陈皮 12 克。煎汁内服，每日一剂。一般 2-3 剂可愈。

12. 30g of dandelion, 20g of whole trichosanthes, 20g of honeysuckle, and 12g of tangerine peel. Decoct the liquid for oral administration. Take one dose daily. Generally, 2-3 doses can achieve a cure.

13. 浙贝母 15 克，当归身 20 克，白芷 10 克，生甘草 9 克，黄酒 30 毫升。

上四味药同煎两遍，后将药液与黄酒混合，煮沸。早晚两次分服，每服以遍身微汗为佳。

13. 15g of Fritillaria thunbergii, 20g of angelica root, 10g of angelica dahurica, 9g of raw licorice, and 30ml of yellow rice wine. Decoct the above four herbs together twice, then mix the herbal liquid with the yellow rice wine and bring to a boil. Divide into two servings in the morning and evening. It is best if the patient breaks out in a mild sweat all over the body after each dose.

14. 将苦楝子连皮带仁，捣碎晒干，炒微黄，研细末，储瓶备用。

14. Take Chinaberry fruits with their skin and seeds intact. Crush them, sun-dry, stir-fry until slightly yellow, grind into fine powder, and store in a bottle for later use.

用法：取苦楝子末 20-50 克，红糖 100 克，以黄酒或开水 100-200 毫升冲服。每日 1-2 次，连服 2-3 天。

Usage: Take 20-50g of Chinaberry fruit powder and 100g of brown sugar. Steep with 100-200ml of yellow rice wine or boiling water and take. Take 1-2 times a day for 2-3 consecutive days.

15. 取砂仁 10-20 克，研成细末，密贮瓶中备用。用时取糯米饭少许和砂仁末拌匀，搓成索条状如花生米大小，外裹以消毒青布（必须是棉织品）塞鼻。左乳腺炎塞右，右乳腺炎塞左，亦可左右交替塞用，每隔 12 小时如法更换一次，直至炎症消失为止。

15. Take 10-20g of cardamom, grind into fine powder, and store in a tightly sealed bottle. When using, take a small amount of glutinous rice, mix evenly with the cardamom powder, and roll it into a rope-like strip the size of a peanut. Wrap it externally with sterilized green cloth (must be cotton fabric) and plug it into the nostril. For left mastitis, plug the right nostril; for right mastitis, plug the left nostril. You can also alternate between left and right. Change it every 12 hours following the same method until the inflammation disappears.

16. 取蒲公英、紫荆皮、芙蓉花（或叶）各 160 克，独活 90 克，赤芍 60 克，石菖蒲 50 克，白芷 30 克，共研极细末。发病 1 至 3 日用热开水调服，4 至 7

日用热酒调敷，皮肤过敏者用温蜜糖水调敷。一般外敷 3-5 天可愈。

16. Take 160g each of dandelion, bauhinia bark, and hibiscus flower (or leaves), 90g of pubescent angelica root, 60g of red peony root, 50g of sweetflag rhizome, and 30g of angelica dahurica. Grind them together into extremely fine powder. For the first 1-3 days of onset, mix and apply with hot boiling water. From the 4th to 7th day, mix and apply with hot liquor. For patients with skin allergies, mix and apply with warm honey water. Generally, topical application for 3-5 days can achieve a cure.

17. 菊叶三七（块根）50 克，内风消 30 克，马鞭草 10 克，见肿消 30 克，蛇含草 20 克（均用鲜品），50 度白酒 10 克，冰片 5 克（碾细）。

17. 50g of chrysanthemum-leaf gynura (tuberous root), 30g of Neifengxiao, 10g of verbena, 30g of Jianzhongxiao, and 20g of snake-moss (all fresh), 10g of 50-degree liquor, and 5g of borneol (crushed into fine powder).

用法：先将上药洗净泥砂，分别用刀切细，然后碾烂再加入冰片粉 5 克，50 度白酒 10 克和匀，外敷乳腺炎肿胀部位，内层用白纸，外层用白色乙烯薄膜包紧，每 12 小时换药 1 次。

Usage: First, wash the mud and sand off the above herbs, cut them finely with a knife separately, then mash them. Add 5g of borneol powder and 10g of 50-degree liquor and mix evenly. Apply topically to the swollen area of mastitis. Wrap the inner layer with white paper and the outer layer tightly with white polyethylene film. Change the dressing once every 12 hours.

《中药科技报》1993 年 3 月 25 日（张亚利）

TCM Science and Technology News, March 25, 1993 (Zhang Yali)

18. 哺乳妇乳汁郁积，乳房红肿硬痛：犁头草 15 克，天花粉 30 克，煎水内服。

18. For nursing mothers with milk retention and red, swollen, hard, and painful breasts: Decoct 15g of violet (ploughshare grass) and 30g of trichosanthes root in water for oral administration.

《民族医药报》1992 年 9 月 4 日（云南 欧永彬）

Ethnic Medicine News, September 4, 1992 (Ou Yongbin, Yunnan)

19. 牛蒡子（又名大力子、鼠粘子、炒牛蒡）90 克，泉水煎 1 小时左右，取其浓汁服，1 日 3 次。此方适用于乳房初起红肿、疼痛，并伴有发热畏寒、坐卧不安、厌食等全身症状患者。

19. Take 90g of burdock seeds (also known as Dali Zi, Shu Nian Zi, or stir-fried burdock). Decoct in spring water for about 1 hour, take the concentrated liquid, and consume 3 times a day. This prescription is suitable for patients in the early stage of breast redness, swelling, and pain, accompanied by systemic symptoms such as fever, chills, restlessness, and loss of appetite.

20. 急性乳腺炎是妇科常见病之一，红肿痛热，患者坐卧不安，甚至并发全身感染。

20. Acute mastitis is one of the common gynecological diseases, characterized by redness, swelling, pain, and heat. Patients are often restless, and it may even be complicated by systemic infections.

民间用面种（即发酵馒头、包子用的面种）或发酵后的面团外敷，有较好的疗效。

Folk remedies using sourdough starter (the starter used for fermenting steamed buns) or fermented dough as a topical application have good therapeutic effects.

用法：将面种或发酵后的面团用适量的冷开水和软（以粘手为度），然后沿乳头周围均匀外敷，覆盖整个患乳，然后用纱布或乳罩固定，每天换药一次。

Usage: Mix the sourdough starter or fermented dough with an appropriate amount of cooled boiled water until soft (to the point of being sticky to the touch). Then, apply it evenly around the nipple to cover the entire affected breast, and secure it with gauze or a bra. Change the dressing once a day.

一般 2-3 天即可消冲，乳汁流畅，症状消失。

Generally, within 2-3 days, the swelling and redness will subside, milk flow will become smooth, and symptoms will disappear.

面种治疗急性乳腺炎的机理是：面团或面种局部外敷后，缓慢发酵释放热量，温通散结，使乳腺管扩张，促进血液循环及乳汁通畅，从而达到消炎、散结、止痛目的。

The mechanism of using sourdough starter to treat acute mastitis is as follows: After topical application, the dough or starter undergoes slow fermentation and releases heat, which warms and unblocks the channels to dissipate nodules. This dilates the mammary ducts, promotes blood circulation and smooth milk flow, thereby achieving the goals of reducing inflammation, dissipating nodules, and relieving pain.

这种疗法仅适用于早期乳腺炎，若局部已形成脓肿，则需到医院进一步治疗。

This therapy is only applicable to early-stage mastitis. If a local abscess has already formed, further treatment at a hospital is required.

《民族医药报》1991 年 11 月 5 日（唐红山 黄月生）

Ethnic Medicine News, November 5, 1991 (Tang Hongshan, Huang Yuesheng)

21. 急性乳腺炎祖国医学称乳痈，是初产妇易患的一种乳房化脓性炎症。

21. In traditional Chinese medicine, acute mastitis is called "Ruyong" (breast abscess). It is a purulent inflammation of the breast that primiparas are prone to.

症见起病时感患侧乳房肿胀疼痛、皮肤红肿，严重的可伴有发热等全身感染中毒症状。

Symptoms include swelling and pain in the affected breast at the onset, along with red and swollen skin. Severe cases may be accompanied by systemic infection and toxic symptoms such as fever.

对于本病的治疗，最近有资料介绍用中药半夏加葱白治疗效果好，早期运用治愈率可达 100%，此法不仅疗效好，还具有经济实用，治疗时痛苦少等优点，笔者运用此法均获良效，现将具体方法介绍如下：

For the treatment of this disease, recent literature reports that using the Chinese herb Pinellia (Banxia) combined with green onion white yields good results, with a cure rate of up to 100% when used in the early stage. This method is not only highly effective but also economical, practical, and causes little pain during treatment. The author has achieved excellent results using this method, and the specific procedure is introduced as follows:

取生半夏和葱白各等量先捣烂成泥糊状，再将其做成枣核状的栓剂，大小以能塞入鼻孔内为准，使用时将做好的栓剂塞入病人健侧鼻孔内，塞入后注意要多喝水，30 分钟后再取出，每日 2 次。

Take equal amounts of raw Pinellia and green onion white, mash them into a paste, and then shape them into suppositories the size and shape of jujube pits (large enough to fit into the nostril). When using, insert the prepared suppository into the healthy nostril of the patient. After insertion, the patient should drink plenty of water. Remove it after 30 minutes. Do this twice a day.

上述方法对于发病在 24 小时之内。一般用药后 1-2 天症状即可消失，如果发病超过 48 小时或已进入酿脓期时，疗效欠佳，须配合应用抗生素或切开引流排脓。

The above method is highly effective for cases that have been developing for less than 24 hours. Generally, symptoms will disappear 1-2 days after medication. If the onset exceeds 48 hours or if it has entered the suppurative stage, the efficacy is poor, and it must be combined with antibiotics or incision and drainage.

《民族医药报》1992 年 5 月 29 日（新疆 宋修伦）

Ethnic Medicine News, May 29, 1992 (Song Xiulun, Xinjiang)

22. 萱草根适量，洗净兑甜酒捣绒，敷患处（忌包乳头），1 日 1 换，有良效。

22. Take an appropriate amount of daylily roots, wash them, mix with sweet wine, and mash into a fluffy pulp. Apply it to the affected area (avoid covering the nipple). Change the dressing once a day. It has good therapeutic effects.

此方适用于乳房呈硬块的突发症患者。若伴有忽冷忽热的全身症状，加蒲公英。

This prescription is suitable for sudden-onset patients with hard lumps in the breast. If accompanied by systemic symptoms of alternating chills and fever, add dandelion.

另取蒲公英适量，兑淘米水捣汁服，1 次 10 毫升为宜。

Additionally, take an appropriate amount of dandelion, mix with rice-washing water, mash and extract the juice, and take it orally. An appropriate dose is 10ml per time.

23. 阳尘（火烟久熏所致的黑色的附梁柱上之物）适量，以鸡蛋清调匀，擦患部，每小时 1 次，3-5 日痊愈。

23. Take an appropriate amount of "Yangchen" (black soot accumulated on beams and pillars from long-term smoke exposure), mix evenly with egg white, and rub it on the affected area. Do this once an hour. It can be cured in 3-5 days.

此方适用于病程长，已溃烂化脓的患者。

This prescription is suitable for patients with a long disease course who have developed ulceration and suppuration.

《民族医药报》（贵州 谢昭齐 文中祥）

Ethnic Medicine News (Xie Zhaoqi, Wen Zhongxiang, Guizhou)

24. 治乳腺炎：牛黄解毒片粉末同酒糟和匀外敷患处。日 2 次，一般 3 天肿块变软，肿消痛除，乳汁通畅。

24. Treating Mastitis: Mix the powder of Niuhuang Jiedu Tablets evenly with distillers' grains and apply it topically to the affected area. Do this twice a day. Generally, after 3 days, the mass will soften, swelling and pain will be eliminated, and milk flow will become smooth.

《民族医药报》1993 年 4 月 2 日（李志民）

Ethnic Medicine News, April 2, 1993 (Li Zhimin)

25. 取韭菜 50 克洗净，杏仁 6 克去皮，一起放入碗中捣烂如泥，外敷患处，每日 2 次，疗效甚佳。

25. Wash 50g of Chinese chives and peel 6g of almonds. Put them together in a bowl and mash them into a mud-like paste. Apply it topically to the affected area twice a day. It has excellent therapeutic effects.

《中医药信息报》1990 年 10 月 6 日（常祖光）

TCM Information News, October 6, 1990 (Chang Zuguang)

三、回乳（24 方）
III. Lactation Suppression (24 Prescriptions)

小儿出生后，母亲无乳、乳少、乳汁不通，全家人为之苦恼。现将治乳汁不通的民间秘方十则介绍如下。

After the birth of a baby, if the mother has no milk, insufficient milk, or blocked milk flow, the whole family is distressed. The following are ten folk secret prescriptions for treating blocked milk flow.

1. 钟乳粉，通草等分共研细末，米汤饮调服一克，日 3 次，用于气少血衰的气血不通。

Mix equal amounts of stalactite powder and tetrapanax pith, and grind them into fine powder. Take 1g mixed with rice soup, 3 times a day. This is used for poor circulation of qi and blood due to qi deficiency and blood depletion.

2. 葵菜籽炒香，缩砂仁等分，研细末，热酒送服 6 克。用于经络凝滞，奶房胀痛的乳汁不通。

2. Stir-fry mallow seeds until fragrant, mix with equal amounts of cardamom, and grind into fine powder. Take 6g with warm liquor. This is used for blocked milk flow caused by meridian stagnation and breast distension and pain.

3. 木莲 2 个，猪前脚 1 个，共煮烂食之，并饮汁尽，一日乳汁即通。

3. Boil 2 fig fruits and 1 pig’s front trotter until soft, eat the meat, and drink all the broth. Milk flow will be unblocked within a day.

4. 赤小豆半斤，煮汁服。或赤小豆 60 克，糯米 120 克，共煮粥食之。或赤小豆 240 克，白糖 90 克，共煮烂分 3 次吃，治乳汁不通。

4. Boil half a jin (250g) of adzuki beans and drink the broth. Alternatively, boil 60g of adzuki beans and 120g of glutinous rice together into porridge and eat it. Or boil 240g of adzuki beans and 90g of white sugar until soft, and eat it in three divided doses to treat blocked milk flow.

5. 丝瓜莲子烧存性研末，酒送服 6 克，盖被子取汗，乳汁即通。

5. Burn loofah and lotus seeds until carbonized but retaining their properties,

and grind into powder. Take 6g with liquor, cover with a blanket to induce sweating, and milk flow will be unblocked.

6. 白僵蚕末 6 克，酒送服，少顷，以脂麻茶一杯投服，用梳子梳奶头数十遍，奶汁即出。

6. Take 6g of white silkworm powder with liquor. After a while, drink a cup of sesame tea. Comb the nipples dozens of times with a comb, and milk will flow out.

7. 穿山甲炮研细末，酒送服 1 克，日 2 次，外以油梳梳乳房，乳汁即通。

7. Roast pangolin scales, grind into fine powder, and take 1g with liquor twice a day. Externally, comb the breasts with an oiled comb, and milk flow will be unblocked.

8. 炒黑芝麻 16 克，研末，以猪蹄汤一次服下，治乳汁不通。

8. Stir-fry 16g of black sesame seeds, grind into powder, and take it all at once with pig’s trotter soup to treat blocked milk flow.

9. 鲤鱼 1 条，冬瓜皮 30 克，共煮烂食之，治无乳汁。

9. Boil 1 carp and 30g of winter melon peel until soft, and eat them to treat the absence of breast milk.

10. 豆腐炖羊肉食之，治乳汁不通。

10. Stew tofu with mutton and eat it to treat blocked milk flow.

《中药科技报》（河南 李平）

TCM Science and Technology News (Li Ping, Henan)

11. 河南新乡市第一人民医院王蕴蕴回乳有良法，一付药即可。适应于各年龄组哺乳妇女。她所治疗的 24-30 岁 30 例；30-45 岁 20 例，共 50 例，均服 1 付药乳汁即回。

11. Wang Yunyun from the First People’s Hospital of Xinxiang, Henan, has an excellent method for lactation suppression, requiring only one dose of medicine. It is suitable for nursing women of all age groups. Among the 50 cases she treated (30 cases aged 24-30 and 20 cases aged 30-45), all achieved lactation suppression after taking just one dose.

方药组成及用法：丹参 5 克，川芎 6 克，木香 6 克，红花 10 克，焦麦芽 60 克，桃仁 9 克，泽膝 15 克，川牛膝 15 克，当归 12 克，赤芍 10 克。取上药一付煎汤温顿服之。

Prescription Composition and Usage: 5g of salvia, 6g of ligusticum, 6g of costus root, 10g of safflower, 60g of scorched malt, 9g of peach seed, 15g of lycopus, 15g of cyathula root, 12g of angelica, and 10g of red peony. Decoct one dose of these herbs into a soup and take it warm all at once.

服药后情况：如若出现乳房胀满，让小孩将其奶液吸完或用吸奶器将其剩余奶汁吸空，乳房即变软而乳汁即回。

Post-medication Condition: If breast fullness occurs, let the baby suck out all the milk or use a breast pump to empty the remaining milk. The breasts will soften, and lactation will be suppressed.

《中医药信息报》（河南 张炎）

TCM Information News (Zhang Yan, Henan)

12. 陈皮 30-40 克，柴胡 10 克，水煎服，每日一剂，连服 2-3 天。

12. Take 30-40g of tangerine peel and 10g of bupleurum. Decoct in water and take. Take one dose daily for 2-3 consecutive days.

13. 焦麦芽 30 克，红花 6 克，桃仁 6 克，泽兰 6 克，怀牛膝 9 克，当归 6 克，赤芍 6 克，川芎 3 克，水煎服，每日一剂，连服 1-2 剂。

13. Take 30g of scorched malt, 6g of safflower, 6g of peach seed, 6g of lycopus, 9g of achyranthes root, 6g of angelica, 6g of red peony, and 3g of ligusticum. Decoct in water and take. Take one dose daily for 1-2 consecutive doses.

《民族医药报》1991 年 7 月 5 日（广东张仲林）

Ethnic Medicine News, July 5, 1991 (Zhang Zhonglin, Guangdong)

在产后哺乳期间，乳汁甚少或全无，称之缺乳，亦称乳汁不行。用方食疗，效果颇佳。

During the postpartum lactation period, if breast milk is extremely scarce or completely absent, it is called “Que Ru” (insufficient milk) or “Ru Zhi Bu Xing” (blocked milk flow). Using dietary therapy prescriptions yields excellent results.

14. 猪蹄二只，花生仁 150 克，猪蹄切碎，加水适量，不加盐炖食。或加黄酒一两对服。

14. Take 2 pig’s trotters and 150g of peanut kernels. Chop the trotters, add an appropriate amount of water, and stew without adding salt. Alternatively, add 1 liang (50g) of yellow rice wine to take together.

15. 鲜鲫鱼约 100 克二条，去肠杂，与豆芽煮适量同炖服，或加通草 10 克，同炖，连汤带肉同食，此方催乳效佳。

15. Take 2 fresh crucian carps (about 100g each), remove the internal organs, and stew them with an appropriate amount of bean sprouts. Alternatively, add 10g of tetrapanax pith and stew together. Eat the meat and drink the soup. This prescription has excellent milk-promoting effects.

16. 活鲜胎盘一只洗净，于新瓦上焙干为末，分四次兑入热黄酒送服。适用于产后血虚者。

16. Wash a fresh placenta, bake it dry on a new tile, and grind into powder. Divide into four doses and take with warm yellow rice wine. This is suitable for postpartum women with blood deficiency.

17. 鲜豆腐一斤，鲜羊肉 250 克，皂角刺 15 克，加水炖服，去皂角刺，喝汤食肉吃豆腐。适用于气血虚弱而乳少者。

17. Take 500g of fresh tofu, 250g of fresh mutton, and 15g of honeylocust spine. Add water and stew. Remove the honeylocust spine, drink the soup, and eat the meat and tofu. This is suitable for those with insufficient milk due to qi and blood deficiency.

18. 黄芪 100 克，炮山甲，通草各 15 克，猪蹄二只切碎，加水适量炖烂，加黄酒一两对服。适用于气血虚弱而乳汁不行者。

18. Take 100g of astragalus, 15g of roasted pangolin scales, and 15g of tetrapanax pith. Chop 2 pig’s trotters, add an appropriate amount of water, and stew until soft. Add 1 liang (50g) of yellow rice wine to take together. This is suitable for those with blocked milk flow due to qi and blood deficiency.

19. 王不留行 15 克，猪蹄两只，同炖饮汤食肉。适用于乳房胀痛，肝郁气滞，乳汁不通者。

19. Take 15g of vaccaria seeds and 2 pig’s trotters. Stew them together, drink the soup, and eat the meat. This is suitable for those with blocked milk flow due to breast distension and pain, and liver qi stagnation.

20. 全瓜蒌一个连壳带仁，切碎，葱白三根，水煎煮兑入黄酒一两服用，每日一次。适用于肝郁气滞乳汁不行。

20. Take 1 whole trichosanthes fruit (including the shell and seeds), chop it, and add 3green onion whites. Decoct in water, add 1 liang (50g) of yellow rice wine, and take once a day. This is suitable for blocked milk flow due to liver qi stagnation.

21. 刺猬皮 10 克，焙干为末，分二次以黄酒冲服，睡卧出汗。

21. Take 10g of hedgehog skin, bake it dry, and grind into powder. Divide into two doses and take with yellow rice wine. The patient should sleep and sweat after taking it.

22. 鲜鲢鱼一条去肠杂约 500 克，路路通 20 个，丝瓜仁 50 克捣碎加水炖烂，喝汤食鱼，治产后无乳，效果极佳。

22. Take 1 fresh silver carp (about 500g after removing the internal organs), 20 liquidambar fruits, and 50g of loofah seeds. Crush them, add water, and stew until soft. Drink the soup and eat the fish. It has excellent effects in treating postpartum agalactia.

23. 黑芝麻 50 克炒焦研末，每次 10 克对入适量黄酒。若加猪蹄炖汤对服芝麻末，效果确切。

23. Stir-fry 50g of black sesame seeds until scorched, and grind into powder. Take 10g each time with an appropriate amount of yellow rice wine. If stewed with pig’s trotter soup and taken together with the sesame powder, the effect is definite.

24. 鲤鱼一尾约 250 克，猪肚一个切碎，顿服。若在内服药汁同时，还应佐以外治。以木梳背浸青油后，轻刮乳房，以刺激乳房有通络下乳之效。如乳房有硬结者，可以干净毛巾局部热敷，有宣通气血，运行乳汁之效。

24. Take 1 carp (about 250g) and 1 pig's stomach, chop them, and take all at once. While taking the oral herbal decoction, external treatment should also be used as an adjunct. Soak the back of a wooden comb in green oil, gently scrape the breasts to stimulate the meridians and promote milk flow. If there are hard lumps in the breasts, apply a warm compress locally with a clean towel to promote the circulation of qi and blood and the flow of milk.

《中药科技报》1992 年 7 月 26 日（虞永水）

TCM Science and Technology News, July 26, 1992 (Yu Yongshui)

四、带症（16 方）

IV. Leukorrhea (16 Prescriptions)

1. 女性由于脾肾生理功能下降，性器官萎缩，性激素分泌障碍，导致肾阳不足，脾虚失运而致水湿下注。其表现为腰膝、小腹冷痛，四肢不温，纳呆，或有便溏，下肢微肿，舌淡苔白，脉沉细。笔者拟用桂术芪防汤治疗一百余例，皆获得疗效。

Due to the decline in the physiological functions of the spleen and kidney, atrophy of sexual organs, and impaired sex hormone secretion, women may suffer from insufficient kidney yang and poor spleen transportation, leading to the downward flow of dampness. The manifestations include cold pain in the lower back, knees, and lower abdomen, cold extremities, poor appetite, loose stools, mild swelling in the lower limbs, pale tongue with white coating, and deep and thready pulse. The author formulated Guishu Qifang Decoction to treat over a hundred cases, all of which achieved therapeutic effects.

处方：肉桂六克，炒白术十五克，炒苍术、防风各九克，破故纸十二克，肉蔻六克，黄芪四十克，一日一剂，水煎服。若是水肿甚者加附片六克，茯苓十五克。

Prescription: 6g of cassia bark, 15g of stir-fried atractylodes macrocephala, 9g each of stir-fried atractylodes lancea and saposhnikovia root, 12g of psoralea fruit,

6g of nutmeg, and 40g of astragalus. Take one dose daily, decocted in water. For severe edema, add 6g of aconite slices and 15g of poria.

本方治疗一百余例患者中，一般服六剂见效，最多服十二剂痊愈。

Among the over a hundred patients treated with this prescription, significant effects were generally seen after taking six doses, and a maximum of twelve doses was required for a complete cure.

《中药科技报》1993 年 3 月 25 日（刘启明）

TCM Science and Technology News, March 25, 1993 (Liu Qiming)

2. 脾气虚弱：可用淮山药（炒）30 克，芡实（炒）18 克，黄柏 6 克，车前子（酒炒）10 克，白果 10 枚（打碎）水煎服，连服 3-5 天。或用炒扁豆 500 克、磨粉，每日早晨冲服 15 克。

2. Spleen Qi Deficiency: Take 30g of stir-fried Chinese yam, 18g of stir-fried euryale seeds, 6g of phellodendron bark, 10g of wine-stir-fried plantain seeds, and 10 crushed ginkgo nuts. Decoct in water and take for 3-5 consecutive days. Alternatively, stir-fry 500g of hyacinth beans, grind them into powder, and take 15g mixed with hot water every morning.

3. 痰湿阻滞：常用法夏、苍术、白术、茯苓各 10 克，陈皮、白芷、甘草、香附各 6 克、水煎服。或用海螵蛸去甲，炙研末 15 克，水煎浓汁服。

3. Phlegm-Dampness Stagnation: Commonly use 10g each of pinellia, atractylodes lancea, atractylodes macrocephala, and poria, and 6g each of tangerine peel, angelica dahurica, licorice, and cyperus. Decoct in water and take. Alternatively, remove the hard shell from cuttlebone, roast it, grind into powder, take 15g, and decoct into a concentrated liquid to take.

4. 肾阳不足：金樱子根 60 克、黑大豆 60 克、葵花梗芯 15 克，水煎温服。也可用红枣、黑豆、白果各 10 克煎水，每日空腹服，连服 10 日。体质虚弱者，每日可加服乌鸡白凤丸一粒。

4. Kidney Yang Deficiency: Take 60g of rosa laevigata root, 60g of black soybeans, and 15g of sunflower stem pith. Decoct in water and take warm. Alternatively, decoct 10g each of red dates, black soybeans, and ginkgo nuts in

water, take on an empty stomach daily for 10 consecutive days. For patients with weak constitutions, one Wujibai Feng Pill can be added daily.

5. 湿热下注：用白鸡冠花 60 克，水煎分两次服，每日一剂，连服 3 天。或用墓头回、椿根皮各 12 克，凤尾草 30 克，水煎服。并可与市售愈带丸同服。

5.Downward Flow of Damp-Heat: Take 60g of white cockscomb flower, decoct in water and divide into two servings. Take one dose daily for 3 consecutive days. Alternatively, take 12g each of heterosmilax root and ailanthus bark, and 30g of maidenhair fern. Decoct in water and take. It can also be taken together with commercially available Yudai Pills.

6. 寒湿内结: 用土硫磺 18 克，鸡蛋六个，将硫磺研为细末再将鸡蛋打开小孔，倒出少量蛋清后，每个装入硫磺末 3 克，其中三个放食盐少许，用面糊封口蒸熟，每日早晚各食一个，病重者可重服一次。

6. Internal Accumulation of Cold-Dampness: Take 18g of native sulfur and 6 eggs. Grind the sulfur into fine powder. Make a small hole in each egg, pour out a little egg white, and fill each with 3g of sulfur powder. Add a little salt to three of them. Seal the holes with dough paste and steam until cooked. Eat one in the morning and one in the evening daily. For severe cases, take another dose.

生活调摄

Lifestyle and Care

对于白带病的防治，必须贯彻"预防为主"的方针，向广大妇女群众大力宣传有关防治白带的知识，实行计划生育，避免早婚、多产，节制性生活。

For the prevention and treatment of leukorrhea, the policy of "prevention first" must be implemented. Vigorous publicity regarding the prevention and treatment of leukorrhea should be carried out among women. Family planning should be practiced to avoid early marriage and excessive childbirth, and sexual activity should be moderated.

要经常保持外阴清洁，宜温水洗涤，勤换内裤。若湿毒致外阴瘙痒，严禁搔抓及热水洗烫。

The vulva should be kept clean regularly. It is advisable to wash with warm water and change underwear frequently. If damp-toxin causes vulvar itching, scratching and washing with hot water are strictly prohibited.

勿久卧湿地，尽量减少水中作业，以免外湿内侵。

Do not lie on damp ground for a long time, and minimize working in water to prevent external dampness from invading the body.

勿过食生冷，以免碍脾助湿，少吃厚味、甜味及刺激性食物，以防蕴湿生热。

Do not eat excessive raw and cold foods to avoid impairing the spleen and promoting dampness. Eat less greasy, sweet, and irritating foods to prevent the accumulation of dampness and the generation of heat.

《中药科技报》1992 年 2 月 26 日

TCM Science and Technology News, February 26, 1992

妇女阴道内平时有少许分泌物，臭味不大称白带。若白带过多，臭味较大，伴有腹痛、腰酸等称“带下”。可选用以下药膳防治。

Women normally have a small amount of vaginal discharge with little odor, which is called leukorrhea. If the discharge is excessive, has a strong odor, and is accompanied by abdominal pain and backache, it is called “Daixia” (abnormal vaginal discharge). The following medicinal diets can be selected for prevention and treatment.

7. 山萸肉粥：山萸肉 20 克，粳米 100 克，白糖适量。制法：将山萸肉洗净，去核，与粳米同入砂锅煮粥，加入白糖即可。每日 1 次，分 2 次服，3-5 天一疗程。功效：补益肝肾，涩精敛汗。适用于肝肾不足，带下，遗尿，小便频数患者。

7. Cornus Porridge: 20g of cornus fruit, 100g of japonica rice, and an appropriate amount of white sugar. Preparation: Wash the cornus fruit, remove the seeds, and cook it with the japonica rice in a clay pot to make porridge. Add white sugar. Take once a day, divided into two servings, for 3-5 days as a course. Efficacy: Tonifies the liver and kidneys, astringes essence, and stops sweating. Suitable for patients with liver and kidney deficiency, leukorrhea, enuresis, and frequent urination.

8. 金樱子粥：金樱子 10-15 克，粳米 60-100 克。先煎金樱子，去渣取汁，同粳米煮粥。日分 2 次服，3 天为一疗程。功效：补肾、固精。适用于妇女带下、子宫脱垂。

8. Rosa Laevigata Porridge: 10-15g of rosa laevigata and 60-100g of japonica rice. Decoct the rosa laevigata first, remove the dregs, and use the liquid to cook porridge with the japonica rice. Divide into two servings daily, with 3 days as one course. Efficacy: Tonifies the kidney and astringes essence. Suitable for women with leukorrhea and uterine prolapse.

9. 鸡冠花茶：鸡冠花 30 克，切碎，煎水。代茶频饮。功效：治妇女赤白带下，对阴道滴虫有杀灭作用。

9. Cockscomb Flower Tea: 30g of cockscomb flower, chopped and decocted in water. Drink frequently as a tea substitute. Efficacy: Treats red and white leukorrhea in women and has a lethal effect on Trichomonas vaginalis.

《民族医药报》1992 年 8 月 7 日（淳朴）

Ethnic Medicine News, August 7, 1992 (Chunpu)

带下病为妇科四大症之一，中药外治具有针对性强无副作用的特点，患者易于接受，便于开展，根据临床综合报道。现介绍几种外治方法，供参考。

Abnormal vaginal discharge is one of the four major gynecological diseases. External treatment with traditional Chinese medicine is highly targeted and has no side effects. It is easily accepted by patients and convenient to carry out. Based on comprehensive clinical reports, several external treatment methods are introduced here for reference.

10. 苦参 60 克，蛇床子、黄柏各 30 克，苍术、薏苡仁各 15 克，水煎 1 小时过滤，洗外阴周围及阴道，每日 2- 3 次，7 日为一疗程，连用 3 个月，适用于阴道炎所致带下。

10. Take 60g of sophora flavescens, 30g each of cnidium fruit and phellodendron bark, and 15g each of atractylodes lancea and coix seed. Decoct in water for 1 hour and filter. Wash the vulva and vagina. Do this 2-3 times a day, with 7 days as one course, continuously for 3 months. Suitable for leukorrhea caused by vaginitis.

11. 六神丸 15 粒，洗净外阴，塞入阴道，每晚一次，经期停用，6 日疗程，二疗程可愈，用于滴虫性带下。

11. Take 15 Liushen Pills. After washing the vulva, insert them into the vagina once every night. Stop during menstruation. 6 days constitute one course, and two courses can achieve a cure. Used for trichomonas leukorrhea.

12. 芡实、桑螵蛸各 30 克，白芷 20 克共研细末，醋调敷脐，一日换一次，一周即愈，用于各种带下。

12. Take 30g each of euryale seeds and mantis egg cases, and 20g of angelica dahurica. Grind them together into fine powder. Mix with vinegar and apply to the navel. Change once a day, and it can be cured in a week. Used for various types of leukorrhea.

13. 艾叶、鲜葱各 500 克，捣烂炒热装袋，置外阴，上用热水袋热慰 1-2 小时，用于虚寒性带下。

13. Take 500g each of mugwort leaves and fresh green onions. Mash them, stir-fry until hot, and put them in a bag. Place it on the vulva and apply a hot water bottle on top for 1-2 hours. Used for leukorrhea due to deficiency-cold.

14. 中药熏洗。取蛇床子、白蘚皮、黄柏各 50 克，荆芥、防风、苦参、龙胆草各 15 克，薄荷（后下）10 克，水煎熏洗外阴，每日 2 次，10-15 日为一疗程，用于霉菌或滴虫所致湿热型带下。

14. Herbal Fumigation and Washing. Take 50g each of cnidium fruit, dictamnus bark, and phellodendron bark, 15g each of schizonepeta, saposhnikovia root, sophora flavescens, and gentian root, and 10g of mint (added later). Decoct in water to fumigate and wash the vulva. Do this twice a day, with 10-15 days as one course. Used for damp-heat leukorrhea caused by fungi or trichomonas.

15. 艾叶 100 克，盐 10 克共炒后，用布包好，热熨肚部和小腹部，日二次。

15. Stir-fry 100g of mugwort leaves and 10g of salt together, wrap them in cloth, and apply hot compresses to the abdomen and lower abdomen twice a day.

《中药科技报》1992 年 5 月 6 日（董万法）

TCM Science and Technology News, May 6, 1992 (Dong Wanfa)

16. 带下症药浴：妇人症见腰腹酸痛，白带特多而且有臭腥味，舌红苔白，脉沉缓者，多为湿热下注所致。方药：艾叶 15 克，苍术 30 克，苦参 50 克，黄柏 20 克，白蘚皮 30 克，木芙蓉 50 克，水煎熏洗阴部可愈。

16. Herbal Bath for Leukorrhea: For women with symptoms of aching in the lower back and abdomen, excessive leukorrhea with a fishy odor, red tongue with white coating, and deep and slow pulse, it is mostly caused by the downward flow of damp-heat. Prescription: 15g of mugwort leaves, 30g of atractylodes lancea, 50g of sophora flavescens, 20g of phellodendron bark, 30g of dictamnus bark, and 50g of hibiscus mutabilis. Decoct in water to fumigate and wash the genital area to achieve a cure.

《民族医药报》1992 年 6 月 5 日

Ethnic Medicine News, June 5, 1992

五、血崩（4 方）

V. Metrorrhagia / Uterine Bleeding (4 Prescriptions)

1. 乌贼骨炖鸡治疗血崩

Cuttlefish Bone Stewed with Chicken for Metrorrhagia

妇女月经经期延长或不规则，经血量多或淋漓不止，中医称为崩漏。若患者还有头昏晕眩、心悸怔忡、失眠多梦，脉细无力等症状，一般属血虚崩漏。可用乌贼骨炖鸡治疗。

Prolonged or irregular menstrual periods, excessive menstrual bleeding, or continuous spotting are referred to as “Beng Lou” (metrorrhagia and uterine bleeding) in traditional Chinese medicine. If the patient also experiences dizziness, palpitations, insomnia with excessive dreaming, and a thready and weak pulse, it is generally classified as metrorrhagia due to blood deficiency. Cuttlefish bone stewed with chicken can be used for treatment.

乌贼骨含大量碳酸钙及少量磷酸钙、氯化钠、镁盐、胶质等，有收涩止血的功效；鸡肉味道鲜美，含有丰富的蛋白质、脂肪、钙、磷、铁、维生素 BI、

B2，烟酸及维生素 A 等，有益精补血的作用。制作时，用乌贼骨（即海螵蛸）30克，鸡肉 90 克、精盐、味精适量。将鸡肉切成 3 公分长、2 公分宽，洗净，乌贼骨打碎。把鸡肉、乌贼骨装在陶罐内加清水 500 毫升，上蒸笼蒸熟（加适量精盐），吃时可加适量味精。连服 3-5 次即可见效。

Cuttlefish bone contains a large amount of calcium carbonate, as well as small amounts of calcium phosphate, sodium chloride, magnesium salts, and gelatin, which have the effect of astringing and stopping bleeding. Chicken is delicious and rich in protein, fat, calcium, phosphorus, iron, vitamins B1 and B2, niacin, and vitamin A, which help nourish essence and tonify blood. For preparation, use 30g of cuttlefish bone (also known as cuttlebone), 90g of chicken meat, and an appropriate amount of refined salt and MSG. Cut the chicken meat into pieces 3 cm long and 2 cm wide, wash them, and crush the cuttlefish bone. Place the chicken and cuttlefish bone in a clay pot, add 500 ml of water, and steam until cooked (add an appropriate amount of refined salt). MSG can be added when eating. Significant effects can be seen after taking it continuously for 3-5 times.

《中药科技报》（孙摘）

TCM Science and Technology News (Sun Zhai)

2. 三陈汤治疗崩漏证

2. Sanchen Decoction for Metrorrhagia and Uterine Bleeding

民间用陈棉花籽、陈蒜杆、陈棕皮各 50 克，烧炭存性，淬水服治疗崩漏，可获良效。

In folk medicine, 50g each of aged cotton seeds, aged garlic stalks, and aged palm bark are charred to retain their properties, quenched in water, and taken to treat metrorrhagia and uterine bleeding, achieving good therapeutic effects.

崩漏是多种妇科疾病所表现的共有症状，如冲任失调性子宫出血、月经过多，甚至五色带下等都属崩漏范畴。近代之论崩漏，多趋向于冲任失调性阴道出血。考陈棉花籽辛温有毒，功能温肾补虚，陈蒜杆辛温有毒，功能暖脾胃温气血，陈棕皮苦涩平，功能收涩止血，再加各药烧炭，既减轻其毒性，又增强止血用，组方有标本兼治之功。此方适宜于中医辨证属肾阳虚崩漏患者，症见血色淡红，质稀，淋漓不断，体胖，脉沉弱等，若出血多时可见数而无力之脉。笔者曾用该法治疗 23 例肾阳虚崩漏患者，均取得满意疗效。

Metrorrhagia and uterine bleeding are common symptoms of various gynecological diseases, such as uterine bleeding due to Chong-Ren (Penetrating and Conception) meridian dysfunction, menorrhagia, and even multi-colored vaginal discharge, all of which fall under the category of Beng Lou. Modern discussions on this condition tend to focus on vaginal bleeding caused by Chong-Ren dysfunction. Aged cotton seeds are pungent, warm, and toxic, functioning to warm the kidney and tonify deficiency. Aged garlic stalks are pungent, warm, and toxic, functioning to warm the spleen and stomach, and warm qi and blood. Aged palm bark is bitter, astringent, and neutral, functioning to astringe and stop bleeding. Charring these herbs not only reduces their toxicity but also enhances their hemostatic effects, making the prescription effective for both the root cause and the symptoms. This prescription is suitable for patients diagnosed with metrorrhagia due to kidney yang deficiency, presenting with pale red blood, thin consistency, continuous spotting, obesity, and a deep and weak pulse. In cases of heavy bleeding, a rapid and weak pulse may be observed. The author has used this method to treat 23 patients with kidney yang deficiency metrorrhagia, all achieving satisfactory therapeutic effects.

《民族医药报》1991 年 7 月 5 日（贵州 卢之分）

Ethnic Medicine News, July 5, 1991 (Lu Zhifen, Guizhou)

3. 妇女月经期经量多而猛称之为“崩漏”。我们拟用《上海中医药》杂志介绍的验方“止崩汤”治疗，经临床验证，效果明显。现介绍如下：

3. Excessive and severe menstrual bleeding during menstruation is called “Beng Lou” (metrorrhagia and uterine bleeding). We plan to use the proven prescription “Zhibeng Decoction” (Metrorrhagia-Stopping Decoction) introduced in the Journal of Shanghai Traditional Chinese Medicine for treatment. Clinical verification has shown significant effects. The details are introduced as follows:

方药组成：金樱子根 30 克，茜草、夏枯草、地榆炭、鸡冠花各 20 克，水灯草、车前草各 15 克，甜酒 30 毫升（另加）。

Prescription Composition: 30g of rosa laevigata root, 20g each of madder root, selfheal spike, garden burnet charcoal, and cockscomb flower, and 15g each of rush pith and plantain herb, with an additional 30 ml of sweet rice wine.

上述药物以鲜品为佳，煎汁后加入甜酒，每日 1 剂，分 3-4 次服用，一般服 1-3 剂即见效，病愈即停药。

Fresh herbs are preferred for the above prescription. After decocting, add the sweet rice wine. Take one dose daily, divided into 3-4 servings. Generally, significant effects are seen after taking 1-3 doses. Stop taking the medication once the disease is cured.

《民族医药报》1992 年 4 月 17 日（南京 孙哲）

Ethnic Medicine News, April 17, 1992 (Sun Zhe, Nanjing)

4. 单味蚕砂治崩漏

4. Single Herb Silkworm Feces for Metrorrhagia and Uterine Bleeding

笔者运用单味蚕砂治疗崩漏症 4 例，全部治愈，现介绍如下。

The author used single-herb silkworm feces to treat 4 cases of metrorrhagia and uterine bleeding, all of which were completely cured. The details are introduced as follows.

方药与用法：取蚕砂适量，炒炭，研极细末，每服 10 克，每日三次，用黄酒送服，5 天为一疗程。

Prescription and Usage: Take an appropriate amount of silkworm feces, char them by stir-frying, and grind into an extremely fine powder. Take 10g each time, 3 times a day, swallowed with yellow rice wine. 5 days constitute one course of treatment.

病例：苟 XX，女，26 岁。人工流产后 1 个月，有经来潮，突然大量下血，其色紫黑有块，下腹疼痛及腰部抽痛明显，舌有紫点，脉沉涩。曾服失笑散，云南白药，痛减而血不止。即给炒蚕砂末 ，每服 10 克，1 日三次，服 6 次而痛消血止，随访半年月经正常。按：蚕砂为蚕蛾科家蚕之粪便，味辛、甘，功能活血止血、行气、和中缓急。《本草纲目》有“治……症结及妇人血崩。”的记载。蚕砂炒炭存性，据现代药理研究有收缩子宫作用，并能缩短出血和凝血时间，增加血小板。临床用之，效果明显，既简便经济，又无毒副作用。

Case Report: Ms. Gou XX, female, 26 years old. One month after an induced abortion, her menstruation occurred, with a sudden massive hemorrhage. The blood was purplish-black with clots, accompanied by obvious lower abdominal pain and spasmodic back pain. Her tongue had purple spots, and her pulse was deep and choppy. She had previously taken Shixiao San and Yunnan Baiyao; the pain was reduced, but the bleeding did not stop. She was immediately given stir-fried silkworm feces powder, 10g each time, 3 times a day. After 6 doses, the pain disappeared and the bleeding stopped. A six-month follow-up showed normal menstruation. Note: Silkworm feces are the excrement of the domestic silkworm of the Bombycidae family. They are pungent and sweet in taste, functioning to promote blood circulation and stop bleeding, regulate qi, harmonize the middle, and relieve spasms. The Compendium of Materia Medica records that it "treats... abdominal masses and metrorrhagia in women." Charring silkworm feces to retain their properties has been shown in modern pharmacological research to have a uterine-contracting effect, shorten bleeding and clotting time, and increase platelets. Clinical application shows significant effects; it is simple, economical, and has no toxic side effects.

《中药科技报》（贵州 姜长贵）

TCM Science and Technology News (Jiang Changgui, Guizhou)

六．月经不调（43 方）

VI. Irregular Menstruation (43 Prescriptions)

痛经是妇女最常见的疾病，可因风寒湿热燥邪气引发，其病机主要是气血运行不畅，经脉瘀滞，不通则痛；其次是气血虚少，经脉失养所致。民间中蕴藏很多治疗痛经的有效验方，现将搜集到的并与之临床应用有显著效果的介绍如下。

Dysmenorrhea is the most common disease in women, which can be triggered by pathogenic factors such as wind, cold, dampness, heat, and dryness. Its main pathogenesis is the poor circulation of qi and blood, and the stagnation of meridians and collaterals, leading to pain due to blockage; secondly, it is caused by a deficiency of qi and blood, resulting in malnutrition of the meridians. There are many effective proven prescriptions for treating dysmenorrhea hidden in folk medicine. The following are collected prescriptions that have shown significant clinical effects.

1. 紫丹参 250 克研末，每次服 9 克，日 2 次，黄酒引。于月经来潮前服 3 天，连用 3 个周期。本方功效：活血化瘀通经。

Grind 250g of red salvia root into powder. Take 9g each time, twice a day, guided by yellow rice wine. Take it for 3 days before menstruation, continuously for 3 cycles. Efficacy: Promotes blood circulation, removes blood stasis, and unblocks menstruation.

2. 元胡 30 克，研末，每服 6 克，日 2 次，用南木香 10 克水煎送服。本方功效：活血化瘀行滞，理气止痛。适用于经期小腹疼痛服用。特别是情志不畅引起的痛经证。

2. Grind 30g of corydalis tuber into powder. Take 6g each time, twice a day, swallowed with a decoction of 10g of costus root. Efficacy: Promotes blood circulation, removes blood stasis, relieves stagnation, regulates qi, and stops pain. Suitable for lower abdominal pain during menstruation, especially for dysmenorrhea caused by emotional depression.

3. 益母草、刘寄奴（鹅舌草）各 60 克水煎服。本方功效：活血通经。适用于经期或月经前后小腹疼痛时急用。

3. Decoct 60g each of motherwort and artemisia anomala (goose tongue grass) in water and take. Efficacy: Promotes blood circulation and unblocks menstruation. Suitable for emergency use when lower abdominal pain occurs during or before and after menstruation.

4. 炒当归、炒白芍各20克，焦艾叶15克，水煎服，连服3剂，连用3个周期。本方功效：养血温经止痛。适用于血虚脉络失养所致的经后小腹疼痛。

4. Take 20g each of stir-fried angelica and stir-fried white peony root, and 15g of scorched mugwort leaf. Decoct in water and take, continuously for 3 doses and 3 cycles. Efficacy: Nourishes blood, warms the meridians, and stops pain. Suitable for lower abdominal pain after menstruation caused by blood deficiency and malnutrition of the meridians.

5. 杜鹃花根、野玫瑰花根各12克，加红糖适量水煎服，每日一剂，连用3剂。本方功效：活血通经。适用于经行不畅，夹有紫暗色血块者。

5. Take 12g each of rhododendron root and wild rose root, add an appropriate amount of brown sugar, decoct in water and take. Take one dose daily for 3 consecutive doses. Efficacy: Promotes blood circulation and unblocks menstruation. Suitable for irregular menstruation accompanied by purplish-dark blood clots.

6. 泽兰、艾叶各12克，加红糖30克，水煎服，连服3剂。本方功效：化瘀行滞，通络除湿。（无淤湿并存者忌用）。

6.Take 12g each of lycopus and mugwort leaf, add 30g of brown sugar, decoct in water and take, continuously for 3 doses. Efficacy: Removes blood stasis, relieves stagnation, unblocks collaterals, and dispels dampness. (Contraindicated for patients without concurrent blood stasis and dampness).

7. 地骨皮30克，丹皮9克，生地15克，水煎服。每于月经前连服3剂。本方功效：滋阴清热，凉血止痛。

7. Take 30g of cortex lycii radicis, 9g of moutan bark, and 15g of rehmannia root. Decoct in water and take. Take 3 consecutive doses before each menstruation. Efficacy: Nourishes yin, clears heat, cools blood, and stops pain.

8. 菟丝子30克，鹿角胶9克（烊），韭菜子15克，水煎服，于经前速服3-5剂。本方功效：补肾助阳，通经止痛。

8. Take 30g of dodder seed, 9g of antler glue (melted), and 15g of chive seed. Decoct in water and take. Quickly take 3-5 doses before menstruation. Efficacy:

Tonifies the kidney, assists yang, unblocks menstruation, and stops pain.

9. 白芷、干姜、桂子各 2 克，研成粉末，用湿布将脐擦净，将药末 1 克撒于脐上，用胶布固定。每晚睡前用药，次晨去掉。连服 8 天。本方功效：祛风散寒，温肾止痛。

9. Take 2g each of angelica dahurica, dried ginger, and cassia twig. Grind them into powder. Wipe the navel clean with a wet cloth, sprinkle 1g of the powder on the navel, and fix it with adhesive tape. Apply the medicine before going to bed every night and remove it the next morning. Use continuously for 8 days. Efficacy: Dispels wind and cold, warms the kidney, and stops pain.

《中药科技报》1992 年 8 月 26 日（刘启明杨淑英）

TCM Science and Technology News, August 26, 1992 (Liu Qiming, Yang Shuying)

10. 痛经：当归 9 克，川芎 4.5 克，红花 4.5 克，肉桂 3 克，元胡 9 克，香附 12 克，五灵脂 9 克，郁金 9 克，水煎服。

10. Dysmenorrhea: Take 9g of angelica, 4.5g of ligusticum, 4.5g of safflower, 3g of cassia bark, 9g of corydalis tuber, 12g of cyperus, 9g of flying squirrel feces, and 9g of turmeric. Decoct in water and take.

月经后期

Delayed Menstruation

11. 益母草、红糖各 30 克，当归 15 克，水煎服，每日 1 剂，连服 3-5 剂。

11. Take 30g each of motherwort and brown sugar, and 15g of angelica. Decoct in water and take. Take one dose daily for 3-5 consecutive doses.

12. 全当归 20 克，干姜 3 片，水煎服，每日 1 剂，连服 3 剂。

12. Take 20g of whole angelica and 3 slices of dried ginger. Decoct in water and take. Take one dose daily for 3 consecutive doses.

13. 酒制虎杖、酒制香附各等分研末，每服 6 克，日 3 次，连服 5-7 天。

13. Take equal amounts of wine-processed giant knotweed and wine-processed cyperus, grind into powder. Take 6g each time, 3 times a day, continuously for 5-7 days.

月经稀少

Scanty Menstruation

14. 月月红 9 克，全当归 30 克，水煎服，每日 1 剂，连用 3 剂。

14. Take 9g of Chinese rose and 30g of whole angelica. Decoct in water and take. Take one dose daily for 3 consecutive doses.

15. 黄荆子、充蔚子、香附子各等分，童便炒，研末，每服 6 克，日 2 次。

15. Take equal amounts of vitex fruit, motherwort fruit, and cyperus. Stir-fry with boy’s urine, grind into powder. Take 6g each time, twice a day.

16. 元胡 3 克，红花 12 克，益母草 30 克，水煎服，每日 1 剂。

16. Take 3g of corydalis tuber, 12g of safflower, and 30g of motherwort. Decoct in water and take, one dose daily.

月经过多

Menorrhagia (Excessive Menstruation)

17. 旱莲草、红糖各 30 克，水煎服，每日 1 剂，连服 3 剂。

17. Take 30g each of eclipta and brown sugar. Decoct in water and take. Take one dose daily for 3 consecutive doses.

18. 仙鹤草、茜草、紫草各 15 克，水煎服，每日 1 剂，连服 3 剂。

18. Take 15g each of agrimony, madder root, and gromwell root. Decoct in water and take. Take one dose daily for 3 consecutive doses.

19. 丹皮、黄柏皮各 9 克，水煎服，每日 1 剂，连服 3 剂。

19. Take 9g each of moutan bark and phellodendron bark. Decoct in water and take. Take one dose daily for 3 consecutive doses.

倒经

Vicarious Menstruation (Retrograde Menstruation)

20. 韭菜汁、童便各半杯，一次服，每日 1-2 次。

20. Take half a cup each of chive juice and boy’s urine, take at once, 1-2 times a day.

21. 鲜藕、鲜侧柏叶各 30 克，捣烂取汁，用黄酒分 3 次冲服。

21. Take 30g each of fresh lotus root and fresh platycladus leaves. Mash them

to extract the juice, and swallow it in 3 divided doses with yellow rice wine.

22. 鲜慈菇捣汁加冰糖适量服，每日 2 次。

22. Mash fresh arrowhead to extract the juice, add an appropriate amount of rock sugar, and take twice a day.

经痛

Dysmenorrhea

23. 元胡、车前子各等分，研末，每服 6 克，日 3 次，黄酒引。

23. Take equal amounts of corydalis tuber and plantain seed, grind into powder. Take 6g each time, 3 times a day, guided by yellow rice wine.

24. 虎杖根 30 克，水酒各半煎服，日 1 次，连服 3 天。

24. Take 30g of giant knotweed root. Decoct with equal parts of water and liquor, take once a day for 3 consecutive days.

25. 白芷 9 克，干姜 3 克，赤芍 15 克，水煎服，每日服 1 剂。

25. Take 9g of angelica dahurica, 3g of dried ginger, and 15g of red peony root. Decoct in water and take, one dose daily.

（刘启明 杨淑英）

(Liu Qiming, Yang Shuying)

闭经

Amenorrhea

26. 月季花 30 克，瘦猪肉适量，二味共煮，吃肉喝汤。

26. Take 30g of Chinese rose and an appropriate amount of lean pork. Boil the two ingredients together, eat the meat, and drink the soup.

月经失调

Menstrual Irregularities

27. 全当归 60 克，浸白酒 1 公斤，瓶装密封 15 天后启用。每服 10 毫升，早晚各 1 次。

27. Take 60g of whole angelica, soak in 1 kg of liquor, seal in a bottle, and use after 15 days. Take 10 ml each time, once in the morning and once in the evening.

28. 酒制香附、炒充蔚子各 30 克，研末，每服 5 克，日 3 次。连服 3 天。

28. Take 30g each of wine-processed cyperus and stir-fried motherwort fruit, grind into powder. Take 5g each time, 3 times a day. Take continuously for 3 days.

29. 益母草 30 克，全当归 15 克，水酒各半煎服，连服 3-5 天。

29. Take 30g of motherwort and 15g of whole angelica. Decoct with equal parts of water and liquor, take continuously for 3-5 days.

30. 刘寄奴不拘量，晒干研末，每服 6 克，日 3 次，黄酒引。

30. Take an appropriate amount of artemisia anomala, sun-dry and grind into powder. Take 6g each time, 3 times a day, guided by yellow rice wine.

月经先期

Premature Menstruation

31. 益母草、红糖各 30 克，酒制黄芩 9 克，水煎服，日 2 次，连服 1 周。

31. Take 30g each of motherwort and brown sugar, and 9g of wine-processed scutellaria. Decoct in water and take, twice a day, continuously for 1 week.

32. 鲜芹菜 100 克，水煎服，每日 1 次，常服。

32. Take 100g of fresh celery. Decoct in water and take once a day. Take it regularly.

33. 丹皮、生地各 15 克，水煎服，每日 1 剂，连服 3-5 剂。

33. Take 15g each of moutan bark and rehmannia root. Decoct in water and take. Take one dose daily for 3-5 consecutive doses.

34. 旱莲草 30 克，水煎服，每日 1 剂。

34. Take 30g of eclipta. Decoct in water and take, one dose daily.

35. 红枣可治更年期综合症

35. Red Dates for Treating Menopausal Syndrome

红枣是一种滋补佳品，含糖 56-80%（100 克干枣），100 克鲜枣中含维生素 380-600 毫克，内含芦丁可治高血压。红枣还可治疗中年妇女心神不宁、失眠、烦躁不安、情绪不能控制等更年期综合症病例。处方是：大枣（去核）10 个，生甘草 12.5 克，小麦 40 克煎水代茶，疗效很好。

Red dates are an excellent tonic, containing 56-80% sugar (per 100g of dried dates). 100g of fresh dates contain 380-600mg of vitamin C, and the rutin contained within can be used to treat hypertension. Red dates can also be used to treat menopausal syndrome in middle-aged women, presenting with restlessness, insomnia, irritability, and uncontrollable emotions. The prescription is: 10 pitted red dates, 12.5g of raw licorice, and 40g of wheat, decocted in water and taken as a tea substitute. The therapeutic effect is very good.

《中医药信息报》（樊常宝）

TCM Information News (Fan Changbao)

中药外治法

External Treatment Methods of Traditional Chinese Medicine

中药外治法在痛经的治疗中，具有简便、实用，疗效显著的特点。特别是对寒凝及血瘀型的痛经，更具独特功效。现介绍几则外治灵验法如下，供参考。

External treatment methods of traditional Chinese medicine are simple, practical, and have significant therapeutic effects in the treatment of dysmenorrhea. They are particularly uniquely effective for dysmenorrhea caused by cold coagulation and blood stasis. Several effective external treatment methods are introduced below for reference.

36. 热熨法。食盐，葱白各 250 克，生姜 125 克共炒热装布袋熨下腹部，药凉炒热再用，一日数次，每次 30 分钟。适用于虚寒为主痛经。

36. Hot Compress Method: Stir-fry 250g each of salt and green onion whites, and 125g of fresh ginger until hot, place them in a cloth bag, and apply as a hot compress to the lower abdomen. When the medicine cools, stir-fry it again to reheat and reuse. Apply several times a day, 30 minutes each time. Suitable for dysmenorrhea mainly caused by deficiency-cold.

37. 涂擦法。清凉油适量外擦神阙穴，一日 2-3 次，痛愈为止，用于各型痛经。

37. Rubbing Method: Apply an appropriate amount of cooling balm externally to the Shenque acupoint (navel), 2-3 times a day, until the pain is completely cured. Used for all types of dysmenorrhea.

38. 点滴法。取肉桂、公丁香、冰片各 30 克，压碎浸入三花酒 500ml 中，一月后去渣，置眼药或滴鼻液中备用。应用时将药 5-10 滴点舌面，先含后咽。3-15

分钟疼痛缓解，用于寒湿凝滞型痛经。

38. Drip Method: Take 30g each of cassia bark, clove, and borneol, crush them, and soak in 500ml of Sanhua liquor. Remove the dregs after one month, and store the liquid in an eye drop or nasal drop bottle for later use. When applying, drop 5-10 drops onto the surface of the tongue, hold it in the mouth first, and then swallow. Pain relief occurs within 3-15 minutes. Used for dysmenorrhea caused by cold-dampness stagnation.

39. 薄贴法。经前三天，取大小适中的关节镇痛膏（痛舒宁），贴关元、中极、三阴交、肾俞、次髎穴。两天换一次，经净停贴，连用三次，适用于各种痛经。

39. Plaster Application Method: Three days before menstruation, apply appropriately sized joint analgesic plasters (Tongshuning) to the Guanyuan, Zhongji, Sanyinjiao, Shenshu, and Ciliao acupoints. Change the plaster once every two days, stop applying after menstruation ends, and use continuously for three cycles. Suitable for various types of dysmenorrhea.

40. 摩擦法。麝香风湿油，按摩气海、关元穴 3-5 分钟至发热内传为止，每日 1 次，经净停止，连用 2-3 月，用于虚寒痛经。

40. Friction Method: Use muscat rheumatism oil to massage the Qihai and Guanyuan acupoints for 3-5 minutes until a warm sensation is felt radiating inward. Do this once a day, stop after menstruation ends, and use continuously for 2-3 months. Used for deficiency-cold dysmenorrhea.

41. 塞耳法。大蒜捣汁，用消毒棉球蘸汁塞耳中，剧痛者，一次即效。

41. Ear Plugging Method: Mash garlic to extract the juice, dip a sterilized cotton ball in the juice, and plug it into the ear. For severe pain, it takes effect after just one application.

42. 耳压豆法。王不留行籽，用胶布贴压子宫、肝、胆、肾、腹、内分泌、肾上腺、降压沟、耳迷根穴位。每日 10 次，越痛越压。

42. Ear Seed Pressing Method: Use vaccaria seeds and adhesive tape to press and stimulate the acupoints of the uterus, liver, gallbladder, kidney, abdomen, endocrine, adrenal gland, antihypertensive groove, and ear vagus root. Press 10

times a day; the more painful it is, the more you should press.

43. 穴位注射法。于经前后 10 天内，取双侧三阴交、内关穴隔日注射 5% 当归注射液 1mI，用于血虚、血瘀型痛经。

43. Acupoint Injection Method: Within 10 days before and after menstruation, inject 1ml of 5% angelica injection into the bilateral Sanyinjiao and Neiguan acupoints every other day. Used for dysmenorrhea due to blood deficiency and blood stasis.

《中药科技报》1992 年 7 月 6 日（山东 董万发）

TCM Science and Technology News, July 6, 1992 (Dong Wanfa, Shandong)

七、子宫脱垂

VII. Uterine Prolapse

1. 气虚子宫脱垂。用紫花地丁 20 克，金银花 20 克，乌梅 15 克，五倍子 10 克，煎水熏洗外阴部，每日一次。也可用棕树根 50 克，老竹根 30 克，枳壳 15 克，棉花子 10 克，水煎分三次服，每日一剂。

Uterine Prolapse due to Qi Deficiency: Take 20g of common violet herb, 20g of honeysuckle, 15g of dark plum, and 10g of Chinese gall. Decoct in water to fumigate and wash the vulva once a day. Alternatively, take 50g of palm tree root, 30g of old bamboo root, 15g of bitter orange, and 10g of cotton seeds. Decoct in water and divide into three servings. Take one dose daily.

2. 肾虚子宫脱垂。取蓖麻籽 15 克，枳壳 15 克，黄柏 5 克，生姜 3 克，将药物捣烂，贴敷于百会穴。或用棉花根 50 克，金樱子根 50 克，丝瓜藤 30 克，红糖 20 克，煎水代茶饮用。

2. Uterine Prolapse due to Kidney Deficiency: Take 15g of castor seeds, 15g of bitter orange, 5g of phellodendron bark, and 3g of fresh ginger. Mash the herbs into a paste and apply it to the Baihui acupoint. Alternatively, take 50g of cotton root, 50g of rosa laevigata root, 30g of loofah vine, and 20g of brown sugar. Decoct in water and take as a tea substitute.

《民族医药报》1992 年 5 月 8 日（湖南 启年）

Ethnic Medicine News, May 8, 1992 (Qi Nian, Hunan)

3. 黄芪三十五克，升麻三十五克，枸杞十八克，茯苓十八克，金樱根九十克，用水加酒共煎，内服，连服五剂可愈。病情较重者，可连服七至十剂。服药期间忌房事，一个月内忌剧烈运动或强烈劳动。

3. Take 35g of astragalus, 35g of cimicifuga, 18g of wolfberry, 18g of poria, and 90g of rosa laevigata root. Decoct in water with liquor and take orally. Taking five consecutive doses can cure the condition. For severe cases, take 7 to 10 consecutive doses. Abstain from sexual intercourse during medication, and avoid strenuous exercise or heavy labor for one month.

4. 枳实一百克，乌梅一百克（火煨），混研为细末，日服二次，每次五至八克，服药期间忌辛辣，并注意休息调养。

4. Take 100g of bitter orange and 100g of dark plum (baked over a fire). Mix and grind them into a fine powder. Take 5 to 8g each time, twice a day. Avoid spicy food during medication, and pay attention to resting and recuperation.

（是明启）(Shi Mingqi)

5. 治子宫脱垂：用蓖麻籽去壳七粒、白胡椒七粒共研如泥、敷贴在肚脐眼上，用纱布胶布固定，三日一换。同时用鱼鳅串全草 50 克、狗儿弯根 50 克加红糖 50 克共水煎内服，一日一剂，连服七天有效。

5. Treatment for Uterine Prolapse: Shell 7 castor seeds and take 7 white peppercorns. Grind them together into a mud-like paste, apply it to the navel, and fix it with gauze and adhesive tape. Change the dressing every three days. At the same time, take 50g of the whole plant of Crepidiastrum sonchifolium (fish loach string) and 50g of Cynanchum root (dog-bending root), add 50g of brown sugar, decoct in water and take orally. Take one dose daily, and it will be effective after taking it continuously for seven days.

《中药科技报》1991 年 2 月 10 日

TCM Science and Technology News, February 10, 1991

6. 敷脐法治疗子宫脱垂

6. Umbilical Plaster Therapy for Uterine Prolapse

子宫脱垂又叫子宫脱出，俗称“吊茄子”。多因气虚下陷或多产、难产时用力过度，伤及胞络而使胞宫失去维系所致。其主要症状是子宫下垂或脱出阴道口外甚则连同阴道壁、膀胱或直肠一并膨出。患了该症，用下述敷脐疗法治疗可获良效。具体是：用五倍子末 3 克，五味子末 2 克，于每晚睡前用食醋适量调制成药饼敷于脐中，另用胶布固定。每日换药一次，3-6 次为一个疗程。

Uterine prolapse, also known as uterine descent, is commonly referred to as "hanging eggplant". It is mostly caused by Qi deficiency and sinking, or excessive exertion during multiple births or difficult labor, which damages the uterine collaterals and causes the uterus to lose its support. The main symptoms include the uterus descending or protruding out of the vaginal opening, and in severe cases, it may be accompanied by the prolapse of the vaginal wall, bladder, or rectum. For this condition, the following umbilical plaster therapy can achieve good therapeutic effects. Specifically: Take 3g of Chinese gall powder and 2g of schisandra powder. Before going to bed every night, mix them with an appropriate amount of edible vinegar to form a medicinal cake, apply it to the navel, and fix it with adhesive tape. Change the medicine once a day, 3 to 6 applications constitute one course of treatment.

《民族医药报》1991 年 8 月 25 日（李修身）

Ethnic Medicine News, August 25, 1991 (Li Xiushen)

八、不孕症
VIII. Infertility

家传不孕店验方

A Family-Inherited Proven Prescription for Infertility

本方为世代家传验方，经笔者临床应用，治疗原发性不孕症及继发性不孕症 40 余例，疗效显著，今介绍如下。

This prescription has been passed down through generations in the author's family. Through clinical application, the author has treated over 40 cases of primary and secondary infertility with significant therapeutic effects. The details are introduced as follows.

处方：鲜桃树根（去皮）30 克，全当归 30 克，益母草 60 克，怀牛膝、川芎各 15 克，元胡、柴胡各 12 克，沙姜 9 克。

Prescription: 30g of fresh peach tree root (peeled), 30g of whole angelica, 60g of motherwort, 15g each of achyranthes root and ligusticum, 12g each of corydalis tuber and bupleurum, and 9g of sand ginger.

服用法：取乌骨雌鸡 1 只，宰后去毛取出内脏，洗净。将以上药物除沙姜外，用白酒炒至微黄（白酒用量以药物湿润为度），装入腹腔内，针线缝合。

Method of Administration: Take one female black-bone chicken, slaughter it, remove the feathers and internal organs, and wash it clean. Except for the sand ginger, stir-fry the above herbs with liquor until slightly yellow (the amount of liquor should be just enough to moisten the herbs). Place them inside the abdominal cavity and suture it with needle and thread.

用 4-5 斤米酒文火蒸至酒干为止，取鸡食肉，一日食完，空腹服。此法宜于经水净后应用，每隔 3-4 天服 1 剂，每月服 2 剂，一般服三个月见效。体质虚弱者慎用，酒过敏者忌用。本方具有补益肝肾、活血化瘀、温经通络功效。

Steam it over low heat with 4 to 5 jin (2-2.5 kg) of rice wine until the wine dries up. Eat the chicken meat, finish it within one day, and consume it on an empty stomach. This method should be applied after menstruation has completely ended. Take one dose every 3 to 4 days, 2 doses per month. Generally, significant effects can be seen after taking it for three months. Use with caution in patients with weak constitutions, and it is strictly contraindicated for those allergic to alcohol. This prescription has the effects of tonifying the liver and kidneys, promoting blood circulation and removing blood stasis, warming the meridians, and unblocking the collaterals.

《中医药信息报》1992 年 2 月 15 日（青海 刘启明）

TCM Information News, February 15, 1992 (Liu Qiming, Qinghai)

九、阴痒
IX. Pruritus Vulvae (Vulvar Itching)

1. 阴痒症药浴：妇人带下或白或黄，有臭味，外阴部或阴道奇痒难忍且有灼热，少腹胀痛或腰酸胀痛，舌红苔白花剥，脉沉缓。此乃湿热盘踞下焦，久蕴生虫为患。方药：苦参 50 克，蛇床子 60 克，土茯苓 100 克，百部 30 克，紫荆皮 30 克，芦荟 5 克，水煎外洗外阴及阴道，一日 3 次，二周可愈。

Herbal Bath for Pruritus Vulvae: In women presenting with white or yellow vaginal discharge with a foul odor, unbearable itching and burning sensation in the vulva or vagina, lower abdominal distension and pain, or lower back soreness and distension, with a red tongue, white coating with peeling, and a deep and slow pulse, the condition is caused by damp-heat lingering in the lower jiao, which over time breeds parasitic pathogens. Prescription: 50g of sophora flavescens, 60g of cnidium fruit, 100g of smilax glabra, 30g of stemona root, 30g of bauhinia bark, and 5g of aloe. Decoct in water for external washing of the vulva and vagina, 3 times a day. It can be cured within two weeks.

（野荐）(Ye Jian)

2. 女性外阴瘙痒症祖国医学称“阴痒”，由浅部霉菌、白色念珠菌或白带、避孕套、避孕药的刺激所引起，少数病人由于神经精神功能异常，内分泌特别是性内分泌失调有关。据资料介绍应用如下药方治疗多例、疗效满意。处方及用法为：芒硝、苦参、蛇床子、黄柏、川椒各 15 克。加水 1500 毫升，煎至 1000 毫升，去渣倒入盆内，至温热适度，坐浴，浸洗 15-20 分钟左右，每日 1-2 次，一般 3-6 次即愈。

2. Vulvar pruritus in women is called “Yin Yang” in traditional Chinese medicine. It is caused by superficial fungi, Candida albicans, or irritation from vaginal discharge, condoms, and contraceptives. In a few patients, it is related to abnormal neuropsychiatric functions and endocrine disorders, especially sex hormone imbalances. According to literature, the following prescription has been

used to treat multiple cases with satisfactory results. Prescription and Usage: 15g each of mirabilite, sophora flavescens, cnidium fruit, phellodendron bark, and Sichuan pepper. Add 1500 ml of water and decoct to 1000 ml. Remove the dregs, pour into a basin, and wait until the temperature is moderately warm. Sit in the bath and soak for about 15-20 minutes, 1-2 times a day. Generally, it can be cured after 3-6 sessions.

《民族医药报》1993 年 4 月 2 日（野荐）

Ethnic Medicine News, April 2, 1993 (Ye Jian)

3. 五倍子、石榴皮、蛇床子、白蘚皮、黄柏及枯矾各 15 克（中药房均有售），加水煎汤，去渣取汁，趁热熏蒸，然后坐浴、冲洗阴道 30 分钟左右，每日 1 剂，每剂复用 2 次，连用 5-7 日即可收效。

3. Take 15g each of Chinese gall, pomegranate peel, cnidium fruit, dictamnus bark, phellodendron bark, and calcined alum (all available at TCM pharmacies). Decoct in water, remove the dregs, and take the juice. While hot, use the steam to fumigate, then sit in the bath and rinse the vagina for about 30 minutes. Take one dose daily, and reuse each dose twice. It will be effective after continuous use for 5-7 days.

《民族医药报》1992 年 3 月 13 日（江西 久春）

Ethnic Medicine News, March 13, 1992 (Jiu Chun, Jiangxi)

4. 柳叶浸剂治外阴湿疹：将柳叶及嫩柳枝晒干，碾后过筛，取柳叶粉 500 克，加纯酒精 0.5 升浸泡七天，过滤，放入樟脑 10 克，利凡诺 1 克，冰片适量，加冷开水 1 升备用。每次使用时先用 1/ 5 液冲洗外阴，再用浸剂涂擦阴道和外阴。每日一次，一般连用 4 天即愈。

4. Willow Leaf Infusion for Vulvar Eczema: Sun-dry willow leaves and tender willow twigs, grind them, and sift. Take 500g of willow leaf powder, add 0.5 liters of pure alcohol, and soak for seven days. Filter the liquid, add 10g of camphor, 1g of rivanol, and an appropriate amount of borneol, then add 1 liter of cooled boiled water for later use. Each time before use, first rinse the vulva with a 1/5 dilution of the liquid, then apply the infusion to the vagina and vulva. Use once a day, and

it generally cures after 4 consecutive days of use.

5.艾叶洗剂治老年性皮肤瘙痒症：艾叶60克，雄黄6克，防风60克，花椒6克。将上药放入脸盆内，加水适量，置火上煎之，沸后20分钟取下，凉至适宜温度，擦洗患处，有奇效。

5. Mugwort Lotion for Senile Pruritus: Take 60g of mugwort leaf, 6g of realgar, 60g of saposhnikovia root, and 6g of Sichuan pepper. Put the herbs in a washbasin, add an appropriate amount of water, and decoct over a fire. Remove from heat 20 minutes after boiling, cool to a suitable temperature, and wipe and wash the affected area. It has miraculous effects.

（陕西 高绪林）

(Gao Xulin, Shaanxi)

6. 老年性阴道炎：当归50克，加芝麻油数滴，水煎，每晚熏洗阴部连用3-5次即愈。

6. Senile Vaginitis: Take 50g of angelica, add a few drops of sesame oil, and decoct in water. Fumigate and wash the vulva every night. It can be cured after continuous use for 3-5 times.

《中药科技报》，1992年3月26日（纪国安）

TCM Science and Technology News, March 26, 1992 (Ji Guo’an)

7. 药物组成：

7. Prescription Composition:

熏洗方：苦参40克，薏苡仁、白癣皮、土茯苓各30克，黄柏、金银花、鹤虱、甘草梢各15克，苍术、萆薢、白芷各10克，蝉蜕4克。

Fumigation and Washing Prescription: 40g of sophora flavescens, 30g each of coix seed, dictamnus bark, and smilax glabra, 15g each of phellodendron bark, honeysuckle, desmodium seed, and licorice tip, 10g each of atractylodes, dioscorea hypoglauca, and angelica dahurica, and 4g of cicada slough.

冲洗方：蛇床子30克，五倍子10克，枯矾9克，雄黄3克。

Vaginal Irrigation Prescription: 30g of cnidium fruit, 10g of Chinese gall, 9g of calcined alum, and 3g of realgar.

适应症：多种阴道炎（如滴虫性、淋病性、霉菌性阴道炎）及各种阴痒症。阴部干涩者慎用冲洗方。

Indications: Various types of vaginitis (such as trichomonas, gonorrheal, and mycotic vaginitis) and various types of pruritus vulvae. Use the vaginal irrigation prescription with caution in patients with vulvar dryness.

用法：熏洗方每日1剂，水煎至1000毫升，先熏后洗，留汤备用，每日2-3次。冲洗方水煎成200-300毫升药液，然后取100毫升用注射器或冲洗器冲洗阴道，仰卧10-30分钟，每晚1次。

Usage: Take one dose of the fumigation and washing prescription daily, decoct in water to 1000 ml, fumigate first and then wash. Keep the decoction for later use, 2-3 times a day. Decoct the irrigation prescription in water to obtain 200-300 ml of liquid, then take 100 ml to irrigate the vagina using a syringe or irrigator. Lie supine for 10-30 minutes, once every night.

疗效观察：该方为湖南籍已故老中医石补天（1906-1984）经验方。自1984年以来，我们运用该方治疗多种阴道炎共67例（其中滴虫性阴道炎43例，霉菌性阴道炎16例，淋病性阴道炎8例），全部治愈（症状消失，妇检正常，镜检未找到病原体），疗程最短3天，最长36天。

Therapeutic Observation: This prescription is an empirical formula from the late senior TCM physician Shi Butian (1906-1984) from Hunan Province. Since 1984, we have used this prescription to treat 67 cases of various vaginitis (including 43 cases of trichomonas vaginitis, 16 cases of mycotic vaginitis, and 8 cases of gonorrheal vaginitis). All cases were completely cured (symptoms disappeared, gynecological examination was normal, and no pathogens were found under microscopic examination). The shortest course of treatment was 3 days, and the longest was 36 days.

注意事项：对肝肾阴虚、阴部干涩者宜加用养血滋阴、润燥生津之品，并配合知柏地黄汤内服，不宜用冲洗方冲洗阴道。治疗期间忌食酸辣刺激饮食，禁烟酒，避免性生活，夫妻双方同时治疗效果更好。因该病易复发，故症状、体征控制后还应继续用药数天，以巩固疗效。

Precautions: For patients with liver and kidney yin deficiency and vulvar dryness, herbs that nourish blood and yin, moisten dryness, and generate fluids should be added, and Zhibai Dihuang Decoction should be taken orally concurrently. Vaginal irrigation with the irrigation prescription is not recommended. During treatment, avoid spicy and sour irritating foods, abstain from smoking and alcohol, and avoid sexual intercourse. Treating both spouses simultaneously yields better results. Since this disease is prone to relapse, medication should be continued for a few days after symptoms and signs are controlled to consolidate the therapeutic effect.

《民族医药报》1992 年 4 月 3 日（唐乾利 蒋秋燕）

Ethnic Medicine News, April 3, 1992 (Tang Qianli, Jiang Qiuyan)

十、子宫肌瘤
X. Uterine Fibroids

笔者拟方桂苓消症丸治疗子宫肌瘤 38 例，取效理想。现做报道。

The author formulated Guiling Xiaozheng Pills to treat 38 cases of uterine fibroids, achieving ideal therapeutic effects. The report is presented as follows.

一般资料 38 例患者均经妇科及 B 型超声波检查而确诊，治疗后疗效评定也以妇科及 B 型超声波检查为主要标准。年龄 25-50 岁，病程（以临床症状为依据）15 天 -10 年。治疗后，痊愈（连续服药 3-6 个月，症状及肌瘤消失，子宫体大小恢复正常）11 例（28.9%），显效（连续服药 6 个月，症状消失，肌瘤明显缩小）8 例（21.1%），有效（连续服药 6 个月，症状消失或明显减轻，宫体及肌瘤较治疗前无明显变化）11 例（28.9%），无效（连续服药 6 个月，症状及肌瘤均无改变）8 例（21.1%）。

General Data: All 38 patients were diagnosed through gynecological and B-mode ultrasound examinations, and the post-treatment efficacy evaluation was also primarily based on these two methods. The patients' ages ranged from 25 to 50 years old, and the disease duration (based on clinical symptoms) ranged from 15 days to 10 years. After treatment, 11 cases (28.9%) were completely cured (after 3-6 months of continuous medication, symptoms and fibroids disappeared, and the size of the uterus returned to normal); 8 cases (21.1%) showed significant effects (after 6 months of continuous medication, symptoms disappeared, and fibroids shrank significantly); 11 cases (28.9%) were effective (after 6 months of continuous medication, symptoms disappeared or significantly alleviated, with no obvious changes in the uterus and fibroids compared to pre-treatment); and 8 cases (21.1%) were ineffective (after 6 months of continuous medication, there were no changes in symptoms and fibroids).

治疗方法桂苓消症丸系由仲景桂枝茯苓丸合当归芍药散加黄芪、山药、陈皮、昆布、夏枯草、三棱、莪术等组成；取桂枝、白芍、桃仁、丹皮、当归、川芎、泽泻、白术、昆布、陈皮、三棱、莪术各 1 份，茯苓、黄芪、夏枯草、山药各 2 份，共研为极细粉末，炼蜜制丸，每丸 10 克，每日服药 2-3 次，每次 10 克。连续治疗 3 个月进行 1 次妇科及 B 型超声波检查。

Treatment Method: Guiling Xiaozheng Pills are composed of Zhang Zhongjing’s Guizhi Fuling Pills combined with Danggui Shaoyao San, supplemented with astragalus, yam, tangerine peel, kelp, selfheal, sparganium, and zedoary. The formulation uses 1 part each of cassia twig, white peony root, peach seed, moutan bark, angelica, ligusticum, alisma, atractylodes, kelp, tangerine peel, sparganium, and zedoary, along with 2 parts each of poria, astragalus, selfheal, and yam. These are ground into an extremely fine powder, refined with honey to make pills weighing 10grams each. The dosage is 10grams per dose, taken 2-3 times daily. A gynecological and B-mode ultrasound examination is conducted after every 3 months of continuous treatment.

用药分析子宫肌瘤属中医妇科学“症瘕”范畴，主要是由正气亏损、气血失调所致。气能统血行津，气能摄血固液，若气虚则血液运行就会壅滞或溢出脉外形成瘀血，津液就会凝聚成痰浊，瘀血痰浊交结于胞宫而形成瘕（子宫肌瘤）。治当益气扶正、活血祛瘀、化痰消症。方中黄芪、茯苓、山药、白术健脾益气化湿，桂枝温通血脉，川芎、桃仁、当归、丹皮、三棱、莪术活血祛瘀破症，白芍养血平肝，泽泻、昆布、夏枯草、陈皮祛湿化痰、软坚散结。使气机调畅，瘀血消散，痰浊得法，进而使子宫肌瘤得以消散。

Medication Analysis: Uterine fibroids belong to the category of "Zheng Jia" (abdominal masses) in TCM gynecology, mainly caused by a deficiency of healthy qi (Zheng Qi) and the imbalance of qi and blood. Qi governs the circulation of blood and body fluids, and controls blood and secures fluids. If qi is deficient, blood circulation will become obstructed or overflow outside the vessels to form blood stasis, and body fluids will condense into phlegm turbidity. When blood stasis and phlegm turbidity intertwine in the uterus, they form a mass (uterine fibroid). The treatment principle should be tonifying qi to support healthy qi, promoting blood circulation to remove stasis, resolving phlegm, and dissipating masses. In this prescription, astragalus, poria, yam, and atractylodes strengthen the spleen, tonify qi, and transform dampness; cassia twig warms and unblocks the blood vessels; ligusticum, peach seed, angelica, moutan bark, sparganium, and zedoary promote blood circulation, remove stasis, and break down masses; white peony root nourishes blood and calms the liver; alisma, kelp, selfheal, and tangerine peel dispel dampness, resolve phlegm, soften hardness, and dissipate nodules. This allows the qi mechanism to flow smoothly, blood stasis to dissipate, and phlegm turbidity to be properly resolved, thereby enabling the uterine fibroids to dissipate.

《中医药信息报》1992 年 8 月 1 日（河南 吴建华 刘燕红）

TCM Information News, August 1, 1992 (Wu Jianhua, Liu Yanhong, Henan)

十一、中药外治妇科病（6 方）

XI. External Treatment of Gynecological Diseases with Traditional Chinese Medicine (6 Prescriptions)

实践证明：使用外治法治疗妇科疾病，不仅简单、价廉、副作用少，而且有较好的疗效。笔者将日常常见妇科疾病的外治法介绍如下：

Practice has proven that using external treatment methods for gynecological diseases is not only simple, inexpensive, and has few side effects, but also yields good therapeutic results. The author introduces the following external treatments for common daily gynecological diseases:

1. 闭经：女子在 18 岁以上尚未来过月经，或过去月经一向正常，而有连续 3 个月以上不来月经者，均称为闭经。治法：

Amenorrhea: If a female over the age of 18 has never had menstruation, or if her previously normal menstruation ceases continuously for more than 3 months, it is called amenorrhea. Treatment methods:

①益母草 150 克，桂枝 10 克，加水 2 千毫升左右，煎汤熏洗小腹部。

① Take 150g of motherwort and 10g of cassia twig, add about 2000 ml of water, decoct, and use the steam and liquid to fumigate and wash the lower abdomen.

②食盐 300 克，热后洒入适量的白酒，再炒片刻，用布包好，热熨小腹，日两次。

② Take 300g of salt, sprinkle an appropriate amount of liquor on it after heating, stir-fry for a moment, wrap it in a cloth, and apply it as a hot compress to the lower abdomen twice a day.

③蜣螂 1 条焙干，威灵仙 10 克烤干，共研细末，用酒调湿，外敷脐部，再用纱布和胶布固定，每晚睡前贴上，次日早晨弃掉。

③ Bake 1 dung beetle and 10g of clematis root until dry, grind them into a fine powder, moisten with liquor, apply externally to the navel, fix with gauze and adhesive tape, apply before going to bed every night, and discard the next morning.

2.痛经：凡月经期前后，或在来月经期间发生较明显的腹痛，称为痛经。治法：

2. Dysmenorrhea: Significant abdominal pain occurring before or after menstruation, or during menstruation, is called dysmenorrhea. Treatment methods:

①大米 500 克，放锅内炒热，然后用布包好，反复热熨小腹和腰骶部。

① Take 500g of rice, stir-fry it in a pan until hot, wrap it in a cloth, and repeatedly apply it as a hot compress to the lower abdomen and lumbosacral region.

②食盐 500 克，葱白 30 克，生姜 100 克，共炒热布包，温熨小腹部。

② Take 500g of salt, 30g of green onion whites, and 100g of fresh ginger, stir-fry them together until hot, wrap in a cloth, and apply as a warm compress to the lower abdomen.

3. 外阴瘙痒：发痒的部位多在阴蒂和小阴唇附近，也有在大阴唇、会阴与肛门附近。瘙痒常在月经期和夜间加重，严重时，可坐立不安。引起瘙痒的原因很多，主要治法应根据：

3. Vulvar Pruritus: The itchy areas are mostly near the clitoris and labia minora, and sometimes near the labia majora, perineum, and anus. Itching often worsens during menstruation and at night, and in severe cases, it can cause restlessness. There are many causes of itching, and the main treatment methods should be based on:

①无破溃者，蛇床子、川椒、明矾、苦参、百部、地肤子各 20 克，煎汤，趁热先熏后坐浴，一日两次，十次为一疗程。

① For cases without skin ulceration: Take 20g each of cnidium fruit, Sichuan pepper, alum, sophora flavescens, stemona root, and kochia fruit. Decoct in water, and while hot, first fumigate and then sit in the bath. Do this twice a day, with 10 times constituting one course of treatment.

②破溃者，蛤粉 3 克，冰片 0.3 克，共研细末，然后用香油调和，涂敷患处。

② For cases with skin ulceration: Grind 3g of clam shell powder and 0.3g of borneol into a fine powder, mix with sesame oil, and apply to the affected area.

4. 急性乳腺炎：可根据炎症的程度选用不同的药物。治法：

4. Acute Mastitis: Different medications can be selected based on the severity of the inflammation. Treatment methods:

①红肿期：鲜紫花地丁、鲜蒲公英、鲜野菊花叶各 50 克，共捣烂，外敷患处。

① Redness and swelling stage: Take 50g each of fresh common violet herb, fresh dandelion, and fresh wild chrysanthemum leaves, mash them together, and apply externally to the affected area.

②成脓期：仙人掌去刺，切成块状，煨热外敷患处。

② Suppuration stage: Remove the thorns from a cactus, cut it into pieces, warm it, and apply it externally to the affected area.

③破溃期：薄荷 30 克，金银花、橘叶各 50 克，煎水去渣，用毛巾浸汁，外涂患处，一日三次。

③ Ulceration stage: Take 30g of mint, and 50g each of honeysuckle and tangerine leaves. Decoct in water, remove the dregs, soak a towel in the juice, apply externally to the affected area, three times a day.

5. 白带过多：正常的白带犹如白色半透明鸡蛋清，是一种无味，又无刺激性半透明物质。如气味、色泽、性质等方面出现异常变化应及时诊断治疗。如属单纯性白带过多治法：

5. Excessive Leukorrhea: Normal leukorrhea is like white semi-transparent egg whites, an odorless and non-irritating semi-transparent substance. If there are abnormal changes in odor, color, or nature, timely diagnosis and treatment should be sought. For simple excessive leukorrhea, treatment methods:

①艾叶 100 克，盐 10 克，共炒熟后，用布包好，热熨肚脐部和小腹部，每日两次。

① Take 100g of mugwort leaf and 10g of salt, stir-fry until cooked, wrap in a cloth, and apply as a hot compress to the navel and lower abdomen twice a day.

②土茯苓 50 克，苦瓜子 30 克，苦楝皮 20 克，白藓皮 30 克，地肤子 30 克，煎水熏洗外阴，一日两次。

② Take 50g of smilax glabra, 30g of bitter melon seeds, 20g of chinaberry bark, 30g of dictamnus bark, and 30g of kochia fruit. Decoct in water to fumigate and wash the vulva, twice a day.

《中药科技报》1992 年 3 月 6 日（江苏 顾荣霞）

TCM Science and Technology News, March 6, 1992 (Gu Rongxia, Jiangsu)

6. 治痛经：将生盐 400 克，放入铁锅炒爆后，即用陈醋（越旧越好）约小半碗洒入盐内，边洒边炒，务求均匀，洒完再略炒一下，趁热倒在一块干净布内包好，熨肚脐两旁及脐下小腹部。待冷后再热再熨。每次 1 小时，每日 1-3 次，直到病愈。此法专治因受寒而致的痛经。

6. Treating Dysmenorrhea: Put 400g of raw salt into an iron pan and stir-fry until it pops. Immediately sprinkle about half a small bowl of aged vinegar (the older, the better) into the salt, stir-frying as you sprinkle to ensure even distribution. After sprinkling, stir-fry briefly, pour it while hot onto a clean cloth, wrap it up, and apply it as a hot compress to both sides of the navel and the lower abdomen below the navel. When it cools, reheat and apply again. Do this for 1 hour each time, 1-3 times a day, until cured. This method specifically treats dysmenorrhea caused by cold exposure.

治带下：取艾叶、鲜葱各 500 克，捣烂后入锅内炒热装入布袋，平铺在下腹部，上用热水袋压盖住，热敷 1-2 小时，每天早晚各 1 次。此法主治子宫虚寒引起的白带增多。

Treating Leukorrhea: Take 500g each of mugwort leaf and fresh green onion, mash them, stir-fry in a pan until hot, put them in a cloth bag, lay it flat on the lower abdomen, cover and press with a hot water bottle, and apply a hot compress for 1-2 hours. Do this once in the morning and once in the evening daily. This method mainly treats excessive leukorrhea caused by uterine deficiency-cold.

治产后腹痛：取陈艾叶 600 克焙干，捣碎铺于脐上，以手绢覆盖，上面加热水袋进行热熨 1 小时左右，每日 2-3 次。此法主治因感寒邪所致的产后腹痛。

Treating Postpartum Abdominal Pain: Bake 600g of aged mugwort leaf until dry, crush it, spread it on the navel, cover with a handkerchief, add a hot water bottle on top to apply a hot compress for about 1 hour, 2-3 times a day. This method mainly treats postpartum abdominal pain caused by cold pathogenic factors.

治盆腔炎包块：将川椒、大茴香、乳香，没药，降香各 20 克共研细末，用干面粉加高粱酒少许调匀，摊铺于湿纱巾，置于下腹部痛处，上用热水袋热熨，每日 2 次。此法主治气滞血瘀所致盆腔炎包块。

Treating Pelvic Inflammatory Masses: Grind 20g each of Sichuan pepper, star anise, frankincense, myrrh, and 降 香 (dalbergia wood) into a fine powder. Mix evenly with dry flour and a little sorghum liquor, spread on a wet gauze towel, place it on the painful area of the lower abdomen, and apply a hot compress with a hot water bottle on top, twice a day. This method mainly treats pelvic inflammatory masses caused by qi stagnation and blood stasis.

治产后尿潴留: 将葱500克切成细末，与食盐500克放锅内微炒热，装入布袋，在患者脐部热熨，每次1小时，每日1-3次。

Treating Postpartum Urinary Retention: Chop 500g of green onion into fine pieces, put them in a pan with 500g of salt, and stir-fry until slightly hot. Put them in a cloth bag and apply as a hot compress to the patient’s navel for 1 hour each time, 1-3 times a day.

《民族医药报》1991年11月5日（陕西 高文）

Ethnic Medicine News, November 5, 1991 (Gao Wen, Shaanxi)

第十一章　儿科
Chapter 11　Pediatrics

一、小儿腹泻（17 方）
I. Pediatric Diarrhea (17 Prescriptions)

1. 儿童腹泻的家庭治疗

1.Home Treatment for Pediatric Diarrhea

先在患者的腹部放一层较厚的棉布，另将适量的食盐放在锅中炒热（温度以不致烫伤患者的皮肤为宜）。然后将炒热后的食盐放置在棉布上，再用适量的大蒜剥皮后打成蒜泥，放在热盐上。最后用布带裹腰一圈将盐和蒜一起固定在腹部疼痛部位。一天更换一次。一般一次见效，三次痊愈。此法最适于 1-12 岁的儿童，对青少年和成年人也有效。

First, place a relatively thick layer of cotton cloth on the patient' s abdomen. Separately, stir-fry an appropriate amount of salt in a pan until hot (the temperature should be warm enough not to burn the patient' s skin). Then, place the hot salt on the cotton cloth. Next, peel an appropriate amount of garlic, mash it into a paste, and place it on top of the hot salt. Finally, wrap a cloth band around the waist to secure both the salt and garlic over the painful area of the abdomen. Change the dressing once a day. Generally, it takes effect after one application and cures the condition after three applications. This method is most suitable for children aged 1 to 12, but it is also effective for adolescents and adults.

《民族医药报》1992 年 4 月 10 日（贵州 罗安君）

Ethnic Medicine News, April 10, 1992 (Luo Anjun, Guizhou)

2. 笔者运用民间验方“银葛散”治疗小儿腹泻四十例，收到较满意的疗效，现简介如下：

2. The author used the folk proven prescription “Yinge San” (Yinge Powder) to treat 40 cases of pediatric diarrhea, achieving relatively satisfactory therapeutic effects. A brief introduction is as follows:

①一般资料：本组病例均为五岁以下小儿，其中男二十四例，女十六例，临床表现为一天腹泻四次至数十次不等，部分患儿伴见发热、呕吐等症状，病程均在一天以上。

① General Data: All cases in this group were children under five years old, including 24 males and 16 females. The clinical manifestations included diarrhea ranging from 4 to dozens of times a day. Some children were accompanied by symptoms such as fever and vomiting. The disease duration in all cases was more than one day.

②方药及用法：金银花四份，茵陈三份，葛根三份，先将金银花用瓦锅炒至焦黄，再加入茵陈略炒即可，葛根用火煨至微黑，上药共研细末，充分混合后备用，一岁以下每次服二克，二至三岁每次服三克，四至五岁每次服四克，每日服三次，温开水送服。三天为一疗程。脱水明显者，可口服含糖、盐、苏打液纠正水、电解质平衡。

② Prescription and Usage: 4 parts of honeysuckle, 3 parts of capillary wormwood, and 3 parts of pueraria root. First, stir-fry the honeysuckle in a clay pot until scorched yellow, then add the capillary wormwood and stir-fry briefly. Roast the pueraria root over a fire until slightly black. Grind all the above herbs into a fine powder and mix them thoroughly for later use. For infants under one year old, take 2g per dose; for children aged 2 to 3, take 3g per dose; for children aged 4 to 5, take 4g per dose. Take it three times a day with warm boiled water. Three days constitute one course of treatment. For patients with obvious dehydration, oral solutions containing sugar, salt, and baking soda can be used to correct water and electrolyte balance.

治疗结果：经一疗程治疗后，痊愈三十一例（大便次数减少，每日一至二次，精神食欲明显改善，大便常规检查正常），好转六例（大便次数减少，精神食欲改善，大便常规检查未正常），无效三例（症状、体征、大便常规检查均无改善），总有效率为百分之九十二点五。

Therapeutic Results: After one course of treatment, 31 cases were completely cured (the frequency of bowel movements decreased to 1-2 times a day, mental state and appetite significantly improved, and routine stool tests were normal); 6 cases showed improvement (the frequency of bowel movements decreased, mental state and appetite improved, but routine stool tests were not yet normal); and 3 cases were ineffective (no improvement in symptoms, signs, or routine stool tests). The total effective rate was 92.5%.

《中药科技报》1992 年 3 月 6 日

TCM Science and Technology News, March 6, 1992

3. 小儿秋季腹泻验方

3. Proven Prescription for Pediatric Autumn Diarrhea

小儿秋季腹泻，现代医学称病毒性肠炎。由轮状病毒感染所致，多发于秋季，其特点是发病急，流行广，大便次数多，泻下急迫，呈水样便，内有蛋花样物及少量黏液，或伴有呕吐；或伴口渴尿少等失水症。多发于6个月至2岁的小儿。小儿生机旺盛，阴液易乏，本病泻下急迫，最易伤阴。急则治其标，宜养阴防衰；再者小儿脏器清灵，病邪易除，故可止泻解毒并用。以“诃子黄连汤”治之，可起涩肠止泻，清热燥湿之功，疗效颇佳。

Pediatric autumn diarrhea is known as viral enteritis in modern medicine. It is caused by rotavirus infection and mostly occurs in autumn. Its characteristics include acute onset, wide spread, frequent bowel movements, and urgent watery diarrhea containing egg-drop-like substances and a small amount of mucus, sometimes accompanied by vomiting, or dehydration symptoms such as thirst and oliguria. It mostly occurs in infants and young children aged 6 months to 2 years. Children have vigorous vitality but are prone to yin fluid deficiency. The urgent diarrhea in this disease easily damages yin. When treating acute symptoms, one should address the symptoms first by nourishing yin to prevent exhaustion. Furthermore, children’s internal organs are delicate and clear, making pathogenic factors easy to eliminate; thus, stopping diarrhea and detoxifying can be used concurrently. Treating it with "Kezi Huanglian Decoction" can achieve the effects of astringing the intestines to stop diarrhea, clearing heat, and drying dampness, with quite good therapeutic effects.

处方：诃子6克，黄连3克，米壳3克，葛根3克，黄柏6克，白头翁6克，木香3克、白术6克，白芍9克，甘草3克。

Prescription: 6g of chebula, 3g of coptis, 3g of poppy husk, 3g of pueraria root, 6g of phellodendron bark, 6g of pulsatilla root, 3g of costus root, 6g of atractylodes macrocephala, 9g of white peony root, and 3g of licorice.

用法：上药加水500毫升，煎至50-70毫升；煎取2次，得滤液合共100-140毫升，少量多次分饮，一日内服完。加减：有表症者加荆芥、防风；呕吐者加竹茹；腹胀甚者加山楂。

Usage: Add 500 ml of water to the above herbs and decoct to 50-70 ml; decoct twice to obtain a total of 100-140 ml of filtrate. Drink in small amounts frequently, and finish it within one day. Modifications: For cases with exterior syndrome, add schizonepeta and saposhnikovia; for vomiting, add bamboo shavings; for severe abdominal distension, add hawthorn.

《民族医药报》1991年11月5日（钟祖仁）

Ethnic Medicine News, November 5, 1991 (Zhu Zuren)

4. 治婴、幼儿顽固性腹泻验方

4. Proven Prescription for Treating Intractable Diarrhea in Infants and Young Children

本病系指排便次数多于平时，粪便稀薄，含水量增加，有时脂肪增多，带有不消化物，或含有脓血，经各种治疗六天以上仍不愈者。

This disease refers to cases where the frequency of bowel movements is higher than usual, stools are loose with increased water content, sometimes with increased fat, undigested matter, or pus and blood, and remain uncured after more than six days of various treatments.

焦白术10-15克，车前子15-25克，米壳3克。以上三味加水100-250毫升，用文火煎水开 15 分钟，将药液倒入奶瓶加少许白糖搅匀，徐饮服，一日四次，脱水重者配合输液。一般用药一天见效，三天即可痊愈。

Take 10-15g of scorched atractylodes macrocephala, 15-25g of plantain seeds, and 3g of poppy husk. Add 100-250 ml of water to the above three ingredients and decoct over low heat for 15 minutes after boiling. Pour the liquid into a baby bottle, add a little white sugar, stir well, and let the child drink it slowly. Take it four times a day. For severe dehydration, combine with intravenous infusion. Generally, it takes effect after one day of medication and can be cured within three days.

（沂南县中医院 孙勇）

(Yinan County Hospital of Traditional Chinese Medicine, Sun Yong)

5. 药物组成：粳米 40 克，茶叶、鸡内金各 15 克。

5. Prescription Composition: 40g of japonica rice, and 15g each of tea leaves and chicken gizzard lining.

适应证：伤食泄泻，脾虚腹泻，外感寒湿水泄，小儿脾虚挟食滞久泻不止等证。

Indications: Diarrhea caused by indigestion, diarrhea due to spleen deficiency, watery diarrhea caused by external cold-dampness, and prolonged diarrhea in children due to spleen deficiency complicated by food retention.

制法：先将粳米、鸡内金放入锅中炒至外表焦黑，内面焦黄为度，再放入茶叶然后加水煎煮 30 分钟，取汁 200-300 毫升，小儿可酌加少量食糖调味。

Preparation: First, put the japonica rice and chicken gizzard lining in a pan and stir-fry until the outside is scorched black and the inside is scorched yellow. Then add the tea leaves, add water, and decoct for 30 minutes. Obtain 200-300 ml of juice. An appropriate amount of sugar can be added to flavor it for children.

用法：每日 1-2 剂，分次当茶饮，效果好。

Usage: Take 1-2 doses daily, drink as tea in divided doses, with good effects.

《民族医药报》1991 年 7 月 5 日（湖南 彭继东）

Ethnic Medicine News, July 5, 1991 (Peng Jidong, Hunan)

6. 婴幼儿腹泻是临床上的一种常见病，表现为大便次数明显增多，每日 5-10

次不等，大便多为蛋花汤样稀便，有时会有不消化食物，严重者可伴有水、电解质紊乱。我院采用民间验方银杏叶浴足治疗婴幼儿腹泻，经临床验证，效果良好，不妨一试。

6. Infantile diarrhea is a common clinical disease, characterized by a significant increase in the frequency of bowel movements, ranging from 5 to 10 times a day. The stools are mostly egg-drop soup-like loose stools, sometimes with undigested food. Severe cases may be accompanied by water and electrolyte disturbances. Our hospital adopted the folk proven prescription of ginkgo leaf foot bath to treat infantile diarrhea. Clinical verification has shown good effects, and it is worth a try.

治疗方法：取银杏叶干品 100 克（或鲜品 150 克），加水 2000 毫升，水煎 20-30 分钟，（鲜品水煎时间稍短），待水温降至不烫手时，浸泡搓洗患儿双足 20 分钟，1 日 2 次，次日即可见效。

Treatment Method: Take 100g of dried ginkgo leaves (or 150g of fresh ones), add 2000 ml of water, and decoct for 20-30 minutes (fresh leaves require a slightly shorter decoction time). When the water temperature drops to a level that does not scald the hands, soak and rub-wash the child’s feet for 20 minutes, twice a day. It will take effect the next day.

《中药科技报》1992 年 12 月 16 日（南京 孙杨）

TCM Science and Technology News, December 16, 1992 (Sun Yang, Nanjing)

7. 取鲜藕一斤，生姜一两。洗净剁碎后，用干净纱布包起来，绞取汁液，一日内分数次服完，对腹泻、发热、烦躁、口渴有较好疗效。

7. Take 500g of fresh lotus root and 50g of fresh ginger. Wash them, chop them into pieces, wrap them in clean gauze, and squeeze out the juice. Drink it in several portions within one day. It has good therapeutic effects on diarrhea, fever, restlessness, and thirst.

8. 大蒜头一个，用火煨热后，剥去外皮内服；或用大蒜头数个，捣烂成泥状，外敷于足心或肚脐处。

8. Take one clove of garlic, roast it over a fire until hot, peel off the skin, and

take it orally; or take several cloves of garlic, mash them into a paste, and apply them externally to the soles of the feet or the navel.

9. 取茄子叶 10 片洗净后切碎，煎水内服，早晚各服一次。

9. Take 10 eggplant leaves, wash them, chop them, decoct in water and take orally, once in the morning and once in the evening.

10. 将黄豆壳用火焙干后研成细末，每次用开水送服 6-9 克，一日二次。

10. Bake soybean shells over a fire until dry, grind them into a fine powder, and take 6-9g each time with boiling water, twice a day.

《民族医药报》（陕西 高绪林）

Ethnic Medicine News (Gao Xulin, Shaanxi)

11. 大蒜捣烂贴脚心或贴肚脐中。

11. Mash garlic into a paste and apply it to the soles of the feet or the navel.

12. 车前子（盐水炒）、炒山药、茯苓各 60 克，炙甘草 6 克，共为细末，每服 6-9 克，日服三次，炒糊米煎水调服。

12. Take 60g each of plantain seeds (stir-fried with salt water), stir-fried yam, and poria, and 6g of honey-fried licorice. Grind them into a fine powder. Take 6-9g each time, three times a day, mixed with water decocted from scorched rice.

13. 芡实、山药各 60 克，入猪肚内蒸熟分数次服。

13. Take 60g each of euryale seeds and yam, put them inside a pig’s stomach, steam until cooked, and take in several portions.

14. 白术、莲肉、车前子各 15 克，水煎服，每日一付，分早晚两次服。

14. Take 15g each of atractylodes macrocephala, lotus seeds, and plantain seeds. Decoct in water and take orally, one dose daily, divided into two servings in the morning and evening.

15. 烧天枢二穴（脐边左右各三寸），气海穴（脐下寸半）用艾绒如黄豆大膈姜片烧三炷。

15. Moxibustion: Apply moxibustion to the bilateral Tianshu acupoints (3 cun on both sides of the navel) and the Qihai acupoint (1.5 cun below the navel). Use mugwort floss the size of a soybean, place a slice of ginger as a partition, and

burn three cones.

16. 柿饼烧红（放木炭火上）放辅平的灶心土上用碗盖住（不盖则成灰无存性）。待冷后研末米汤调服。此方治小儿久泄完谷不化效果更佳，成人每次两个。日服三次小儿酌减。

16. Roast a dried persimmon until red hot (over a charcoal fire), place it on leveled hearth soil, and cover it with a bowl (if not covered, it will turn to ash and lose its medicinal properties). After it cools, grind it into powder and mix with rice soup to take. This prescription has better effects on treating prolonged diarrhea with undigested food in children. For adults, take two each time, three times a day. Reduce the dosage appropriately for children.

《中药科技报》1992 年 4 月 17 日（济宁 乔健）

TCM Science and Technology News, April 17, 1992 (Qiao Jian, Jining)

17. 上海中医学院附属岳阳医院著名老中医朱锡祺治疗“小儿脂性腹泻”疗效较好。其具体方法如下：山楂炭 15 克、青皮 4 克、陈皮 4 克共研细末，加水及红糖调匀，隔水蒸熟。每次让患儿服 1-2 小匙，日服 3 次。一般一周即愈。

17. The famous senior TCM physician Zhu Xiqi from Yueyang Hospital affiliated to Shanghai College of Traditional Chinese Medicine achieved good therapeutic effects in treating “pediatric fatty diarrhea”. The specific method is as follows: Grind 15g of hawthorn charcoal, 4g of green tangerine peel, and 4g of aged tangerine peel into a fine powder. Add water and brown sugar, mix well, and steam over a water bath. Let the child take 1-2 teaspoons each time, 3 times a day. It generally cures within one week.

《民族医药报》（陈烈辉）

Ethnic Medicine News (Chen Liehui)

二、小儿厌食、疳积（19 方）

II. Pediatric Anorexia and Infantile Malnutrition (19 Prescriptions)

1. 小儿厌食症是指小儿（以 1-6 岁为多见）较长时期见食不贪，食欲不振，甚则拒食的一种常见病证。近年来临床研究证明，部分中药对治疗小儿厌食症有良好疗效，现采菁验方三则介绍如下。

Pediatric anorexia refers to a common condition in children (mostly aged 1-6) characterized by a long-term lack of appetite for food, poor appetite, or even refusal to eat. Recent clinical studies have proven that some traditional Chinese medicines have good therapeutic effects on pediatric anorexia. Three selected proven prescriptions are introduced as follows:

温胆汤加味：陈皮、竹茹各10克，茯苓、半夏各12克，枳实、鸡内金各6克，鱼鳅串、焦三仙、隔山消各15克，甘草3克。口苦、大便黏滞不爽加黄连3克，吐奶加苏叶6克，腹胀加莱菔子12克。水煎服，3-5剂为一疗程。

Modified Wendan Decoction: 10g each of tangerine peel and bamboo shavings, 12g each of poria and pinellia, 6g each of immature bitter orange and chicken gizzard lining, 15g each of yuqiechuan, scorched sanxian, and geshanxiao, and 3g of licorice. For bitter taste in the mouth and sticky, unsmooth bowel movements, add 3g of coptis; for milk regurgitation, add 6g of perilla leaf; for abdominal distension, add 12g of radish seeds. Decoct in water and take orally. 3-5 doses constitute one course of treatment.

解肝煎：白芍12克，苏叶、清半夏、茯苓、陈皮、川朴各6克，砂仁、甘草各3克。腹胀加山楂、谷麦芽；大便滞涩加槟榔、木香；夹虫积加使君子；烦渴寝汗去川朴、砂仁，加乌梅、银柴胡。水煎服，每日1剂。药中病机后，可守方易为散剂调理巩固。

Jiegan Decoction: 12g of white peony root, 6g each of perilla leaf, processed pinellia, poria, tangerine peel, and magnolia bark, and 3g each of cardamom and licorice. For abdominal distension, add hawthorn, malt, and barley malt; for unsmooth bowel movements, add betel nut and costus root; for parasitic accumulation, add quisqualis fruit; for restlessness, thirst, and night sweats, remove magnolia bark and cardamom, and add mume fruit and silver bupleurum. Decoct in water and take orally, 1 dose daily. Once the medication matches the pathogenesis, the prescription can be maintained but changed into a powder form for conditioning and consolidation.

小儿厌食方：太子参、山药、炒扁豆、鸡内金各 5-10 克，生麦芽 8-12 克，莱菔子、陈皮各 3-6 克。血虚者加龙眼肉 5-10 克；有瘀血者加生楂片 8-12 克，丹参 5-10 克；内有蕴热者加连翘 5-10 克；伤暑者加佩兰、藿香 5-10 克；有疳积者加胡黄连、蚕沙各 3-5 克。水煎服，每 2 日剂，每日三四次不等。

Pediatric Anorexia Prescription: 5-10g each of pseudostellaria root, yam, stir-fried hyacinth bean, and chicken gizzard lining, 8-12g of raw malt, and 3-6g each of radish seeds and tangerine peel. For blood deficiency, add 5-10g of longan flesh; for blood stasis, add 8-12g of raw hawthorn slices and 5-10g of salvia root; for internal latent heat, add 5-10g of forsythia; for summer-heat injury, add 5-10g each of eupatorium and agastache; for infantile malnutrition, add 3-5g each of pseudo-coptis and silkworm excrement. Decoct in water and take orally. One dose is taken over 2 days, divided into 3-4 doses daily.

以上三方，药物剂量可随年龄酌情增减。

For the above three prescriptions, the dosage of herbs can be adjusted according to the child’s age.

《中医药信息报》（张仲林 林忠）

TCM Information News (Zhang Zhonglin, Lin Zhong)

2. 生蛤蚧一对焙干（最好是一公一母），炒鸡内金 30 克，共研成粉末，每日用药粉 3 克和塘角鱼蒸服。

2. Bake a pair of fresh geckos (preferably one male and one female) until dry, and 30g of stir-fried chicken gizzard lining. Grind them together into a powder. Take 3g of the powder daily and steam it with a local catfish for consumption.

3. 五谷虫 15 克，炒麦芽、炒内金、炒神曲、槟榔各 10 克，炒山楂 15 克，太子参 12 克，共研末成粉，每天用药 3 克蒸猪肝服用。

3. Take 15g of pentastomum, 10g each of stir-fried malt, stir-fried chicken gizzard lining, stir-fried medicated leaven, and betel nut, 15g of stir-fried hawthorn, and 12g of pseudostellaria root. Grind them together into a powder. Take 3g of the powder daily and steam it with pig liver for consumption.

4. 莪术 8 克，鸡内金、土炒白术、陈皮各 15 克，黑芝麻 20 克，研末成粉，早晚各服一次，每次 1-1.5 克，用米汤送服。

4. Take 8g of zedoary, 15g each of chicken gizzard lining, earth-stir-fried atractylodes macrocephala, and tangerine peel, and 20g of black sesame. Grind them into a powder. Take 1-1.5g each time in the morning and evening, taken with rice soup.

5. 生黄芪、党参、茯苓、白术各 9 克，甘草 6 克，鸡内金 10 克，陈皮 5 克，以上药味煎水服用，每天每剂可分 2-3 次服用。

5. Take 9g each of raw astragalus, codonopsis, poria, and atractylodes macrocephala, 6g of licorice, 10g of chicken gizzard lining, and 5g of tangerine peel. Decoct the above herbs in water and take orally. Each daily dose can be divided into 2-3 servings.

注意事项：在服药治疗期间，禁吃零食和糖类。忌酸、辣和动物油（可吃花生油）。在每日进餐时应少吃多餐，最好是能吃半流汁的食物为宜。

Precautions: During the medication treatment, avoid eating snacks and sugary foods. Avoid sour, spicy foods, and animal fats (peanut oil can be consumed). For daily meals, eat small and frequent meals, preferably semi-liquid foods.

《民族医药报》1992 年 3 月 13 日（广西 谭荣登）

Ethnic Medicine News, March 13, 1992 (Tan Rongdeng, Guangxi)

6. 笔者多年来在临床治疗小儿疳积病方治疗共有门诊登记的小儿疳积病。在 52 例患儿中有 46 例不超过两周痊愈，好转 4 例，无效 2 例。现将该方献出供病者及同行参考，在临床运用时，若酌情加减功效亦佳。

6. Over the years, the author has treated pediatric infantile malnutrition in clinical outpatient settings. Among 52 pediatric patients, 46 were cured within no more than two weeks, 4 showed improvement, and 2 were ineffective. This prescription is now shared for the reference of patients and peers. When applied clinically, appropriate modifications can also yield good effects.

本方由雷丸 6 克（后下）石榴皮 9 克，芦荟 3 克，焦山楂 12 克，神曲 10 克，炙内金 3 克，炒苍术 7.5 克七味药组成，水煎分两次服。

This prescription consists of seven herbs: 6g of omphalia (added later), 9g of pomegranate peel, 3g of aloe, 12g of scorched hawthorn, 10g of medicated leaven, 3g of honey-fried chicken gizzard lining, and 7.5g of stir-fried atractylodes. Decoct in water and take in two divided doses.

加减：口渴甚者加花粉 9 克、乌梅 5 克以止渴生津，增强其驱虫之功；脾土虚弱者加太子参 6 克、炒白术 6 克。

Modifications: For severe thirst, add 9g of trichosanthes root and 5g of mume fruit to quench thirst, generate fluids, and enhance the anthelmintic effect; for weak spleen earth, add 6g of pseudostellaria root and 6g of stir-fried atractylodes macrocephala.

（汪荣喜）

(Wang Rongxi)

7.治小儿疳积方: 采一枝黄花(别名蛇头王)鲜草 30 克，洗净晒干，大米 25 克，置锅内用文火炒黄，新鲜猪肝 50 克，洗净切片。将一枝黄花、炒大米与猪肝共置瓷碗内，加清水适量，上笼蒸 30 分钟，取出吃猪肝饮药汁。每天一剂，连服 3-5 剂即可见效，患儿食欲明显改善。

7. Prescription for Treating Pediatric Infantile Malnutrition: Pick 30g of fresh goldenrod (also known as shetouwang), wash and sun-dry it. Take 25g of rice and stir-fry it in a pan over low heat until yellow. Take 50g of fresh pig liver, wash and slice it. Place the goldenrod, stir-fried rice, and pig liver together in a porcelain bowl, add an appropriate amount of water, and steam in a steamer for 30 minutes. Remove and eat the pig liver while drinking the medicinal juice. Take one dose daily. It will take effect after 3-5 consecutive doses, and the child' s appetite will significantly improve.

8. 小儿疳积（即小儿营养不良）主要表现为：食欲差、烦躁、喜哭闹、消瘦、腹胀等。好发于断奶后的小婴儿及炎热的夏季。笔者在儿科临床工作中每遇此症，嘱其按下述方法之一治疗，均获满意疗效。如小儿腹胀明显（尤其是农村小儿），经检查为蛔虫病则须先行驱蛔虫治疗，然后再按小儿疳积治疗。

8. Pediatric infantile malnutrition (i.e., pediatric malnutrition) is mainly

characterized by poor appetite, restlessness, frequent crying, emaciation, and abdominal distension. It is common in infants after weaning and during hot summers. In my pediatric clinical practice, whenever I encounter this condition, I advise treating it with one of the following methods, all of which have achieved satisfactory results. If a child has obvious abdominal distension (especially rural children) and is diagnosed with ascariasis through examination, anthelmintic treatment must be administered first, followed by treatment for infantile malnutrition.

方药：独脚疳（独脚金），全草 10 克（干）、（鲜草 20 克），瘦猪肉 50 克。用法：将瘦猪肉剁碎成肉饼状，装入一小碗内，再把独脚疳切 2-3 节放入肉上面，加水适量，隔水蒸 30-40 分钟，然后将药渣去掉，加少许食盐，以能食为度，吃猪肉及汤。每晚睡前服一次，连服 5-7 次，隔 3-5 天，再服 5-7 次即可。

Prescription: Dujiaogan (Monochasma savatieri), 10g of the whole dried herb (or 20g of fresh herb), and 50g of lean pork. Usage: Mince the lean pork into a patty shape, place it in a small bowl, cut the Monochasma savatieri into 2-3 sections and place it on top of the meat. Add an appropriate amount of water and steam over a water bath for 30-40 minutes. Remove the herbal dregs, add a little salt to taste, and eat the pork and drink the soup. Take it once every night before bed, continuously for 5-7 times. After an interval of 3-5 days, take it again for 5-7 times.

方药：饿蚂蟥 15 克，猪肝 50 克（切成片状）或鸡肝一个（可不用切）。

Prescription: 15g of emahuan (a local herb), and 50g of pig liver (sliced) or one chicken liver (can be left uncut).

《民族医药报》1992 年 7 月 3 日（广西 梁晓）

Ethnic Medicine News, July 3, 1992 (Liang Xiao, Guangxi)

疳积是儿科四大证之一，中药外治多以敷药为主，疗效肯定，患儿易于接受。其中以脐疗效果最优，因脐在胚胎发育过程中为腹壁最后闭合处，该处无皮下脂肪，表面角质层最薄，屏障功能较弱，药物易吸收。兹将疳积外治验方数则，介绍于后。

Infantile malnutrition is one of the four major pediatric syndromes. External treatment with traditional Chinese medicine mainly involves applying herbal pastes, which has definite therapeutic effects and is easily accepted by children. Among them, umbilical therapy has the best effect because the umbilicus is the last part of the abdominal wall to close during embryonic development. This area has no subcutaneous fat, the thinnest stratum corneum on the surface, and a weaker barrier function, making it easy for drugs to be absorbed. Several proven external prescriptions for infantile malnutrition are introduced below.

9. 桃仁、杏仁、生山栀、冰片各等分，研极细末，用鸡蛋清适量调成糊状，敷于双侧内关穴，纱布包扎，24小时后去之，疳证初、中期，多1次见效。不愈者，间隔 2-3 天再治。

9. Take equal amounts of peach seed, apricot seed, raw gardenia, and borneol. Grind them into an extremely fine powder, mix with an appropriate amount of egg white to form a paste, and apply to the bilateral Neiguan acupoints. Bandage with gauze and remove after 24 hours. For infantile malnutrition in the early and middle stages, it often takes effect after one application. For cases that are not cured, repeat the treatment after an interval of 2-3 days.

10. 白矾、陈醋各适量调成糊状，敷于涌泉穴，每日换 1 次，连用 3-5 次为一疗程。适用于虚寒型的疳积。

10. Mix an appropriate amount of alum and aged vinegar into a paste, apply to the Yongquan acupoint, change once daily, and use continuously for 3-5 times as one course of treatment. Suitable for infantile malnutrition of the deficiency-cold type.

11. 五倍子焙黄研极细末，用醋捣为膏，摊布外贴囟门。

11. Roast Chinese gallnuts until yellow and grind into an extremely fine powder. Mash with vinegar to form a paste, spread on a cloth, and apply externally to the fontanelle.

12. 蓖麻子仁 1 至 2 粒，杏仁 1 粒，朱砂少许，共研为细末，外贴印堂穴，1 至 3 日去掉，留有粟米大的小水泡。

12. Take 1-2 castor seeds, 1 apricot seed, and a small amount of cinnabar.

Grind them together into a fine powder, apply externally to the Yintang acupoint, remove after 1-3 days. It will leave small blisters the size of millet grains.

13. 鲜野麻草 15 克，生姜、小葱各 30 克，上药捣烂，用鸡蛋清适量，搅匀外敷脚心一夜，隔 3 日一次，连用 5 至 7 次。

13. Take 15g of fresh wild nettle grass, and 30g each of fresh ginger and small green onions. Mash the above herbs into a paste, mix evenly with an appropriate amount of egg white, apply externally to the soles of the feet overnight. Repeat once every 3 days, continuously for 5-7 times.

14. 皮硝 30-60 克，放于布袋内，敷于脐上，每日一换，连用 2-3 次。

14. Take 30-60g of mirabilite, place it in a cloth bag, apply it to the navel, change once daily, and use continuously for 2-3 times.

15. 桃仁、杏仁、小枣各 7 个，栀子 30 克，朴硝、川军各 9 克，鸡蛋 3 个，蜜 30 克。将前 6 味药共研细末，用鸡蛋清、蜜调匀，摊于布上，贴脐中，七日一换，连贴 3 次。

15. Take 7 each of peach seeds, apricot seeds, and small dates, 30g of gardenia, 9g each of mirabilite and rhubarb, 3 eggs, and 30g of honey. Grind the first six herbs into a fine powder, mix evenly with egg whites and honey, spread on a cloth, and apply to the navel. Change once every seven days, and apply continuously for 3 times.

16. 玄胡粉 3 克，胡椒粉 0.5 克，蛋清适量调为糊状，敷于脐中，每日一换。

16. Take 3g of corydalis powder and 0.5g of pepper powder. Mix with an appropriate amount of egg white to form a paste, apply to the navel, and change once daily.

17. 将艾叶适量捣烂、加酒、胡椒调成糊状，敷于脐部，用于虚寒型疳积。

17. Mash an appropriate amount of mugwort leaves, add liquor and pepper to form a paste, and apply to the navel. Used for infantile malnutrition of the deficiency-cold type.

18. 山栀子、山楂、大枣（去核）各 7 粒，葱头 9 个，芒硝 30 克，共研细末，用醋调成糊状，敷贴神阙，两足涌泉穴。一日换药 2 次，连敷 3 天见效。

18. Take 7 each of gardenia, hawthorn, and dates (pitted), 9 scallion bulbs, and 30g of mirabilite. Grind them into a fine powder, mix with vinegar to form a paste, and apply to the Shenque (navel) and bilateral Yongquan acupoints on the soles of the feet. Change the medication twice a day. It will take effect after continuous application for 3 days.

《中药科技报》1992 年 5 月 6 日（周丹）

TCM Science and Technology News, May 6, 1992 (Zhou Dan)

19. 治小儿厌食症方

19. Prescription for Treating Pediatric Anorexia

小儿厌食症是指小儿较长时期食欲不振甚至拒食的一种常见病症，多发于 1-6 岁小儿，尤以城镇儿童为多见。如不及时治疗，常可导致小儿营养不良，影响小儿正常生长发育。许多家长遇到小儿患厌食症时往往不知所措，甚为烦恼。现介绍 1 则治小儿厌食症有效验方。取土炒白术、鸡内金、陈皮各等份，共研为细末与芝麻炒后捣末）、红糖各酌量混匀。4 岁以下小儿每次服 1-3 克，5 岁以上小儿每次服 3-6 克，每日服 2-3 次。一般在用药 3-5 周后显效。本方能健脾和胃、消食化积。此外，在进行药物治疗的同时，平素家长应注意培养小儿正确的饮食习惯。

Pediatric anorexia refers to a common condition where children have a long-term lack of appetite or even refuse to eat. It mostly occurs in children aged 1-6, especially in urban children. If not treated promptly, it often leads to pediatric malnutrition and affects normal growth and development. Many parents are often at a loss and very troubled when their children suffer from anorexia. An effective proven prescription for treating pediatric anorexia is now introduced. Take equal amounts of earth-stir-fried atractylodes macrocephala, chicken gizzard lining, and tangerine peel. Grind them into a fine powder, mix with an appropriate amount of roasted and crushed sesame seeds and brown sugar. For children under 4 years old, take 1-3g each time; for children over 5 years old, take 3-6g each time, 2-3 times daily. It generally shows significant effects after 3-5 weeks of medication. This prescription can invigorate the spleen and harmonize the stomach, promote digestion, and resolve food accumulation. In addition, while undergoing drug treatment, parents should usually pay attention to cultivating correct eating habits in children.

（河南 吴建华）

(Wu Jianhua, Henan)

三、小儿便秘（9 方）

III. Pediatric Constipation (9 Prescriptions)

婴幼儿便秘，这对于年轻的父母来说是常遇到的事。由于大便秘结，腹部胀痛不适，常致使幼儿食欲减退，睡眠不安、啼哭不止，从而影响其正常的生长发育和生活，也给年轻的父母增添了不少烦恼。为此，下面介绍几种简便易行的家庭治疗方法，孩子的父母们不妨一试。

Infantile constipation is a common issue for young parents. Due to hard and impacted stools accompanied by abdominal distension and pain, young children often experience a loss of appetite, restless sleep, and incessant crying. This affects their normal growth, development, and daily life, while also causing considerable distress to their parents. Therefore, the following simple and easy-to-implement home treatment methods are introduced, which parents may wish to try.

1. 用蜂蜜适量兑温开水冲服，每次不得少于 60-90 毫升，每日饮 2-4 次。

1. Mix an appropriate amount of honey with warm boiled water and drink. The volume for each dose should be no less than 60-90 ml. Drink 2-4 times a day.

2. 取莱菔子（萝卜子）适量炒黄研末瓶装备用。每晚睡前取 5-20 克（视年龄大小而定）拌蜂蜜或白糖，用温开水送服。

2. Take an appropriate amount of radish seeds (laifuzi), stir-fry until yellow, grind into a powder, and store in a bottle for later use. Every night before going to bed, take 5-20g (depending on the child’s age), mix with honey or white sugar, and swallow with warm boiled water.

3. 取蜂蜜适量，微火煎熬放温后，手捻作锭，纳入肛门之中，每日一次。

3. Take an appropriate amount of honey, simmer over low heat until warm, shape it into a suppository-like stick by hand, insert it into the anus, and do this once a day.

4. 取大枣适量，蒸煮之后剥皮，研为枣泥，然后再取芝麻适量，炒后研为末，拌入枣泥之中，每次食 2 匙，每日 3-4 次。

4. Take an appropriate amount of red dates, steam or boil them, peel off the skin, and mash them into a date paste. Then, take an appropriate amount of sesame seeds, stir-fry them, grind them into a powder, and mix them into the date paste. Take 2 spoonfuls each time, 3-4 times a day.

5. 将桃仁和黑芝麻按 2:1 的比例取适量，用文火炒熟，然后研细末调匀，每日清晨取一汤匙用温开水送服。

5. Take an appropriate amount of peach seeds and black sesame seeds in a 2:1 ratio, stir-fry them over low heat until cooked, then grind them into a fine powder and mix well. Take one tablespoon with warm boiled water every morning.

6. 患儿仰卧，家长右手四指并拢放于小儿脐部，以顺时针方向作环形按摩，用力均匀，不轻不重按摩三百次左右，每日早晚各一次。

6. Have the child lie on their back. The parent should place four fingers of their right hand together on the child’s navel and perform circular massage in a clockwise direction. Apply even pressure—not too light and not too heavy—for about 300 times. Do this once in the morning and once in the evening every day.

《中医科技报》1992 年 8 月 26 日（四川 郭晓明）

TCM Science and Technology News, August 26, 1992 (Guo Xiaoming, Sichuan)

7. 胖大海为梧桐科落叶乔木胖大海树的叶子，味甘淡性凉，归肺与大肠经。具有宣上导下，润燥解结，通便泄热之功，对于婴幼儿肺热肠燥而致的大便不通，用之效果甚佳。笔者曾用胖大海泡茶治疗婴幼儿大便不通 43 例，均收显效。用法：取胖大海 3 枚，放在茶杯或碗里，沸水约 150 毫升冲泡 15 分钟，待其发大后，少量分次频频饮服，一般饮服一天即可大便畅通。如治刘 xx，男，3 岁半，1991 年 5 月 13 日初诊。其母代诉：大便不通 4 日，食少腹胀，用开塞露则便通，药停如故。遂用上法治疗，次日来告，大便畅通。随访一旬，大便每日一行。

7. Sterculia seed (pangdahai) is the seed of the deciduous tree Sterculia lychnophora of the Sterculiaceae family. It is sweet and bland in taste, cool in nature, and enters the Lung and Large Intestine meridians. It has the effects of diffusing the upper and guiding the lower, moistening dryness and resolving nodules, relieving constipation, and clearing heat. It has excellent effects on treating constipation in infants and young children caused by lung heat and intestinal dryness. The author once used sterculia seed tea to treat 43 cases of infantile constipation, all of which achieved significant therapeutic effects. Usage: Take 3 sterculia seeds, place them in a teacup or bowl, and brew with about 150 ml of boiling water for 15 minutes. After they expand, drink in small amounts frequently. Generally, the bowels will be unblocked after one day of drinking. For example, in the treatment of a male patient surnamed Liu, aged 3.5 years, who had his first visit on May 13, 1991. His mother reported: The child had been constipated for 4 days, with poor appetite and abdominal distension. Using glycerin enema (Kaisailu) relieved the constipation, but the condition returned once the medication was stopped. The above method was then used for treatment. The next day, the mother reported that the child’s bowels were unblocked. After a ten-day follow-up, the child had one bowel movement daily.

《中药科技报》（江苏 秦亮）

TCM Science and Technology News (Qin Liang, Jiangsu)

13 岁以下的儿童常因饮食等原因而导致便秘。如遇此情况家长不必过于紧张，可用下述方法通便，常可收到理想效果。

Children under the age of 13 often suffer from constipation due to diet and other reasons. In such cases, parents do not need to be overly anxious. The following methods can be used to relieve constipation, and they often achieve ideal results.

8. 将肥皂的一头用刀削成 2.5-3.5 厘米长，直径 1.5 厘米，顶端尖的小圆锥体，用温水搓出泡沫后，插入肛门并轻轻旋转一会，一般抽出后不久大便即通。

8.Shave one end of a bar of soap with a knife into a small cone measuring 2.5

to 3.5 cm in length and 1.5 cm in diameter, with a pointed tip. Rub it with warm water to create a lather, then insert it into the anus and gently rotate it for a while. Generally, the bowels will be unblocked shortly after it is removed.

9. 将晒软或腌咸的胡萝卜削成上述形状的小圆锥体。涂上菜籽油或花生油或肥皂沫，插入肛门，轻轻转动，不久即可通便。

9.Peel a sun-dried softened or salt-pickled carrot into a small cone of the aforementioned shape. Coat it with rapeseed oil, peanut oil, or soap lather, insert it into the anus, and gently rotate it. The bowels will be unblocked shortly.

《民族医药报》1992 年 8 月 7 日（贵州 罗安君）

Ethnic Medicine News, August 7, 1992 (Luo Anjun, Guizhou)

四、小儿夜啼（10 方）

IV. Pediatric Nocturnal Crying (10 Prescriptions)

小儿夜啼，系指小儿白天正常，入夜则啼哭或梦中惊啼的病证。祖国医学认为，小儿为“纯阳”之体，阳热有余而神气不足。若喂养不当，过食乳汁或恣食肥甘厚味，以致心脾积热，夜间烦躁而啼哭。或因白天偶受惊吓，或耳闻异声，眼看异物，使心神不宁，而梦中惊啼。

Pediatric nocturnal crying refers to a condition where a child is normal during the day but cries at night or cries out in fright during sleep. Traditional Chinese medicine believes that children have a “pure yang” constitution, with excessive yang-heat and insufficient mental energy (shen qi). If fed improperly, such as consuming excessive milk or overindulging in rich, sweet, and greasy foods, it can lead to accumulated heat in the heart and spleen, causing nighttime restlessness and crying. Alternatively, if a child is accidentally frightened during the day, hears strange noises, or sees unusual objects, it can cause mental restlessness, leading to crying out in fright during sleep.

1. 蝉蜕 5-7 只，去足洗净水煎取汁约 100 毫升，稍加白糖，待温后一日分 3-5 次喂完。大多在 3 日内见效。

1. Take 5-7 cicada sloughs, remove the legs, wash them, and decoct in water to obtain about 100 ml of juice. Add a little white sugar, wait until it is warm, and feed it to the child in 3-5 divided doses within a day. It mostly takes effect within 3 days.

2. 全虫、胆星各 1 克，荆芥、蝉蜕、钩藤、防风各 1.5 克，薄荷 0.5 克，水煎服。

2. Take 1g each of whole scorpion and arisaema with bile, 1.5g each of schizonepeta, cicada slough, uncaria, and saposhnikovia, and 0.5g of mint. Decoct in water and take orally.

3. 青黛，研为细末，每次冲服 1.5 克，睡前服。

3. Take indigo naturalis, grind it into a fine powder, and take 1.5g each time with hot water before going to bed.

4. "钱窜子" 1 个，足全者为宜。抓住后用针扎住，在瓦上烧黄后，研为细末，睡前一次冲服。

4. Take 1 "qianchuanzi" (centipede), preferably with all its legs intact. Hold it and pierce it with a needle, roast it on a tile until yellow, grind it into a fine powder, and take it all at once with hot water before going to bed.

5. 朱砂安神丸 10 粒，研碎，加食醋调成糊状，敷贴于脐部，外盖纱布固定，每日换药一次，连用 3 天。

5. Take 10 pills of Zhusha Anshen Pills, crush them, add edible vinegar to form a paste, apply it to the navel, cover with gauze to secure it, change the medication once a day, and use it continuously for 3 days.

《中药科技报》1992 年 2 月 26 日（郑俊芝）

TCM Science and Technology News, February 26, 1992 (Zheng Junzhi)

6. 小儿夜间哭闹不宁，而又无其它疾病所致者，称为小儿夜啼。笔者用下述方法治疗，有较好的疗效，现予介绍。

6. When a child cries and is restless at night without being caused by any other diseases, it is called pediatric nocturnal crying. The author has achieved good therapeutic effects by treating it with the following methods, which are now introduced.

基本方：淡竹叶 8 克、灯芯一小团、大枣 4 枚、夜交藤 5 克、麦冬 6 克、蝉蜕 3 只、柴胡 4 克、炙甘草 6 克。（本方功效：清心安神、解郁除烦）

Basic Prescription: 8g of lophatherum, a small tuft of rush pith, 4 red dates, 5g of polygonum multiflorum vine, 6g of ophiopogon, 3 cicada sloughs, 4g of bupleurum, and 6g of honey-fried licorice. (The effects of this prescription are to clear the heart and calm the mind, relieve depression, and eliminate restlessness.)

加减：

Modifications:

小儿舌苔黄燥、小便短黄者为心经有热，加薄荷 3 克，重用淡竹叶至 12 克。

If the child has a yellow and dry tongue coating and short, yellow urine, indicating heat in the heart meridian, add 3g of mint, and increase the dosage of lophatherum to 12g.

小儿烦躁易怒，睡眠不安者加柏子仁 5 克，合欢花 4 克。

If the child is irritable and has restless sleep, add 5g of platycladus seeds and 4g of albizia flowers.

由于受惊吓而夜啼者加枣仁 4 克，朱砂 0、5 克（冲服）。

If the child cries at night due to being frightened, add 4g of sour jujube seeds and 0.5g of cinnabar (to be taken by brewing with hot water).

用法：每日一剂水煎服，睡前加服一次。

Usage: Decoct one dose in water daily and take orally. Take an additional dose before going to bed.

《民族医药报》1992 年 5 月 15 日（广西）

Ethnic Medicine News, May 15, 1992 (Guangxi)

治小儿夜啼方

Prescription for Treating Pediatric Nocturnal Crying

7. 蝉蜕 3 克、薄荷 1 克、槟榔 3 克、枳壳 3 克、灯芯草 6 克，共煎水，分三次喂下，连服 7 天。

7. Take 3g of cicada slough, 1g of mint, 3g of betel nut, 3g of bitter orange, and 6g of rush pith. Decoct them together in water, divide the liquid into three

portions to feed the child, and take it continuously for 7 days.

8. 用朱砂 3 克、黄连 3 克、钩藤 6 克，共研成细粉装瓶，每次取 0.5 克药粉撒于母乳头上，让小儿吸吮；断奶的孩子用开水冲服。

8. Take 3g of cinnabar, 3g of coptis, and 6g of uncaria. Grind them together into a fine powder and store in a bottle. Each time, take 0.5g of the powder and sprinkle it on the mother's nipple for the child to suckle; for weaned children, brew it with boiling water and take orally.

9. 黑丑（黑色牵牛子）7 粒，研细后，用温开水调成糊状，于睡前敷于小儿肚脐上覆盖纱布，用胶布固定。第二早晨取之，每天一次，连用 7 天。

9. Take 7 black morning glory seeds (heichou). After grinding them finely, mix with warm boiled water to form a paste. Apply it to the child's navel before going to bed, cover with gauze, and secure it with medical tape. Remove it the next morning. Do this once a day, continuously for 7 days.

10. 灯芯草单味煎水喂。按年龄给药，1-6 个月的 6 克，6-12 个月的 9 克，均加水煎至一半后，分三次给小儿服之，三天为一个疗程，连用 2-3 个疗程，即可使“夜哭郎”一觉睡到大天亮矣！

10. Decoct only rush pith in water to feed the child. Administer the dosage according to age: 6g for infants aged 1-6 months, and 9g for those aged 6-12 months. In both cases, add water and decoct until the liquid is reduced by half, then divide it into three portions for the child to take. Three days constitute one course of treatment. After continuously using 2-3 courses, the "night crier" will be able to sleep soundly until daybreak!

《中医药信息报》1992 年 1 月 25 日（刘永志）

TCM Information News, January 25, 1992 (Liu Yongzhi)

五、小儿遗尿（16 方）

V. Pediatric Enuresis (16 Prescriptions)

1. 本方来源于我区名老中医邱老先生几十年的临床经验。我在临床十多年的运用中，收到较好的效果。时近冬季，特整理如下，供同仁参考。

1. This prescription originates from the decades of clinical experience of Mr. Qiu, a renowned senior TCM practitioner in our region. Through my own clinical application over the past decade, it has achieved good therapeutic effects. As winter approaches, I have specifically compiled this for the reference of my colleagues.

药物组成：黄芪 30 克，党参 30 克，山药 30 克，鸡内金 7 克，桑螵蛸 10 克，补骨脂 15 克，覆盆子 20 克，益智仁 10 克，乌药 5 克。

Composition: 30g of astragalus, 30g of codonopsis, 30g of yam, 7g of chicken gizzard lining, 10g of mantis egg case, 15g of psoralea fruit, 20g of raspberry, 10g of alpinia oxyphylla, and 5g of lindera root.

加减：口渴，自汗气阴虚者加麦冬、五味子；气坠便溏脾虚者加白术、升麻。

Modifications: For patients with thirst, spontaneous sweating, and qi-yin deficiency, add ophiopogon and schisandra fruit; for those with spleen deficiency characterized by bearing-down sensation and loose stools, add atractylodes macrocephala and cimicifuga.

煎服法：用猪尿胞三个、洗净，与上药同放有盖小锅内，加水适量同煮，肉熟后加适量食盐调味，早上，中午各喝汤一小盅，晚上食肉〈不喝汤〉，3-5 日食完〈每次服药前必须加热〉。

Preparation and Usage: Wash three pig bladders thoroughly. Place them in a small pot with a lid together with the above herbs, add an appropriate amount of water, and boil together. After the meat is cooked, add an appropriate amount of salt for seasoning. Drink a small cup of the soup in the morning and at noon, and eat the meat in the evening (do not drink the soup). Finish consuming it within 3-5 days (the medication must be heated before each dose).

如猪尿胞不易得，可将药改为散剂亦可，将药物全部碾为极细末，每日早、晚各用药粉末 7-10 克、调入鸡蛋（1-2 个中），加适量食盐，蒸熟食之。

If pig bladders are not easily available, the herbs can be changed into a powder form. Grind all the herbs into an extremely fine powder. Take 7-10g of the powder in the morning and evening, mix it into 1-2 eggs, add an appropriate amount of salt, and steam it before eating.

按：小儿遗尿病，在农村中较为常见，每入冬季，时有患儿家长上门求治，本病虽然不太严重，亦不会影响生命，但长期尿床，不仅患儿精神苦闷，且影响其父母睡眠。

Note: Pediatric enuresis is relatively common in rural areas. Every winter, parents often bring their children for treatment. Although this disease is not very serious and does not affect life, prolonged bedwetting not only causes mental distress to the child but also affects the parents' sleep.

对本病前人分为湿热和肾气不足两类，前者临床不多见，且病短而易治，湿热一去，遗尿即止；后者，入冬后，每晚必尿床 1-2 次，且一时不易治愈。对此病，曾遵前人之法用缩泉丸桑螵蛸散温肾为主，终感疗效不佳，改用针灸，患儿又不易接受，且农村就医也不容易。

Previous generations classified this disease into two types: damp-heat and kidney qi deficiency. The former is rarely seen clinically, has a short disease course, and is easy to treat; once the damp-heat is cleared, the enuresis stops. In the latter type, after the onset of winter, the child inevitably wets the bed 1-2 times every night, and it is not easily cured in a short time. For this disease, I once followed the traditional method of using Suoquan Pill and Sangpiaoxiao Powder to warm the kidney as the main treatment, but ultimately felt the therapeutic effect was not ideal. Switching to acupuncture and moxibustion was not easily accepted by children, and seeking medical care in rural areas is also not easy.

本方以桑螵蛸散，缩泉丸合方加减组成，方中重用黄芪党参大补肺气为主，因其水之上源；山药鸡内金健脾为辅；培土以生金；佐以覆盆子，桑螵蛸，补骨脂，益智仁温补肾气而缩小便；使以通行三焦之乌药理气以防参芪之滞。全方共奏益气温肾缩泉止遗之功。如是肺气治节于上，肾气因摄于下，膀胱约而遗尿自止。该方多数病人服一剂尿床即可停止。

This prescription is composed of modified combinations of Sangpiaoxiao Powder and Suoquan Pill. In this formula, astragalus and codonopsis are heavily used as the main ingredients to greatly tonify lung qi, because the lung is the upper source of water; yam and chicken gizzard lining serve as secondary ingredients to invigorate the spleen, cultivating earth to generate metal; raspberry, mantis egg case, psoralea fruit, and alpinia oxyphylla are used as adjuvants to warm and tonify kidney qi and reduce urination; lindera root is used as a guiding drug to regulate qi and unblock the triple energizer, preventing the stagnation caused by codonopsis and astragalus. The whole formula works together to tonify qi, warm the kidney, reduce urination, and stop enuresis. Thus, when lung qi regulates above and kidney qi grasps below, the bladder is restrained and enuresis naturally stops. For most patients, bedwetting stops after taking just one dose of this prescription.

《中医药信息报》1992 年 10 月 17 日（贵州 先全祥）

TCM Information News, October 17, 1992 (Xian Quanxiang, Guizhou)

2. 河南省宁陵县中医院王建海医师等近年采用简便方法治疗遗尿，获满意效果。取关节止痛膏 1 张，贴于以关元穴为中心的下腹部，2 日换 1 次，无皮损可连续贴敷，一般 10-15 日即可痊愈。

2. In recent years, Dr. Wang Jianhai and others at Ningling County TCM Hospital in Henan Province have used a simple and convenient method to treat enuresis with satisfactory results. Take one piece of joint analgesic plaster and apply it to the lower abdomen centered on the Guanyuan acupoint. Change it once every two days. If there is no skin damage, it can be applied continuously. Generally, it can be cured within 10-15 days.

（计惠民）

(Ji Huimin)

3. 取木瓜粗末 30 克，装于四层纱布口罩内，每天傍晚让患儿戴口罩两小时左右；或以木瓜 30 克粗末，装入一小布袋中，置于枕旁，让患儿在睡眠时闻其气。此法可经嗅觉吸入药气，提高中枢对膀胱充盈的“警觉”。一般连用一周见效。

3. Take 30g of coarse papaya powder, put it into a four-layer gauze mask, and have the child wear the mask for about two hours every evening; alternatively,

put 30g of coarse papaya powder into a small cloth bag and place it beside the pillow so that the child can inhale its aroma during sleep. This method allows the medicinal aroma to be inhaled through the olfactory sense, enhancing the central nervous system ’ s “alertness” to bladder fullness. Generally, it takes effect after continuous use for one week.

4. 用五倍子研成细末，取适量填入患儿肚脐眼内，并用纱布覆盖，胶布固定。此法可使药气经脐部透入膀胱，提高膀胱括约肌的收缩能力。一般连用五天见效。

4. Grind Chinese gallnuts into a fine powder, take an appropriate amount and fill it into the child ’ s navel, cover it with gauze, and secure it with medical tape. This method allows the medicinal properties to penetrate into the bladder through the umbilicus, enhancing the contractile ability of the bladder sphincter. Generally, it takes effect after continuous use for five days.

5. 用猪膀胱一只洗净，加桑螵蛸 15-30 克，覆盆子 15-30 克，山萸肉 5 克，石菖蒲 5 克，将诸药用纱布袋包在一起，与猪膀胱一道放入砂罐或铁锅内，用水炖熟，饮汁吃肉。此法可使中枢神经与植物神经、膀胱逼尿肌与括约肌的机能协调。每隔三天吃一次，一般连吃三次就可收到显著效果。

5. Wash one pig bladder thoroughly. Add 15-30g of mantis egg case, 15-30g of raspberry, 5g of Asiatic cornelian cherry fruit, and 5g of grass-leaved sweetflag. Wrap these herbs together in a gauze bag, place them together with the pig bladder into a clay pot or iron pan, and stew them in water until cooked. Drink the broth and eat the meat. This method can coordinate the functions of the central nervous system and autonomic nervous system, as well as the detrusor muscle and sphincter of the bladder. Eat it once every three days. Generally, significant effects can be achieved after eating it three consecutive times.

（江苏 吉联军）

(Ji Lianjun, Jiangsu)

6. 药用：太子参、黄芪、条参、菟丝子、益智仁、芡实各 9 克，白果 6 克，猪脬 1 只。将上药装入猪脬中，细线扎口，加入适量水文火煎 20 分钟。饮汤食脬肉，日一剂。

6. Medicinal ingredients: 9g each of pseudostellaria root, astragalus, codonopsis, dodder seed, alpinia oxyphylla, and euryale seed, 6g of ginkgo nut, and one pig bladder. Put the above herbs into the pig bladder, tie the opening tightly with a thin thread, add an appropriate amount of water, and decoct over low heat for 20 minutes. Drink the soup and eat the bladder meat. Take one dose a day.

一般说来，小儿遗尿多系肾气不足，下元虚寒，或脾肺气虚，水道失约所致。本方具有培元益气，固摄止溺之效。笔者先后用之治疗小儿遗尿 30 余例，每服 2-5 剂即愈。

Generally speaking, pediatric enuresis is mostly caused by insufficient kidney qi, deficiency-cold in the lower jiao, or deficiency of spleen and lung qi leading to uncontrolled water passages. This prescription has the effects of cultivating primordial qi, tonifying vital qi, consolidating retention, and stopping enuresis. The author has used it to treat over 30 cases of pediatric enuresis, and patients were cured after taking 2-5 doses each time.

《民族医药报》1992 年 5 月 22 日（广西 韦金星）

Ethnic Medicine News, May 22, 1992 (Wei Jinxing, Guangxi)

7. 近年来，笔者拟用升陷汤为主治疗小儿遗尿症，均获满意疗效。现介绍如下。

7. In recent years, the author has used Shengxian Decoction as the main prescription to treat pediatric enuresis, and all cases have achieved satisfactory therapeutic effects. The details are introduced as follows.

一般资料：共观察 12 例，男 8 例，女 4 例，年龄在 3-9 岁之间；夜尿次数 2-6 次，尿量 30-60 毫升，实验室检查无阳性发现。

General Data: A total of 12 cases were observed, including 8 males and 4 females, aged between 3 and 9 years old. The frequency of nocturnal enuresis was 2-6 times per night, with a urine volume of 30-60 ml. Laboratory tests showed no positive findings.

治疗方法：患者服用“遗尿升陷汤”。药用黄芪、党参各 15 克，炒山药 12 克，益智仁、菟丝子、桑螵蛸各 9 克，肉桂 3 克。

Treatment Method: Patients took "Yiniao Shengxian Decoction". The medicinal ingredients were: 15g each of astragalus and codonopsis, 12g of stir-fried yam, 9g each of alpinia oxyphylla, dodder seed, and mantis egg case, and 3g of cinnamon bark.

加减法：脾胃虚弱加焦三仙，气虚明显者重用参芪，肾阳虚明显者加补骨脂，遗尿次数超过3次以上者加覆盆子。每剂药水煎2次，取汁60-100毫升，分3次服，每日一剂。

Modifications: For weak spleen and stomach, add scorched sanxian; for obvious qi deficiency, increase the dosage of codonopsis and astragalus; for obvious kidney yang deficiency, add psoralea fruit; for enuresis occurring more than 3 times, add raspberry. Decoct each dose twice in water, obtain 60-100 ml of liquid, divide it into 3 servings, and take one dose daily.

治疗效果：12例患者服3剂后遗尿次数明显减少，服至6剂后遗尿基本治愈，无需再服。本组 12 例患儿经一年随访，未见复发。

Therapeutic Effects: After taking 3 doses, the frequency of enuresis in the 12 patients significantly decreased. After taking 6 doses, the enuresis was basically cured and no further medication was needed. After a one-year follow-up of the 12 children in this group, no relapse was observed.

体会：升陷汤为清末名医张锡纯经验方，具有补中益气、升阳举陷功效。小儿"稚阴稚阳"之体，脏腑娇嫩，禀赋不足，肾气未充，膀胱约束无力，故而睡眠中遗尿。本方党参、黄芪、山药合用，益肺补脾，升阳举陷，调畅气机；益智仁、菟丝子、桑螵蛸及肉桂，暖肾壮阳固精，促进膀胱功能正常，开阖有度。肺为水之上源，调畅水道，脾主运化而制水，肾是水之大主，且肺脾肾精气互生，水道通畅，气化正常，膀胱约束有力，排尿自能控制。

Experience: Shengxian Decoction is an empirical prescription by Zhang Xichun, a famous doctor in the late Qing Dynasty, which has the effects of tonifying the middle and replenishing qi, raising yang, and lifting prolapse. Children have a "tender yin and yang" constitution, with delicate zang-fu organs, insufficient innate endowment, unfulfilled kidney qi, and weak bladder control, thus leading to enuresis during sleep. In this prescription, the combination of codonopsis, astragalus, and yam tonifies the lung and spleen, raises yang, lifts prolapse, and regulates qi mechanism; alpinia oxyphylla, dodder seed, mantis egg case, and cinnamon bark warm the kidney, invigorate yang, and consolidate essence, promoting normal bladder function with proper opening and closing. The lung is the upper source of water and regulates water passages; the spleen governs transportation and transformation to control water; the kidney is the master of water. Moreover, the essence and qi of the lung, spleen, and kidney mutually generate each other. When the water passages are unobstructed and qi transformation is normal, the bladder has strong restraint, and urination can be naturally controlled.

《民族医药报》（青海省 刘启明 张世梅）

Ethnic Medicine News (Liu Qiming, Zhang Shimei, Qinghai Province)

8. 对患有遗尿症的小儿，可用普通香烟在其至阴穴（足小趾外侧趾甲角旁约 0.1 寸）温灸，每次 10-15 分钟，一日 2 次，数日即可见效。

8. For children suffering from enuresis, a regular cigarette can be used to apply warm moxibustion to the Zhiyin acupoint (located about 0.1 cun lateral to the outer corner of the toenail of the little toe). Do this for 10-15 minutes each time, twice a day. Therapeutic effects can usually be seen within a few days.

《中医药信息报》1993 年 4 月 24 日（宁蔚夏）

TCM Information News, April 24, 1993 (Ning Weixia)

9.食疗法：鸡肠一具，洗净切成小块。在瓦片上焙干后碾碎，加入200克面粉、适量的油、盐和水和成面团，烙成饼，作为食品给小儿常服用。

9. Dietary Therapy: Take one set of chicken intestines, wash them thoroughly, and cut them into small pieces. Bake them dry on a tile, then crush them into a powder. Add 200g of flour, an appropriate amount of oil, salt, and water to knead into a dough, and pan-fry them into flatbreads. Serve these as a regular food for the child.

10. 食饴糖法：桂枝 3 克，白芍、甘草各 6 克，黄芪 9 克，煎汤去渣，与饴糖适量冲服，每日 2 次，可治脾肺气虚之小儿遗尿。

10. Maltose Therapy: Take 3g of cinnamon twig, 6g each of white peony root and licorice, and 9g of astragalus. Decoct them in water, discard the residue, and mix the liquid with an appropriate amount of maltose to drink. Take this twice a day. It can treat pediatric enuresis caused by spleen and lung qi deficiency.

11. 敷肚脐法：将葱白 7-8 根，硫磺 50 克，共捣成糊状，在小儿临睡前敷于肚脐处，用胶布固定，连用 3 夜。

11. Navel Application Method: Pound 7-8 scallion whites and 50g of sulfur together into a paste. Apply it to the child' s navel right before going to bed, secure it with medical tape, and use it continuously for three nights.

12. 升麻、附片（先煎 30 分钟）、菟丝子各 10 克，熟地 12 克，党参 15 克，黄芪、生山药各 20 克，柴胡 16 克，肉桂 3 克，水煎服。用于肾阳不足型（其症状为肢凉畏冷、大便溏泄、小便清长）小儿遗尿。连服 5-10 剂可愈。

12. Take 10g each of cimicifuga, aconite slices (decocted 30 minutes in advance), and dodder seed, 12g of prepared rehmannia root, 15g of codonopsis, 20g each of astragalus and raw yam, 16g of bupleurum, and 3g of cinnamon bark. Decoct in water and take orally. This is used for pediatric enuresis of the kidney yang deficiency type (symptoms include cold limbs, aversion to cold, loose stools, and copious clear urine). Taking 5-10 consecutive doses can cure the condition.

《民族医药报》1993 年 2 月 26 日（河北 辛化乙）

Ethnic Medicine News, February 26, 1993 (Xin Huayi, Hebei)

3 岁以上小儿，夜间睡熟时常不能自主排尿而尿床者，可视为遗尿症。在治疗上除于睡前不要大量喝水，夜间定时叫醒小儿排 1-2 次小便外，选用下述方法。

Children over the age of three who frequently wet the bed due to an inability to urinate voluntarily during deep sleep at night can be diagnosed with enuresis. In addition to avoiding drinking large amounts of water before bedtime and waking the child up at scheduled times at night to urinate 1-2 times, the following methods can be selected for treatment.

13. 白果红枣糖水：取白果仁（银杏）30 粒，红枣 10 个，白糖适量。将红枣去核，加水煎白果仁、红枣，取浓汤，加糖调匀后于白天服。

13. Ginkgo Nut and Red Date Sugar Soup: Take 30ginkgo nut kernels and 10 red dates, along with an appropriate amount of white sugar. Pit the red dates, add water to decoct the ginkgo nut kernels and red dates, and obtain a thick soup. Add sugar, mix well, and take it during the daytime.

14. 白果苡仁猪膀胱汤：取白果仁 30 克，苡仁 15 克，猪膀胱 1 个。将猪膀胱洗净，加白果仁、苡仁一起煮汤，调味后于白天服。

14. Ginkgo Nut, Coix Seed, and Pig Bladder Soup: Take 30g of ginkgo nut kernels, 15g of coix seeds, and one pig bladder. Wash the pig bladder thoroughly, add the ginkgo nut kernels and coix seeds, and boil them together into a soup. Season it and take it during the daytime.

15. 桑螵蛸核桃仁汤：取桑螵蛸 10 克，核桃仁 2 个，水煎后，去桑螵蛸，服汤和核桃仁。

15. Mantis Egg Case and Walnut Kernel Soup: Take 10g of mantis egg case and two walnut kernels. Decoct them in water, remove the mantis egg case, and consume the soup along with the walnut kernels.

《民族医药报》1992 年 2 月 28 日（李子云）

Ethnic Medicine News, February 28, 1992 (Li Ziyun)

七、小儿杂症

VI. Miscellaneous Pediatric Diseases

（一）小儿癫痫中西医结合防治研究（1 方）

(1) Research on the Integrated Traditional Chinese and Western Medicine Prevention and Treatment of Pediatric Epilepsy (1 Prescription)

小儿癫痫系一种病因较为复杂的神经系统综合征，其发病率较高，据国内文献报告约占人群之 0.78-1.75%。若不及时治疗，本病可严重影响小儿精神及智能发育。近年来，中西医结合防治小儿癫痫出现了可喜的苗头，兹简要介绍如下：

Pediatric epilepsy is a neurological syndrome with a relatively complex etiology. It has a high incidence rate, with domestic literature reporting it accounts for approximately 0.78%-1.75% of the population. If left untreated, this disease can severely affect a child's mental and intellectual development. In recent years, encouraging progress has been made in the integrated prevention and treatment of pediatric epilepsy using both traditional Chinese and Western medicine. A brief introduction is as follows:

①中西药优势相加。西药苯妥英钠等在控制癫痫发作方面起着重要的作用，但对肝、肾、造血系统均有一定毒副作用。中医认为本病多与风痰郁闭或心脾肾俱虚有关，辨证论治每能获效。中西药取各自长处联合运用其疗效明显比单用要好，且症情稳定后尚可酌减西药，避免其毒副作用。有学者报告以紫金锭及紫参片（紫金锭加苦参）与西药联用（治疗过程中递减西药），收治 105 例，治愈 41 例，有效率达 70% 以上。张树臣等以丹参、败酱草、珍珠粉、樟脑、冰片、甘草、苯巴比妥、士的宁、溴化钠混合浸膏制成"治痫灵"观察表明对多年服用西药无效者尚有较好的治疗作用。而以丹参、月石、苯妥英钠共研细末敷脐亦是一种有益的尝试。

① Combining the advantages of Chinese and Western medicines. Western medicines such as phenytoin sodium play an important role in controlling epileptic seizures, but they have certain toxic side effects on the liver, kidneys, and hematopoietic system. Traditional Chinese medicine (TCM) believes that this disease is mostly related to wind-phlegm stagnation or deficiency of the heart, spleen, and kidneys, and syndrome differentiation and treatment can often achieve good results. Combining the respective strengths of Chinese and Western medicines yields significantly better therapeutic effects than using either alone. Furthermore, once the condition stabilizes, the dosage of Western medicine can be appropriately reduced to avoid its toxic side effects. Some scholars have reported using Zijin Ding (Purple Gold Pill) and Zishen Tablets (Zijin Ding plus Sophora flavescens) in combination with Western medicine (with a gradual reduction of Western medicine during treatment). Among 105 treated cases, 41 were cured, achieving an effective rate of over 70%. Zhang Shuchen and others created "Zhixianling" (Epilepsy Treatment Pill) using a mixed extract of red sage root, patrinia, pearl powder, camphor, borneol, licorice, phenobarbital, strychnine, and sodium bromide. Observations showed it had a good therapeutic effect on patients who had been unresponsive to Western medicine for years. Additionally, grinding red sage root, borax, and phenytoin sodium into a fine powder and applying it to the navel is also a beneficial attempt.

②中医辨证与西医辨病相结合。这种中西医结合研究思路已逐渐趋于成熟，临床运用上主要表现为结合中药现代药理研究，在辨证论治基础上选用具有抗癫痫效应有关中药。或专病专方，其组方既切中癫痫主要病机又吻合药理研究。其次是中医辨证与西医分型相对应。如吕学泰氏把本病分为风痰壅盛，清窍闭阻；风痰上逆，神明受扰；气血两亏、筋脉失养；肝火暴胀、风痰上壅等四型，其分别相当于西医之大发作、小发作、局限性发作、神经运动发作。

② Combining TCM syndrome differentiation with Western disease diagnosis. This integrated research approach has gradually matured. In clinical application, it mainly involves integrating modern pharmacological research of Chinese herbs, selecting anti-epileptic herbs based on syndrome differentiation. Alternatively, specific prescriptions for specific diseases are used, where the formulation targets the main pathogenesis of epilepsy while aligning with pharmacological research. Secondly, TCM syndrome differentiation corresponds to Western medical classifications. For example, Lu XueTai classified this disease into four types: abundant wind-phlegm with blocked clear orifices; upward counterflow of wind-phlegm disturbing the mind; deficiency of both qi and blood with malnourished tendons and vessels; and hyperactive liver fire with upward surging of wind-phlegm. These correspond respectively to grand mal, petit mal, focal seizures, and psychomotor seizures in Western medicine.

③中药现代药理研究，目前主要是单味中药药效学研究及有效成分提取。

方剂学研究正亟待起步。文献资料表明：胆南星、川芎、钩藤、柴胡、僵蛹有抗惊厥作用；桂枝具有增强血液循环及镇静作用，石菖蒲除镇静作用外，尚能显著延长戊巴比妥钠麻醉作用。α-细辛醚则是从石菖蒲中提取的一种活性成分，其有抑制乙酰胆碱、组织胺和 5- 羟色胺生成作用。

③ Modern pharmacological research on Chinese herbs currently focuses mainly on pharmacodynamic studies of single herbs and the extraction of active ingredients. Research on herbal formulas urgently needs to be initiated. Literature indicates that bile-processed arisaema, ligusticum wallichii, uncaria, bupleurum, and stiff silkworm pupae have anticonvulsant effects; cassia twig enhances blood circulation and has a sedative effect. In addition to its sedative effect, grass-leaved sweetflag can significantly prolong the anesthetic effect of sodium pentobarbital. α-asarone is an active ingredient extracted from grass-leaved sweetflag, which has the effect of inhibiting the production of acetylcholine, histamine, and 5-hydroxytryptamide (serotonin).

《中医药信息报》（江苏 葛志奇）

TCM Information News (Ge Zhiqi, Jiangsu)

（二）治小儿暑热症（1 方）

(2) Treating Pediatric Summer Heat Syndrome (1 Prescription)

小儿暑热症亦称夏季热，是 1-3 岁的幼儿常患的一种疾病。中医认为该病为小儿元气未充，脏气未盛，肺脾两虚，暑热内蕴所致。

Pediatric summer heat syndrome, also known as summer fever, is a common disease in toddlers aged 1-3. TCM believes that this disease is caused by a child’s insufficient primordial qi, underdeveloped zang-fu organ qi, deficiency of both the lung and spleen, and the internal retention of summer heat.

孩子患了暑热症，表现为持续发热（体温 37.5C-39.5C，月余不退，甚至迁延 2-3 个月，一般天气越热，体温越高。并常伴有口渴、多尿、少汗、烦躁、厌食等症状。患儿面色苍白而口唇红，心率快，体重也日渐下降。如果发现小儿长期发热不退，全身检查和化验检查又没有发现异常，就应该想到暑热症的可能。

When a child suffers from summer heat syndrome, it manifests as continuous fever (body temperature of 37.5 ° C-39.5 ° C) that does not subside for over a month, and can even linger for 2-3 months. Generally, the hotter the weather, the higher the body temperature. It is often accompanied by symptoms such as thirst, frequent urination, scanty sweating, restlessness, and loss of appetite. The child' s face is pale while the lips are red, the heart rate is fast, and body weight gradually decreases. If a child has a prolonged fever without any abnormalities found during physical and laboratory examinations, the possibility of summer heat syndrome should be considered.

笔者临证 20 余载，用自拟方“清暑解热汤”治疗小儿暑热症，屡验显效。处方：童参 9 克，银花 6 克，枇杷叶 6 克，苡仁 9 克，竹叶 6 克，鲜荷叶 1 张，西瓜翠衣 30 克，甘草 6 克。用法：上药加水 500 毫升，浸泡半小时左右，煎至 200 毫升左右，加冰糖适量，分 3-4 次服完，每日一剂，一般连用 5-7 剂可愈。

In over 20 years of clinical practice, the author has used a self-formulated prescription called “Qingshu Jiere Tang” (Summer Heat-Clearing and Fever-Relieving Decoction) to treat pediatric summer heat syndrome, with repeatedly proven significant effects. Prescription: 9g of ginseng radix, 6g of honeysuckle, 6g of loquat leaf, 9g of coix seed, 6g of bamboo leaf, 1 fresh lotus leaf, 30g of watermelon rind (green outer layer), and 6g of licorice. Usage: Add 500 ml of water to the above herbs, soak for about half an hour, and decoct until about 200 ml remains. Add an appropriate amount of rock sugar, divide into 3-4 servings, and take one dose daily. Generally, continuous use of 5-7 doses can cure the condition.

《民族医药报》1992 年 6 月 5 日（山东 梁兆松）

Ethnic Medicine News, June 5, 1992 (Liang Zhaosong, Shandong)

（三）治婴儿惊恐（1 方）

(3) Treating Infantile Fright (1 Method)

我是《民族医药报》的一名忠实读者，并且将每一期的验方剪下来贴在自己制作的《百科知识剪报》本上。今年元月初我刚满四个月的小女，受到惊吓，晚上睡眠不安，神情恐惧，全身发抖、大声哭喊，连续几个晚上扰得大家不能入眠。我按照 1991 年 11 月 25 日《民族医药报》上刊登的“治婴儿惊恐一法”试了一次，真是不试不知道，一试真奇妙，小女儿当晚便能安然入睡，不再吵闹。

I am a loyal reader of Ethnic Medicine News, and I cut out the effective prescriptions from each issue and paste them into my self-made “Encyclopedia Knowledge Clippings” notebook. In early January this year, my daughter, who had just turned four months old, was frightened. She slept restlessly at night, looked terrified, trembled all over, and cried loudly, keeping everyone awake for several consecutive nights. I tried the “Method for Treating Infantile Fright” published in the November 25, 1991 issue of Ethnic Medicine News. It was truly miraculous; my little daughter slept soundly that very night and stopped crying.

按摩脊椎 1-2 次，然后用双手大拇指、食指掐提脊椎肌肉，提起即松开，由胸椎至尾椎，只需一次，患儿即可好转。（该法原载于本报 1991 年 11 月 25 日 2 版“小验方”栏目。）

Massage the spine 1-2 times, then use the thumbs and index fingers of both hands to pinch and lift the muscles along the spine. Lift and immediately release, moving from the thoracic vertebrae down to the coccyx. Only one session is needed for the child to improve. (This method was originally published in the “Little Effective Prescriptions” column on page 2 of this newspaper on November 25, 1991.)

八、《民族医药报》1992 年 2 月 14 日（湖北 曹长江）
Ethnic Medicine News, February 14, 1992 (Cao Changjiang, Hubei)

（四）治腮腺炎方（1 方）

(4) Prescription for Treating Mumps (1 Prescription)

初起。处方：芙蓉叶、赤小豆各 30 克，白芨 15 克。用法：将上三味药共研为细末调匀（上述为一料，可分为 5-6 次）。用鸡蛋清调敷患处，每天 2-3 次，轻者一料可愈。注意不可碰损皮肤，以免感染。

For the initial stage. Prescription: 30g each of hibiscus leaves and adzuki beans, and 15g of pseudobulbus bletillae seu striatae. Usage: Grind the above three herbs together into a fine powder and mix well (the above amount is one batch, which can be divided into 5-6 uses). Mix the powder with egg white and apply it to the affected area 2-3 times a day. Mild cases can be cured with one batch. Be careful not to damage the skin to avoid infection.

重症。处方：雄黄15克，明矾12克，冰片3克。用法：以上3味共研为细末，加75%酒精或醋适量调匀，用消毒棉签蘸药液搽患处，每日3-4次。

For severe cases. Prescription: 15g of realgar, 12g of alum, and 3g of borneol. Usage: Grind the above three ingredients together into a fine powder, add an appropriate amount of 75% alcohol or vinegar to mix evenly, dip a sterile cotton swab into the liquid, and apply it to the affected area 3-4 times a day.

处方及用法：吴茱萸12克，浙贝母、大黄各9克，胆南星3克，共研为细末。以上药末用米醋调成糊状外敷足心（涌泉穴），患左敷右，患右敷左，双侧患病，左右均敷，每日换药1次。轻者1-3次可愈，较重者可配合内服银花、菊花等清热解毒药物。

Prescription and usage: 12g of evodia fruit, 9g each of thunberg fritillary bulb and rhubarb, and 3g of arisaema with bile. Grind them together into a fine powder. Mix the powder with rice vinegar to form a paste and apply it externally to the soles of the feet (Yongquan acupoint). Apply to the right foot if the left side is affected, and vice versa. If both sides are affected, apply to both feet. Change the medication once a day. Mild cases can be cured after 1-3 applications. For more severe cases, it can be combined with oral heat-clearing and detoxifying herbs such as honeysuckle and chrysanthemum.

取中成药防风通圣散一粒，血竭2克，二味均研末与食醋调成糊状外涂患处，每日5-6次，很快可愈。具有消肿化瘀的作用。

Take one pill of Fangfeng Tongsheng San (a Chinese patent medicine) and 2g of dragon’s blood. Grind both into a powder, mix with edible vinegar to form a paste, and apply it externally to the affected area 5-6 times a day. It can cure the condition quickly. It has the effects of reducing swelling and resolving blood stasis.

《民族医药报》1992 年 11 月 17 日（晴荐）

Ethnic Medicine News, November 17, 1992 (Recommended by Qing)

（五）中药益智方（2 方）

(5) TCM Prescriptions for Enhancing Intelligence (2 Prescriptions)

1. 益智丸。功效及适应证：能补肾、健脑、益智。适用于智能低下儿童，健康儿童服用亦佳。药物组成及制法与服法：益智仁、合欢花、菖蒲、女贞子、炒杜仲、牛膝、莲子心、竹叶、楮实子、旱莲草、瓦松、黄精、神曲各 9 克，何首乌 30 克。上药研细，炼蜜为丸，每丸重 1.6 克。每日服用量：1 岁 2 丸，三岁 4 丸，6 岁 6 丸，分 2-3 次服下。

Yizhi Pill (Intelligence-Enhancing Pill). Efficacy and indications: It can tonify the kidney, invigorate the brain, and enhance intelligence. It is suitable for children with low intelligence, and it is also beneficial for healthy children. Composition, preparation, and usage: 9g each of alpinia oxyphylla, albizia flowers, grass-leaved sweetflag, glossy privet fruit, fried eucommia bark, achyranthes root, lotus plumule, bamboo leaves, paper mulberry fruit, eclipta prostrata, orostachys fimbriata, polygonatum, and medicated leaven, and 30g of fleece-flower root. Grind the above herbs finely, refine honey to make pills, with each pill weighing 1.6g. Daily dosage: 2 pills for 1-year-olds, 4 pills for 3-year-olds, and 6 pills for 6-year-olds, taken in 2-3 divided doses.

2. 儿童智力晶：能健胃、安神、开窍、益智，提高大脑功能。药物组成及制法：人参 30 克，肉豆蔻 90 克，菖蒲、远志、补骨脂各 120 克。上药研细，加入蜂蜜、白糖适量，制成结晶颗粒。服法：儿童每次取一匙（约 9 克）温水溶后服，日服 2 次。

2. Children’s Intelligence Crystals: It can invigorate the stomach, calm the mind, open the orifices, enhance intelligence, and improve brain function. Composition and preparation: 30g of ginseng, 90g of nutmeg, and 120g each of grass-leaved sweetflag, polygala root, and psoralea fruit. Grind the above herbs finely, add an appropriate amount of honey and white sugar, and make them into

crystalline granules. Usage: Children take one teaspoon (about 9g) each time, dissolved in warm water, twice a day.

《民族医药报》1992 年 6 月 5 日（广东 陈烈辉）

Ethnic Medicine News, June 5, 1992 (Chen Liehui, Guangdong)

（六）小儿流涎验方（2 方）

(6) Effective Prescriptions for Pediatric Drooling (2 Prescriptions)

1. 生白术 10 克。用法：将药捣碎，加水和白糖适量，放锅蒸汁，分次口服，每日一剂，连服 3-5 天即可奏效。

10g of raw atractylodes macrocephala. Usage: Crush the herb, add an appropriate amount of water and white sugar, steam it in a pot to extract the juice, and take it orally in divided doses. Take one dose daily, and it will take effect after 3-5 consecutive days of use.

2. 吴茱萸 3 份，胆南星 1 份。用法：将上药研细粉混匀，贮瓶密封，备用。睡前取上药 15 克，用陈米醋调成粘厚糊状饼，敷贴双脚底涌泉穴，外用纱布扎紧。每次贴 12 小时，3-4 次即可治愈。

2. 3 parts of evodia fruit and 1 part of arisaema with bile. Usage: Grind the above herbs into a fine powder, mix well, store in a sealed bottle for future use. Before going to bed, take 15g of the powder, mix it with aged rice vinegar to form a thick, sticky paste cake, apply it to the Yongquan acupoints on the soles of both feet, and wrap it tightly with gauze. Apply for 12 hours each time, and the condition can be cured after 3-4 applications.

《中医药信息报》（王廷兆）

TCM Information News (Wang Tingzhao)

七、小儿脐疗（30 方）

VII. Pediatric Umbilical Therapy (30 Prescriptions)

敷脐是中医一种独特的治疗方法。肚脐在经络学说中属任脉的神阙穴，为人体元气之海，维系着全身的经脉。脐部皮肤又有薄且多皱的特点，最利于药物的吸收，故敷脐疗法具有疗效好、方法简单易行等特点。现介绍几种常见儿科疾病的敷脐疗法，供选用。

Umbilical application is a unique therapeutic method in Traditional Chinese Medicine (TCM). In meridian theory, the navel is the Shenque acupoint of the Conception Vessel (Ren Meridian), which serves as the sea of primordial qi in the human body and maintains the meridians throughout the body. The skin of the umbilical area is thin and highly wrinkled, making it most conducive to drug absorption. Therefore, umbilical therapy is characterized by good therapeutic effects and simple, easy-to-implement methods. Several umbilical therapies for common pediatric diseases are now introduced for selection.

1. 新生儿脐炎取云南白药适量。先用生理盐水或新洁尔灭溶液将患儿脐部的分泌物清洗干净，然后将云南白药敷在患儿的肚脐处，并盖上一块无菌纱布，再用绷带将其包扎好。隔日换药一次。一般用药 2 次即可痊愈。

1. For neonatal omphalitis, take an appropriate amount of Yunnan Baiyao (a well-known Chinese patent medicine). First, use normal saline or benzalkonium bromide solution to thoroughly clean the secretions around the infant' s umbilicus. Then, apply Yunnan Baiyao to the navel, cover it with a piece of sterile gauze, and bandage it properly. Change the medication every other day. Generally, two applications can cure the condition.

2. 小儿遗尿鲜葱白 10 段（2 寸长）与硫磺 12g 捣烂成饼状，在小儿睡前将药饼敷在肚脐中，以纱布覆盖固定，2 日换药 1 次，可连用 2 周左右，遗尿可愈。

2. For pediatric enuresis, take 10 pieces of fresh scallion whites (2 cun long) and 12g of sulfur, and pound them into a cake shape. Before the child goes to bed, apply the herbal cake to the navel, cover it with gauze, and secure it. Change the medication once every two days. It can be used continuously for about two weeks to cure enuresis.

3. 小儿口舌生疮取细辛 2.5g，将细辛研为细末，然后用适量的面粉及温开水将细辛末调成直径为 3-4cm，厚度为 0.5cm 的面饼，并将此药饼敷在患儿的肚脐处。在药饼上盖层塑料薄膜，一块无菌纱布。再用胶布固定好。每日早晚各换药 1 次。3 天为 1 疗程。多数患儿在经过 1 个疗程治疗后即可痊愈。

3. For pediatric oral and tongue ulcers, take 2.5g of asarum and grind it into a fine powder. Then, use an appropriate amount of flour and warm boiled water to mix the asarum powder into a dough cake with a diameter of 3-4 cm and a thickness of 0.5 cm. Apply this herbal cake to the child’s navel. Cover the cake with a layer of plastic film and a piece of sterile gauze, and then secure it with medical tape. Change the medication once in the morning and once in the evening. Three days constitute one course of treatment. Most children can be cured after one course of treatment.

4. 小儿流涎症取益智仁 9g，车前子 6g，甘草 3g。将上药共研成细末备用。每次用药时，将适量的药末用少许食醋调成稀糊状，敷于患儿肚脐处，再用伤湿止痛膏固定。敷药期间可间断地用热水袋热敷肚脐处。每天换药 1 次，一般 3-5 天即可见效。

4. For pediatric drooling, take 9g of alpinia oxyphylla, 6g of plantain seeds, and 3g of licorice. Grind the above herbs together into a fine powder for later use. Each time the medication is applied, mix an appropriate amount of the powder with a little edible vinegar to form a thin paste, apply it to the child’s navel, and secure it with a rheumatism-relieving analgesic plaster. During the application period, a hot water bottle can be used to apply intermittent warm compresses to the navel. Change the medication once a day; generally, it will take effect within 3-5 days.

5. 小儿便秘取生大黄适量，将生大黄烘干后研成细末备用。每次取生大黄粉末 10g，用适量的白酒将其调成糊状，敷于患儿肚脐上，再盖上一块无菌纱布，并用胶布固定好，然后用热水袋热敷肚脐处 10 分钟，每天换药 1 次，一般 3-5 天可见效。

5. For pediatric constipation, take an appropriate amount of raw rhubarb, dry it, and grind it into a fine powder for later use. Each time, take 10g of raw rhubarb powder, mix it with an appropriate amount of liquor to form a paste, and apply it to the child’s navel. Cover it with a piece of sterile gauze and secure it with

medical tape. Then, use a hot water bottle to apply a warm compress to the navel for 10 minutes. Change the medication once a day; generally, it will take effect within 3-5 days.

6. 婴幼儿腹泻取白胡椒 2g，研成细末备用。先将患儿的神阙穴及长强穴（在尾骨尖下 0.5 寸处，相当于尾骨尖与肛门的中点）清洗干净，然后分别将白胡椒粉 1g 置于神阙穴和长强穴上，再盖上一块无菌纱布，并用胶布固定好。每天换药 1 次，3 天为 1 疗程。

6. For infantile diarrhea, take 2g of white pepper and grind it into a fine powder for later use. First, clean the child's Shenque acupoint and Changqiang acupoint (located 0.5 cun below the tip of the coccyx, which is the midpoint between the coccyx tip and the anus). Then, place 1g of white pepper powder on the Shenque acupoint and 1g on the Changqiang acupoint respectively. Cover them with a piece of sterile gauze and secure them with medical tape. Change the medication once a day, with three days constituting one course of treatment.

7. 小儿盗汗取五倍子适量研成细末备用。每晚临睡前取适量的药末用温水调成软面状，敷于患儿肚脐处，再盖上一块无菌纱布，并用胶布固定，于第二天清晨将药面饼除掉。每日换药 1 次，一般 3-5 天可见效。

7. For pediatric night sweats, take an appropriate amount of Chinese gallnuts and grind them into a fine powder for later use. Every night before going to bed, take an appropriate amount of the powder and mix it with warm water into a soft dough-like consistency. Apply it to the child's navel, cover it with a piece of sterile gauze, and secure it with medical tape. Remove the herbal dough cake the next morning. Change the medication once a day; generally, it will take effect within 3-5 days.

8. 小儿睾丸鞘膜积液取丁香 40g，研成细末备用。每次用药前将患儿的脐周洗净擦干。然后取丁香粉 2g 敷在患儿的肚脐处，让药粉高于周围的皮肤约 0.2cm，再盖上一块无菌纱布，并用胶布固定。每隔 2 天换药 1 次，20 天为 1 疗程。如第 1 个疗程结束后，患儿的病情仍未痊愈，可间隔 5-10 天再进行第 2 个疗程的治疗。多数患儿在经过 2-3 个疗程治疗后，会收到明显的疗效。

8. For pediatric hydrocele of the tunica vaginalis, take 40g of cloves and grind them into a fine powder for later use. Before each application, wash the area around the child' s navel and wipe it dry. Then, apply 2g of clove powder to the child' s navel so that the powder is about 0.2 cm higher than the surrounding skin. Cover it with a piece of sterile gauze and secure it with medical tape. Change the medication every two days, with 20 days constituting one course of treatment. If the child' s condition is not cured after the first course, the second course can be administered after an interval of 5-10 days. Most children will achieve significant therapeutic effects after 2-3 courses of treatment.

《健康报》

Health News

遗溺，又名尿床，系患儿在睡眠中不知不觉地小便，多见于 5-14 岁儿童。我根据辨证施治原则，采用脐疗法，进行治疗获得了满意的疗效。

Enuresis, also known as bedwetting, refers to the involuntary urination of a child during sleep without their awareness. It is most commonly seen in children aged 5 to 14. Based on the principle of syndrome differentiation and treatment, I have applied umbilical therapy to treat this condition and achieved satisfactory therapeutic effects.

9. 龙倍散，方用煅龙骨、五倍子各等份，研细末，以冷开水调成厚糊状，涂满肚脐，外以小红布膏药或肤疾宁贴紧，两天换药一次，两周一疗程。主治小儿肾虚，膀胱失约，夜间尿床。亦治大人遗精、自汗、盗汗。龙骨煅用，功能收敛固涩，五倍子含 70-80% 鞣质，有很强的收敛作用。二药合用，固涩止遗的效果得到了加强。

9. Longbei Powder: The prescription uses equal parts of calcined dragon bone and Chinese gallnuts, ground into a fine powder. Mix them with cold boiled water into a thick paste, apply it to completely fill the navel, and cover it tightly with a small red cloth plaster or Fujining (a medicated plaster). Change the medication once every two days, with two weeks constituting one course of treatment. It is mainly used for pediatric kidney deficiency and loss of bladder control leading

to bedwetting at night. It also treats adult nocturnal emission, spontaneous sweating, and night sweats. Calcined dragon bone has the function of astringency and consolidation. Chinese gallnuts contain 70-80% tannins and have a strong astringent effect. The combination of these two herbs enhances the effect of consolidation and stopping enuresis.

10. 葱硫饼方用鲜葱白七段，与适量硫磺共捣如泥状，每晚睡前将脐部洗净，将药饼敷上，纱布覆盖，胶布固定，次晨除去，连敷 5 日，遗尿即止。以后改为隔日晚间敷药一次，以巩固疗效。主治年龄较大的遗尿患儿，用固涩收敛药不效，同时伴有恶寒背冷，腰疼、腿软、小便清长等下元虚冷证象的。葱白辛温，能散寒通阳；硫磺温热，能补火壮阳。二药合用，共奏振奋肾阳，恢复封藏的功能。

10. Congliu Cake (Scallion and Sulfur Cake): The prescription uses seven pieces of fresh scallion whites and an appropriate amount of sulfur, pounded together into a mud-like paste. Wash the navel every night before going to bed, apply the herbal cake, cover it with gauze, and secure it with medical tape. Remove it the next morning. Apply it continuously for 5 days to stop enuresis. Afterwards, change to applying the medication once every other night to consolidate the therapeutic effect. It is mainly used for older children with enuresis who do not respond to astringent and consolidating herbs, and who are accompanied by symptoms of deficiency-cold in the lower jiao, such as aversion to cold and cold back, lumbago, weak legs, and copious clear urine. Scallion whites are pungent and warm, which can dispel cold and unblock yang; sulfur is warm and hot, which can tonify fire and invigorate yang. The combination of these two herbs works together to invigorate kidney yang and restore the function of storing and retaining essence.

《健康报》1990 年 10 月 6 日

Health News, October 6, 1990

11. 治小儿夏季热：丝瓜叶、苦瓜叶、南瓜叶、荷叶各 2 片，井青台 1 小撮，捣烂后敷于肚脐，每日两次。

11. For treating pediatric summer heat: Take 2 leaves each of loofah, bitter gourd, pumpkin, and lotus, along with a small pinch of Jingqingtai (a type of moss). Pound them into a paste and apply it to the navel twice a day.

12. 治小儿泄泻：干姜、白芷各 5 克，共研细末，酒调敷脐上，每日两次。

12. For treating pediatric diarrhea: Take 5g each of dried ginger and dahurian angelica root, and grind them together into a fine powder. Mix the powder with liquor and apply it to the navel twice a day.

13. 治小儿感冒发热：雄黄 3 克，天南星 20 克，共研细末，与适量面粉调成饼状，敷足底涌泉穴，包扎好，每日换 1 次，一般 2-3 次可愈。

13. For treating pediatric cold and fever: Take 3g of realgar and 20g of arisaema, and grind them together into a fine powder. Mix the powder with an appropriate amount of flour to form a cake, apply it to the Yongquan acupoint on the sole of the foot, and bandage it properly. Change the medication once a day; generally, 2-3 applications can cure the condition.

14. 治小儿惊风：

14. For treating pediatric convulsions:

过墙风 30 克，鸡蛋适量，捣烂后共煎，微热包肚脐，每日 1 次。

Take 30g of Guoqiangfeng (a climbing herb) and an appropriate amount of eggs. Pound them together and decoct them. While slightly warm, wrap the mixture around the navel once a day.

燕子巢捣烂，加入适量鸭蛋清再捣烂如泥，敷于肚脐上，每日一换。

Pound a swallow’ s nest into a pulp, add an appropriate amount of duck egg white, and pound again until it becomes a mud-like paste. Apply it to the navel and change the medication once a day.

15. 治小儿夜啼：丁香 5 克，米饭适量。先将丁香研末再同米饭捣烂作饼，贴肚脐上。

15. For treating pediatric nocturnal crying: Take 5g of cloves and an appropriate amount of cooked rice. First, grind the cloves into a powder, then pound it together with the rice to form a cake, and apply it to the navel.

16. 治小儿疳积：山栀 10 克，将栀子研末加面粉，与鸡蛋清调成 3 个饼，分别敷贴于肚脐和两足足底涌泉穴。每日 1 次，3-4 次可愈。

16. For treating pediatric malnutrition (infantile malnutrition): Take 10g of gardenia fruit. Grind the gardenia into a powder, add flour, and mix with egg white to form 3 cakes. Apply them to the navel and the Yongquan acupoints on the soles of both feet respectively. Apply once a day; 3-4 applications can cure the condition.

17. 治小儿消化不良：胡椒、丁香各 10 克，共研细末，调和成饼，敷肚脐上，每日换 1 次，连续 3-4 次可愈。

17. For treating pediatric indigestion: Take 10g each of black pepper and cloves, and grind them together into a fine powder. Mix them to form a cake and apply it to the navel. Change the medication once a day; continuous application for 3-4 times can cure the condition.

18. 治小儿呕吐：将明矾 15 克研细末用米汤调成浆敷足底涌泉穴，每日 2 次，2-3 日可愈。

18. For treating pediatric vomiting: Grind 15g of alum into a fine powder, mix it with rice soup to form a slurry, and apply it to thc Yongquan acupoint on the sole of the foot. Apply twice a day; it can be cured within 2-3 days.

《民族医药报》1992 年 8 月 7 日（湖南 杨玉钊）

Ethnic Medicine News, August 7, 1992 (Yang Yuzhao, Hunan)

19. 敷脐 治婴幼儿泄泻：秋季腹泻多为病毒感染，婴幼儿发病率较高，轻症每日 5-6 次，多可达 10 余次，水样便，呈黄或黄绿色、白色，有的呕吐，益乳，食欲减退，有低热。治疗方法：胡椒 10 克，用嘴嚼碎后放于肚脐，然后用一块长 8 厘米、宽 3 厘米胶布贴于肚脐固定，以免胡椒散失，24 小时更换 1 次，3-4 次即愈。

19. Umbilical Application for Treating Infantile Diarrhea: Autumn diarrhea is mostly caused by viral infections, with a high incidence rate in infants and toddlers. In mild cases, bowel movements occur 5-6 times a day, and can often reach over 10 times. The stool is watery, appearing yellow, yellowish-green, or

white. Some patients experience vomiting, increased milk intake, loss of appetite, and low-grade fever. Treatment method: Take 10g of black pepper, chew it into pieces, and place it in the navel. Then, apply an 8 cm long and 3 cm wide piece of medical tape over the navel to secure it and prevent the pepper from spilling out. Change the medication every 24 hours; 3-4 applications can cure the condition.

祖国医学认为泄泻为湿盛脾虚，婴幼儿阳常有余，脾常不足，此药具有祛湿，除寒、温中健脾之功，脐的皮肤筋膜与腹膜相连，故使药直达病所。

Traditional Chinese Medicine believes that diarrhea is caused by excessive dampness and spleen deficiency. Infants and toddlers often have an excess of yang and a deficiency of the spleen. This herb has the effects of dispelling dampness, eliminating cold, warming the middle jiao, and invigorating the spleen. The skin and fascia of the navel are connected to the peritoneum, allowing the medicinal properties to directly reach the affected area.

《民族医药报》1992 年 4 月 17 日

Ethnic Medicine News, April 17, 1992

20. 三黄煎剂湿敷治新生儿脐疮

20. Wet Compress with Sanhuang Decoction for Treating Neonatal Umbilical Ulcers

方药：黄连、黄柏、黄芩、生大黄各 20 克，苦参、地榆、五倍子各 15 克。

Prescription: 20g each of coptis, phellodendron, scutellaria, and raw rhubarb; 15g each of sophora flavescens, garden burnet, and Chinese gallnuts.

用法：加水 500 毫升煎取 200 毫升，装入消毒瓶备用。以消毒敷料浸药汁外敷脐部，早、晚各一次，若渗出液多则可酌情增加换药次数。

Usage: Add 500 ml of water to decoct the herbs until 200 ml remains, and store it in a sterilized bottle for later use. Soak a sterile dressing in the medicinal liquid and apply it externally to the umbilical area once in the morning and once in the evening. If there is excessive exudate, the frequency of dressing changes can be increased as appropriate.

疗效分析：中医认为，新生儿脐疮由脐湿不干，湿与热邪互结，日久溃烂所致。

笔者运用清热燥湿、活血凉血、生肌收敛之三黄煎剂湿敷脐部，使药物直中病位，易于吸收，发挥药效，且利于炎症分泌物排泄，使疮面干燥，有利炎症创面修复；同时避膏散之类易形成脓痂，不利炎症创面修复之嫌。

Therapeutic Analysis: Traditional Chinese Medicine (TCM) believes that neonatal umbilical ulcers are caused by prolonged umbilical dampness, where dampness and heat pathogens intertwine, leading to ulceration over time. The author uses the Sanhuang decoction for wet compresses, which has the effects of clearing heat and eliminating dampness, promoting blood circulation and cooling the blood, as well as generating flesh and astringency. This allows the medicine to directly target the lesion, be easily absorbed, and exert its therapeutic effects. It also facilitates the drainage of inflammatory secretions and dries the ulcer surface, promoting the repair of the inflammatory wound. At the same time, it avoids the potential drawbacks of pastes and powders, which easily form purulent scabs and hinder the repair of inflammatory wounds.

《民族医药报》1992 年 3 月 13 日（广西 韦金星）

Ethnic Medicine News, March 13, 1992 (Wei Jinxing, Guangxi)

21. 小儿寒泻，常因年轻父母对小儿护理不周，孩子肚子受凉而引起。主要症状是，大便稀薄，偶有泡沫，绿色。近年来，笔者用艾绒肚兜治疗该疾，收效甚佳，故介绍如下。

21. Pediatric cold diarrhea is often caused by inadequate care from young parents, leading to the child's abdomen catching a cold. The main symptoms are thin stools, occasionally with foam, and a green color. In recent years, the author has used an Artemisia (mugwort) floss belly pouch to treat this condition with excellent results, which is introduced as follows.

方法：取艾绒约 30 克，烘去潮气（如无艾绒，也可用艾叶去茎梗杂质，揉成绒状），用棉布或纱布做一只兜，夹层内铺入艾绒，用线缝好，然后固定在患儿的肚脐上。晨起就可摘下。一般兜一夜腹泻即止。该法无副作用。

Method: Take about 30g of Artemisia floss and bake it to remove moisture (if Artemisia floss is unavailable, mugwort leaves can be used by removing the stems and impurities, then rubbing them into a floss-like texture). Make a pouch using cotton cloth or gauze, spread the Artemisia floss in the interlayer, sew it up, and then fix it on the child' s navel. It can be removed in the morning. Generally, wearing it overnight can stop the diarrhea. This method has no side effects.

《民族医药报》1992 年 6 月 5 日（湖南 兰家长）

Ethnic Medicine News, June 5, 1992 (Lan Jiazhang, Hunan)

药兜，是民间防治疾病的疗法之一。其制法是以柔软的棉布，摺成大小能覆盖脐腹部的兜肚形，内层铺少许棉花，把所用药物研成细末均匀置于棉花上，再盖上稍厚的棉花，经过纵横缝纫，使药末固定在网状小格中以免堆积，佩戴在脐腹上，使药物缓缓发生作用。现介绍一些小儿疾病的中药兜肚方法如下。

Medicinal pouches are one of the folk therapies for preventing and treating diseases. The preparation method involves folding soft cotton cloth into a belly-covering pouch large enough to cover the umbilical and abdominal area. A small amount of cotton is laid in the inner layer, and the medicinal herbs are ground into a fine powder and evenly placed on the cotton. Then, a slightly thicker layer of cotton is placed on top. Through crisscross stitching, the medicinal powder is fixed in a grid-like pattern to prevent clumping. When worn over the umbilical and abdominal area, the medicine exerts its effects gradually. Some TCM medicinal pouch methods for pediatric diseases are introduced as follows.

22. 治小儿厌食：

22. For treating pediatric anorexia:

可将黄芪、黄精、砂仁各 10 克，鸡内金、苍术、青黛、二丑、皮硝各 6 克、麝香 0.15 克，研为细末，做成兜肚，佩戴在脐部，10-15 天换药 1 次。

Take 10g each of astragalus, polygonatum, and amomum fruit; 6g each of chicken gizzard lining, atractylodes, indigo naturalis, morning glory seeds, and mirabilite; and 0.15g of musk. Grind them into a fine powder, make a medicinal pouch, wear it over the navel, and change the medication once every 10-15 days.

23. 治小儿疳证：

23. For treating pediatric malnutrition:

取五谷虫、麦芽、神曲、苍术、炒鸡内金、槟榔、香附、砂仁、肉果各 10 克、冰片 3 克，研为细末，做成兜肚，经常佩戴，半月换药 1 次。

Take 10g each of grain fly larvae, malt, medicated leaven, atractylodes, fried chicken gizzard lining, betel nut, cyperus, amomum fruit, and nutmeg; and 3g of borneol. Grind them into a fine powder, make a medicinal pouch, wear it regularly, and change the medication once every half month.

24. 治小儿每在睡中遗尿：

24. For treating pediatric enuresis during sleep:

可将乌贼骨 20 克，枯矾 10 克，肉桂 5 克研为细末，做在兜肚，每天晚上佩戴，睡前先用热水袋热敷药兜 15-20 分钟，每 2 天换药 1 次。

Take 20g of cuttlebone, 10g of calcined alum, and 5g of cinnamon bark, and grind them into a fine powder. Make a medicinal pouch and wear it every night. Before going to bed, use a hot water bottle to apply a warm compress to the pouch for 15-20 minutes, and change the medication once every two days.

25. 治小儿夜啼，下半夜尤甚：

25. For treating pediatric nocturnal crying, especially in the second half of the night:

取丁香、肉桂、吴茱萸各 15 克，研为细末，做成药物兜肚，每天晚上佩戴，睡前用热水袋热敷药兜 15-20 分钟，每 3 天换药 1 次。

Take 15g each of cloves, cinnamon bark, and evodia fruit, and grind them into a fine powder. Make a medicinal pouch and wear it every night. Before going to bed, use a hot water bottle to apply a warm compress to the pouch for 15-20 minutes, and change the medication once every three days.

26. 治小儿脘腹胀满，昼轻夜重：

26. For treating pediatric abdominal distension and fullness, which is milder during the day and worse at night:

用炒白术、枳实各 20 克，研为细末，与麝香 0.15 克混匀，做成药物兜肚，经常佩戴，每天晚上用热水袋热敷药兜 10 分钟，5 天换药 1 次。

Take 20g each of fried atractylodes macrocephala and bitter orange, and grind them into a fine powder. Mix them evenly with 0.15g of musk, make a medicinal pouch, wear it regularly, use a hot water bottle to apply a warm compress to the pouch for 10 minutes every night, and change the medication once every five days.

27. 治小儿久泻不止，便有不消化食物：

27. For treating prolonged pediatric diarrhea with undigested food in the stool:

用干姜、艾叶、小茴香各 20 克，川椒 15 克，共研为细末，做成兜肚，佩戴在脐腹部，每晚用热水袋热敷药兜 15 分钟，10 天换药 1 次。

Take 20g each of dried ginger, mugwort leaves, and fennel; and 15g of Sichuan pepper. Grind them together into a fine powder, make a medicinal pouch, wear it over the umbilical and abdominal area, use a hot water bottle to apply a warm compress to the pouch for 15 minutes every night, and change the medication once every ten days.

28. 小儿急惊风：

28. For pediatric acute convulsions:

将人参、白术、茯神、琥珀、天麻、白僵蚕、胡椒、防风、胆南星、生白附子、乌梢蛇（酒焙）各 3 克、艾叶 15 克，麝香 0.1 克研为细末，做成药兜，经常佩戴，10 天换药 1 次。

Take 3g each of ginseng, atractylodes macrocephala, poria with hostwood, amber, gastrodia, stiff silkworm, black pepper, saposhnikovia, arisaema with bile, raw pinellia, and Zaocys dhumnades (baked with wine); and 15g of mugwort leaves. Grind them together with 0.1g of musk into a fine powder, make a medicinal pouch, wear it regularly, and change the medication once every ten days.

《民族医药报》1992 年 5 月 22 日（河北 刘健英）

Ethnic Medicine News, May 22, 1992 (Liu Jianying, Hebei)

29. 用 2% 碘酒在患儿脐周消毒（半径约为 5 厘米范围），然后用 75% 酒精脱碘，再用 75% 酒精将云南白药的药粉调成糊状，并以 4 厘米半径在脐周敷盖，最后用消毒纱布固定，24 小时后除药更换。一般连用 3 天左右即可收到理想效果。该方法简单易行，疗效肯定，易被患儿接受。

29. Disinfect the area around the child’s navel (with a radius of about 5 cm)

using 2% iodine tincture, then remove the iodine with 75% alcohol. Next, use 75% alcohol to mix Yunnan Baiyao powder into a paste, and apply it around the navel with a radius of 4 cm. Finally, secure it with sterile gauze and remove and replace the medication after 24 hours. Generally, continuous use for about three days can achieve ideal results. This method is simple, easy to implement, has definite therapeutic effects, and is easily accepted by children.

《民族医药报》1992 年 8 月 21 日（吉林 张英俊）

Ethnic Medicine News, August 21, 1992 (Zhang Yingjun, Jilin)

30. 婴幼儿腹泻是 2 岁以下小儿常见病，河南驻马店市医院徐文清医师等近年采用白胡椒粉敷贴神阙、长强二穴治疗 214 例，获效满意。

30. Infantile diarrhea is a common disease in children under the age of two. In recent years, Dr. Xu Wenqing and others at Zhumadian City Hospital in Henan Province have used white pepper powder applied to the Shenque and Changqiang acupoints to treat 214 cases, achieving satisfactory results.

将患儿神阙及长强穴局部洗净，每穴每次敷贴研细的白胡椒粉一克，用胶布固定于穴位上。每日更换 1 次，连用 3 次为一疗程，经治疗 214 例有效率为 97.2%，结果优于常规西药对照组。

Wash the local areas of the Shenque and Changqiang acupoints of the child, apply 1g of finely ground white pepper powder to each acupoint each time, and secure it to the acupoints with medical tape. Change the medication once a day, with three consecutive applications constituting one course of treatment. Among the 214 treated cases, the effective rate was 97.2%, and the results were superior to those of the conventional Western medicine control group.

《中医药信息报》1992 年 1 月 25 日（计惠民）

TCM Information News, January 25, 1992 (Ji Huimin)

第十二章 肿瘤
Chapter 12 Tumors

一、治癌验方（25 方）
I. Effective Prescriptions for Treating Cancer (25 Prescriptions)

1. 旋复花（包）15 克，蒲公英 30 克，海藻、昆布各 15 克，煨三棱、煨莪术、赤芍、川贝各 10 克，炒橘核、牡蛎粉各 24 克，紫花地丁、夏枯草各 30 克，白花蛇舌草 90 克。水煎去渣，加蜂蜜 60 克熬和，分 2 日 6 次服。禁忌一切发疮动火之物。

1. 15g of inula flower (wrapped in gauze), 30g of dandelion, 15g each of seaweed and kelp, 10g each of baked sparganium, baked zedoary, red peony root, and Fritillaria cirrhosa, 24g each of fried tangerine seeds and oyster shell powder, 30g each of violet and common selfheal fruit spike, and 90g of oldenlandia. Decoct the herbs in water, remove the dregs, add 60g of honey, and simmer to mix well. Take the decoction in six divided doses over two days. Avoid all foods that can induce sores or generate internal heat.

湖北中医学院张梦依先生治疗唐某，男，26 岁。确诊为前上纵隔瘤。患者不愿手术，遂以上方治之。连续服药 2 个月，X 线拍片对照："前上纵隔瘤已完全消失"。患者自觉无任何症状，惟身体虚弱未复，再以滋阴润燥，败毒消肿法善其后。方用太子参、南沙参、山药、玉竹各 15 克，麦冬、天冬、茯苓、生甘草各 10 克，白花蛇舌草、白茅根各 60 克。水煎服，每日 1 剂。2 月后，再次拍片，肿块消失，一切正常，已上班工作。

Mr. Zhang Mengyi from Hubei College of Traditional Chinese Medicine treated a 26-year-old male patient surnamed Tang, who was diagnosed with an anterior superior mediastinal tumor. The patient refused surgery, so the above prescription was used. After taking the medication continuously for two months, a follow-up X-ray showed: "The anterior superior mediastinal tumor has completely disappeared." The patient had no symptoms but still felt physically weak. To consolidate the treatment, a method of nourishing yin, moistening dryness, eliminating toxins, and reducing swelling was applied. The prescription used was 15g each of pseudostellaria root, adenophora root, Chinese yam, and polygonatum odoratum; 10g each of ophiopogon, asparagus root, poria, and raw licorice; and 60g each of oldenlandia and cogongrass rhizome. Decocted in water and taken one dose daily. Two months later, another X-ray showed the mass had disappeared and everything was normal, and the patient had returned to work.

2. 核桃树枝，每次 200-250 克，鲜、干均可，煮鸡蛋（每次 3 个，带壳煮），小火煮 4 小时后，吃蛋及部分汤汁，余汁亦分次服完。

2. 200-250g of walnut tree branches (fresh or dried) are boiled with 3 eggs (with shells) over low heat for 4 hours. Eat the eggs and drink part of the soup; the remaining soup should be consumed in divided doses.

《江苏中医杂志》（1980.2）报告：以此方长期服用，治愈 一例胃淋巴肉瘤患者。

Jiangsu Journal of Traditional Chinese Medicine (February 1980) reported: Long-term use of this prescription cured a patient with gastric lymphosarcoma.

3. 攻坚丸：马钱子 5 克、蝎牛 2.5 克、蜈蚣 7.5 克、乳香 2.5 克、带子蜂房 2.5 克、全蝎 1.5 克。马钱子用井水泡渍 24 小时后换清水，连续泡 7-10 天，每 24 小时换水一次。取出去皮晒干，用麻油炒黄，研为细末。将蜈蚣、全蝎、蜂房炒微黄研末。将蝎牛捣烂晒干，研末。然后把以上各种细末，和乳香粉末充分混合，制成小水丸，每 20 粒约 5 克左右。治疗胃癌每次 10 粒，每日 2 次。本方若同时配合化疗进行，则效果会更加显著。

3. Jiangong Pills (Tumor-Resolving Pills): 5g of nux vomica, 2.5g of scorpion cattle, 7.5g of centipede, 2.5g of frankincense, 2.5g of wasp nest with larvae, and 1.5g of scorpion. Soak the nux vomica in well water for 24 hours, then change

to fresh water. Continue soaking for 7-10 days, changing the water once every 24 hours. Remove, peel, sun-dry, fry in sesame oil until yellow, and grind into a fine powder. Fry the centipede, scorpion, and wasp nest until slightly yellow, then grind into powder. Pound the scorpion cattle into a pulp, sun-dry, and grind into powder. Thoroughly mix all the above fine powders with the frankincense powder, and make small water pills, with 20 pills weighing about 5g. For treating gastric cancer, take 10 pills each time, twice a day. If this prescription is used in combination with chemotherapy, the effect will be more significant.

4. 粘液腺癌方：半枝莲 60 克，山豆根、制鳖甲、制牡蛎各 30 克，夏枯草、女贞子各 15 克，天南星、枳实各 12 克，党参、白术、茯苓、制甘草、陈皮、半夏、地龙各 9 克，水煎服，每日 1 剂。

4. Prescription for Mucinous Adenocarcinoma: 60g of scutellaria barbata, 30g each of subprostrate sophora root, processed turtle shell, and processed oyster shell, 15g each of common selfheal fruit spike and glossy privet fruit, 12g each of arisaema and bitter orange, and 9g each of codonopsis, atractylodes, poria, processed licorice, tangerine peel, pinellia, and earthworm. Decoct in water and take one dose daily.

上海市肿瘤医院用本方配合针刺，主穴：章门、痞根；配穴：内关、足三里及胸背部反应点。治疗腹壁广泛转移性粘液腺癌病人，取得一定疗效。

Shanghai Cancer Hospital used this prescription combined with acupuncture. Main acupoints: Zhangmen and Pigen; Auxiliary acupoints: Neiguan, Zusanli, and reactive points on the chest and back. This treatment achieved certain therapeutic effects in patients with extensive metastatic mucinous adenocarcinoma of the abdominal wall.

5. 胸腺肿瘤方：丹参、红花、白术、黄花、党参、山药各 25 克。清半夏、白芍、三棱、莪术、柴胡各 15 克。水煎服，每日一剂。

5. Prescription for Thymic Tumors: 25g each of salvia miltiorrhiza, safflower, atractylodes, astragalus, codonopsis, and Chinese yam; 15g each of processed pinellia, white peony root, sparganium, zedoary, and bupleurum. Decoct in water

and take one dose daily.

《新中医》（1983.11）报告：周耀群以此方加减治疗本病取得效果。

Journal of New Traditional Chinese Medicine (November 1983) reported: Zhou Yaoqun achieved therapeutic effects by modifying this prescription to treat this disease.

《中医药信息报》1992年5月30日（浙江 常敏毅）

TCM Information News, May 30, 1992 (Chang Minyi, Zhejiang)

肿瘤效验方

Effective and Verified Prescriptions for Tumors

6. 口腔黏膜白斑 I 方：蜂胶提纯后制成 50% 蜂胶复合药膜，用药时将药膜剪成相等于白斑的大小，将含蜂胶的药面贴在病变黏膜上，厚的白斑每日贴 2-3 次，薄的白斑每日贴 1-2 次。2 周为 1 疗程，如白斑未退，可继续用药，一般用药 2 个疗程后可酌情停用数天至 1 周后再继续用药。

6. Prescription I for Oral Leukoplakia: Purified propolis is made into a 50% propolis composite medicinal film. When using, cut the film to the size of the leukoplakia, and apply the propolis-containing side to the diseased mucosa. For thick leukoplakia, apply 2-3 times a day; for thin leukoplakia, apply 1-2 times a day. Two weeks constitute one course of treatment. If the leukoplakia does not subside, continue the medication. Generally, after two courses, the medication can be paused for a few days to a week as appropriate before resuming.

《中西医结合杂志》（1985.8）报告：以本方治疗癌前病变 --- 口腔黏膜白斑病人 45 例，痊愈 28 例，显效 14 例，好转 3 例。痊愈病例的治疗时间最短为 1疗程，最长为4疗程。有较好的疗效。蜂胶为蜜蜂科昆虫中华蜜蜂 Apis cerana 下，或意大利蜜蜂 A.mell：fera L. 所分泌的黄褐色或黑褐色的黏性物质，有使角化组根软化脱落及止痛等多种作用。

Journal of Integrated Traditional and Western Medicine (August 1985) reported: This prescription was used to treat 45 patients with precancerous lesions—oral leukoplakia. 28 cases were cured, 14 showed marked improvement, and 3 showed improvement. The shortest treatment time for cured cases was one course, and the longest was four courses, demonstrating good therapeutic efficacy. Propolis is a yellowish-brown or dark-brown viscous substance secreted by the honeybee Apis cerana or the Italian bee Apis mellifera L. It has multiple effects, including softening and shedding keratinized tissues and relieving pain.

7. 声带息肉癌变方：蛇莓、石见穿、开金锁各 25g，龙葵、白毛藤各 50g，金杯茶匙、麦冬各 20g。水煎服，每天 2 剂。

7. Prescription for Malignant Transformation of Vocal Cord Polyps: 25g each of snake berry, Salvia chinensis, and Fagopyrum cymosum; 50g each of black nightshade and Solanum lyratum; 20g each of Odontites vulgaris and ophiopogon. Decoct in water and take two doses daily.

此为上海民间验方。方中石见穿为唇形科的紫参 Sa1via chinsis B.，有清热解毒，活血定痛作用；开金锁为蓼科植物金荞麦 Fagopyrum Cymosum（T.）M.，有清热解毒，活血止瘀的功效。

This is a folk prescription from Shanghai. Salvia chinensis B. in the Lamiaceae family has the effects of clearing heat and detoxifying, promoting blood circulation, and relieving pain; Fagopyrum cymosum (T.) M. in the Polygonaceae family has the effects of clearing heat and detoxifying, promoting blood circulation, and resolving blood stasis.

8. 声带肿瘤方：黄毛耳草、龙葵、白毛藤、开金锁根各 50g，蛇果草 40g，小石苇 25g，米冬 20g（亦可加玄参 15g）。水煎服，每日 1 剂。

8. Prescription for Vocal Cord Tumors: 50g each of Hedyotis chrysotricha, black nightshade, Solanum lyratum, and Fagopyrum cymosum root; 40g of Potentilla anserina; 25g of Lepisorus ussuriensis; and 20g of ophiopogon (15g of scrophularia can also be added). Decoct in water and take one dose daily.

此亦为上海民间方。方中黄毛耳草又名石打穿，系茜草科植物，学名为 HedyotisichrysotrichaCP.JM.，药用全草，有清热利湿、消肿解毒的作用。

This is also a folk prescription from Shanghai. Hedyotis chrysotricha in the prescription, also known as Shidachuan, belongs to the Rubiaceae family, with the scientific name Hedyotis chrysotricha C.P.JM. The whole plant is used

medicinally, having the effects of clearing heat and eliminating dampness, reducing swelling, and detoxifying.

9. 听神经纤维瘤方：土茯苓、牡蛎（先煎）各 30g，夏枯草、丹参、玄参、钩藤、忍冬藤各 12g，昆布、海藻、防风、白芷、苍耳、荆芥各 9g，红花、旱莲草、三七粉（冲）各 3g，干地黄 18g。水煎服，每日 1 剂。

9. Prescription for Acoustic Neuroma: 30g each of smilax glabra and oyster shell (decocted first); 12g each of common selfheal fruit spike, salvia miltiorrhiza, scrophularia, uncaria, and honeysuckle stem; 9g each of kelp, seaweed, saposhnikovia, dahurian angelica root, xanthium, and schizonepeta; 3g each of safflower, eclipta, and notoginseng powder (stirred in); and 18g of dried rehmannia root. Decoct in water and take one dose daily.

《中国抗癌报》

China Anti-Cancer News

白英的药用

Medicinal Uses of Solanum lyratum

贵报一九九二年二月十五日（第六期）介绍《白英的药用》，据我所知，尚有以下的用途：国内外药理研究表明，白英含有白英硷等多种生物硷。白英硷中的 B- 苦茄碱对小鼠肉瘤 180 和瓦克癌 256 均有显著的抑制作用，日本已用于临床。我国民间用白英配伍他药治疗癌症：

Your newspaper introduced the “Medicinal Uses of Solanum lyratum” in Issue 6 on February 15, 1992. As far as I know, it has the following additional uses: Pharmacological studies both domestically and internationally have shown that Solanum lyratum contains multiple alkaloids, including solalyrine. Beta-solamarine in solalyrine has a significant inhibitory effect on mouse sarcoma 180 and Walker carcinoma 256, and it has been used clinically in Japan. In China, folk medicine uses Solanum lyratum in combination with other herbs to treat cancer:

10. 治声带癌：白英、龙葵、蛇莓、石见穿、野荞麦、麦冬、石苇。

10. For treating vocal cord cancer: Solanum lyratum, black nightshade, snake berry, Salvia chinensis, wild buckwheat, ophiopogon, and Lepisorus ussuriensis.

11. 子宫颈癌：白英配伍大枣。白英配伍苦荞麦。白英配伍龙葵、马尾伸筋草、枫树根。

11. For cervical cancer: Solanum lyratum combined with jujubes; Solanum lyratum combined with tartary buckwheat; Solanum lyratum combined with black nightshade, horse-tail clubmoss, and maple tree roots.

12. 肺癌：白英、垂盆草。

12. For lung cancer: Solanum lyratum and stringy stonecrop.

13. 膀胱癌：白英、蛇莓、龙葵。

13. For bladder cancer: Solanum lyratum, snake berry, and black nightshade.

14. 肝硬化腹水：白英、猪肝。

14. For liver cirrhosis with ascites: Solanum lyratum and pig liver.

15. 淋巴结核：白英、紫背天葵、猪瘦肉。白英、萝卜、猪瘦肉。

15. For lymphatic tuberculosis: Solanum lyratum, purple-backed amaranth, and lean pork; or Solanum lyratum, radish, and lean pork.

16. 肝脓肿：白英、蒲公英、银花、败酱草、生苡仁、冬瓜子、柴胡、丹皮、赤芍、焦山栀、生甘草。

16. For liver abscess: Solanum lyratum, dandelion, honeysuckle, patrinia, raw coix seed, winter melon seeds, bupleurum, moutan bark, red peony root, scorched gardenia, and raw licorice.

《中国抗癌报》（高闽）

China Anti-Cancer News (Gao Min)

17. 多发性神经瘤方：半枝莲、六耳棱、野菊花各 30g，当归尾 12g，象皮（先下）、炮山甲各 9g，蜈蚣 2 条，全蝎 6g，水煎服，每日 1 剂。

17. Prescription for Multiple Neuromas: 30g each of scutellaria barbata, Eupatorium chinense, and wild chrysanthemum; 12g of tail of angelica sinensis; 9g each of elephant skin (decocted first) and processed pangolin scales; 2 centipedes; and 6g of scorpion. Decoct in water and take one dose daily.

广西南宁反修医院治疗某女，19 岁。全身多处结节，疼痛，已 10 余年。经病理切片确诊为多发性神经瘤。1990 年初，先用半枝莲、六耳棱、野菊花各

30g，水煎，服药 5 剂后，疼痛减轻。即改以上方，共用 30 余剂，疼痛消失，各处结节肿块均明显缩小。

A 19-year-old female patient was treated at Fanxiu Hospital in Nanning, Guangxi. She had multiple nodules all over her body accompanied by pain for over 10 years. She was diagnosed with multiple neuromas via pathological section. In early 1990, she was first given a decoction of 30g each of scutellaria barbata, Eupatorium chinense, and wild chrysanthemum. After taking 5 doses, her pain was relieved. She was then switched to the above prescription. After taking more than 30 doses in total, her pain disappeared, and the nodules and masses in various parts of her body significantly shrank.

18. 神经系统纤维瘤方：天南星、生半夏各 80g ，苍耳草、白蒺藜各 15g，加生姜适量，水煎服，每日 1 剂。

18. Prescription for Nervous System Fibromas: 80g each of arisaema and raw pinellia; 15g each of xanthium herb and puncturevine caltrop fruit; with an appropriate amount of fresh ginger added. Decoct in water and take one dose daily.

此方出自《实用抗癌手册》。方中天南星和半夏都是生用，大大超过常规剂量。但肿瘤病人用之，多无中毒等反应，反而有疗效。

This prescription comes from the Practical Anti-Cancer Handbook. Both arisaema and pinellia in this prescription are used in their raw form, which greatly exceeds the conventional dosage. However, when used in cancer patients, they mostly do not cause poisoning or other adverse reactions, but instead produce therapeutic effects.

19. 放射性口腔炎方：生地、天冬、麦冬、金银花、连翘各 15g，玄参、沙参、石斛各 12g，花芩 10g，生甘草 5g。咽喉红肿疼痛伴溃疡者加山豆根、板蓝根各 15g；恶心呕吐，舌苔白滑或黏腻者，原方去生地、玄参、甘草，加藿香、佩兰各 6g，陈皮 5g，生薏苡仁 30g；伴咳嗽痰血者，加仙游草、旱莲草各 12g。

19. Prescription for Radiation-induced Stomatitis: 15g each of raw rehmannia, asparagus root, ophiopogon, honeysuckle, and forsythia; 12g each

of scrophularia, adenophora, and dendrobium; 10g of scutellaria; and 5g of raw licorice. For patients with red, swollen, and painful throat accompanied by ulcers, add 15g each of subprostrate sophora root and isatis root. For patients with nausea, vomiting, and a white, slippery, or sticky tongue coating, remove raw rehmannia, scrophularia, and licorice from the original prescription, and add 6g each of patchouli and eupatorium, 5g of tangerine peel, and 30g of raw coix seed. For patients accompanied by coughing with blood-tinged sputum, add 12g each of Aster tataricus and eclipta.

《江苏中医》（1989.10）报告：本方对舌体癌、鼻咽癌、恶性淋巴瘤，扁桃体瘤、肺癌、喉癌等病人，放疗后出现口腔炎，以本方治疗，效果很好。结果口腔炎及溃疡均于用药后 3 -14 日消退。在水煎服本方同时，尚可加用珠黄散外用。珠黄散成分为珍珠、牛黄各等份，研极细粉，吹入口腔中。有清热解毒止痛之效。

Jiangsu Journal of Traditional Chinese Medicine (October 1989) reported: This prescription has very good effects on patients with tongue cancer, nasopharyngeal carcinoma, malignant lymphoma, tonsillar tumors, lung cancer, and laryngeal cancer who develop stomatitis after radiotherapy. As a result, both stomatitis and ulcers subsided 3 to 14 days after medication. While taking this decoction orally, Zhuhuang Powder can also be used topically. Zhuhuang Powder consists of equal parts of pearl and ox-bezoar, ground into an extremely fine powder and blown into the oral cavity. It has the effects of clearing heat, detoxifying, and relieving pain.

20. ①藤梨根 100g，野葡萄根 25g，水杨梅 25g，凤尾草 25g，黄药子 50g，七叶一枝花 25g，半枝莲 25g，半边莲 25g，土贝母 25g，白茅根 50g。水煎服，每日 1 剂。脓血加白头翁 25g，秦皮 20g。②藤梨根 20g，瞿麦 20g，瘦猪肉 20g。食肉饮汤，早晚分服。①和②方交替服用。③全鸦胆子研碎，水煎 2 次，浓缩后加乙醇处理，回收乙醇，浓缩，加水稀释至 20 % 浓度，分装成 2ml 安瓶，消毒后备用。每次 4 ml，加温水 10ml，保留灌肠，用一般导尿管，注入瘤体上方。

20. ① 100g of Actinidia chinensis root, 25g each of wild grape root, water

globeflower, and brake fern; 50g of Dioscorea bulbifera; 25g each of Paris polyphylla, scutellaria barbata, Lobelia chinensis, and Bolbostemma paniculatum; and 50g of cogongrass rhizome. Decoct in water and take one dose daily. If there is pus and blood in the stool, add 25g of pulsatilla and 20g of ash bark. ② 20g of Actinidia chinensis root, 20g of dianthus, and 20g of lean pork. Eat the meat and drink the soup, divided into morning and evening doses. Prescriptions ① and ② are taken alternately. ③ Crush the whole Brucea javanica seeds, decoct in water twice, concentrate, add ethanol for processing, recover the ethanol, concentrate again, and dilute with water to a 20% concentration. Dispense into 2ml ampoules, sterilize, and store for later use. Each time, take 4ml, add 10ml of warm water, and administer as a retention enema. Using a standard urinary catheter, inject the solution above the tumor mass.

据报告：以上法治疗直肠癌 11 例（其中 9 例确诊为腺癌），临床治愈 2 例，有效 3 例，无效 6 例：其中存活 2 年以上者 2 例，1 年以上者 1 例。在治疗的过程中，未见有不良反应。

According to reports: The above method was used to treat 11 cases of rectal cancer (9 of which were confirmed as adenocarcinoma). 2 cases were clinically cured, 3 were effective, and 6 were ineffective. Among them, 2 cases survived for more than 2 years, and 1 case survived for more than 1 year. No adverse reactions were observed during the treatment process.

21. 髓母细胞瘤方：猫爪草 40g，虎杖 20g，菝葜 50g，冬虫夏草 3g，水煎服，每日 1 剂，3 个月为一疗程。

21. Prescription for Medulloblastoma: 40g of cat's claw grass, 20g of giant knotweed rhizome, 50g of greenbrier rhizome, and 3g of cordyceps. Decoct in water and take one dose daily, with three months constituting one course of treatment.

此为：西南昌市中草药研究所所长陈茂梧副主任医师治疗髓母细胞瘤及间皮瘤验方。有化瘀散结的作用。

This is a verified prescription for treating medulloblastoma and mesothelioma by Deputy Chief Physician Chen Maowu, Director of the Southwest Nanchang Institute of Chinese Herbal Medicine. It has the effects of resolving blood stasis and dissipating nodules.

22. 牙龈癌方：蒲公英、夏枯草、白毛藤、紫花地丁、白花蛇舌草各 50g，水煎浓液，频口、含漱后咽下。每日至少饮服 5 次。若同时送服六神丸，则效果更佳。

22. Prescription for Gingival Cancer: 50g each of dandelion, common selfheal fruit spike, Solanum lyratum, violet, and oldenlandia. Decoct the herbs in water to make a concentrated liquid, take frequent sips, gargle, and then swallow. Drink and take at least 5 times a day. If taken concurrently with Liushen Pills, the therapeutic effect will be even better.

23. 硬腭肿瘤方：蒲公英、金银花各 50g，连翘 15g，天花粉、土花苓各 20g，山慈菇 45g，水煎服，每日 1 剂。

23. Prescription for Hard Palate Tumors: 50g each of dandelion and honeysuckle, 15g of forsythia, 20g each of trichosanthes root and Bolbostemma paniculatum, and 45g of pseudobulbus Cremastrae seu Pleiones. Decoct in water and take one dose daily.

我曾以此方加女贞子 30g，治疗某女、81 岁，确诊为硬腭肿瘤，服用达 9 个月之久，临床效果十分满意。

I once used this prescription with the addition of 30g of glossy privet fruit to treat an 81-year-old female patient diagnosed with a hard palate tumor. After taking the medication for up to nine months, the clinical outcome was highly satisfactory.

24. 纤维肉瘤方：生黄花、党参、白术、熟地、枸杞、山药、天冬各 15g，茯苓 12g，甘草、木香各 4.5g，首乌、黄精各 9g，白花蛇舌草 30g，大枣 5 个。水煎服，每日 1 剂。

24. Prescription for Fibrosarcoma: 15g each of raw astragalus, codonopsis, atractylodes, prepared rehmannia, wolfberry, Chinese yam, and asparagus root; 12g of poria; 4.5g each of licorice and costus root; 9g each of fleece-flower root

and polygonatum; 30g of oldenlandia; and 5 jujubes. Decoct in water and take one dose daily.

福州市第一人民医院用此方治疗纤维肉瘤取得疗效。如魏某，女，35 岁。确诊为左髂窝深部纤维瘤。服用本方配合化疗一年多，原发灶及转移灶均消失。患者已恢复正常工作。

Fuzhou First People’s Hospital achieved therapeutic effects using this prescription to treat fibrosarcoma. For example, a 35-year-old female patient surnamed Wei was diagnosed with a deep fibroma in the left iliac fossa. After taking this prescription in combination with chemotherapy for over a year, both the primary and metastatic lesions disappeared. The patient has since returned to normal work.

《中国抗癌报》1992 年 7 月 20 日（毅敏常）

China Anti-Cancer News, July 20, 1992 (Yi Minchang)

25. 乳腺癌：贝母、人参、香附、茯苓、陈皮、熟地、川芎、当归、白芍各 10g，白术 12g，桔梗、甘草各 6g，生姜三片，大枣二枚，煎服。

25. Breast Cancer: 10g each of fritillaria, ginseng, cyperus, poria, tangerine peel, prepared rehmannia, ligusticum wallichii, angelica sinensis, and white peony root; 12g of atractylodes; 6g each of platycodon and licorice; 3 slices of fresh ginger; and 2 jujubes. Decoct in water and take orally.

《中医肿瘤学》

TCM Oncology

二、癌症疼痛的中药外治（5 方）

II. External Application of Traditional Chinese Medicine for Cancer Pain (5 Prescriptions)

癌性疼痛，多采用镇痛剂，有时还需作持续硬外麻来止痛，其副作用明显，而用中药外治无毒副作用，也无一般剧麻药的成瘾性，是值得推广的一种有效方法。根据临床综合报道，现辑录几则有效的外治方法：

Cancer pain is mostly treated with analgesics, and sometimes continuous epidural anesthesia is required for pain relief, which has obvious side effects. In contrast, external application of TCM has no toxic side effects and no addiction like general severe anesthetics. It is an effective method worth promoting. Based on comprehensive clinical reports, several effective external treatment methods are compiled as follows:

1. 敷脐法外方：穿山甲末 100 克，乳香、没药各 20 克，鸡矢藤挥发油 0.5ml，冰片少许，乙醇 500ml。治法：取没药、乳香浸入乙醇溶液中 20 天备用；取穿山甲 100 克研末，喷入乳香、没药液 70ml（醇溶液），烘干，再加入鸡矢藤挥发油，少许冰片。用食醋调敷脐部。

1. Umbilical Application Method: 100g of pangolin scales powder, 20g each of frankincense and myrrh, 0.5ml of Paederia foetida volatile oil, a small amount of borneol, and 500ml of ethanol. Treatment method: Soak the myrrh and frankincense in the ethanol solution for 20 days for later use. Grind 100g of pangolin scales into powder, spray 70ml of the frankincense and myrrh liquid (alcohol solution) into it, dry it, then add the Paederia foetida volatile oil and a small amount of borneol. Mix with edible vinegar and apply to the umbilical area.

2. 外贴法：用琥珀止痛膏贴于疼痛部位每日换药一次，可连用 10-20 天。取蟾酥膏敷于疼处，每日换药一次，7 天为一疗程，用药 15-30 分钟即可见效。

2. External Plaster Method: Apply Amber Analgesic Plaster to the painful area and change the dressing once a day, which can be used continuously for 10-20 days. Apply Toad Venom Plaster to the painful area, change the dressing once a day, with 7 days as one course of treatment. It can take effect within 15-30 minutes after application.

3. 涂擦法：用朱砂、乳香、没药各 15 克，冰片 30 克捣碎装盛有 500ml 米酒的小瓶，密封两天取上清液入小瓶备用；用棉签或毛笔蘸药水涂痛处，稍干后再用 3-4 遍，一般的中药外治用药 10-15 分钟疼痛消失，维持 2-3 小时，不等疼痛再用药。

3. Smearing and Rubbing Method: Take 15g each of cinnabar, frankincense,

and myrrh, and 30g of borneol, crush them, and put them in a small bottle containing 500ml of rice wine. Seal it for two days, then take the supernatant liquid into a small bottle for later use. Use a cotton swab or a brush to dip the medicinal liquid and apply it to the painful area. After it dries slightly, apply it 3-4 more times. Generally, with external TCM treatment, the pain disappears in 10-15 minutes and lasts for 2-3 hours. Do not wait for the pain to return before applying the medication again.

4. 热罨法：取樟脑，阿丁粉（阿魏、丁香、山柰、白蚤休），藤黄等量，分别研成细末备用，依肿块大小和疼痛部位，按以上用药次序分别撒在胶膏上，敷贴于患处，随即用 60℃热毛巾在胶膏上敷 30 分钟，每日 3 次，5-7 日换药一次，可反复使用。

4. Hot Compress Method: Take equal amounts of camphor, Ading powder (asafoetida, clove, sand ginger, and Paris polyphylla), and gamboge, and grind them into fine powders separately for later use. Depending on the size of the mass and the painful area, sprinkle them on the adhesive plaster in the above medication order, and apply it to the affected area. Immediately apply a hot towel at 60℃ on the plaster for 30 minutes, 3 times a day. Change the medication once every 5-7 days, and it can be used repeatedly.

5. 注射法。穴位注射法：仔细扪压寻求压痛点和常用穴位，找出最敏点在皮内注射 0.1ml，（注射用水）每次 2-4 点，1 日 1 次，5 日为一疗程。肌肉注射：常规操作，肌注蟾酥注射液 20-40m1，每日 1-2 次，2 周为一疗程。

5. Injection Method. Acupoint Injection Method: Carefully palpate and press to find the tender points and common acupoints, identify the most sensitive points, and inject 0.1ml intradermally (water for injection). Inject 2-4 points each time, once a day, with 5 days as one course of treatment. Intramuscular Injection: Follow routine procedures to intramuscularly inject 20-40ml of toad venom injection, 1-2 times a day, with 2 weeks as one course of treatment.

《中医药信息报》1992 年 5 月 9 日（山东 董万法）

TCM Information News, May 9, 1992 (Dong Wanfa, Shandong)

三、中医抗癌食谱（64 味）

III. TCM Anti-Cancer Dietary Recipes (64 Ingredients)

大蒜 芦笋 白菜 香菇 蘑菇 黑木耳 苦瓜 胡萝卜 黄瓜 南瓜 扁豆

Garlic, asparagus, Chinese cabbage, shiitake mushrooms, common mushrooms, black fungus, bitter melon, carrots, cucumbers, pumpkins, and flat beans.

玉米 绿豆 马齿苋 荸荠 菱角 苦参 海带 龙眼 萝卜 百合 薏米 黄芪

Corn, mung beans, purslane, water chestnuts, water caltrops, lightyellow sophora root, kelp, longan, radishes, lily bulbs, Job’s tears, and astragalus.

银耳 枸杞 蟑螂 桑葚 鱼腥草 芡实 蛇舌草 人参 灵芝 小白菜 圆白菜

Tremella, wolfberries, cockroaches, mulberries, heartleaf houttuynia, Gordon euryale seeds, oldenlandia, ginseng, reishi mushrooms, bok choy, and green cabbage.

油菜 大头菜 荠花 菜花 绿茶 牛蒡 山药 冬虫草 佛手 番茄 甘薯 茯苓

Rapeseed greens, turnips, shepherd’s purse, cauliflower, green tea, burdock, Chinese yam, cordyceps, bergamot, tomatoes, sweet potatoes, and poria.

莲藕 火龙果 五谷 麦麸皮 黄豆 粗米 红枣 葡萄 猕猴桃 嫩芽 香蕉

Lotus roots, dragon fruit, five grains, wheat bran, soybeans, unpolished rice, red dates, grapes, kiwis, sprouts, and bananas.

红豆 苹果 甘蓝 洋葱 豆腐 桔子 柠檬 菠菜

Adzuki beans, apples, kale, onions, tofu, tangerines, lemons, and spinach.

一定要多吃水果、蔬菜等碱性食品，少吃脂肪肉类等酸性食品，少吃熏肉，腌制食品，少吸烟少饮酒。

It is essential to eat more alkaline foods such as fruits and vegetables, and consume fewer acidic foods like fatty meats. Additionally, one should eat less smoked and pickled foods, and reduce smoking and alcohol consumption.

第十三章 皮肤科
Chapter 13 Dermatology

一、带状疱疹（44 方）
I. Herpes Zoster (44 Prescriptions)

1. 瓜子菜治带状疱疹

Treating Herpes Zoster with Guazicai (Purslane)

瓜子菜又名马齿苋、马齿菜。具有清热祛湿解毒之功效。笔者经多年临床实践，运用瓜子菜治疗带状疱疹多例，每每疗效满意，现介绍如下：

Guazicai, also known as purslane（马 齿 苋）or machicai, has the effects of clearing heat, eliminating dampness, and detoxifying. Based on many years of clinical practice, the author has treated multiple cases of herpes zoster with purslane, achieving satisfactory therapeutic effects, which are introduced as follows:

具体方法：取新鲜瓜子菜一把洗净加少许冰片，二味共捣烂榨取药汁涂抹患处，每日数次。也可取新鲜瓜子菜适量加冰片少许共捣烂外敷患处，1 日 1 换。还可取新瓜子菜适量煎水内服外洗，1 日 1 剂。一般 3-5 天可愈。

Specific Method: Take a handful of fresh purslane, wash it, add a small amount of borneol, and crush them together to extract the medicinal juice. Apply the juice to the affected area several times a day. Alternatively, take an appropriate amount of fresh purslane, add a little borneol, crush them together, and apply the mixture externally to the affected area, changing the dressing once a day. It can also be decocted in water for both oral intake and external washing, taking one dose a day. It generally takes 3 to 5 days to cure.

《民族医药报》（广西 肖祖镒）

Ethnic Medicine News (Xiao Zuyi, Guangxi)

2. 取雄黄、白矾各等份研为细末，茶水调敷患处，厚约2毫米，每日4次。

2. Take equal amounts of realgar and alum, grind them into a fine powder, mix with tea water, and apply to the affected area to a thickness of about 2 mm, four times a day.

3. 口服六神丸10粒，每日3次。外用根据病患部位大小，每次取六神丸30-60粒，研细末，用适量食醋调成糊状，用棉签蘸药涂于患处，每日1-2次。

3. Take 10 Liushen Pills orally, three times a day. For external use, depending on the size of the affected area, take 30-60 Liushen Pills each time, grind them into a fine powder, mix with an appropriate amount of edible vinegar to form a paste, dip a cotton swab in the medicine, and apply it to the affected area 1-2 times a day.

4. 取青黛10克，雄黄10克，冰片8克，共研细末，过100目筛后混合浸入75%乙醇175克中备用，每日用浸液外涂患处3次。

4. Take 10g of natural indigo, 10g of realgar, and 8g of borneol, grind them into a fine powder together, pass through a 100-mesh sieve, mix, and soak in 175g of 75% ethanol for later use. Apply the soaking liquid to the affected area externally three times a day.

《民族医药报》1991年7月5日（旻坚）

Ethnic Medicine News, July 5, 1991 (Min Jian)

5. 带状疱疹，祖国医学称为“蛇串疮”“缠腰火丹”等。笔者临床应用草药瓜子金治疗本病，获良效，兹介绍如下：

5. Herpes zoster is referred to as “shechuanchuang” (snake-creeping sore) or “chanyaohuodan” (waist-wrapping fire elixir) in traditional Chinese medicine. The author has achieved good therapeutic effects by clinically applying the herbal medicine Polygala japonica (瓜子金) to treat this disease, which is introduced as follows:

取洗净的鲜瓜子金根30-50克，晾干水，切碎，放入小茶杯或小碗内，倒入白酒 30-50 毫升，浸泡一小时后便可使用。先将患处洗净，后用棉签蘸上药酒涂搽其病变部位，一天搽 4-5 次。搽药之后，疼痛便会随之减轻，一般 1-2 天可愈。

Take 30-50g of fresh Polygala japonica roots, wash them, air-dry, chop them into pieces, and put them in a small teacup or bowl. Pour in 30-50 ml of white liquor (baijiu), and it can be used after soaking for one hour. First, wash the affected area, then use a cotton swab to dip the medicinal wine and apply it to the diseased area 4-5 times a day. After applying the medicine, the pain will be relieved accordingly, and it generally takes 1-2 days to cure.

《民族医药报》1992 年 1 月 31 日（湖南 兰家长）

Ethnic Medicine News, January 31, 1992 (Lan Jiachang, Hunan)

6. 取雄黄 10 克，大黄 10 克，白矾 6 克共研细末，加入 75% 酒精 100 毫升混合，每日用浸液搽敷患处 3 次。

6. Take 10g of realgar, 10g of rhubarb, and 6g of alum, grind them into a fine powder together, add 100ml of 75% alcohol, and mix well. Apply the soaking liquid to the affected area 3 times a day.

7. 取雄黄 4 克，季得胜蛇药片 4 片共研细末，加入 75% 酒精适量调敷患处，每日 3 次。

7. Take 4g of realgar and 4 Jidesheng Snake Medicine Tablets, grind them into a fine powder together, add an appropriate amount of 75% alcohol to form a paste, and apply it to the affected area 3 times a day.

8. 先用梅花针叩击疱疹处，再施拔罐 20 分钟，一日一次。另用雄黄 3 克、冰片 0.5 克共研细末，用 75% 酒精适量调敷患处，每日 2-3 次。

8. First, tap the herpes area with a plum-blossom needle, and then apply cupping for 20 minutes, once a day. In addition, take 3g of realgar and 0.5g of borneol, grind them into a fine powder together, add an appropriate amount of 75% alcohol to form a paste, and apply it to the affected area 2-3 times a day.

《民族医药报》1991 年 8 月 25 日（方伟平 李永春 张国彪）

Ethnic Medicine News, August 25, 1991 (Fang Weiping, Li Yongchun, Zhang

Guobiao)

9. 生明矾 4.5 克，杭菊花、板蓝根、神曲各 10 克，钩藤、地草丁各 15 克，生甘草 3 克，每日一剂，水煎服。外用黄黑膏涂患处（明雄黄 6 克，烟膏 10 克，杵泥调麻油外涂）。

9. 4.5g of raw alum; 10g each of Hangzhou chrysanthemum, isatis root, and medicated leaven; 15g each of uncaria and Viola yedoensis; and 3g of raw licorice. Decoct in water and take one dose daily. For external use, apply Huanghei (Yellow-Black) Paste to the affected area (6g of realgar and 10g of tobacco paste, pounded into mud and mixed with sesame oil for external application).

10. 生大黄、黄柏、黄连各 30 克，制乳香、没药各 15 克，共研细末加细茶叶泡浓汁适量调成糊状，外敷患处，干则易之。1-2 日后结痂，疼痛消失，4-6 日痊愈。

10. 30g each of raw rhubarb, phellodendron bark, and coptis root; and 15g each of processed frankincense and myrrh. Grind them into a fine powder together, add an appropriate amount of strong tea brewed from fine tea leaves to form a paste, and apply it externally to the affected area. Change the dressing when it dries. Scabs will form after 1-2 days, and the pain will disappear. The patient will recover in 4-6 days.

11. 用紫金锭片、季德胜蛇药片各一片，加板蓝根注射液 4 毫升，白醋 10 毫升，冷开水适量，调成稀糊状，用消毒棉签蘸药涂擦患处，每日 4-5 次。

11. Take 1 Zijin Ding Tablet and 1 Jidesheng Snake Medicine Tablet, add 4ml of isatis root injection, 10ml of white vinegar, and an appropriate amount of cooled boiled water, and mix them into a thin paste. Dip a sterilized cotton swab in the medicine and apply it to the affected area 4-5 times a day.

（河南 是明启）

(Shi Mingqi, Henan)

12. 带状疱疹方是病毒引起的急性皮肤病，祖国医学称为“缠腰火丹”“蛇窜疮”“蜘蛛疮”等，一年四季均可发病。患者一般都有轻度发热、疲乏无力及患处皮肤灼热、疼痛等症状。皮疹的特点多沿着一侧躯体某一周围神经分布，排列成带状、群簇状水疱本病采用中药外治疗效颇佳。

12. Herpes zoster is an acute skin disease caused by a virus. In traditional Chinese medicine, it is referred to as "chanyaohuodan" (waist-wrapping fire elixir), "shechuanchuang" (snake-creeping sore), and "zhizhuchuang" (spider sore), and it can occur in all four seasons. Patients generally have symptoms such as mild fever, fatigue, and a burning sensation and pain in the affected skin. The characteristic of the rash is that it is mostly distributed along a certain peripheral nerve on one side of the body, arranged in a band-like, clustered vesicular pattern. The external application of traditional Chinese medicine has a very good therapeutic effect on this disease.

具体方法：取王不留行、雄黄各等份、冰片少许，研成细末，瓶装备用。用时取药粉适量，加醋调成糊状敷于患处，每日换药 2-3 次，绝大多数患者用药 3 天局部疼痛及皮疹消失。

Specific Method: Take equal amounts of vaccaria seeds and realgar, and a small amount of borneol, grind them into a fine powder, and store them in a bottle for later use. When using, take an appropriate amount of the powder, add vinegar to form a paste, and apply it to the affected area. Change the dressing 2-3 times a day. For the vast majority of patients, the local pain and rash disappear after 3 days of medication.

《民族医药报》1991 年 6 月 26 日（柳州 潘彦清）

Ethnic Medicine News, June 26, 1991 (Pan Yanqing, Liuzhou)

13. 七厘散 应用七厘散治疗带状疱疹的报道近年较多，疗效都很好。患者一般在服药第 2-3 天疼痛减轻，水疱不再增加；第 4 天水疱干瘪，第 5-6 天结痂而愈。方法：取七厘散 1.2 克（1 支），每天 1 次，温开水送服，如用蜂蜜冲服更好。

13. Qili San (Seven-Cent Powder): In recent years, there have been many reports on the application of Qili San for treating herpes zoster, and the therapeutic effects are all very good. Patients generally experience pain relief and no new blisters appear on the 2nd to 3rd day of taking the medication; the blisters

shrivel on the 4th day, and scabs form with healing by the 5th to 6th day. Method: Take 1.2g (1 vial) of Qili San once a day, swallowed with warm water. It is even better to brew it with honey.

14. 六神丸 六神丸对本病亦有极好的疗效。方法：按六神丸 5 粒、醋 1 克比例配制，研末调和，以干净毛笔蘸药液涂擦患处，一日 3 次，同时内服本品，一日 3 次，再次 5-10 粒，一般用药后当晚疼痛减轻，第二日患处颜色变暗，3-5 日后可愈。

14. Liushen Pills (Six-God Pills): Liushen Pills also have an excellent therapeutic effect on this disease. Method: Prepare according to a ratio of 5 Liushen Pills to 1g of vinegar, grind them into a powder, and mix. Use a clean brush to dip the medicinal liquid and apply it to the affected area 3 times a day. At the same time, take the pills orally 3 times a day, 5-10 pills each time. Generally, the pain is relieved on the night after taking the medication, the color of the affected area darkens on the second day, and the patient can recover in 3-5 days.

15. 云南白药 以伤科名药云南白药治疗带状疱疹，疗效颇优。方法：取白药粉末用白酒适量和麻油（菜油）数滴配成稀糊状，涂患处，每日 3-5 次，用量视皮损范围大小增减；同时内服白药 0.3 克 / 次，每日 4 次，对病情较重者，适当增加服药次数或加量至 0.5 克 / 次，保险留在早晨服下，15 岁以下患者药量酌减。

15. Yunnan Baiyao (Yunnan White Medicine): Using the famous traumatology medicine Yunnan Baiyao to treat herpes zoster yields excellent therapeutic effects. Method: Take the powder of Yunnan Baiyao, mix it with an appropriate amount of white liquor (baijiu) and a few drops of sesame oil (or rapeseed oil) to form a thin paste, and apply it to the affected area 3-5 times a day. Adjust the dosage according to the size of the skin lesion. At the same time, take 0.3g of Yunnan Baiyao orally each time, 4 times a day. For severe cases, appropriately increase the frequency of medication or increase the dosage to 0.5g each time. Take the "insurance pill" (a special safety pill included in the package) in the morning. Reduce the dosage appropriately for patients under 15

years old.

16. 南通蛇药片 每次取蛇药 6-10 片，以 50-60 度白酒适量融散，搅拌调成稀糊状，以此搽疱疹，每天 4-8 次不等；并内服蛇药片，5 片 / 次，3 次 / 日，直至痊愈。据报道，用此法治疗 50 例带状疱疹患者，治愈 46 例，好转 2 例，无效 2 例，平均见效时间 1.2 天，痊愈天数平均 4.5 天，治愈后不出现后遗性神经痛。

16. Nantong Snake Medicine Tablets: Take 6-10 snake medicine tablets each time, dissolve them in an appropriate amount of 50-60 degree white liquor, and stir to form a thin paste. Apply this to the herpes 4-8 times a day. Also, take the snake medicine tablets orally, 5 tablets each time, 3 times a day, until fully recovered. According to reports, this method was used to treat 50 patients with herpes zoster. 46 cases were cured, 2 cases improved, and 2 cases were ineffective. The average time to see effects was 1.2 days, and the average number of days to full recovery was 4.5 days. No postherpetic neuralgia occurred after recovery.

《中药科技报》1991 年 6 月 26 日（广州 贺振泉）

Chinese Medicine Science and Technology News, June 26, 1991 (He Zhenquan, Guangzhou)

17. 带状疱疹：中成药解毒消炎丸适量加水研磨溶化外擦疾患部位，每天涂擦 2-3 次，每天口服本药两次，每次成人 10 粒，小儿、老年人酌减。一般七天左右结痂痊愈。

17. Herpes Zoster: Take an appropriate amount of Jiedu Xiaoyan Pills (Detoxifying and Anti-inflammatory Pills, a proprietary Chinese medicine), add water, grind, and dissolve it to externally rub the affected area 2-3 times a day. Take this medicine orally twice a day, 10 pills each time for adults, with reduced dosages for children and the elderly. Generally, scabs form and the patient recovers in about seven days.

《中药科技报》1993 年 3 月 26 日

Chinese Medicine Science and Technology News, March 26, 1993

18. 带状疱疹：蛇倒退（杠板归）叶、虎耳草、红浮漂（红浮萍）各适量熬水回搽洗患处，一般用药 2-3 次即愈。

18. Herpes Zoster: Take an appropriate amount of Polygonum perfoliatum (shedou tui) leaves, saxifrage, and red duckweed (hong fuping), boil them in water, and use the water to wash and rub the affected area. Generally, it can be cured after 2-3 applications.

带状疱疹，又名蛇患疮，中医亦称缠腰火丹，乃情志内伤以致肝胆火盛，或因脾湿郁久湿热内蕴，外受毒邪而发。皮损于腰背部，夏季多发，儿童易罹患。临床主要表现为神经痛和渗出及出血性疱疹。中医治疗效果颇佳，下面辑录数则行之有效的单验方，以供参考。

Herpes zoster, also known as shehuanchuang, is referred to as "chanyaohuodan" (waist-wrapping fire elixir) in traditional Chinese medicine. It is caused by internal emotional injuries leading to hyperactive fire in the liver and gallbladder, or by long-standing spleen dampness transforming into internal damp-heat, which is then triggered by external toxic pathogens. The skin lesions mainly occur on the lower back and back, are most common in summer, and children are highly susceptible. The main clinical manifestations are neuralgia, exudation, and hemorrhagic blisters. Traditional Chinese medicine has a very good therapeutic effect. Several effective single-ingredient and verified prescriptions are compiled below for reference.

19. 菟丝子烘干碾碎，加香油调成糊状。外敷于患处，每日 2-3 次，一般 4-5 次可愈。

19. Dry and crush dodder seeds, and add sesame oil to form a paste. Apply it externally to the affected area 2-3 times a day. Generally, it can be cured after 4-5 applications.

20. 雄黄、白芷等量，碾碎成细末，瓶装备用。患者有疹出时，可将药末直接撒在患处，若无疹出，用陈醋调和外敷，每日 2-3 次。

20. Take equal amounts of realgar and dahurian angelica root, crush them into a fine powder, and store them in a bottle for later use. When the patient has a rash, the powder can be directly sprinkled on the affected area. If there is no rash,

mix it with aged vinegar for external application, 2-3 times a day.

21. 二味拔毒散（雄黄、明矾）5 克，冰片 5 克，乳没粉 5 克，加 75% 酒精调配成混悬液外敷于患处，每日 4-6 次，一般 2-8 日便可痊愈。

21. Erwei Badu San (Two-Ingredient Toxin-Extracting Powder: realgar and alum) 5g, borneol 5g, and frankincense and myrrh powder 5g. Add 75% alcohol to prepare a suspension and apply it externally to the affected area 4-6 times a day. Generally, the patient can recover in 2-8 days.

22. 生大黄、黄柏、黄连、红枣及二味拔毒散各等份，碾碎用陈醋调成糊状外用。

22. Take equal amounts of raw rhubarb, phellodendron bark, coptis root, red dates, and Erwei Badu San (Two-Ingredient Toxin-Extracting Powder). Crush them and mix with aged vinegar to form a paste for external use.

23. 千里光、白芷各 30 克、薄荷 15 克，冰片 5 克，碾碎成粉，有疹出时直接撒在皮损处，无疹出时可用 75% 酒精或陈醋调匀外用。

23. 30g each of Senecio scandens (qianliguang) and dahurian angelica root, 15g of mint, and 5g of borneol. Crush them into a powder. When a rash appears, sprinkle it directly on the skin lesions. When there is no rash, mix it evenly with 75% alcohol or aged vinegar for external use.

24. 取云南白药用菜油或鲜菜汁调和糊状，每日 1-2 次外敷，一周皮损恢复如常。

24. Take Yunnan Baiyao and mix it with rapeseed oil or fresh vegetable juice to form a paste. Apply it externally 1-2 times a day. The skin lesions will return to normal within a week.

25. 蛇皮，用文火炒存性为末，用香油调和外用，每日 2 次，2-3 日可愈。

25. Snake skin: Roast snake skin over a gentle fire until carbonized but retaining its properties, then grind it into a powder. Mix it with sesame oil for external application, twice a day. It can generally be cured in 2-3 days.

26. 取五倍子、雄黄各 30 克，碾碎成细面，外擦于患处，可用香油调匀外涂。

26. Take 30g each of Chinese gallnut and realgar, crush them into a fine

powder, and rub it externally on the affected area. It can also be mixed evenly with sesame oil for external application.

27. 生南星、半夏、半边莲、白芷各 15-30 克研为细末，用香油调和外敷。

27. Take 15-30g each of raw jack-in-the-pulpit tuber, pinellia tuber, half-edge lotus, and dahurian angelica root, grind them into a fine powder, mix with sesame oil, and apply externally.

28. 龙胆泻肝汤加桔梗或板蓝根、蚤休，煎汁内服，一般 5 剂可愈。

28. Longdan Xiegan Decoction (Gentian Liver-Draining Decoction) with the addition of platycodon or isatis root and Paris polyphylla: Decoct the herbs in water for oral intake. Generally, 5 doses can cure the disease.

29. 蚤休、生柏叶各 15 克，雄黄 3 克，捣碎成末，用蜂蜜调糊外敷。

29. 15g each of Paris polyphylla and raw arborvitae leaves, and 3g of realgar. Crush them into a powder, mix with honey to form a paste, and apply externally.

30. 取新鲜蒲公英或鲜地黄，洗净甩干，捣烂或泥状，敷于患处，每日 2-3 次。

30. Take fresh dandelion or fresh rehmannia root, wash them, shake dry, and mash them into a paste or mud-like consistency. Apply to the affected area 2-3 times a day.

31. 黄连膏加 30% 雄黄粉调匀外敷，若水疱未破溃，可用三棱针刺之，以减胀痛。

31. Mix Coptis Ointment with 30% realgar powder evenly for external application. If the blisters have not ruptured, they can be pricked with a three-edged needle to relieve distension and pain.

32. 沙参、地黄、寸冬、当归、枸杞、川楝、黄连、醋白芍各适量，煎汁内服，疼痛较甚者可加延胡索、乳香、没药等。一般 3-5 剂便可治愈。

32. Take an appropriate amount of glehnia root, rehmannia, dwarf lilyturf tuber, angelica sinensis, wolfberry, chinaberry fruit, coptis root, and vinegar-fried white peony root. Decoct the herbs in water for oral intake. For patients with severe pain, add corydalis, frankincense, and myrrh. Generally, 3-5 doses can cure the disease.

《中药科技报》1990 年 10 月 6 日（济南 王洪道）

Chinese Medicine Science and Technology News, October 6, 1990 (Wang Hongdao, Jinan)

带状疱疹是一种病毒所致疾病，中医称缠腰蛇丹，以疱疹、局部疼痛较剧、发痒为主症，病程亦较长，西医目前除使用抗病毒药物，局部使用炉甘石洗剂，锌氧糊膏或神经根封闭外，尚无特效药物。而中药治疗本病疗效迅捷。现辑验方八则供选用。

Herpes zoster is a viral disease. In traditional Chinese medicine, it is called "chanyaoshedan" (waist-wrapping snake elixir). Its main symptoms are blisters, severe local pain, and itching, and its course of disease is relatively long. Currently, besides using antiviral drugs, topical calamine lotion, zinc oxide paste, or nerve root blocks, Western medicine has no specific cure for it. In contrast, traditional Chinese medicine has a rapid and effective therapeutic effect on this disease. Eight verified prescriptions are now compiled for selection.

33. 七厘散成人每日三次，每次 1.2 克，用温开水或黄酒送服，儿童酌减。服后 1-2 天疼痛减退，2-3 天丘疹消退，4-6 天水泡变干结痂。

33. Qili San (Seven-Cent Powder): For adults, take 1.2g each time, three times a day, swallowed with warm water or yellow rice wine. Reduce the dosage appropriately for children. After taking the medication, the pain will subside in 1-2 days, the papules will recede in 2-3 days, and the blisters will dry up and form scabs in 4-6 days.

34. 冰硼散 4 支加凡士林膏，以 1:3 调成糊状，敷于患处，每日 1 次，一般 3-4 天即愈。

34. Bingpeng San (Borneol and Borax Powder): Add 4 vials of Bingpeng San to Vaseline ointment, mix them into a paste at a ratio of 1:3, and apply it to the affected area once a day. It generally takes 3-4 days to cure.

35. 川乌 10 克，冰片 5 克，分别研成细粉末，混匀后加麻油适量，呈稀糊状，涂于皮损疼痛及区域，涂后用薄层纱布覆盖，严禁入口，每日涂搽 3-5 次。一般 2 天痛减，3 天部分皮损开始结痂，一周痊愈。

35. 10g of Sichuan aconite root and 5g of borneol. Grind them into fine powders separately, mix them evenly, and add an appropriate amount of sesame oil to form a thin paste. Apply it to the painful skin lesion areas, cover with a thin layer of gauze after application. Strictly forbidden for oral ingestion. Apply 3-5 times a day. Generally, the pain is reduced in 2 days, some skin lesions begin to form scabs in 3 days, and the patient recovers in a week.

36. 雄黄 50 克捣为粉末，95% 酒精 50 毫升，2.5% 利多卡因 4 毫升，置一密封器皿混匀，在疱疹周围用毛刷或棉签涂擦，每日 5-10 次，一般 3-5 天即愈。

36. Pound 50g of realgar into a powder, add 50ml of 95% alcohol and 4ml of 2.5% lidocaine, place them in a sealed container, and mix well. Use a brush or cotton swab to apply the mixture around the herpes 5-10 times a day. It generally takes 3-5 days to cure.

37. 青黛 10 克，冰片 5 克，鲜仙人掌 100 克左右，将冰片与青黛共研细末，将仙人掌刮刺，与上药共捣为膏即成。将患部消毒，有水泡者轻轻将水泡刺破，待泡液自然流尽后，放上膏一薄层，外用纱布固定，每日换药 1 次。一般 5-7 天即愈。

37. 10g of natural indigo, 5g of borneol, and about 100g of fresh cactus. Grind the borneol and natural indigo together into a fine powder. Scrape off the thorns of the cactus, and pound it together with the above-mentioned herbs into a paste. Disinfect the affected area. If there are blisters, gently prick them and wait for the blister fluid to drain naturally. Apply a thin layer of the paste and secure it with gauze. Change the dressing once a day. It generally takes 5-7 days to cure.

38. 荞麦面、小麦面、硫磺各等份，共研细面，浓茶叶水调和抹患处，一日 6 次，一般 3-5 天即愈。

38. Take equal amounts of buckwheat flour, wheat flour, and sulfur, grind them into a fine powder, mix with strong tea water, and apply it to the affected area 6 times a day. It generally takes 3-5 days to cure.

39. 取半边莲一大把洗净泥土，捣烂如泥敷于患处，盖上纱布，胶布固定。若干时用冷开水湿润之，每日换药 1-2 次，一般一周即愈。

39. Take a large handful of half-edge lotus, wash off the dirt, mash it into a mud-like paste, and apply it to the affected area. Cover it with gauze and secure it with medical tape. Moisten it with cooled boiled water when it dries. Change the dressing 1-2 times a day. It generally takes a week to cure.

40. 鲜马齿苋适量捣烂成糊状，敷于患处。一日换 2 次，一般 2 天痛止，5-7 天痊愈。

40. Take an appropriate amount of fresh purslane, mash it into a paste, and apply it to the affected area. Change the dressing twice a day. Generally, the pain stops in 2 days, and the patient recovers in 5-7 days.

《民族医药报》（张宏俊 王道俊）

Ethnic Medicine News (Zhang Hongjun, Wang Daojun)

41. 鲜韭菜根 30 克，地龙泥（地龙排泄物）15 克。共入碗内捣烂，加少量香油，调匀备用。用时洗净患处，将药泥薄施（0.5 厘米厚）于疹面，用纱布覆盖。一日一至二次，五至七日即愈。

41. Take 30g of fresh Chinese chive roots and 15g of earthworm mud (earthworm excrement). Put them in a bowl, mash them together, add a small amount of sesame oil, and mix well for later use. When using, wash the affected area clean, apply a thin layer of the medicinal mud (0.5 cm thick) on the rash, and cover it with gauze. Apply once or twice a day, and it can be cured in five to seven days.

42. 雄黄、白芷等分。共为细末，香油调搽患处，一日数次，一般一周左右即愈。

42. Take equal amounts of realgar and dahurian angelica root. Grind them into a fine powder together, mix with sesame oil, and apply it to the affected area several times a day. It generally takes about a week to cure.

43. 青黛 20 克，蒲黄 30 克，滑石粉 30 克。共研末均匀备用。患处如有渗液可用干粉外扑，无渗液者用香油调搽，一日三至五次。其它湿疹症，效果也很好。

43. Take 20g of natural indigo, 30g of cattail pollen, and 30g of talcum powder. Grind them together into a fine powder and mix evenly for later use.

If there is exudation on the affected area, the dry powder can be dusted on it. If there is no exudation, mix it with sesame oil and apply it 3 to 5 times a day. It also has a very good effect on other types of eczema.

《中药科技报》1992 年 8 月 26 日

Chinese Medicine Science and Technology News, August 26, 1992

44. 取干柏树枝 50 克，烧灰，加入大黄、雄黄各 15 克，研末。先取菜油适量放在勺内加热，待沸后倒入上药，搅匀，凉后再加入冰片末 3 克，拌匀。涂搽患处，每日 2 次。

44. Take 50g of dry cypress branches and burn them into ashes. Add 15g each of rhubarb and realgar, and grind them into a powder. First, heat an appropriate amount of rapeseed oil in a spoon, pour in the above-mentioned medicinal powder after it boils, and stir well. After it cools down, add 3g of borneol powder and mix well. Apply it to the affected area twice a day.

《民族医药报》

Ethnic Medicine News

二、慢性湿疹（4 方）

II. Chronic Eczema (4 Prescriptions)

1. 治疗慢性湿疹的复方中草药

Compound Herbal Medicine for Treating Chronic Eczema

湿疹是一种过敏性皮肤病，多发生在暴露部位。初为红斑，血疹，后发水疱，甚至糜烂有渗出液，刺痒难忍。

Eczema is an allergic skin disease that mostly occurs on exposed areas. It initially presents as erythema and blood papules, which later develop into blisters, and may even become eroded with exudate, accompanied by unbearable itching.

治疗方法较多，有口服药和外用药，但都较易复发。根据临床病例观察，除特别严重者加用内服药外，均可使用复方中药煎剂，泡洗患处，对慢性湿疹能免除复发，以达根治。

There are many treatment methods, including oral and topical medications, but they are prone to relapse. Based on clinical case observations, except for particularly severe cases that require additional oral medications, a compound traditional Chinese medicine decoction can be used to soak and wash the affected area. This can prevent the relapse of chronic eczema and achieve a radical cure.

处方：大皂角 10 克，蛇床子 15 克，蛇蜕 6 克，白鲜皮 15 克，五加皮 15 克，透骨草 30 克，大青盐 6 克。

Prescription: 10g of large soap pod, 15g of common cnidium fruit, 6g of snake slough, 15g of dictamnus bark, 15g of acanthopanax bark, 30g of Clerodendranthus spicatus (tougucao), and 6g of large rock salt.

用法：以上数种药水煎为一剂，滤过后存放。同时反复加热泡洗患部。每日1-2次，每次15分钟。

Usage: Decoct the above herbs in water as one dose, filter it, and store it. Repeatedly heat the liquid to soak and wash the affected area. Do this 1-2 times a day, 15 minutes each time.

《中药科技报》1992 年 8 月 26 日（川秀）

Chinese Medicine Science and Technology News, August 26, 1992 (Chuan Xiu)

2. 蛇床子、苦参、芜荑各 30 克，雄黄 15 克，枯矾 45 克，硫磺、轻粉、樟脑各 10 克，川椒 15 克，大枫子（取肉）15 克，为末，生猪油调敷患处。[按] 本方聚多味有毒猛烈之品，杀虫医疮、燥湿止痒之力极强。用于疥疮有神效。对妇女阴蚀（外阴溃疡）、外阴白斑、湿疹及各种顽癣恶疮亦有很好疗效。

2. Take 30g each of common cnidium fruit, lightyellow sophora root, and elm seed; 15g of realgar; 45g of calcined alum; 10g each of sulfur, calomel, and camphor; 15g of Sichuan pepper; and 15g of chaulmoogra seed (pulp only). Grind them into a powder and mix with fresh raw lard to apply to the affected area. [Note] This prescription combines many highly toxic and fierce ingredients, possessing extremely strong effects of killing parasites, healing sores, drying dampness, and relieving itching. It has miraculous effects on scabies. It also has very good therapeutic effects on vulvar erosion (vulvar ulcers), vulvar leukoplakia, eczema,

and various intractable tinea and malignant sores in women.

（卢世秀）

(Lu Shixiu)

3. 湿疹：鲜虎耳草适量煎水洗或捣烂取汁涂搽患处，一日数次。

3. Eczema: Take an appropriate amount of fresh saxifrage, decoct it in water to wash the affected area, or mash it to extract the juice and apply it to the affected area several times a day.

4. 治疗湿疹：捕捉活蟾蜍（癞蛤蟆）3-5 只，用清水将其洗净，把蟾蜍之背皮剥下，用针刺数孔以排出毒气，然后用此皮涂擦患处。每日 2-3 次，连用 4-7 日。

4. Treating Eczema: Catch 3-5 live toads, wash them clean with water, peel off the skin on their backs, prick several holes in the skin with a needle to discharge the toxic substances, and then use this skin to rub the affected area. Do this 2-3 times a day continuously for 4-7 days.

三、痱子（8 方）
III. Prickly Heat / Miliaria (8 Prescriptions)

1. 鱼腥草，系三白草科植物，治疗痱子效果很好。用法：将鲜品捣汁涂敷，或干品适量煎汤口服，日服 2-3 次，均能起到清热消肿，除痱止痒的作用。此外亦可用鱼腥草注射液搽抹患处，一般连用数次，痱子便可结痂消去。

1. Houttuynia cordata (heartleaf houttuynia), a plant of the Saururaceae family, has a very good effect on treating prickly heat. Usage: Mash the fresh herb to extract the juice and apply it topically, or decoct an appropriate amount of the dried herb in water for oral intake, 2-3 times a day. Both methods can clear heat, reduce swelling, eliminate prickly heat, and relieve itching. In addition, Houttuynia cordata injection can be applied to the affected area. Generally, after continuous application for several times, the prickly heat will form scabs and disappear.

《民族医药报》（广西 刘伟祥）

Ethnic Medicine News (Liu Weixiang, Guangxi)

2. 苦瓜汁治痱子有奇效 鲜苦瓜一条，洗净去仁，切碎瓜肉，捣烂取汁，将汁直接涂在痱子上，每日早晚各一次，一般 2-3 日便可痊愈。

2. Bitter Melon Juice Has Miraculous Effects on Treating Prickly Heat: Take one fresh bitter melon, wash it, remove the seeds, chop the flesh, and mash it to extract the juice. Apply the juice directly to the prickly heat, once in the morning and once in the evening. It generally takes 2-3 days to cure.

（樊常宝）

(Fan Changbao)

3. 六一散（成药）15 克，开水冲泡服，每日二次，也可外用敷涂患处。

3. Take 15g of Liuyi San (Six-One Powder, a proprietary Chinese medicine), brew it with boiling water for oral intake, twice a day. It can also be applied topically to the affected area.

4. 鲜嫩黄瓜一条，切圈片，涂患处擦患处每日数次。

4. Take one fresh and tender cucumber, cut it into round slices, and rub it on the affected area several times a day.

5. 鲜丝瓜叶捣烂挤汁涂患处，每日数次。

5. Mash fresh loofah leaves to extract the juice and apply it to the affected area several times a day.

6. 黄连 30 克，加水 250 克，煎至 100 克，滤渣，涂患处，每日数次。

6. Take 30g of coptis root, add 250g of water, decoct until 100g of liquid remains, filter out the dregs, and apply the liquid to the affected area several times a day.

7. 香瓜蒂轻轻在痱子上涂擦，每日数次。

7. Gently rub the stem of a muskmelon on the prickly heat, several times a day.

8. 绿豆 120 克，微炒研成细粉，滑石粉 15 克，拌均匀用纱布包好扎紧，洗澡后或清洁皮肤后，揩干扑在痱子上。

8. Take 120g of mung beans, lightly roast them, and grind them into a fine powder. Add 15g of talcum powder, mix evenly, wrap the mixture tightly in a gauze bag. After bathing or cleaning the skin, wipe the area dry and pat the

powder onto the prickly heat.

《民族医药报》（上海 何悦飞）

Ethnic Medicine News (He Yuefei, Shanghai)

四、治褥疮方（3 方）
IV. Prescriptions for Treating Bedsores (3 Prescriptions)

1. 处方及用法：当归 60 克，白芷 15 克，白蜡 12 克，甘草 30 克，紫草 6 克，血竭 12 克，轻粉 12 克，银花 30 克，麻油 500 克。先将当归、白芷、甘草、紫草加入麻油内浸泡三天，然后以慢火煎成糊状，取出药渣，加入血竭、银花（研粉）、白蜡、轻粉混合成药膏。用时以消毒纱布蘸取药膏填敷褥疮面，每天换药一次，填敷时先将疮面消毒清洗干净。一般用药一周褥疮基本愈合；重者用药 20-30 天痊愈。笔者在临床上常以此方治疗无名肿毒伤口久溃不敛、蛇伤溃疡、疮疖等，屡试屡效。此方具有取材容易、炮制简便、见效快、愈合后创面不留明显疤痕等优点，同道们不妨试。

1. Prescription and Usage: 60g of angelica sinensis, 15g of dahurian angelica root, 12g of white wax, 30g of licorice, 6g of gromwell root, 12g of dragon’s blood, 12g of calomel, 30g of honeysuckle flower, and 500g of sesame oil. First, soak the angelica sinensis, dahurian angelica root, licorice, and gromwell root in sesame oil for three days, then decoct over a gentle fire into a paste. Remove the herbal dregs, and add the dragon’s blood, honeysuckle flower (ground into powder), white wax, and calomel, mixing them into an ointment. When using, dip a sterilized gauze in the ointment and pack it onto the bedsore surface. Change the dressing once a day, and disinfect and clean the sore surface before packing. Generally, the bedsore basically heals after one week of medication; severe cases can be cured in 20-30 days. In clinical practice, the author often uses this prescription to treat unexplained toxic swellings with long-standing unhealed wounds, snakebite ulcers, and sores/boils, with consistent success. This prescription has the advantages of easy access to materials, simple preparation,

rapid effects, and no obvious scarring on the wound after healing. Fellow practitioners might as well give it a try.

《民族医药报》1993 年 1 月 1 日（广西 秦祥仁）

Ethnic Medicine News, January 1, 1993 (Qin Xiangren, Guangxi)

2. 褥疮、伤口久不愈合：麦饭石不拘多少，研成粉末，置于锅炒热，冷却后瓶贮备用。先将伤口用双氧水洗净，撒布麦饭石粉末，再用复方鱼肝油软膏纱布覆盖，胶布固定，每隔两天换药一次。

2. Bedsores and Long-standing Unhealed Wounds: Take an appropriate amount of maifan stone (maifanite), grind it into a powder, stir-fry it in a pan until hot, and store it in a bottle for later use after cooling. First, wash the wound clean with hydrogen peroxide, sprinkle the maifan stone powder on it, cover it with gauze containing compound cod liver oil ointment, and secure it with medical tape. Change the dressing every two days.

3. 用滑石 10 克，冰片 0.5 克，炉甘石 0.5 克，共研细末混匀，装瓶备用。使用前，先将褥疮清洗干净，然后撒上药粉，再用敷料包扎（避免用胶布，防止损伤皮肤）。每天两次。一般用药 1-3 天褥疮结痂，4-5 天痊愈。笔者用此法治疗 28 例褥疮患者，疗效颇佳。

3. Take 10g of talcum powder, 0.5g of borneol, and 0.5g of calamine. Grind them into a fine powder, mix evenly, and store in a bottle for later use. Before use, clean the bedsore first, then sprinkle the medicinal powder on it, and bandage it with a dressing (avoid using medical tape to prevent skin damage). Do this twice a day. Generally, the bedsore forms scabs after 1-3 days of medication and heals in 4-5 days. The author used this method to treat 28 patients with bedsores, achieving excellent therapeutic effects.

《民族医药报》1992 年 5 月 26 日（湖南 兰家长 王艳）

Ethnic Medicine News, May 26, 1992 (Lan Jiachang, Wang Yan, Hunan)

五、治癣方（16 方）

V. Prescriptions for Treating Tinea and Psoriasis (16 Prescriptions)

1. 大蒜韭菜泥：取大蒜、韭菜各 50 克，将大蒜去皮，韭菜洗净，2 味共捣如泥状，置火上烘热，用力涂擦患处，每日 2-3 次，连续数日。主治：牛皮癣，对过敏性皮炎也有效。

1. Garlic and Chive Mud: Take 50g each of garlic and Chinese chives. Peel the garlic and wash the chives. Mash the two ingredients together into a mud-like paste, heat it over a fire, and vigorously rub it onto the affected area 2-3 times a day for several consecutive days. Indications: Psoriasis; also effective for allergic dermatitis.

2. 花椒硫磺膏：取花椒、明矾各 30 克，食盐、硫磺、火硝各 120 克，猪油适量。先将前药研为细末，过筛后调入猪油成膏，涂擦患处，1 日 2 次，治愈为止。该方有解毒燥湿、杀虫止痒的功效。主治：牛皮癣。

2. Sichuan Pepper and Sulfur Ointment: Take 30g each of Sichuan pepper and alum; 120g each of table salt, sulfur, and saltpeter; and an appropriate amount of lard. First, grind the aforementioned herbs into a fine powder, sift them, and mix them with lard to form an ointment. Rub the ointment onto the affected area twice a day until cured. This prescription has the effects of detoxifying, drying dampness, killing parasites, and relieving itching. Indications: Psoriasis.

3.荸荠陈醋糊: 取鲜荸荠 15 枚，陈醋 100 毫升，将荸荠去皮，切成片浸入醋中，2 味放锅内以文火煎煮 10 多分钟，待醋干后，将荸荠出锅捣成糊即成。用时，先将患处涂上少量糊，用纱布轻轻摩擦，至局部发红时，再敷上药糊，每日 1 次，至愈为止。主治：牛皮癣。

3. Water Chestnut and Aged Vinegar Paste: Take 15 fresh water chestnuts and 100ml of aged vinegar. Peel the water chestnuts, cut them into slices, and soak them in the vinegar. Put both ingredients in a pot and decoct over a gentle fire for more than 10 minutes. After the vinegar dries up, take the water chestnuts out of the pot and mash them into a paste. When using, first apply a small amount of the paste to the affected area, gently rub it with gauze until the local area turns red,

and then apply the medicinal paste. Do this once a day until cured. Indications: Psoriasis.

《民族医药报》（湖南 兰家长）

Ethnic Medicine News (Lan Jiachang, Hunan)

4. 治疗牛皮癣：采回鲜苧麻枝尖嫩叶，捣烂敷于患处，一日一次。

4. Treating Psoriasis: Pick fresh tender leaves from the tips of ramie branches, mash them, and apply them to the affected area once a day.

5. 银屑病：石榴树皮（炒炭，研细末）1 份，麻油 3 份，调成稀糊状，涂患处，每日 2 次。

5. Psoriasis: Take 1 part of pomegranate bark (stir-fried into charcoal and ground into a fine powder) and 3 parts of sesame oil. Mix them into a thin paste and apply it to the affected area twice a day.

6. 头癣：蜂房 1 个，蜈蚣 2 条，明矾适量。烤焦共研为末，麻油调敷。

6. Tinea Capitis: Take 1 wasp nest, 2 centipedes, and an appropriate amount of alum. Roast them until scorched, grind them into a powder together, and mix with sesame oil for external application.

（燕子堂）

(Yan Zi Tang)

7. 治疗头癣验方

7. Verified Prescription for Treating Tinea Capitis

单用川楝子（12 克）一味。将川楝子加热使之烤黄（不要烧焦或炭化），研成极细粉，取麻油少许与川楝粉混合调成糊状，将此糊状物，涂于患处每日 2-3 次，有速效。

Use only one ingredient: 12g of chinaberry fruit. Heat the chinaberry fruit until it turns yellow (do not scorch or carbonize it), and grind it into an extremely fine powder. Take a small amount of sesame oil, mix it with the chinaberry powder to form a paste, and apply this paste to the affected area 2-3 times a day. It has a rapid effect.

《中医药信息报》

Traditional Chinese Medicine Information News

8.头癣：鲜野菊花全草500克，洗净泥土置于锅内水煮一小时后加苦矾10克，取药汁洗头，每日2次，一般连用3天。

8. Tinea Capitis: Take 500g of fresh wild chrysanthemum whole plant, wash off the dirt, put it in a pot, and boil it in water for one hour. Add 10g of bitter alum, use the medicinal liquid to wash the hair twice a day, and generally use it continuously for 3 days.

9.将土大黄（鲜品）切碎后加食用醋浸泡一昼夜，去渣用其液。用前先以温水将脚洗净，用洁净毛刷或棉花蘸药液涂擦患处，每日1-2次，至治愈。

9. Chop fresh Rumex madaio (tu da huang), soak it in edible vinegar for a day and a night, remove the dregs, and use the liquid. Before use, wash the feet with warm water, dip a clean brush or cotton swab in the medicinal liquid, and rub it onto the affected area 1-2 times a day until cured.

10.将萹蓄、白鲜皮、蛇床子各15克水煎沸后30分钟，把明矾30克打碎放入，边放边搅拌，使明矾溶化，然后将药水倒入瓷盆，先用热气熏患处，后浸泡半小时，每日1次，一般泡7天治愈。尤对湿性脚癣，效果更好。

10. Decoct 15g each of common knotweed, dictamnus bark, and common cnidium fruit in water for 30 minutes after boiling. Break 30g of alum and add it to the liquid, stirring continuously until the alum dissolves. Then, pour the medicinal liquid into a porcelain basin. First, fumigate the affected area with the hot steam, and then soak it for half an hour. Do this once a day, and it generally takes 7 days to cure. It is especially effective for wet tinea pedis.

11.将地肤子、蛇床子、重楼、明矾各30克，用冷开水200毫升浸泡1周。去渣，将此药与1000毫升醋混合，装入瓶中备用。每天取用，浸泡脚癣2次，每次15分钟，连治5天可愈。

11. Soak 30g each of Kochia fruit, common cnidium fruit, Paris polyphylla, and alum in 200ml of cooled boiled water for 1 week. Remove the dregs, mix the medicinal liquid with 1000ml of vinegar, and store it in a bottle for later use. Use it daily to soak the tinea pedis twice a day, 15 minutes each time. Continuous

treatment for 5 days can cure it.

12. 先采集指甲花茎叶 200 克，洗净并切碎，浸入浓度为 5% 的水醋酸液体 1000毫升中，4-6小时后将其药渣拧干弃去，配方即成。同时将患脚浸泡该溶液中，每次 20-30 分钟，每日 1-2 次，一般治疗 2-4 次即可痊愈。

12. First, collect 200g of henna stems and leaves, wash and chop them, and soak them in 1000ml of 5% acetic acid solution. After 4-6 hours, wring out and discard the herbal dregs, and the prescription is ready. Soak the affected foot in this solution for 20-30 minutes each time, 1-2 times a day. Generally, it can be cured after 2-4 treatments.

《中药科技报》1992 年 9 月 26 日（河南 是明启）

Chinese Medicine Science and Technology News, September 26, 1992 (Shi Mingqi, Henan)

六、黄水疮方（9 方）

VI. Prescriptions for Treating Impetigo (9 Prescriptions)

1. 苦杏仁适量，火炙成炭存性，研成细末，用香油或豆油熬开调成稀糊状备用。用时，先用淡盐水将污痂洗净，然后将上药涂患处薄薄一层，可用干净纱布或软布覆盖，以防药物脱落和污染衣被。一般每日或隔日涂 1 次，1-2 次脱痂，3-4 次痊愈。

1. Take an appropriate amount of bitter apricot kernels, roast them over a fire until carbonized but retaining their properties, and grind them into a fine powder. Boil sesame oil or soybean oil, mix it with the powder to form a thin paste, and set it aside for later use. When using, first wash away the dirty scabs with light salt water, then apply a thin layer of the medicine to the affected area. It can be covered with clean gauze or soft cloth to prevent the medicine from falling off and contaminating clothes and bedding. Generally, apply it once a day or every other day. The scabs will fall off after 1-2 applications, and it will be cured after 3-4 applications.

2. 熟鸡蛋黄 5 个，用铁锅文火焙干出油为止，涂抹患处。随疮面大小涂药多少，每日 5-6 次。

2. Take 5 hard-boiled egg yolks, bake them in an iron pan over a gentle fire until they dry out and release their oil, and apply the oil to the affected area. Adjust the amount of medicine according to the size of the sore. Apply it 5-6 times a day.

3. 大黄 15 克，枯矾 5 克，冰片 1.5 克，青黛 3 克，麻油适量。将大黄研极细面，再加后 3 味药共为细面，装瓶密封备用。流黄水者，用药面外敷；不流水者，用麻油调匀外敷。每日 2-3 次。

3. Take 15g of rhubarb, 5g of calcined alum, 1.5g of borneol, 3g of natural indigo, and an appropriate amount of sesame oil. Grind the rhubarb into an extremely fine powder, then add the other three ingredients and grind them together into a fine powder. Store it in a sealed bottle for later use. For oozing yellow fluid, apply the dry powder topically; if there is no exudation, mix it evenly with sesame oil for external application. Do this 2-3 times a day.

4. 松香、枯矾、野菊花粉各适量。先采集野菊花秧的嫩梢洗净晒干，研为细末。后取上三味药末等分，过筛，瓶装备用。用温盐开水洗净患处，取此药加青油调成清糊状，涂擦患处，每日 3 次。

4. Take an appropriate amount of rosin, calcined alum, and wild chrysanthemum powder. First, collect the tender shoots of wild chrysanthemum seedlings, wash them, dry them in the sun, and grind them into a fine powder. Then, take equal amounts of the aforementioned three powdered herbs, sift them, and store them in a bottle for later use. Wash the affected area with warm salted boiled water, take this powder, add some vegetable oil to form a thin paste, and apply it to the affected area 3 times a day.

5. 青蒿、鲜藿香、鲜佩兰、连翘、车前子（包）、六一散（包）、赤芍、山栀各 9 克，银花、蒲公英各 12 克，水煎服。

5. Take 9g each of sweet wormwood, fresh patchouli, fresh eupatorium, forsythia, plantain seed (wrapped), Liuyi San (Six-One Powder, wrapped), red

peony root, and gardenia; and 12g each of honeysuckle flower and dandelion. Decoct them in water for oral intake.

6. 轻粉、铝粉、胡石各 30 克，冰片 15 克，银朱 6 克。先将胡石火煅辗细，加入轻粉再辗，后入冰片轻轻辗，待极细后再同银朱、铝粉和匀备用。黄水多时，用干粉撒布患处，黄水少时，加适量芝麻油或菜油调匀搽之，每日 2-3 次。

6. Take 30g each of calomel, aluminum powder, and Hushi (a type of mineral); 15g of borneol; and 6g of cinnabar. First, calcine Hushi over a fire and grind it finely, then add calomel and grind again. After that, add borneol and grind gently. Once it is extremely fine, mix it evenly with cinnabar and aluminum powder for later use. When there is a lot of yellow exudate, sprinkle the dry powder on the affected area. When there is little exudate, add an appropriate amount of sesame oil or vegetable oil, mix evenly, and apply it 2-3 times a day.

7. 鲜灯笼草、鲜马齿苋各适量。将上药洗净，晾干、捣烂，用纱布绞取鲜汁，装瓶。用时，以棉球或毛笔蘸药水涂患处，每日数次。

7. Take an appropriate amount of fresh Physalis angulata (lantern grass) and fresh purslane. Wash the herbs, air-dry them, and mash them. Squeeze out the fresh juice using gauze and store it in a bottle. When using, dip a cotton ball or a brush in the medicinal liquid and apply it to the affected area several times a day.

8. 蚕豆荚煅灰干扑，每日 2-3 次；或野菊花适量，煎汤洗，并捣烂外敷日 3 次。

8. Calcine broad bean pods into ashes and apply the dry powder to the affected area 2-3 times a day; or take an appropriate amount of wild chrysanthemum, decoct it in water to wash the area, and mash it for external application 3 times a day.

9. 锅底灰、枯矾、黄柏各等量。上药共研细末备用。用时，将患处用生理盐水或淡盐水洗净，取适量香油调药末成膏状，外涂疮面，每日 2-3 次。

9. Take equal amounts of soot from the bottom of a wok, calcined alum, and phellodendron bark. Grind the aforementioned herbs together into a fine powder for later use. When using, wash the affected area with normal saline or light salt water, take an appropriate amount of sesame oil to mix the powder into a paste,

apply it externally to the sore, 2-3 times a day.

《民族医药报》（四川 刘驰）

Ethnic Medicine News (Liu Chi, Sichuan)

七、下肢溃疡久不收口（8 方）

VII. Chronic Non-healing Lower Limb Ulcers (8 Prescriptions)

臁疮，俗称“老烂腿”，又称慢性下肢溃疡，是一种病程缠绵难愈的疾病。为此特辑验方七则，供患者选用。

Varicose ulcers, commonly known as “old rotten leg” and also referred to as chronic lower limb ulcers, are a disease with a prolonged and difficult-to-cure course. For this reason, seven verified prescriptions are specially compiled here for patients to choose from.

1. 鸡蛋黄油。选新鲜鸡蛋 5 枚煮熟，剥去蛋白，取蛋黄放在热锅中爆炒至黑，然后将黑油涂在患处，每日一次，一般三次即取效。

1. Egg Yolk Oil: Boil 5 fresh eggs, peel off the egg whites, and take the egg yolks. Stir-fry the yolks in a hot pan until they turn black, then apply the black oil to the affected area once a day. It generally takes effect after three applications.

2. 油调甘草粉。炙甘草粉，用香油调成膏状，外敷患部，一日换一次，二天症减，一周即愈。

2. Licorice Powder Mixed with Oil: Mix honey-fried licorice powder with sesame oil to form a paste, apply it externally to the affected area, and change the dressing once a day. Symptoms will alleviate in two days, and it will be cured in a week.

3. 马应龙麝香痔疮膏。用生理盐水清洗疮面后，外敷本膏，一日两次直至愈合。

3. Mayinglong Musk Hemorrhoids Ointment: After cleaning the ulcer surface with normal saline, apply this ointment externally twice a day until it heals.

4. 桑白皮贴法。采用鲜桑白皮洗净去赤层备用，使用前用等溶盐水清洗患部，将桑白皮扎在小腿，自溃疡上缘 2cm 处开始呈叠瓦状向下把疮面封住，直到疮面下缘 2cm 为止，包扎稍用力，使中段正贴疮面，三至四天更换一次，一般几次即愈。

4. Mulberry Root Bark Application Method: Wash fresh mulberry root bark, peel off the reddish outer layer, and set it aside for later use. Before use, wash the affected area with isotonic saline. Tie the mulberry root bark around the lower leg, starting from 2 cm above the upper edge of the ulcer and overlapping it downwards like roof tiles to seal the ulcer surface until 2 cm below the lower edge. Bandage it with moderate force so that the middle part fits tightly against the ulcer. Change it every three to four days. It generally takes a few applications to cure.

5. 五倍枯金散。五倍子、石榴皮、枯矾各 30 克，鸡内金、青黛各 20 克、冰片 5 克。先将五倍子、石榴皮、鸡内金焙黄研末，枯矾、冰片研粉，加入青黛，上药和匀，过 100 目筛，高压消毒后贮瓶备用，用时先用生理盐水清洗疮面，并用消毒纱布拭干，然后取本散均匀地撒在疮面上，每日一次，一般三天即取效。

5. Wubei Kujin Powder: Take 30g each of Chinese gallnut, pomegranate peel, and calcined alum; 20g each of chicken gizzard lining and natural indigo; and 5g of borneol. First, roast the Chinese gallnut, pomegranate peel, and chicken gizzard lining until yellowish, then grind them into a powder. Grind the calcined alum and borneol into a powder as well, add the natural indigo, mix all the herbs evenly, and sift through a 100-mesh sieve. Sterilize it under high pressure and store it in a bottle for later use. When using, first clean the ulcer surface with normal saline, wipe it dry with sterilized gauze, and then evenly sprinkle this powder on the ulcer surface once a day. It generally takes effect in three days.

6. 密陀僧散。密陀僧 10 克，炉甘石 30 克，雄黄 10 克，朱砂 3 克，共研末，用猪油和白糖调匀，摊在油纸上，包扎患处，每日一次，一般一周即取效。

6. Mituoseng Powder: Take 10g of litharge, 30g of calamine, 10g of realgar, and 3g of cinnabar. Grind them into a powder together, mix evenly with lard and white sugar, spread it on oil paper, bandage the affected area once a day. It

generally takes effect in a week.

7. 维痢粉。将维生素 B6、痢特灵共研成粉外撒患处一般 3 次即效。

7. Weili Powder: Grind Vitamin B6 and Furazolidone into a powder together and sprinkle it externally on the affected area. It generally takes effect after three applications.

（江苏 张宏俊 王道俊）

(Zhang Hongjun, Wang Daojun, Jiangsu)

8. 治下肢溃疡日久不收口效方

8. Effective Prescription for Treating Chronic Non-healing Lower Limb Ulcers

下肢溃疡是一种常见的皮肤病，多因湿热下注，瘀血凝聚，经络阻滞，气血不通，肌肤破溃而成，用桉叶糊剂治疗有特效。其方法如下：将新鲜桉树叶切碎放入砂锅加水煎 3 小时，去渣再煎成糊剂备用。擦药前先用艾叶煎水反复清洗创面，洗净后，用消毒棉签蘸桉叶糊剂涂于患处，再用消毒纱布包扎好。每日换药一次，一般半月可愈。

Lower limb ulcers are a common skin disease, mostly caused by the downward flow of damp-heat, blood stasis accumulation, meridian blockage, poor circulation of qi and blood, and subsequent skin breakdown. Treating it with eucalyptus leaf paste has a special effect. The method is as follows: Chop fresh eucalyptus leaves, put them in a clay pot, add water, and decoct for 3 hours. Remove the dregs and continue to decoct until it forms a paste for later use. Before applying the medicine, repeatedly wash the wound with mugwort leaf decoction. After washing, use a sterilized cotton swab to dip the eucalyptus leaf paste and apply it to the affected area, then bandage it with sterilized gauze. Change the dressing once a day, and it generally takes half a month to cure.

《民族医药报》1993 年 4 月 2 日（福建 李志民）

Ethnic Medicine News, April 2, 1993 (Li Zhimin, Fujian)

八、氟尿嘧啶在皮肤科的应用（6方）

VIII. Dermatological Applications of Fluorouracil (6 Prescriptions)

氟脲嘧啶（5-Fu）是早在50年代就用于临床治疗肿瘤的药物，至今仍是常用的抗肿瘤药物之一。近年来发现该药治疗一些皮肤病也有一定的功效。

Fluorouracil (5-Fu) has been used clinically for tumor treatment since the 1950s and remains one of the commonly used anti-tumor drugs today. In recent years, it has been discovered that this drug also has certain therapeutic effects on some skin diseases.

1. 尖锐湿疣系人类乳头瘤病毒感染引起的生殖器会阴和肛门部位的表皮瘤样增生，属于性传播疾病。该病传统的治疗药物足叶草脂刺激性大，用量过大吸收后还可引起全身毒性反应。氟脲嘧啶是脱氧胸苷酸合成酶抑制剂，能破坏病毒的核糖核酸及蛋白质合成，从而阻止人类乳头瘤病毒的生长繁殖，加之其局部皮肤黏膜外用有一定的腐蚀剥脱作用，可使尖锐湿疣萎缩脱落痊愈。用2.5%氟脲嘧啶霜每日4次外涂男性尿道口尖锐湿疣，两周为一疗程，有效率达90%。

1. Condyloma acuminatum is an epidermal tumor-like proliferation in the genital, perineal, and anal areas caused by human papillomavirus (HPV) infection, and it belongs to sexually transmitted diseases. The traditional treatment drug, podophyllin, is highly irritating, and excessive absorption can cause systemic toxic reactions. Fluorouracil is a thymidylate synthase inhibitor that can destroy viral RNA and protein synthesis, thereby preventing the growth and reproduction of HPV. In addition, its topical application to local skin and mucous membranes has a certain corrosive and exfoliating effect, which can cause condyloma acuminatum to atrophy, shed, and heal. Applying 2.5% fluorouracil cream to condyloma acuminatum at the male urethral meatus four times a day, with a two-week course of treatment, achieves an effective rate of 90%.

2. 白色念珠菌感染 应用本品0.25克加生理盐水20毫升超声雾化吸入，每天一次，或本药0.25克加生理盐水40毫升口腔局部涂擦治疗口腔白色念珠菌感染，收到显著效果。

2. Candida albicans Infection: Administering 0.25g of this drug with 20ml of normal saline via ultrasonic nebulization inhalation once a day, or applying 0.25g of this drug mixed with 40ml of normal saline topically to the oral cavity, has yielded significant results in treating oral Candida albicans infections.

3. 血管性紫癜 应用 5- Fu 0.5 克、氢化可的松 0.1 克加入 10% 葡萄糖 500 毫升内静脉滴注，每天一次，10-12 天为一疗程，治愈 7 例血管性紫癜，一般在用药 4-5 天紫癜开始消退，7-8 天全部消失。采用 2.5% 的 5- Fu 软膏涂擦治疗脂溢性角化病。结果：痊愈 23 例，显效 7 例，有效 6 例，总有效率 97. 3%。

3. Angiopathic Purpura: Intravenous infusion of 0.5g of 5-Fu and 0.1g of hydrocortisone in 500ml of 10% glucose solution once a day, with a 10-12 day course of treatment, cured 7 cases of angiopathic purpura. The purpura generally began to subside after 4-5 days of medication and completely disappeared within 7-8 days. Additionally, applying 2.5% 5-Fu ointment was used to treat seborrheic keratosis. Results: 23 cases were cured, 7 cases showed significant improvement, and 6 cases were effective, resulting in a total effective rate of 97.3%.

4. 瘢痕疙瘩 应用 2.5% 的 5-Fu 4 毫升、利多卡因 2 毫升、泼尼松龙混悬液 1 毫升（25 毫克）混合注入瘢痕组织内，每 6 天 1 次，5 次为 1 疗程。治疗 18 例，结果患者痊愈 10 例，有效 8 例。

4. Keloids: A mixture of 4ml of 2.5% 5-Fu, 2ml of lidocaine, and 1ml (25mg) of prednisolone suspension was injected into the scar tissue once every 6 days, with 5 injections constituting one course of treatment. Among 18 treated cases, 10 patients were cured and 8 showed effectiveness.

5. 扁平疣 先将扁平疣用手轻搓，局部发红后用 2.5%5-Fu 霜，每天两次外涂，皮损结痂后停药，结果 87 例患者全部痊愈。

5. Verruca Plana (Flat Warts): First, gently rub the flat warts by hand. After the local area turns red, apply 2.5% 5-Fu cream topically twice a day. Stop the medication after the skin lesions form scabs. As a result, all 87 patients were completely cured.

6. 白癜风和外阴白斑 有人用 5%5- Fu 霜局部贴敷，结果：7-9 天皮损发生糜烂，经 10 天渐愈合，并在愈合后 1-2 周开始出现色素沉着，两个月内皮损完全发生色素沉着。共治疗 28 例，其中 18 例全部色素再生，5 例部分再生，5 例无效。

6. Vitiligo and Vulvar Leukoplakia: Some individuals applied 5% 5-Fu cream topically. Results: Skin lesions developed erosions within 7-9 days, gradually healed over 10 days, and began to show pigmentation 1-2 weeks after healing. Complete pigmentation of the skin lesions occurred within two months. A total of 28 cases were treated, among which 18 cases achieved complete pigment regeneration, 5 cases achieved partial regeneration, and 5 cases were ineffective.

《中国医药报》

China Medical News.

第十四章　其他科
Chapter 14　Other Departments

一、失眠（16 方）
I. Insomnia (16 Prescriptions)

1.“镇心安神汤”治疗重症失眠

1. “Zhengan Anshen Decoction” (Sedating the Heart and Calming the Spirit Decoction) for Treating Severe Insomnia

失眠为临床常见病证之一。由于病因不同，体质差异，病程久等因素，失眠的程度也轻重不等。患者紧张、焦虑、恐惧、求治心越切，越是卧下辗转难眠，如此恶性循环，甚至通宵目不交睫，造成严重失眠症。我们在临床自拟“镇心安神汤”治疗严重失眠症，收到满意疗效，曾对 157 例患者进行疗效观察，结果治疗显效 98 例，占 62%；好转 55 例，占 35%，总有效率为 97%。兹介绍方药如下：生龙骨 10-30 克，生牡蛎 30 克，染茯苓 12 克，紫丹参 30 克，炒枣仁 30 克，合欢皮 12 克，夜交藤 30 克。

Insomnia is one of the common clinical syndromes. Due to different causes, physical constitutions, and prolonged disease courses, the severity of insomnia varies. The more anxious, fearful, and eager for treatment the patients are, the more they toss and turn in bed, creating a vicious cycle. They may even stay awake all night, leading to severe insomnia. We formulated the “Zhengan Anshen Decoction” in our clinical practice to treat severe insomnia and achieved satisfactory results. A clinical observation of 157 patients showed that 98 cases (62%) had significant effects, 55 cases (35%) showed improvement, with a total effective rate of 97%. The prescription is as follows: 10-30g of raw dragon bone (longgu), 30g of raw oyster shell (muli), 12g of dyed poria (fuling), 30g of red salvia root (danshen), 30g of stir-fried ziziphus seeds (suanzaoren), 12g of albizia bark (hehuanpi), and 30g of polygonum multiflorum vine (yejiaoteng).

辨证加味：阴血虚，加当归身、白芍、生地、龙眼肉；气阴虚，加太子参、麦冬、五味子；阴虚火旺，加生地、麦冬、川连；心火偏亢，加川连（或莲子芯）、黄芩、麦冬；心肝火旺，加川连、麦冬、山栀、丹皮；惊吓，加酒炒郁李仁、生龙齿；肝郁，加四逆散。

Syndrome Differentiation and Modifications: For Yin and blood deficiency, add angelica sinensis (root center), white peony root (baishao), rehmannia root (shengdi), and longan aril (longyanrou); for Qi and Yin deficiency, add pseudostellaria root (taizishen), ophiopogon tuber (maidong), and schisandra fruit (wuweizi); for Yin deficiency with hyperactive fire, add rehmannia root, ophiopogon tuber, and coptis rhizome (chuanlian); for hyperactive heart fire, add coptis rhizome (or lotus plumule/lianxixin), scutellaria root (huangqin), and ophiopogon tuber; for hyperactive heart and liver fire, add coptis rhizome, ophiopogon tuber, gardenia fruit (shanzhi), and moutan bark (danpi); for fright and palpitations, add wine-fried bush cherry seed (yuliren) and raw dragon teeth (longchi); for liver stagnation, add Sini Powder (Four Reversal Powder).

服法：每日一剂，下午或傍晚先服二煎药，头煎药留在睡前服；若早醒者，入睡前服头煎药，二煎药等醒来后继服。

Administration: One dose per day. Take the second decoction in the afternoon or evening, and reserve the first decoction to be taken before going to bed; for those who wake up too early, take the first decoction before sleep, and take the second decoction after waking up.

疗程：以三天为一疗程。不愈可再服第二疗程。

Course of Treatment: Three days constitute one course. If not cured, a second course can be taken.

《民族医药报》1992 年 2 月 7 日（江苏 吴自强）

Ethnic Medicine News, February 7, 1992 (Wu Ziqiang, Jiangsu)

2. 调整阴阳节规，治疗失眠顽症

2. Regulating Yin-Yang Circadian Rhythms to Treat Intractable Insomnia

失眠症在中老年脑力劳动者和大、中专学生中的发生率近年来日趋增加，而且目前治疗方法仍停留在服用镇静、催眠药物阶段。由于服用这些药物容易产生耐药性、成瘾性等副作用。因此，探索一种较好的自我疗法，成为医务人员的科研课题。

The incidence of insomnia among middle-aged and elderly mental workers, as well as college and secondary school students, has been increasing in recent years. Currently, treatment methods still rely on the use of sedative and hypnotic drugs. Since taking these drugs easily leads to side effects such as drug resistance and addiction, exploring a better self-therapy method has become a research topic for medical personnel.

宁夏医学院生理教研室贺义讲师等根据祖国医学阴阳睡眠学说，认为人一日之中，睡眠和觉醒的过程是阴阳进退消长、潜藏出入的过程。他们模拟睡眠觉醒概日节规为本校 50 名失眠症大学生采取①调兴奋：花茶 20 克，每天上午 9 时、14 时饮浓茶 1-2 杯，连服 10 天。②调抑制：午休和晚间睡前 30 分钟先进行渐进性松弛训练后入睡。③调脏腑、平衡阴阳：每天 16 时左右进行热身锻炼 1 次，约 30 分正钟。经过 10 天的疗程治疗，患者平均睡眠时间由 5.6 小时增加到 7 小时，睡眠质量也好于过去。

Based on the traditional Chinese medicine theory of Yin-Yang and sleep, Lecturer He Yi and others from the Physiology Teaching and Research Office of Ningxia Medical College believe that the process of sleeping and waking throughout the day is a process of the advance and retreat, waxing and waning, and hiding and emerging of Yin and Yang. Simulating the circadian rhythm of sleep and wakefulness, they applied the following methods to 50 university students with insomnia: 1. Regulating Excitement: Drink 1-2 cups of strong tea (20g of flower tea) at 9:00 AM and 2:00 PM daily for 10 consecutive days. 2. Regulating Inhibition: Perform progressive relaxation training 30 minutes before the afternoon nap and before going to bed at night, then go to sleep. 3. Regulating

Zang-Fu Organs and Balancing Yin-Yang: Do warm-up exercises once a day at around 4:00 PM for about 30 minutes. After a 10-day course of treatment, the patients' average sleep time increased from 5.6 hours to 7 hours, and their sleep quality was better than before.

《中医药信息报》1993 年 4 月 24 日（张毅）

Traditional Chinese Medicine Information News, April 24, 1993 (Zhang Yi)

3. 酸枣仁粥治失眠

3. Ziziphus Seed Porridge for Treating Insomnia

酸枣仁 10 克，洗净，捣碎，加水适量，煎汤取汁；粳米 100 克，洗净，以药汁煎煮，必要时中途可添开水。粥内，略加白糖调味服食。

Take 10g of ziziphus seeds, wash them, crush them, add an appropriate amount of water, and decoct to extract the liquid. Wash 100g of japonica rice and boil it in the medicinal liquid, adding boiling water midway if necessary. Add a little white sugar to the porridge for flavoring before eating.

（戴廷荣）

(Dai Tingrong)

4. 莲子二十粒和龙眼肉 20 克，于临睡前用水炖吃。

4. Stew 20 lotus seeds and 20g of longan arils in water and consume them before going to bed.

5. 将橘树鲜叶 30 克洗净，水煎十分钟，在药液中加白糖适量，每晚临睡前饮服，可治失眠。

5. Wash 30g of fresh tangerine leaves, decoct them in water for 10 minutes, add an appropriate amount of white sugar to the liquid, and drink it before going to bed every night to treat insomnia.

6. 对于心烦意乱引起的失眠症，可用百合 6 克，莲藕 10 克煎水服，多则三服，少则一服即可见效。

6. For insomnia caused by restlessness and vexation, 6g of lily bulbs and 10g of lotus roots can be decocted in water for oral intake. It will take effect after a minimum of one dose and a maximum of three doses.

7. 小麦 60 克、大枣 15 枚、甘草 30 克与四杯的水同煎，取汁一杯，分两次服用，对于神经衰弱引起的失眠有较好的疗效。

7. Decoct 60g of wheat, 15 red dates, and 30g of licorice with four cups of water. Extract one cup of the liquid and take it in two divided doses. It has a good therapeutic effect on insomnia caused by neurasthenia.

8. 酸枣仁 6 克，加白糖适量同研，临睡前用温开水冲服。

8. Grind 6g of ziziphus seeds together with an appropriate amount of white sugar into a powder, and dissolve it in warm water to drink before going to bed.

9. 每晚于临睡前喝蜂蜜水一杯，亦有助于睡眠。

9. Drinking a cup of honey water before going to bed every night is also conducive to sleep.

10. 生百合 6 克，蜂蜜一至二匙，一同蒸熟，临睡前服用，对睡眠不宁，惊惕易醒有效。

10. Steam 6g of raw lily bulbs together with one to two teaspoons of honey until cooked, and take it before going to bed. It is effective for restless sleep, fright, and easy awakening.

11. 睡前端坐床上，用右手掌拍打左脚涌泉穴 120 次，力度以感到微微胀痛为宜，再换用左手拍打右脚涌泉。此法可以治疗失眠，且可强壮身体，使人精力充沛。

11. Before going to bed, sit upright on the bed and use the right palm to pat the Yongquan acupoint on the left foot 120 times. The intensity should be enough to cause a slight feeling of distension and soreness. Then switch to the left hand to pat the Yongquan acupoint on the right foot. This method can treat insomnia, strengthen the body, and make people energetic.

失眠患者除用上面介绍的方法治疗外，还需注意有规律的生活，睡前不宜吃有刺激性的食物如咖啡、茶、酒等；晚餐不要吃得过饱；保持大小便通畅，因为便秘也可引起失眠。

In addition to the methods mentioned above, insomnia patients should also maintain a regular lifestyle. They should avoid eating stimulating foods such as coffee, tea, and alcohol before bed; avoid overeating at dinner; and maintain smooth bowel and urinary movements, as constipation can also cause insomnia.

《民族医药报》1991 年 11 月 5 日（新荐）

Ethnic Medicine News, November 5, 1991 (Xin Jian)

凡病后体虚，或心神被扰，或心火亢盛时出现心烦意乱、头晕耳鸣、五心烦热、梦遗滑泄、心悸健忘、多梦易醒、均为失眠的表观。失眠是健康的大敌，应及时治疗。下列介绍几则镇静安神的有效良方，供选用。

Whenever there is physical weakness after an illness, disturbance of the heart spirit, or hyperactive heart fire, accompanied by restlessness, dizziness, tinnitus, heat in the palms, soles, and chest, nocturnal emission, palpitations, poor memory, excessive dreaming, and easy awakening, these are all manifestations of insomnia. Insomnia is a major enemy of health and should be treated promptly. The following are several effective prescriptions for sedating and calming the spirit for selection.

12. 夜交藤方：夜交藤 50 克、大枣 50 克，加水煎服。此方补养心脾、和胃安神。

12. Polygonum Multiflorum Vine Prescription: Decoct 50g of polygonum multiflorum vine and 50g of red dates in water for oral intake. This prescription nourishes the heart and spleen, harmonizes the stomach, and calms the spirit.

13. 灯芯草方：灯芯草 50 克，鲜淡竹叶 50 克，水煎服。此方治热病烦渴、心烦不寐、小儿惊痛、咳逆等症。

13. Rush Pith Prescription: Decoct 50g of rush pith and 50g of fresh lophatherum leaves in water for oral intake. This prescription treats febrile diseases with vexation and thirst, restlessness and insomnia, infantile convulsions and pain, and coughing and vomiting.

14. 酸枣仁方：酸枣仁 20 克，焙焦为末，水煎服。此方治虚烦不眠、惊悸怔忡、烦渴虚汗。

14. Ziziphus Seed Prescription: Roast 20g of ziziphus seeds until scorched, grind them into a powder, and decoct in water for oral intake. This prescription

treats deficiency-type restlessness and insomnia, palpitations, and fright, as well as vexation, thirst, and night sweats.

15. 桑椹方：桑葚 15 克、远志 5 克，水煎服。此方滋补肾阴、清心降火。

15. Mulberry Fruit Prescription: Decoct 15g of mulberry fruits and 5g of polygala root in water for oral intake. This prescription nourishes kidney Yin, clears the heart, and reduces fire.

16. 莲子心方：莲子心 30 个，加少许盐煎汁，每晚临睡前顿服。此方益气、镇惊、安神。

16. Lotus Plumule Prescription: Decoct 30 lotus plumules with a little salt, and take the entire dose before going to bed every night. This prescription tonifies Qi, relieves fright, and calms the spirit.

《中药科技报》1992 年 5 月 16 日（黄海平）

Chinese Medicine Science and Technology News, May 16, 1992 (Huang Haiping)

二、神经衰弱（10 方）

II. Neurasthenia (10 Prescriptions)

蒙古族民间治神经衰弱方五则：

Five folk prescriptions for treating neurasthenia from the Mongolian ethnic group:

1. 广枣 50 克，豆蔻 40 克，白苣子 30 克，荜茇 20 克，石决明（煅）20 克。碎成细粉过筛，混匀备用。每日 2-3 次，每次 3-4 克，牛奶为引，开水送服。

1. Take 50g of hackberry fruit, 40g of cardamom, 30g of white lettuce seeds, 20g of long pepper, and 20g of calcined abalone shell. Grind them into a fine powder, sift, and mix evenly for later use. Take 3-4g each time, 2-3 times a day, using milk as a guiding medium and taking it with boiled water.

2. 酸枣仁（炒）50 克，白檀香 30 克，肉豆蔻 20 克，佛手参 20 克。碎粉过筛，混匀备用。每日 2-3 次，每次 3-5 克，开水送服。

2. Take 50g of stir-fried ziziphus seeds, 30g of white sandalwood, 20g of nutmeg, and 20g of gymnadenia orchid root. Grind into a powder, sift, and mix evenly for later use. Take 3-5g each time, 2-3 times a day, with boiled water.

3. 五味子 50 克，广枣 50 克，肉豆蔻 30 克，柏子仁 50 克，朱砂 10 克。朱砂另研外，其余碎成细粉过筛混匀，再兑入朱砂，研细备用。每日 2-3 次，每次 3-4 克，开水送服。

3. Take 50g of schisandra fruit, 50g of hackberry fruit, 30g of nutmeg, 50g of arborvitae seeds, and 10g of cinnabar. Grind the cinnabar separately. Grind the other ingredients into a fine powder, sift, and mix evenly, then add the cinnabar and grind finely for later use. Take 3-4g each time, 2-3 times a day, with boiled water.

4. 远志 50 克，石决明（制）40 克，沉香 40 克，肉豆蔻 30 克，广枣 30 克，木香 30 克，诃子、草阿魏、红盐、五灵脂各 20 克。碎成细粉过筛混匀备用。每日 2-3 次，每次 2-4 克，开水送服。

4. Take 50g of polygala root, 40g of processed abalone shell, 40g of agarwood, 30g of nutmeg, 30g of hackberry fruit, 30g of costus root, and 20g each of chebula fruit, assafoetida, red salt, and flying squirrel feces. Grind them into a fine powder, sift, and mix evenly for later use. Take 2-4g each time, 2-3 times a day, with boiled water.

5. 刺人参 100 克，广枣 30 克，白苣子 30 克，肉豆蔻 20 克，荜茇 20 克。碎成细粉过筛混匀备用。每日 1-2 次，每次 3-4 克，服前饮热牛奶 1 杯，后开水送服。

5. Take 100g of oplopanax root, 30g of hackberry fruit, 30g of white lettuce seeds, 20g of nutmeg, and 20g of long pepper. Grind them into a fine powder, sift, and mix evenly for later use. Take 3-4g each time, 1-2 times a day. Drink a cup of hot milk before taking the medication, and then take it with boiled water.

《民族医药报》1993 年 4 月 2 日（内蒙古 王曙霞）

Ethnic Medicine News, April 2, 1993 (Wang Shuxia, Inner Mongolia)

神经衰弱属神经官能症的一种，以失眠、多梦、头晕、健忘、耳鸣、眼花等为常见症状，除药物治疗、体育锻炼外，可选用下面介绍的食疗方进行辅助治疗。

Neurasthenia is a type of neurosis, with common symptoms including insomnia, excessive dreaming, dizziness, poor memory, tinnitus, and blurred vision. In addition to medication and physical exercise, the following dietary therapy prescriptions can be used as auxiliary treatments.

6. 甘麦大枣汤：取小麦 60 克，甘草 15 克，大枣 10 个。煎汤服，每日一剂。

6. Licorice, Wheat, and Jujube Soup: Take 60g of wheat, 15g of licorice, and 10 red dates. Decoct them into a soup for oral intake, one dose per day.

7. 淮杞炖猪脑：取淮山 50 克，杞子 20 克，猪脑 2 具。先将猪脑膜上红筋挑去，洗净，一起加水炖 1-2 小时后调味服。

7. Stewed Pig Brain with Chinese Yam and Wolfberry: Take 50g of Chinese yam, 20g of wolfberries, and 2 pig brains. First, remove the red blood vessels on the pig brain membrane, wash them clean, add water, and stew together for 1-2 hours. Season and consume.

8. 莲子百合瘦肉汤：取莲子、百合各 50 克，猪瘦肉 200 克，一起煎汤至莲子熟透后，调味服。

8. Lean Pork Soup with Lotus Seeds and Lily Bulbs: Take 50g each of lotus seeds and lily bulbs, and 200g of lean pork. Decoct them into a soup until the lotus seeds are thoroughly cooked. Season and consume.

9. 核桃芝麻膏：取核桃仁、黑芝麻各 250 克，红砂糖 500 克。先将红砂糖放锅中，加水溶解糖后，用慢火熬至成稠膏，加入炒熟的黑芝麻、核桃仁，调匀后趁热将上述各物一起倒入表面涂过麻油的大盘中，待稍冷后压平整，切成小块，随意取服。

9. Walnut and Black Sesame Paste: Take 250g each of walnut kernels and black sesame seeds, and 500g of brown sugar. First, put the brown sugar in a pan, add water to dissolve it, and simmer over low heat until it forms a thick paste. Add the roasted black sesame seeds and walnut kernels, mix evenly, and while still hot, pour the mixture into a large plate coated with sesame oil. When it cools

slightly, press it flat, cut it into small pieces, and consume as desired.

10. 桑椹膏：取桑椹子 500 克，加水煮至极烂，另加冰糖 200 克，用文火收膏，每日服二次，每次两汤匙，开水冲服。

10. Mulberry Fruit Paste: Take 500g of mulberry fruits, add water, and boil until they are extremely soft. Add 200g of rock sugar, and simmer over a gentle fire to form a paste. Take it twice a day, two tablespoons each time, dissolved in boiled water.

《中药科技报》1993 年 1 月 14 日（南宁市 李子云）

Chinese Medicine Science and Technology News, January 14, 1993 (Li Ziyun, Nanning City)

三、烧烫伤（11 方）

III. Burns and Scalds (11 Prescriptions)

1. 药物制备：紫草、白芷、忍冬藤、黄蜡各 320g，冰片 16g，麻油 1000g。将冰片研为细粉，紫草、白芷、忍冬藤分别切碎备用。取麻油加热，将白芷、忍冬藤入锅炸至白芷变黄色，去渣，再加入紫草，用微火炸枯至油呈紫红色时，捞除残渣，滤过，油液备用。制膏时，取黄蜡加入上述药油内熔化，倾入容器中，待温度降至 40-50℃时，兑入冰片细粉，搅匀至冷凝状即得。本品为紫红色软膏，具有特殊的油腻气味和冰片香气。功效：清热、消炎、止痛，用于治疗Ⅱ度烧烫伤。外用，涂敷于患处，每日 2-3 次。

1.Preparation of the Medicine: Take 320g each of gromwell root (zicao), angelica root (baizhi), and honeysuckle stem (ren dong teng); 16g of borneol; and 1000g of sesame oil. Grind the borneol into a fine powder, and chop the gromwell root, angelica root, and honeysuckle stem separately for later use. Heat the sesame oil, add the angelica root and honeysuckle stem to the pan, and fry them until the angelica root turns yellow. Remove the dregs, then add the gromwell root and fry it over a gentle fire until it is scorched and the oil turns purplish-red. Remove the remaining dregs, filter the oil, and set it aside. To make the ointment, add yellow beeswax to the aforementioned medicated oil and melt it. Pour it into a container, and when the temperature drops to 40-50℃ , mix in the fine borneol powder and stir evenly until it cools and solidifies. This product is a purplish-red ointment with a special greasy odor and the fragrance of borneol. Effects: Clears heat, reduces inflammation, and relieves pain; used for treating second-degree burns and scalds. For external use, apply it to the affected area 2-3 times a day.

（湖北 刘峥嵘）

(Liu Zhengrong, Hubei)

炎热的夏天单衣薄裳，稍有不慎就会触及沸水、热火，引起皮肤烫伤。笔者根据多年的临床经验，总结出验方四则，供患者选用。

In the hot summer when people wear thin clothing, a slight carelessness may lead to touching boiling water or open flames, causing skin scalds. Based on years of clinical experience, the author has summarized four verified prescriptions for patients to choose from.

2. 取新鲜的小蓟 300 克，用清水洗净吹干，放在容器内捣烂，滤渣取汁，用时先用冷开水将烫伤部位洗净，用纱布蘸小蓟汁外涂于患处，干者即涂。适用于Ⅱ度烫伤，面积稍大，水疱较多而未破的病人，用后，一般 3-5 小时疼痛即可缓解，12-24 小时水疱即可消失，2-3 天即愈。

2. Take 300g of fresh field thistle, wash it with clean water, air-dry it, put it in a container, and mash it. Filter out the dregs and extract the juice. When using, first wash the scalded area with cooled boiled water, dip gauze in the field thistle juice, and apply it externally to the affected area. Reapply when it dries. It is suitable for patients with second-degree scalds, slightly large areas, and many unruptured blisters. After application, the pain can generally be relieved within 3-5 hours, the blisters will disappear within 12-24 hours, and the patient will be cured in 2-3 days.

3. 取生大黄 30 克、生地榆 330 克、冰片 15 克，共研细末，加入麻油 500 克，搅成糊状涂于患处，每日 1-2 次。适用于各种烫伤，尤宜局部红肿热痛、糜烂、滋水淋漓的病人。

3. Take 30g of raw rhubarb, 30g of raw garden burnet root, and 15g of borneol. Grind them together into a fine powder, add 500g of sesame oil, stir into a paste, and apply it to the affected area 1-2 times a day. It is suitable for various scalds, especially for patients with local redness, swelling, heat, pain, erosion, and profuse exudation.

4. 取石灰50克、放入清水2000毫升，冷却澄淀后，取其液体，加适量的麻油，外搽患处，每日2-3次。适用于急性浅表性烫伤，能较有效地减轻痛苦、减少水疱。

4. Take 50g of quicklime, add 2000ml of clean water, and after it cools and settles, take the clear liquid, add an appropriate amount of sesame oil, and apply it externally to the affected area 2-3 times a day. It is suitable for acute superficial scalds and can effectively relieve pain and reduce blisters.

5. 取新鲜鸡蛋6-7枚，煮熟，去蛋白，留蛋黄，放在武火锅内爆炒至黑成油，外涂于患处。适于烫伤后肉芽组织不新鲜，久不收口的病人。一般3-5天即可获效。

5. Take 6-7 fresh eggs, boil them, peel off the egg whites, keep the egg yolks, put them in a hot pan over high heat, and stir-fry until they turn black and release oil. Apply the oil externally to the affected area. It is suitable for patients whose granulation tissue is not fresh after a scald and whose wounds do not heal for a long time. It generally takes effect within 3-5 days.

《中医药信息报》（张宏俊 王道俊）

Traditional Chinese Medicine Information News (Zhang Hongjun, Wang Daojun)

仡佬族治水火烫伤：

Treatments for burns and scalds from the Gelao ethnic group:

6. 生石灰适量（根据伤面大小而定），以泉水调成糊状涂擦伤处。每日数次，可防伤面起水疱和化脓，愈后不留下疤痕。

6. Take an appropriate amount of quicklime (depending on the size of the wound), mix it with spring water into a paste, and apply it to the wound. Apply it several times a day to prevent blisters and suppuration on the wound surface, and it will heal without leaving scars.

7. 土石膏（俗名水凝硼）适量，研细末撒伤面，每日数次，愈后无痕。此方适用于已化脓者，新伤不宜用。

7. Take an appropriate amount of native gypsum (commonly known as water coagulation boron), grind it into a fine powder, and sprinkle it on the wound surface several times a day. It will heal without leaving traces. This prescription is suitable for wounds that have already suppurated; it should not be used for fresh wounds.

8. 鼠仔（未生毛者）、桐油（菜油亦可）将二味同放入玻璃瓶中泡作汁备用，用鸡鸭翅羽蘸取药汁涂搽患处，每日数次，数日痊愈。此方适宜于新、旧伤者。

8. Take hairless baby mice and tung oil (rapeseed oil can also be used). Put both ingredients into a glass bottle and soak them to extract the juice for later use. Use a chicken or duck wing feather to dip in the medicinal juice and apply it to the affected area several times a day. It will be cured in a few days. This prescription is suitable for both fresh and old wounds.

注以上三方在使用期间忌食青菜、南瓜、辣椒，以防患部发痒。水火烫伤需治多久一般视伤势而定。

Note: During the use of the above three prescriptions, avoid eating green vegetables, pumpkins, and chili peppers to prevent itching in the affected area. The duration of treatment for burns and scalds generally depends on the severity of the injury.

《民族医药报》1992 年 5 月 13 日（贵州 谢昭齐 谢卓芳）

Ethnic Medicine News, May 13, 1992 (Xiao Zhaoqi, Xiao Zhuofang, Guizhou)

9. 白糖、蚯蚓治疗水火烫伤。被沸水或火烫伤后，先用米醋冲洗患部，可起到止痛和预防起泡的效果，然后速取活蚯蚓 50 克左右，用清水洗净泥沙。盛装在碗或瓶内，加入白糖，以 1：1.5 的比例混合，让其蠕动，慢慢形成粘液，用棉签或洁净的鸡鸭羽毛，蘸取其粘液涂患处，每日 4 次，可止痛消肿，对于Ⅰ度烧伤效果较好；Ⅱ度烧伤范围小，处理及时同样有效。如果为大面积烧伤且病情较重，应及时送医院诊治。

9. White Sugar and Earthworms for Treating Burns and Scalds. After being

scalded by boiling water or burned by fire, first rinse the affected area with rice vinegar, which can relieve pain and prevent blisters. Then quickly take about 50g of live earthworms and wash away the mud with clean water. Put them in a bowl or bottle, add white sugar in a ratio of 1:1.5, let them wriggle, and slowly form mucus. Use a cotton swab or a clean chicken or duck feather to dip in the mucus and apply it to the affected area 4 times a day. It can relieve pain and reduce swelling. It has a good effect on first-degree burns; for second-degree burns with a small area, timely treatment is equally effective. If the burns are large in area and the condition is severe, the patient should be promptly sent to a hospital for treatment.

《民族医药报》1992 年 5 月 26 日

Ethnic Medicine News, May 26, 1992

10. 田螺白矾治疗烧烫伤

10. River Snails and Alum for Treating Burns and Scalds

在日常生活中，由于种种原因导致人体被水火烫伤之病症时有发生。若患者一时找不到较为理想的方法治疗，可取活田螺 10 枚左右（视烧伤面积大小而定具体个数）、白矾 10 克（研极细末）。先将活田螺外壳洗净，再用清水漂养 20-30 分钟，然后用针刺破田螺外壳，并加入白矾细末。待 30 分钟后除去田螺外壳，用洁净之羽毛或棉花蘸取其汁涂擦患处，烧伤者每日涂 2 次，烫伤者每日用 1 次。用该法治疗症状不是很重的烧烫伤患者，一般 3 天可愈。若症情较为严重，应在医师指导下用药治疗。

In daily life, burns and scalds caused by water or fire occur from time to time due to various reasons. If patients cannot find an ideal treatment method temporarily, they can take about 10 live river snails (the specific number depends on the size of the burn area) and 10g of alum (ground into an extremely fine powder). First, wash the shells of the live river snails, then soak them in clean water for 20-30 minutes, pierce the shells with a needle, and add the fine alum powder. After 30 minutes, remove the river snail shells, use a clean feather or cotton to dip in the juice and apply it to the affected area. Burn patients should apply it twice a day, and scald patients should apply it once a day. Using this method to treat patients with mild burns and scalds generally cures them in 3 days. If the condition is more severe, medication should be used under the guidance of a doctor.

《民族医药报》1991 年 7 月 5 日

Ethnic Medicine News, July 5, 1991

11. 烫伤：酸汤杆（虎杖）磨菜油搽患处，一天多次，几天后痊愈。虎杖老根效果显著。

11. Scalds: Grind sour soup stems (giant knotweed) with rapeseed oil and apply it to the affected area several times a day. It will be cured after a few days. The old roots of giant knotweed have a significant effect.

四、冻疮（41 方）
IV. Chilblains (41 Prescriptions)

1. 多年来，笔者用活血化瘀、通络止痛的当归桂枝芍药汤治疗冻疮，取得了显著效果，一般 3 剂即可见红肿消退，溃烂创面在一周内愈合。方药：当归 12 克，桂枝 10 克，赤芍 9 克，生姜 5 克，大枣 10 枚，甘草 5 克。水煎服。每日 1 剂。

1.For many years, the author has used the Danggui Guizhi Shaoyao Decoction, which promotes blood circulation, removes blood stasis, unblocks collaterals, and relieves pain, to treat chilblains with remarkable results. Generally, redness and swelling subside after 3 doses, and ulcerated wounds heal within a week. Prescription: 12g of angelica sinensis (danggui), 10g of cassia twig (guizhi), 9g of red peony root (chishao), 5g of fresh ginger (shengjiang), 10 red dates (dazao), and 5g of licorice (gancao). Decoct in water for oral intake, one dose per day.

《民族医药报》1998 年 1 月 23 日（杜连生）

Ethnic Medicine News, January 23, 1998 (Du Liansheng)

2. 生萝卜1个洗净，切成大块，轻擦患处，以自己感觉患处皮肤变得温热为度。每日数次，直至痊愈。冻疮已破溃者不宜用此法。

2. Wash 1 fresh radish, cut it into large pieces, and gently rub the affected area until the skin feels warm. Do this several times a day until cured. This method should not be used if the chilblains have already ulcerated.

3. 大蒜杆250克，棉籽50克，加水适量煎半小时，温热时洗患处，每日1次，连用5日。

3. Take 250g of garlic stalks and 50g of cotton seeds, add an appropriate amount of water, and decoct for half an hour. Wash the affected area with the warm liquid once a day for 5 consecutive days.

4. 萝卜1个，橘皮9克，煎汤外洗患处，再用蟹壳2个焙干研末，香油调涂患部。

4. Take 1 radish and 9g of tangerine peel, decoct them in water, and wash the affected area externally. Then, roast 2 crab shells until dry, grind them into a powder, mix with sesame oil, and apply to the affected area.

5. 用醋洗涤局部后，将鲜藕捣烂，敷于受冻部位，或将藕蒸熟后捣烂敷于患处。

5. After washing the local area with vinegar, mash fresh lotus roots and apply them to the frostbitten area; alternatively, steam the lotus roots until cooked, mash them, and apply to the affected area.

6. 干净蜂蜜75克，和炼过的猪油25克混合，搅匀后为油膏状，外涂患处，每日数次。

6. Mix 75g of clean honey with 25g of refined lard, stir evenly to form an ointment, apply it externally to the affected area several times a day.

7. 花椒15克浸入30毫升白酒中，7天后捞去花椒，取生姜6片切碎绞汁，与甘油6毫升一同加入酒内，摇匀，外涂患处。

7. Soak 15g of Sichuan peppercorns in 30ml of liquor. After 7 days, remove the peppercorns. Chop 6 slices of fresh ginger, extract the juice, and add it to the liquor along with 6ml of glycerin. Shake well and apply externally to the affected area.

8. 老丝瓜烧成炭，研成细末，拌在动物油里，涂搽患处，每日 2 次。

8. Burn old loofahs into charcoal, grind them into a fine powder, mix with animal fat, and apply to the affected area twice a day.

9. 杏仁 10 个，芝麻 15 克，花椒 9 克，分别炒香研末后混匀，香油调涂患处。

9. Take 10 almonds, 15g of sesame seeds, and 9g of Sichuan peppercorns. Roast them until fragrant separately, grind into a powder, mix evenly, and apply to the affected area mixed with sesame oil.

10. 大蒜 15 克去皮捣烂，花椒 15 克研末，放入炼好的 70 克猪油中搅匀，制成膏剂，敷于受冻未破皮处，每日 1 次，用纱布包好。

10. Peel and mash 15g of garlic, and grind 15g of Sichuan peppercorns into a powder. Add them to 70g of refined lard, stir evenly to make a paste, and apply it to the frostbitten but unbroken skin once a day, then wrap it with gauze.

11. 生姜 50 克捣烂，加入白酒 50 毫升浸泡，搅匀后外擦患处，每日 3 次，也可用鲜生姜 1 块，煨热后切成片，趁热擦涂患部。

11. Mash 50g of fresh ginger, add 50ml of liquor to soak, stir evenly, and rub it externally on the affected area 3 times a day. Alternatively, take a piece of fresh ginger, roast it until warm, cut it into slices, and rub the affected area while it is still hot.

12. 红辣椒 10 克去籽切碎，加入白酒 60 毫升中浸泡 7 天，再加入樟脑 2.5 克，用时摇匀，用棉花蘸药水涂患处，每日 2 次。

12. Remove the seeds from 10g of red chili peppers, chop them, and soak them in 60ml of liquor for 7 days. Then add 2.5g of camphor. Shake well before use, dip cotton in the medicinal liquid, and apply it to the affected area twice a day.

《中药科技报》1992 年 12 月 16 日（刘永连）

Chinese Medicine Science and Technology News, December 16, 1992 (Liu Yonglian)

13. 轻度冻疮，皮肤红肿，可将伤湿止痛膏贴于患处，两天换一次，一周后便可消失。

13. For mild chilblains with red and swollen skin, apply a Shangshi Zhitong

Gao (rheumatism and pain-relieving plaster) to the affected area, change it every two days, and it will disappear after a week.

14. 荆芥 30 克，苏叶、桂枝各 15 克，加水 2000-3000 毫升，煮后温洗，每日 1-2 次。

14. Take 30g of schizonepeta, 15g of perilla leaves, and 15g of cassia twigs. Add 2000-3000ml of water, boil, and wash the affected area with the warm liquid 1-2 times a day.

15. 把尖辣椒切成丝，放进 60 度的白酒中浸泡 10 天左右，再用它擦患处，每天 5 次，疗效特别好，适用于未破溃的冻疮。

15. Cut hot chili peppers into shreds, soak them in 60-degree liquor for about 10 days, and then rub the affected area with the liquid 5 times a day. This has a particularly good effect and is suitable for unruptured chilblains.

16. 用十滴水擦洗患处，每日 3 次。

16. Wipe and wash the affected area with Shidishui (Ten Drops Water, a traditional Chinese liquid medicine for heatstroke), 3 times a day.

17. 用生姜一块，在火上煨热后，切片，擦红肿处，每天 2 次，每次 15 分钟。

17. Take a piece of fresh ginger, roast it over a fire until warm, cut it into slices, and rub the red and swollen area for 15 minutes each time, twice a day.

18. 冻疮已溃烂者，可用螃蟹烧灰，蜂蜜适量调成糊状，外涂患处，一周左右可治愈。

18. For ulcerated chilblains, burn crabs into ash, mix with an appropriate amount of honey to form a paste, apply it externally to the affected area, and it can be cured in about a week.

19. 山楂数个，烧熟去核，捣成膏状，敷于患处，用于冻疮破溃久不收口者，疗效甚好。

19. Take several hawthorns, roast them until cooked, remove the pits, mash them into a paste, and apply to the affected area. This has a very good effect on ulcerated chilblains that fail to heal for a long time.

20. 用棉花的花焙焦研成细末，撒在布上外敷患处，每日 1 次，对已破溃者疗效更佳。

20. Roast cotton flowers until scorched, grind them into a fine powder, sprinkle them on a piece of cloth, and apply it externally to the affected area once a day. This has an even better effect on ruptured chilblains.

《民族医药报》1996 年 12 月 25 日（江苏 纪国安）

Ethnic Medicine News, December 25, 1996 (Ji Guo' an, Jiangsu)

21. 把新鲜鸡蛋煮熟，剥去蛋壳、蛋白，留下蛋黄，盛在铁勺内放在火上烤，蛋黄油渗出，冷却后敷用。先用 3 % 的双氧水溶液清洗患处，然后再敷上鸡蛋黄油，并用干净纱布包扎，一般 3-5 天后伤口即可愈合。

21. Boil fresh eggs, peel off the shells and egg whites, and keep the egg yolks. Place the yolks in an iron spoon and roast them over a fire until the yolk oil seeps out. Let it cool before applying. First, clean the affected area with a 3% hydrogen peroxide solution, then apply the egg yolk oil, and bandage it with clean gauze. Generally, the wound will heal after 3-5 days.

22. 橘子皮两个、干姜片适量煮汤洗患处。

22. Boil 2 tangerine peels and an appropriate amount of dried ginger slices in water, and use the soup to wash the affected area.

23. 黑胡椒 5 克或干辣椒 25-50 克，研末或切碎，开水泡后浸洗患处。

23. Take 5g of black pepper or 25-50g of dried chili peppers, grind them into a powder or chop them, steep in boiling water, and soak/wash the affected area with the liquid.

24. 冬瓜皮、茄子杆各 50 克，水煮洗患处。

25. Take 50g each of winter melon peel and eggplant stems, boil them in water, and wash the affected area with the liquid.

25. 萝卜切厚片煮熟，捞出待片刻，趁热敷患处，每次 10 分钟。

25. Cut radishes into thick slices, boil them until cooked, take them out, wait for a moment, and apply them to the affected area while still warm for 10 minutes each time.

26. 取米制陈醋 500 克，中药当归 20 克，共放入陶制品内用小火煮开，时间不得少于 20 分钟，然后取出当归放入少许白糖，倒入另一容器，趁热浸泡或用纱布擦洗冻疮患处，直至皮肤松皱为止（皮肤有溃烂者应用擦的方法）。一般连续治疗 4 天即愈。

26. Take 500g of rice vinegar and 20g of angelica sinensis (danggui). Put them together in a ceramic container and bring to a boil over low heat for no less than 20 minutes. Then remove the angelica sinensis, add a little white sugar, and pour the liquid into another container. While still hot, soak or scrub the chilblain-affected area with gauze until the skin becomes loose and wrinkled (for patients with ulcerated skin, use the scrubbing method). Generally, continuous treatment for 4 days will cure the condition.

《民族医药报》1991 年 3 月 5 日（赵艳）

Ethnic Medicine News, March 5, 1991 (Zhao Yan)

27. 在夏天吃西瓜的时候，将西瓜皮稍留厚一些，用它在冬天患过冻疮的皮肤处来回轻擦十几下，这样续擦三至五次，便可起到预防冻疮的作用。

27. When eating watermelons in summer, leave the rind slightly thick. Gently rub it back and forth over the skin that had chilblains in winter about a dozen times. Repeat this process three to five times to prevent chilblains.

28. 取适量的鲜芝麻叶或新鲜的芝麻花十几朵，放在生过冻疮的皮肤上，用手来回搓擦约二十分钟，然后将其叶汁或花汁留在皮肤上，不要急于洗去，待一小时以后再用水洗净。这样反复几次亦可收到预防之效。

28. Take an appropriate amount of fresh sesame leaves or a dozen fresh sesame flowers, place them on the skin that has had chilblains, and rub back and forth with your hands for about 20 minutes. Leave the leaf or flower juice on the skin without washing it off immediately. Wash it clean with water after an hour. Repeating this process several times can also achieve a preventive effect.

29. 在大伏天，选一些独头紫皮大蒜，去皮捣烂后，放在烈日下曝晒一小时左右，然后取大蒜汁，涂搽患过冻疮的皮肤处，每天三至四次，连涂四至五天即可。

29. During the dog days of summer, select some single-clove purple-skinned garlic, peel and mash it, and expose it to the blazing sun for about an hour. Then,

extract the garlic juice and apply it to the skin that has had chilblains, three to four times a day, for four to five consecutive days.

（湖南 李凤发）

(Li Fengfa, Hunan)

局部治疗：

Local Treatment:

30. 早期：指局部结节、痒痛未破溃者。治疗：外涂樟脑酒精剂；该剂组成：樟脑：75% 酒精 =1:10（单位：克）按此比例混合。70% 蜂蜜、30% 猪油混合制成软膏厚搽患处。

30. Early stage: Refers to local nodules with itching and pain that have not yet ulcerated. Treatment: Apply camphor alcohol solution externally. Composition of the solution: Mix camphor and 75% alcohol in a ratio of 1:10 (in grams). Alternatively, mix 70% honey and 30% lard to make an ointment, and apply it thickly to the affected area.

31. 晚期：指疮溃破、出血。溃破出血者，按溃疡处理。如用氯霉素、黄连素软膏外涂，合并感染严重者应选用适应的抗生素治疗。

31. Late stage: Refers to ruptured and bleeding chilblains. Treat ruptured and bleeding cases as ulcers. For example, apply chloramphenicol or berberine ointment externally. For severe cases with concurrent infection, appropriate antibiotics should be used for treatment.

32. 中药外洗：药方组成如下：宽筋藤 30 克，威灵仙 15 克，红花 15 克，鸡血藤 30 克，三棱 15 克，苏木 12 克，牛膝 30 克，海桐皮 20 克，莪术 12 克，桃仁 10 克，水煎外泡洗患处。

32. External Herbal Wash: The prescription consists of the following: 30g of wide-tendon vine (kuanjinteng), 15g of clematis root (weilingxian), 15g of safflower (honghua), 30g of spatholobus stem (jixueteng), 15g of sparganium rhizome (sanleng), 12g of sappanwood (sumu), 30g of achyranthes root (niuxi), 20g of erythrina bark (haitongpi), 12g of zedoary rhizome (ezhu), and 10g of peach seed (taoren). Decoct in water and soak/wash the affected area.

33. 局部按摩：局部按摩可促进周围血液循环，对冻疮的治疗有一定作用，不要用力挤压结节；紫外线、红外线照射均有利于冻疮治疗。

33. Local Massage: Local massage can promote peripheral blood circulation and has a certain therapeutic effect on chilblains. Do not squeeze the nodules forcefully. Ultraviolet and infrared irradiation are also beneficial for the treatment of chilblains.

《民族医药报》1992 年 1 月 31 日（广西 蓝日程）

Ethnic Medicine News, January 31, 1992 (Lan Richeng, Guangxi)

34. 鲜茄根 50 克，水煎洗烫，每日 1 次。

34. Take 50g of fresh eggplant roots, decoct in water, and wash/soak the affected area once a day.

35. 干红辣椒少许，加水煮沸，待水不烫时泡洗，每日 1 次。

35. Take a small amount of dried red chili peppers, add water and boil. Wait until the water is no longer scalding hot, then soak and wash the affected area once a day.

36. 辣椒柴、松树叶各等份，水煎洗烫，每日 1 次。

36. Take equal amounts of chili pepper branches and pine needles, decoct in water, and wash/soak the affected area once a day.

37. 冬青叶 15 克，加水煮沸，待水不烫时泡洗，每日 1 次。

37. Take 15g of holly leaves, add water and boil. Wait until the water is no longer scalding hot, then soak and wash the affected area once a day.

38. 中药木瓜、白茄秧、艾叶适量煎水浸泡，每次 10-15 分钟，每日 1-2 次。

38. Take an appropriate amount of Chinese medicinal papaya, white eggplant seedlings, and mugwort leaves. Decoct them in water and soak the affected area for 10-15 minutes each time, 1-2 times a day.

39. 姜叶一把，剪碎，用豆腐水煎之，局部洗烫，每日 2 次。

39. Take a handful of ginger leaves, cut them into pieces, and decoct them in tofu water. Wash/soak the local affected area with the liquid twice a day.

40. 樱桃叶适量，食盐少许，捣烂取汁，每日 2 次涂擦。

40. Take an appropriate amount of cherry leaves and a small amount of table salt, mash them to extract the juice, and apply/rub it on the affected area twice a day.

《民族医药报》1992 年 9 月 4 日（湖南 李凤发）

Ethnic Medicine News, September 4, 1992 (Li Fengfa, Hunan)

41. 冻疮一般较难根除，严冬到来之际，容易复发。如采用下述方法，可达到治愈的目的，患者不妨一试。

41. Chilblains are generally difficult to eradicate completely and tend to relapse when the severe winter arrives. Using the following method can achieve a cure, and patients might as well give it a try.

方法是：取米制陈醋 500 克，中药当归 20 克，共放入陶制品内用文火煮沸，20 分钟以上，然后连当归一起倒入容器内，若是手足部患冻疮者，可趁热将患处浸泡于药液中；若患处位于耳部等处不便浸泡，可用纱布或毛巾蘸醋药液涂擦患处，一直浸涂擦到患处皮肤松皱为止，每天 3 至 4 次，一般连续数天可愈。

Method: Take 500g of rice vinegar and 20g of angelica sinensis (danggui). Put them together in a ceramic container and bring to a boil over a gentle fire for more than 20 minutes. Then, pour the liquid along with the angelica sinensis into a container. If the chilblains are on the hands or feet, soak the affected area in the hot medicinal liquid. If the affected area is on the ears or other places where soaking is inconvenient, use gauze or a towel dipped in the vinegar medicinal liquid to wipe and rub the affected area until the skin becomes loose and wrinkled. Do this 3 to 4 times a day, and it generally takes several consecutive days to cure.

《民族医药报》1993 年 1 月 1 日（贵州 胡定绶）

Ethnic Medicine News, January 1, 1993 (Hu Dingshou, Guizhou)

五、脚气（18 方）
V. Athlete’s Foot (18 Prescriptions)

1. 一九八九年六月以来，笔者配以“苦桃液”外用治疗脚气病（足趾缝间出小泡，脱皮，奇痒）八十余例，均收满意效果，现介绍如下：

1. Since June 1989, the author has used the externally applied "Kutao Liquid" to treat over 80 cases of athlete's foot (characterized by small blisters, peeling, and severe itching between the toes), with satisfactory results. The details are as follows:

方药与制法：取苦参 20 克，青核桃五六枚，百分之九十五酒精 300 毫升，将苦参研末，青核桃刮剥取皮，兑入酒精内，密封一星期后，酒精即变为棕褐色，滤去药渣，备用。

Ingredients and Preparation: Take 20g of sophora flavescens root (kushen), 5-6green walnuts, and 300ml of 95% alcohol. Grind the sophora flavescens root into a powder, peel the green walnuts, and soak them in the alcohol. Seal the container for one week until the alcohol turns brownish. Filter out the medicinal dregs and set aside for later use.

用法：把患脚用温开水洗净擦干，用棉球浸药液擦抹患处，立即止痒，每日二至三次，二至三天即愈。无任何副作用。

Usage: Wash the affected foot with warm boiled water and dry it. Dip a cotton ball in the medicinal liquid and apply it to the affected area. It can relieve itching immediately. Apply 2-3 times a day, and it will be cured in 2-3 days. There are no side effects.

《中医药信息报》（河南 王君洲）

Traditional Chinese Medicine Information News (Wang Junzhou, Henan)

2. 取韭菜一把，洗净捣烂放在脚盆内，再倒入热开水小半盆，然后加盖。过 10 分钟左右，待水稍凉后，将患脚浸泡在水中搓擦。半小时后将脚擦干，换穿干净鞋袜即可。每日一次，一般数次可愈。

2. Take a handful of Chinese chives, wash and mash them, put them in a footbath, and then pour in a little less than half a basin of hot boiled water. Cover the basin. After about 10 minutes, when the water cools slightly, soak the affected foot in the water and rub it. After half an hour, dry the foot and put on clean shoes and socks. Do this once a day, and it generally takes several times to cure.

3. 用茄秧根 5 个，以水煮沸 5 分钟，晾温后浸泡患脚 15 分钟，2 天浸泡 3 次，3 天为 1 疗程。

3. Take 5 eggplant seedling roots, boil them in water for 5 minutes, and wait until the liquid is warm. Soak the affected foot for 15 minutes, 3 times in 2 days. Three days make one course of treatment.

4. 用嫩柳树叶数片，揉成小丸，夹在脚趾腐烂处。如果患处面积大，可用柳树叶熬水洗脚。

4. Take several tender willow leaves, rub them into small balls, and place them between the decayed toes. If the affected area is large, you can boil willow leaves in water to wash the feet.

5. 醋精加水少许，进行擦拭，每日 1-2 次，连续 5 天。

5. Add a small amount of water to glacial acetic acid (vinegar essence), wipe the affected area with it 1-2 times a day, and continue for 5 consecutive days.

6. 把患脚用热水洗净后，浸泡在山西老陈醋当中，把脚掌全部浸泡过来，每次浸泡半小时至四十分钟，每日三次，用过的醋下次再用，数天后可愈。

6. After washing the affected foot with hot water, soak it entirely in Shanxi mature vinegar. Soak for 30 to 40 minutes each time, 3 times a day. The used vinegar can be reused for the next time, and it can be cured in a few days.

《民族医药报》1992 年 6 月 5 日（北京 马宝山）

Ethnic Medicine News, June 5, 1992 (Ma Baoshan, Beijing)

除脚臭妙法

Effective Methods for Eliminating Foot Odor

7. 取 2-3 粒卫生球，将其研成粉末，均匀地撒在洗干净的鞋内，再垫上一块鞋垫，这样穿鞋时就不易产生脚臭。

7. Take 2-3 mothballs, grind them into a powder, and sprinkle them evenly inside the clean shoes. Then place an insole over it. This can effectively prevent foot odor when wearing the shoes.

8. 每日洗脚后，滴 1-2 滴风油精在脚上，并将其搓匀，稍等片刻后再以清水冲洗一次，即可将脚上的汗臭除去。

8. After washing your feet every day, drop 1-2 drops of Fengyoujing (balm) on your feet, rub evenly, wait for a moment, and then rinse with clean water. This can eliminate the sweaty foot odor.

9. 取食醋适量，加水 3-5 倍稀释，待每日睡前洗脚后，将稀释液涂擦于脚底、趾缝等处，异味即可消除。

9. Take an appropriate amount of edible vinegar and dilute it with 3-5 times the amount of water. After washing your feet before bed every day, apply the diluted liquid to the soles and between the toes to eliminate the odor.

10. 取中药煅龙骨 30 克，煅牡蛎 30 克，枯矾 30 克，将其研末调匀细筛后备用。每次洗脚后将药粉在脚底涂抹一次，长期坚持，有良好的效果。

10. Take 30g each of calcined dragon bone, calcined oyster shell, and exsiccated alum. Grind them into a powder, mix evenly, and sift for later use. After washing your feet each time, apply the powder to the soles once. Long-term adherence will yield good results.

《民族医药报》（四川 郭晓明）

Ethnic Medicine News (Guo Xiaoming, Sichuan)

11. 治足汗方：取白矾 25 克（打碎），芒硝 25 克，萹蓄根 30 克，水煎取煎液 2000 毫升，倒在盒内。将患脚浸泡在药液里，每次 30 分钟，每日 3 次，在每次浸泡前加温，每剂用 2 日，连用 4-6 日。

11. Prescription for Hyperhidrosis of the Feet: Take 25g of alum (crushed), 25g of mirabilite, and 30g of knotweed root. Decoct them in water to obtain 2000ml of liquid, and pour it into a basin. Soak the affected feet in the medicinal liquid for 30 minutes each time, 3 times a day. Warm the liquid before each soaking. Use one dose for 2 days, and continue for 4-6 consecutive days.

12. 香港脚（烂脚丫）：杨梅树皮磨醋搽，随磨随搽，1-2 天见效。

12. Athlete’s Foot (Erosive Type): Grind bayberry bark with vinegar and apply it to the affected area. Grind and apply simultaneously. It will take effect in 1-2 days.

13. 白矾 20 克，水 1000 克，混合溶解后浸患脚 10 分钟，让其自然晾干，每晚 1 次，连洗 5 天。

13. Take 20g of alum and 1000g of water. Mix and dissolve, then soak the affected foot for 10 minutes. Let it air dry naturally. Do this once a night for 5 consecutive days.

14. 大白萝卜适量，洗净切片加水煎煮，以煎液洗烫患脚，每日 2 次。

14. Take an appropriate amount of large white radish, wash, slice, and boil in water. Use the decoction to wash and soak the affected feet twice a day.

15. 干姜 15 克，白矾 15 克，煎水洗患脚，连洗数日。

15. Take 15g of dried ginger and 15g of alum. Decoct them in water and wash the affected feet. Continue for several days.

《民族医药报》1998 年 1 月 23 日（马宝山）

Ethnic Medicine News, January 23, 1998 (Ma Baoshan)

16. 取中药煅龙骨 30 克，煅牡蛎 30 克，枯矾 30 克，将其研末调匀细筛后备用。每次洗脚后将药粉在脚底敷抹一次，长期坚持，有良好的效果。

16. Take 30g each of calcined dragon bone, calcined oyster shell, and exsiccated alum. Grind them into a powder, mix evenly, and sift for later use. After washing your feet each time, apply the powder to the soles once. Long-term adherence will yield good results.

17. 鲜侧柏叶 60 克，苦参 100 克，花椒 30 克，诸药共浸泡于 300 毫升陈醋中 5 天后即可备用。使用前先将脚用温水浸泡洗净，再用棉球蘸药液涂搽脚掌部，每日早晚各一次。

17. Take 60g of fresh platycladus leaves, 100g of sophora flavescens root, and 30g of Sichuan peppercorns. Soak all the ingredients in 300ml of mature vinegar for 5 days for later use. Before use, soak and wash the feet with warm water, then dip a cotton ball in the medicinal liquid and apply it to the soles twice a day, in the morning and evening.

《中医药信息报》（郭晓明）

Traditional Chinese Medicine Information News (Guo Xiaoming)

18. 药物组成：滑石、海螵蛸（刮去背面一层硬壳）、制炉甘石各 15 克，赤石脂、蛤壳各 10 克，轻粉、雄黄、黄丹、枯矾各 6 克，冰片 3 克。

18. Ingredients: 15g each of talcum, cuttlebone (with the hard shell on the back scraped off), and processed calamine; 10g each of halloysite and clam shell; 6g each of calomel, realgar, minium, and exsiccated alum; and 3g of borneol.

制作及用法: 将以上药物共研粉、和匀，贮藏于瓶内，用时先将患足洗净擦干，再把药粉撒于足癣处即可。

Preparation and Usage: Grind all the above ingredients into a powder and mix evenly. Store in a bottle. When using, first wash and dry the affected foot, and then sprinkle the medicinal powder on the tinea pedis area.

《民族医药报》1992 年 8 月 14 日（杭州 张亦华）

Ethnic Medicine News, August 14, 1992 (Zhang Yihua, Hangzhou)

六、解酒方

VI. Remedies for Hangovers and Alcohol Intoxication

1.“陈皮散”醒酒疗效甚佳，现介绍如下：

1. “Chenpi San” (Tangerine Peel Powder) has excellent efficacy in relieving hangovers. The details are as follows:

药物组成与剂量：陈皮、青皮各 50 克，食盐（炒） 30 克。檀香 20 克、人参、白豆蔻仁各 10 克，绿豆花、葛花各 2.5 克，以上药物共研细末，装瓶备用。

Ingredients and Dosage: 50g each of tangerine peel (chenpi) and green tangerine peel (qingpi); 30g of roasted salt; 20g of sandalwood; 10g each of ginseng and white cardamom seeds; and 2.5g each of mung bean flowers and kudzuvine flowers. Grind all the above ingredients into a fine powder, store in a bottle, and set aside for later use.

功能与主治：降低血中乙醇浓度、止呕、除烦渴等功效。用于解酒毒。

Functions and Indications: Reduces blood ethanol concentration, relieves vomiting, and alleviates restlessness and thirst. Used for detoxifying alcohol.

用法与特点：每日 1-2 次，每次 3-5 克，以白开水调服。服药后临床诸证能迅速缓解，多数服药 2-4 次后即可痊愈。

Usage and Characteristics: Take 3-5g each time, 1-2 times a day, mixed with plain boiled water. After taking the medicine, clinical symptoms can be relieved rapidly, and most patients can be cured after taking it 2-4 times.

《民族医药报》（内蒙古 徐青）

Ethnic Medicine News (Xu Qing, Inner Mongolia)

2. 柑子皮适量，食盐 1 克。用法：上药焙干，研为细末，加入食盐，温开水冲服。

2. Take an appropriate amount of tangerine peel and 1g of salt. Usage: Roast the tangerine peel until dry, grind it into a fine powder, add the salt, and take it with warm boiled water.

3. 枳椇子果 60 克（或其种子 30 克）。用法：随意嚼服。

3. Take 60g of raisin tree fruits (or 30g of its seeds). Usage: Chew and swallow at will.

4. 葛花 20 克。用法：开水泡服。

4. Take 20g of kudzuvine flowers. Usage: Steep in boiling water and drink.

5. 党参、葛花、白术、泽泻（盐水炒）茯苓、白蔻仁、砂仁各 3 克，猪苓、陈皮、青皮各 2.1 克，神曲（炒）、木香各 1.5 克，生姜 3 片。

5. Take 3g each of codonopsis root (dangshen), kudzuvine flowers, atractylodes macrocephala (baizhu), alisma rhizome (zexie, stir-fried with salt water), poria (fuling), white cardamom seeds, and cardamom (sharen); 2.1g each of polyporus (zhuling), tangerine peel (chenpi), and green tangerine peel (qingpi); 1.5g each of medicated leaven (shenqu, stir-fried) and costus root (muxiang); and 3 slices of fresh ginger.

用法：上药水煎服。此法适于饮酒过多呕吐。

Usage: Decoct the above ingredients in water for oral intake. This method is suitable for vomiting caused by excessive drinking.

6. 甘蔗汁适量。用法：饮服数次。此方用于酒后干呕。

6. Take an appropriate amount of sugarcane juice. Usage: Drink it several

times. This prescription is used for dry retching after drinking.

《中药科技报》（郭广）

Chinese Medicine Science and Technology News (Guo Guang)

7. 吃些豆腐或其他豆制品，不仅对身体有很大好处，而且是解酒佳品。

7. Eating some tofu or other soy products is not only highly beneficial to the body but also an excellent remedy for relieving alcohol intoxication.

8. 鲜柑皮煮水，再加少许细盐，服后可醒酒。

8. Boil fresh tangerine peel in water, add a little fine salt, and drink it to relieve hangovers.

9. 西红柿、苹果、梨等水果，可以冲淡血液中的酒精浓度，加速排泄，因而吃水果可以解酒。

9. Fruits such as tomatoes, apples, and pears can dilute the alcohol concentration in the blood and accelerate excretion; therefore, eating fruits can relieve hangovers.

10. 将白菜心和萝卜切成细丝，加醋、糖拌匀吃用，可解酒。

10. Cut the hearts of Chinese cabbages and radishes into fine shreds, add vinegar and sugar, mix well, and eat to relieve hangovers.

11. 味道清淡的汤菜，如清炖冬瓜汤等，能促使酒精随汗或尿迅速排出。

11. Lightly flavored soups, such as clear stewed winter melon soup, can promote the rapid excretion of alcohol through sweat or urine.

12. 用酸枣仁或葛根 10-15 克，加水同煎，饮服可以解酒。

12. Take 10-15g of sour jujube seeds or pueraria roots, decoct them together with water, and drink to relieve hangovers.

13. 将两小块樟树皮洗净，置口中咀嚼 1 分钟吐出，或用樟木 100 克，加水同煎饮服，可以解酒。如果酒精中毒严重，应该及时送医院治疗。

13. Wash two small pieces of camphor tree bark, chew them in the mouth for 1 minute, and spit them out; alternatively, take 100g of camphor wood, decoct it with water, and drink to relieve hangovers. If alcohol poisoning is severe, the patient should be promptly sent to a hospital for treatment.

《民族医药报》1993 年 1 月 15 日（湖南 李凤发）

Ethnic Medicine News, January 15, 1993 (Li Fengfa, Hunan)

14. 白萝卜汁加红糖，每次饮用一杯。

14. Mix white radish juice with brown sugar and drink one cup each time.

15. 用鸡毛扫其喉部或用其它方法促使醉酒者呕吐，这样就可吐出很多的酒，减轻醉酒程度。

15. Use a chicken feather to tickle the drunk person’s throat or use other methods to induce vomiting. This allows them to vomit a large amount of alcohol and reduce the severity of intoxication.

16. 陈醋 30 克、红糖 15 克，生姜 3 片，共煎水服，有较明显的解酒效果。

16. Take 30g of mature vinegar, 15g of brown sugar, and 3 slices of fresh ginger. Decoct them together in water and drink. This has a relatively obvious effect in relieving hangovers.

17. 清炖冬瓜汤给醉酒者饮服亦能解酒。

17. Giving clear stewed winter melon soup to a drunk person to drink can also relieve hangovers.

七、蛲虫（9 方）

VII. Pinworms (9 Prescriptions)

蛲虫病是小儿最常见的一种肠道寄生虫病，这种病不仅给小儿带来痛苦，而且还会影响健康。

Pinworm infection is the most common intestinal parasitic disease in children. This condition not only causes suffering to children but also affects their health.

病从口入，如饭前便后不洗手，爱在潮湿泥土间游戏，爱吮手指，吃未经洗净的瓜果生冷食物等，都容易使蛲虫卵进入人体而致病。

The infection is transmitted via the oral route. Factors such as not washing hands before meals and after using the toilet, playing in damp soil, sucking fingers, and eating unwashed raw fruits and melons can easily allow pinworm eggs to enter the human body and cause disease.

当虫卵进入人体后，在胃及十二指肠内进行孵化，然后在小肠下端及大肠内发育为成虫。雌虫每到夜间爬至肛门产卵，刺激局部，引起肛门及阴部发痒，此时在肛门口可见到白线样成虫。由于肛门、会阴奇痒，用手搔抓时，虫卵沾染于手指及指甲上，带入口内吞下，又在肠内发育繁殖。

After entering the human body, the eggs hatch in the stomach and duodenum, and then develop into adult worms in the lower small intestine and large intestine. Female worms crawl to the anus at night to lay eggs, stimulating the local area and causing itching in the anus and genital region. At this time, white thread-like adult worms can be seen at the anal opening. Due to the severe itching in the anus and perineum, scratching with hands causes the eggs to contaminate the fingers and nails. When the hands are brought to the mouth and the eggs are swallowed, they develop and multiply in the intestines again.

蛲虫病的临床症状以夜间肛门及阴部奇痒为其主要特征。其他尚有食欲不振、消瘦、烦躁不安、夜间惊叫啼哭及尿频、遗尿等。由于蛲虫在肠道内引起机械性刺激，故在临床上亦可出现胃肠道症状，如恶心呕吐、腹痛腹泻、严重时有脱肛现象。如皮肤搔破，还可引起疮疹。女孩患者常可因虫体钻入阴道而发生阴道炎，出现阴道瘙痒。

The clinical symptoms of pinworm infection are mainly characterized by severe itching in the anus and genital region at night. Other symptoms include loss of appetite, weight loss, restlessness, nocturnal screaming and crying, frequent urination, and bedwetting. Because pinworms cause mechanical irritation in the intestinal tract, gastrointestinal symptoms such as nausea, vomiting, abdominal pain, and diarrhea may also appear clinically; in severe cases, rectal prolapse may occur. If the skin is scratched open, it can also cause sores and rashes. In female patients, the worms often enter the vagina, causing vaginitis and vaginal itching.

家长对蛲虫病，应随时注意，积极防治，要使小孩养成良好的卫生习惯。饭前、便后要洗手，不吃未洗净的食物。勤剪指甲，勤洗澡，勤换衣被，纠正小孩吮手指的不良习惯。若发现小儿患者有蛲虫病后，应及时治疗。现笔者介绍几则简便有效而又易为小儿接受的治疗方药，供选用。

Parents should always pay attention to pinworm infections, actively prevent and treat them, and help children develop good hygienic habits. They should wash their hands before meals and after using the toilet, and avoid eating unwashed food. Nails should be trimmed frequently, and children should bathe and change clothes and bedding regularly to correct the bad habit of sucking fingers. If a child is found to have a pinworm infection, timely treatment should be administered. The author now introduces several simple, effective, and easily acceptable treatment prescriptions for children' s reference.

1. 取大蒜一个，约 5-10 克左右，去皮捣汁，加温开水 50 毫升，直肠灌注，每晚 1 次，一般 3-4 次即愈。亦可用脱脂棉蘸此汁塞入肛门。

1.Take one clove of garlic (about 5-10g), peel and mash it to extract the juice, and add 50ml of warm boiled water. Administer it as a rectal enema once a night. It generally takes 3-4 times to cure. Alternatively, dip absorbent cotton in this juice and insert it into the anus.

2. 取槟榔 30 克研细，加水 500 毫升，煎至 100 毫升，加蜂蜜适量，空腹 1 次服。连服 2-3 天 。

2. Take 30g of betel nut, grind it into a fine powder, add 500ml of water, and decoct until it reduces to 100ml. Add an appropriate amount of honey and take it once on an empty stomach. Take it continuously for 2-3 days.

3. 每晚睡前用脱脂棉蘸浓醋（食醋 100 毫升煎至 50 毫升），塞入肛门。浓醋能抑制蛲虫。

3. Before going to bed every night, dip absorbent cotton in concentrated vinegar (100ml of edible vinegar decocted to 50ml) and insert it into the anus. Concentrated vinegar can inhibit pinworms.

《民族医药报》1992 年 7 月 10 日（广西 李子云）

Ethnic Medicine News, July 10, 1992 (Li Ziyun, Guangxi)

4. 取苦杏仁 5 克晒干或炒干研成细面，放到干净瓶内，加干净凉开水 30 克，猛摇瓶子1-3分钟。然后静放1-2小时备甲。用法：用干净脱脂棉球蘸表层上清液，待棉球基本湿透后取出，轻放入肛门内。每晚一次，一般2-5次痊愈。

4. Take 5g of bitter almonds, sun-dry or stir-fry until dry, and grind into a fine powder. Put them in a clean bottle, add 30g of clean cool boiled water, and shake the bottle vigorously for 1-3 minutes. Then let it stand for 1-2 hours for preparation. Usage: Dip a clean absorbent cotton ball into the supernatant liquid on the surface. After the cotton ball is basically soaked, take it out and gently insert it into the anus. Do this once a night, and it generally takes 2-5 times to cure.

5. 枯矾、冰片各1克，香油10克。上药共放到干净器皿内，用干净小棒拌成稀膏状备用。用法：用干净棉签蘸药液，涂于肛门近周一圈，宽度约3cm，并另取棉球蘸少许药液，轻送入肛门内。每晚一次，用5-7天即可。

5. Take 1g each of exsiccated alum and borneol, and 10g of sesame oil. Put all the ingredients in a clean container and mix them with a clean small stick to form a thin paste for later use. Usage: Dip a clean cotton swab in the medicinal liquid and apply it in a circle around the anus with a width of about 3cm. Also, take another cotton ball, dip it in a little medicinal liquid, and gently insert it into the anus. Do this once a night, and it takes 5-7 days.

《中药科技报》1990年12月26日

Chinese Medicine Science and Technology News, December 26, 1990

6. 治蛲虫熏洗方

6. Fumigation and Washing Prescription for Pinworms

苦楝树根皮25克，鹤虱、蛇床子、百部、野菊花各15克，生甘草5克。共放在砂罐中，加水2公斤，煮沸30分钟，去药渣，倒入洁净盆中，趁热先熏，待温度适宜时以药液洗涤肛门，每晚临睡前洗1次。次日痒感减轻，3次后痒感消失，连用5日可愈。

Take 25g of chinaberry tree root bark, 15g each of fleabane fruit, cnidium fruit, stemona root, and wild chrysanthemum, and 5g of raw licorice. Put them all in a clay pot, add 2kg of water, and boil for 30 minutes. Remove the dregs, pour the liquid into a clean basin, and fumigate the area while it is hot. When the temperature is appropriate, wash the anus with the medicinal liquid. Wash once a night before going to bed. The itching will be reduced the next day and disappear after 3 washes. Continuous use for 5 days can cure the condition.

《民族医药报》1998 年 1 月 23 日（陈青林）

Ethnic Medicine News, January 23, 1998 (Chen Qinglin)

7. 烟袋油灌肛：取烟袋油少许，用 5-10 毫升生理盐水稀释，每晚睡前用注射器注入肛门保留灌肠，连用 1-2 次。

7. Tobacco Pipe Oil Enema: Take a small amount of tobacco pipe oil, dilute it with 5-10ml of normal saline, and use a syringe to inject it into the anus as a retention enema before going to bed every night. Use it continuously for 1-2 times.

8. 盐酸左旋咪唑片肛门塞入：将盐酸左旋咪唑片研成粉末（按每公斤体重 5 毫克计算），装入空心胶囊中，趁小儿入睡之际，塞入肛门深部 2 厘米处即可，如需要者 1 个月后重复 1 次。

8. Rectal Insertion of Levamisole Hydrochloride Tablets: Grind levamisole hydrochloride tablets into a powder (calculated at 5mg per kilogram of body weight), put it into empty capsules, and while the child is asleep, insert it 2cm deep into the anus. If necessary, repeat once after 1 month.

9. 百部酒精浸液擦肛门：取生百部 30 克，加入 55% 酒精 150 毫升浸泡三天后，收集药液贮瓶备用。使用时，用棉球蘸百部酒精浸液，擦肛门附近皱襞。擦时最好于晚上临睡前，用温水清洗后擦。一般擦用三个疗程，每疗程 7 天，每晚一次。

9. Wiping the Anus with Stemona Alcohol Extract: Take 30g of raw stemona root, add 150ml of 55% alcohol, and soak for three days. Collect the medicinal liquid and store it in a bottle for later use. When using, dip a cotton ball in the stemona alcohol extract and wipe the folds around the anus. It is best to wipe after washing with warm water before going to bed at night. Generally, three courses of treatment are required, each lasting 7 days, applied once a night.

《民族医药报》1992 年 4 月 3 日（广东 张仲林）

Ethnic Medicine News, April 3, 1992 (Zhang Zhonglin, Guangdong)

八、防治流脑验方（7方）
VIII. Proven Prescriptions for the Prevention and Treatment of Epidemic Cerebrospinal Meningitis (7 Prescriptions)

1. 中草药防治：取芦根18克、连翘12克、菊花9克、桑叶9克、桔梗6克、薄荷3克、甘草3克。水煎服，一日一剂分两次服。可防治流脑。

1.Herbal Medicine for Prevention and Treatment: Take 18g of reed rhizome (lugen), 12g of forsythia fruit (lianqiao), 9g each of chrysanthemum flower (juhua) and mulberry leaf (sangye), 6g of platycodon root (jiegeng), 3g of peppermint (bohe), and 3g of licorice (gancao). Decoct in water for oral intake, one dose a day divided into two servings. This can prevent and treat epidemic cerebrospinal meningitis.

2. 早期治法：如发现症状，抢时间治疗。服黄胺类药物和等量的碳酸氢钠。成年人每天服上述两味药各二克，分两次服完，小儿每公斤体重一百毫克，分二次服完，此方剂对早期效果较好。

2. Early-stage Treatment: If symptoms are detected, seek treatment immediately. Administer sulfonamides and an equal amount of sodium bicarbonate. Adults should take 2g of each of the above two medicines daily, divided into two doses. Children should take 100mg per kilogram of body weight, divided into two doses. This prescription has a good effect in the early stage.

3. 食物预防：取生橄榄7个、白萝卜250克（切片）水煎代茶饮。一日一剂，连饮七日，可预防流脑。

3. Dietary Prevention: Take 7 fresh olives and 250g of white radish (sliced), decoct them in water, and drink as a tea substitute. Take one dose a day and drink continuously for seven days to prevent epidemic cerebrospinal meningitis.

4. 食盐漱口：在流脑流行时期，饭前饭后用泡好的浓盐水漱口，或每天生嚼大蒜，每次半瓣。

4. Salt Water Gargle: During the epidemic period of cerebrospinal meningitis, gargle with strong salt water before and after meals, or chew raw garlic daily, half

a clove each time.

5. 贯众甘草汤：取贯众 30 克，甘草 9 克，水煎服，连服七天，无病能防，有病早治。

5. Guanzhong and Licorice Decoction: Take 30g of cyrtomium rhizome (guanzhong) and 9g of licorice (gancao). Decoct in water for oral intake and take continuously for seven days. It can prevent the disease in healthy individuals and treat it early in infected individuals.

6. 荸荠石膏汤：取鲜荸荠、生石膏各等量，共煎汤服或代茶饮，连服七日，可预防流脑。

6. Water Chestnut and Gypsum Decoction: Take an equal amount of fresh water chestnuts and raw gypsum. Decoct them together and drink, or use as a tea substitute. Drink continuously for seven days to prevent epidemic cerebrospinal meningitis.

7. 中药五味汤：大青叶 15 克、野菊花 15 克、金银花 9 克、板蓝根 9 克、贯众 9 克，每日一剂，水煎服或代茶饮，七天为一个疗程，对早期流脑治愈率较高，预防效果更佳。

7. Five-Ingredient Herbal Decoction: Take 15g each of isatis leaf (daqingye) and wild chrysanthemum (yejuhua), and 9g each of honeysuckle flower (jinyinhua), isatis root (banlangen), and cyrtomium rhizome (guanzhong). Take one dose daily, either decocted in water or as a tea substitute. Seven days make one course of treatment. It has a high cure rate for early-stage epidemic cerebrospinal meningitis and an even better preventive effect.

《中药科技报》1992 年 3 月 16 日

Chinese Medicine Science and Technology News, March 16, 1992

九、防治中暑（10 方）

IX. Prevention and Treatment of Heatstroke (10 Prescriptions)

1. 蒲公英 20 克，马齿苋 20 克，青蒿 10 克，薄荷 3 克，水煎服，一日数次。

1.Take 20g of dandelion, 20g of purslane, 10g of sweet wormwood, and 3g of peppermint. Decoct in water for oral intake, several times a day.

2. 香薷叶 20 克，荷叶 30 克，扁豆 21 克，蜂蜜 12 克，煎后，灌服昏迷患者。

2. Take 20g of elsholtzia leaves, 30g of lotus leaves, 21g of hyacinth beans, and 12g of honey. After decocting, administer it to unconscious patients via gavage.

3. 桑叶 20 克，鱼腥草 20 克，金果榄 14 克，野菊花 14 克，水煎服，一日三次。

3. Take 20g of mulberry leaves, 20g of houttuynia cordata, 14g of tinospora root, and 14g of wild chrysanthemum. Decoct in water for oral intake, three times a day.

4. 石菖蒲 12 克，苍术 10 克，公丁香 6 克，地胡椒 8 克，牙皂 6 克，水煎服，一日三次。

4. Take 12g of sweetflag rhizome, 10g of atractylodes lancea, 6g of clove, 8g of ground pepper, and 6g of Chinese honeylocust fruit. Decoct in water for oral intake, three times a day.

5. 石膏 20 克，知母 12 克，金银花 14 克，连翘 12 克，竹叶心 20 克，水煎服，一日二次。

5. Take 20g of gypsum, 12g of anemarrhena rhizome, 14g of honeysuckle flower, 12g of forsythia fruit, and 20g of bamboo leaf hearts. Decoct in water for oral intake, twice a day.

6. 苦爹菜 20 克，金银花 20 克，鱼腥草 30 克，香薷 8 克，水煎后加入冰块、紅糖，常饮用。

6. Take 20g of false daisy, 20g of honeysuckle flower, 30g of houttuynia cordata, and 8g of elsholtzia. After decocting in water, add ice cubes and brown sugar, and drink frequently.

7. 鲜丝瓜叶 60 克，升麻 3 克，滑石 20 克，鲜萝卜叶 30 克，水煎服，一日二次。

7. Take 60g of fresh loofah leaves, 3g of cimicifuga rhizome, 20g of talcum, and 30g of fresh radish leaves. Decoct in water for oral intake, three times a day.

8. 荷叶 30 克，香薷 14 克，扁豆 6 克，冬瓜皮 6 克，水煎后。调拌蜂蜜冲服，一日数次。

8. Take 30g of lotus leaves, 14g of elsholtzia, 6g of hyacinth beans, and 6g of winter melon peel. After decocting in water, mix with honey and take as a beverage, several times a day.

9. 鲜鸡矢藤 30 克，虎杖 20 克，穿心莲 6 克，鲜葎草 30 克，水煎后，加入冰糖食盐、冰块，常饮用。

9. Take 30g of fresh paederia scandens, 20g of giant knotweed rhizome, 6g of andrographis paniculata, and 30g of fresh Japanese hop. After decocting in water, add rock sugar, salt, and ice cubes, and drink frequently.

10. 冬瓜子 12 克，莱菔子 12 克，蒲公英 20 克，西瓜子 6 克。将药物研细末，谓拌蜂蜜冲服，一日三次。

10. Take 12g of winter melon seeds, 12g of radish seeds, 20g of dandelion, and 6g of watermelon seeds. Grind the ingredients into a fine powder, mix with honey, and take as a beverage, three times a day.

《民族医药报》（叶德松）

Ethnic Medicine News (Ye Desong)

十、治红斑狼疮（5 方）

X. Treatment of Lupus Erythematosus (5 Prescriptions)

1. 土茯苓 25-50 克，金银花 10-20 克。水煎服，服后再将药渣煎汁熏洗患处，每日一次。

1.Take 25-50g of smilax glabra (tufuling) and 10-20g of honeysuckle flower (jinyinhua). Decoct in water for oral intake. After taking the decoction, boil the remaining dregs again to extract the liquid, and use it to fumigate and wash the affected area once a day.

2. 青黛粉 25-50 克（根据感染面积决定用量）调菜油涂抹患处，每日数次。

2. Take 25-50g of natural indigo powder (qingdaifen) (the dosage depends on

the size of the infected area), mix it with vegetable oil, and apply it to the affected area several times a day.

3. 用紫草 25-50 克煎菜油涂患处。

3. Take 25-50g of gromwell root (zicao) and decoct it in vegetable oil, then apply the oil to the affected area.

4. 如狼疮已破，可干煎鸡蛋黄，待蛋黄出油后，用蛋黄油兑冰片擦患处，每日数次。

4. If the lupus lesions have ulcerated, dry-fry egg yolks. Once the oil is extracted from the yolks, mix the yolk oil with borneol (bingpian) and apply it to the affected area several times a day.

5. 如属湿疹性质，可用防风 12 克，地肤子 9 克，白癣皮 9 克，银花 30 克，蒲公英 12 克，薄荷 6 克，生甘草 6 克，煎汁擦洗患处。两日一副，每日擦洗数次。

5. If it is eczematous in nature, take 12g of saposhnikovia root (fangfeng), 9g of Kochia fruit (difuli), 9g of dictamnus bark (baixianpi), 30g of honeysuckle flower (yinhua), 12g of dandelion (pugongying), 6g of peppermint (bohe), and 6g of raw licorice (shenggancao). Decoct them in water and use the liquid to wash and wipe the affected area. Use one dose every two days, and wash and wipe several times a day.

《民族医药报》1992 年 6 月 26 日（广东 林伟）

Ethnic Medicine News, June 26, 1992 (Lin Wei, Guangdong)

十一、流行性腮腺炎（11 方）
XI. Epidemic Parotitis (11 Prescriptions)

1. 仙人掌 120 克，生石膏 45 克，天花粉 15 克，芒硝 5 克，以上药物混合捣烂成糊状外贴局部，干后即换，连用 3 天即可。

1.Take 120g of cactus, 45g of raw gypsum, 15g of trichosanthes root, and 5g of mirabilite. Mash these ingredients together into a paste and apply it to the affected area. Replace the paste when it dries. Continuous use for 3 days is sufficient.

2. 鲜白花蛇舌草、鲜木芙蓉叶各适量捣烂敷患处，3-4 天即愈。

2. Take an appropriate amount of fresh oldenlandia herb and fresh cotton rose leaves, mash them, and apply the paste to the affected area. It will be cured in 3-4 days.

3. 马鞭草 60 克，板兰板 15 克，蒲公英 20 克，水煎服，每天 2 次，连用 3 天。

3. Take 60g of verbena, 15g of isatis root, and 20g of dandelion. Decoct them in water for oral intake, twice a day, and continue for 3 consecutive days.

4. 仙人掌、白矾、牛蒡子各 10 克，土豆一枚共研如泥状，贴敷患部。

4. Take 10g each of cactus, alum, and burdock fruit, along with one potato. Grind them together into a mud-like paste and apply it to the affected area.

5. 金银花 6 克，七叶一枝花 10 克（水磨成浓汁），冰片 10 克，板蓝根 10 克，共研细末调匀涂于局部，每天 3-4 次，2-3 天即行。

5. Take 6g of honeysuckle flower, 10g of paris polyphylla (ground into a thick juice with water), 10g of borneol, and 10g of isatis root. Grind them into a fine powder, mix evenly, and apply the mixture to the affected area 3-4 times a day. It will take effect in 2-3 days.

6. 鲜车前草、鲜鱼腥草、鲜蒲公英各 100 克捣汁加入绿豆粉 60 克敷患部，亦可煎服。

6. Take 100g each of fresh plantain herb, fresh houttuynia cordata, and fresh dandelion. Mash them to extract the juice, add 60g of mung bean powder, and apply the mixture to the affected area. Alternatively, it can be decocted and taken orally.

7. 雄黄 40 克，白矾 45 克，川芦贝 10 克，冰片 5 克共研细末装瓶备用，每用取 5 克，以 95% 酒精调糊涂于患处。

7. Take 40g of realgar, 45g of alum, 10g of Sichuan fritillary bulb, and 5g of borneol. Grind them into a fine powder, store in a bottle for later use. Each time, take 5g of the powder, mix it with 95% alcohol into a paste, and apply it to the affected area.

8. 吴茱萸、大黄、黄连各 10 克，紫花地丁 6 克，胆南星 6 克研末调匀贴紧双足涌泉穴，次晨取下，一般 3 晚即可。

8. Take 10g each of evodia fruit, rhubarb, and coptis root, and 6g each of violet herb and arisaema with bile. Grind them into a powder, mix evenly, and apply the paste firmly to the Yongquan acupoints on the soles of both feet. Remove it the next morning. Generally, applying it for 3 nights is sufficient.

9. 季德胜蛇药片或六神丸调糊涂患处皆有效。

9. Applying a paste made by mixing Jidesheng Snake Medicine Tablets or Liushen Pills and applying it to the affected area is also effective.

《民族医药报》1993 年 4 月 2 日（安徽 胡宪华）

Ethnic Medicine News, April 2, 1993 (Hu Xianhua, Anhui)

10. 治腮腺炎：用米醋调牛黄解毒片粉末外敷患处（两腮部），每日 2 次，一般 2 日可愈。

10. Treating Parotitis: Mix the powder of Niuhuang Jiedu Tablets with rice vinegar to form a paste, and apply it externally to the affected area (both cheeks). Do this twice a day, and it generally takes 2 days to cure.

11. 腮腺炎外治法：

11. External Treatment for Parotitis:

此病一年四季均有发生，多见冬春两季，状见腮部肿胀疼痛，肿胀呈弥漫性边缘不清，有压痛。处方及用法：青黛粉 15 克，生石膏 30 克，冰片 3 克，七叶一枝花 15 克。以上药共研为细末，以米醋适量调为糊状，外敷患处，每日 4-6 次，一般 2-3 天即可治愈。此药具有疏风清热、消肿散结。

This disease can occur in all four seasons, but is most common in winter and spring. The symptoms include swelling and pain in the cheeks, with diffuse swelling, unclear edges, and tenderness upon pressure. Prescription and Usage: Take 15g of natural indigo powder, 30g of raw gypsum, 3g of borneol, and 15g of paris polyphylla. Grind the above ingredients into a fine powder, add an appropriate amount of rice vinegar to form a paste, and apply it externally to the affected area 4-6 times a day. It generally takes 2-3 days to cure. This medicine has the effects of dispelling wind, clearing heat, reducing swelling, and dissipating nodules.

（广西 阳离萍）

(Yang Liping, Guangxi)

十二、中药治落枕（2 方）
XII. Treating Stiff Neck with Traditional Chinese Medicine (2 Prescriptions)

1. 中药治落枕

1.Treating Stiff Neck with Traditional Chinese Medicine

落枕又称失枕、失颈，多因睡眠姿势不当或颈部当风受寒所致。其主要症状是颈部酸痛不适，屈伸转侧受限；重者疼痛延及患侧肩背部及上肢，头向一侧歪斜，患侧颈肩部位有明显压痛。本病采用中药治疗疗效甚好，其方药组成及用法是：

Stiff neck, also known as "shizhen" or "shijing," is mostly caused by improper sleeping posture or exposure of the neck to wind and cold. Its main symptoms include soreness and discomfort in the neck, with restricted flexion, extension, and turning. In severe cases, the pain extends to the shoulder, back, and upper limbs on the affected side; the head tilts to one side, and there is obvious tenderness upon pressure in the neck and shoulder area on the affected side. This condition responds very well to Traditional Chinese Medicine treatment. The ingredients and usage of the prescription are as follows:

葛根 45 克，桂枝 9 克，生黄芪 18 克，炙甘草 12 克，大枣 5 枚，防风 9 克，麻黄 9 克，白芍 30 克，每日一剂，水煎分 2 次温服，服药后若能盖被至全身微出汗，则效果更佳。

Take 45g of pueraria root (gegen), 9g of cassia twig (guizhi), 18g of raw astragalus root (shenghuangqi), 12g of honey-fried licorice (zhigancao), 5 pieces of jujube (dazao), 9g of saposhnikovia root (fangfeng), 9g of ephedra (mahuang), and 30g of white peony root (baishao). Take one dose daily, decocted in water and taken warm in two divided doses. After taking the medicine, covering up with a blanket to induce slight sweating all over the body will yield even better results.

《民族医药报》1992 年 5 月 22 日（广西 韦礼贵）

Ethnic Medicine News, May 22, 1992 (Wei Ligui, Guangxi)

2. 笔者自拟治落枕方治疗落枕 38 例，均取得满意疗效，现介绍如下。

2. The author formulated a self-devised prescription for treating stiff neck and applied it to 38 cases, all of which achieved satisfactory results. The details are introduced as follows.

处方及用法：葛根 30 克，菊花 15 克，生白芍 24 克，柴胡 12 克，生甘草 9 克，水煎取药液再加红糖 30 克调服，一次服下，服药后卧床休息一小时取微汗，每日一剂，一般 2-4 剂即愈。

Prescription and Usage: Take 30g of pueraria root (gegen), 15g of chrysanthemum flower (juhua), 24g of raw white peony root (shengbaishao), 12g of bupleurum root (chaihu), and 9g of raw licorice (shenggancao). Decoct them in water to extract the liquid, then add 30g of brown sugar to mix and take it in one go. After taking the medicine, rest in bed for one hour to induce slight sweating. Take one dose daily, and it generally takes 2-4 doses to cure.

《民族医药报》1992 年 7 月 10 日（河南 陈勇）

Ethnic Medicine News, July 10, 1992 (Chen Yong, Henan)

十三、眩晕（2 方）
XIII. Vertigo (2 Prescriptions)

1. 反复发作性眩晕，中医认为多系痰凝血瘀所致。临床表现为反复眩晕、心慌胸闷、耳鸣目花、恶心呕吐等症，用燥湿运脾化痰，活血通络清经之法治疗，可收到良好效果。

1. Recurrent vertigo is considered in Traditional Chinese Medicine to be mostly caused by phlegm accumulation and blood stasis. Clinical manifestations include recurrent vertigo, palpitations, chest tightness, tinnitus, blurred vision, nausea, and vomiting. Treating it with the methods of drying dampness, activating the spleen, resolving phlegm, promoting blood circulation, unblocking collaterals, and clearing the meridians can achieve good results.

药物组成：天麻、白术、姜半夏、枳实、黄芩、石菖蒲各10克，白芍、茯苓各12克，竹茹15克，胆星、橘红、甘草各5克，每日一剂，水煎服，7日为1疗程。

Ingredients: Take 10g each of gastrodia rhizome (tianma), atractylodes macrocephala (baizhu), ginger-processed pinellia (jiangbanxia), immature bitter orange (zhishi), scutellaria root (huangqin), and sweetflag rhizome (shichangpu); 12g each of white peony root (baishao) and poria (fuling); 15g of bamboo shavings (zhuru); and 5g each of arisaema with bile (dannanxing), tangerine peel (juhong), and licorice (gancao). Take one dose daily, decocted in water for oral intake. Seven days make one course of treatment.

《民族医药报》1992年5月22日（南京 孙哲）

Ethnic Medicine News, May 22, 1992 (Sun Zhe, Nanjing)

2. 眩晕：千针万线草根30克、紫丹参30克。水煎加红糖10克为引。1日1剂，分3次服，连服10日为1疗程。

2. Vertigo: Take 30g of Qianzhen Wanxiancao (a type of herb root) and 30g of red salvia root (zidanshen). Decoct them in water and add 10g of brown sugar as a guiding ingredient. Take one dose daily, divided into three servings. Continuous use for 10 days makes one course of treatment.

十四、腋臭（12方）

XIV. Body Odor / Bromhidrosis (12 Prescriptions)

1. 青蒿治狐臭

1. Treating Body Odor with Sweet Wormwood

青蒿药源广泛，味苦性寒入肝胆经，有清热、退黄、解暑之功效。余少时常目睹外祖母用之治疗狐臭患者，疗效确切，现介绍如下。

Sweet wormwood (Artemisia annua) is widely available as a medicinal herb. It is bitter and cold in nature, and enters the liver and gallbladder meridians. It has the effects of clearing heat, reducing jaundice, and relieving summer heat. In my youth, I often saw my maternal grandmother use it to treat patients with body odor, and the efficacy was definite. The method is introduced as follows.

每天采摘新鲜青蒿 60 克左右，洗净晾干，再用热的熟米饭或糯米饭团一个，加樟脑 3 克，拌匀捣烂，在不烫伤皮肤的情况下，左右腋下各夹一个，约 15 分钟后即可去掉。上法连用 3 天，短期效果明显，没有副作用。对某些使用香露及除臭液皮肤过敏者，尤其适用。

Pick about 60g of fresh sweet wormwood daily, wash and air-dry it. Then, take a hot ball of cooked rice or glutinous rice, add 3g of camphor, mix and mash them evenly. Without scalding the skin, clamp one ball under each armpit and remove it after about 15 minutes. Using this method continuously for 3 days yields obvious short-term effects with no side effects. It is especially suitable for those who are allergic to perfumes and deodorants.

疗效分析：青蒿的化学成分中含挥发油，药理研究表明嫩青蒿的水浸剂（1：3）在试管内对皮肤真菌有抑制作用；樟脑外用能刺激皮肤黏膜，改善局部血液循环，促进黏膜分泌并具有防腐作用；配以饭团可促进药物的黏附与渗透。

Efficacy Analysis: The chemical components of sweet wormwood contain volatile oils. Pharmacological studies have shown that the aqueous extract (1:3) of tender sweet wormwood has an inhibitory effect on dermatophytes in vitro. Topical application of camphor can stimulate the skin mucosa, improve local blood circulation, promote mucosal secretion, and has an antiseptic effect. Combining it with a rice ball can promote the adhesion and penetration of the medicine.

《民族医药报》1992 年 4 月 3 日（广州 罗国良）

Ethnic Medicine News, April 3, 1992 (Luo Guoliang, Guangzhou)

2. 紫丁香 1 克、石膏 2 克、滑石粉 2 克、明矾 1.5 克，研细末混合拌匀即成。早晚用肥皂水洗净患处，敷上药末，如汗液过多，可把药末放在纱袋内，系牢挟腋下，每日一次，轻者半月，重者坚持 1-2 月可愈。

2. Take 1g of lilac, 2g of gypsum, 2g of talcum powder, and 1.5g of alum. Grind them into a fine powder and mix evenly. Wash the affected area with soapy

water in the morning and evening, and apply the powder. If there is excessive sweating, put the powder in a gauze bag, tie it securely, and clamp it under the armpit once a day. Mild cases can be cured in half a month, while severe cases can be cured by persisting for 1-2 months.

《民族医药报》1991 年 8 月 25 日（江苏 吴自强）

Ethnic Medicine News, August 25, 1991 (Wu Ziqiang, Jiangsu)

3. 治疗方法：取雄黄、密陀僧各 30 克，枯矾、樟脑各 10 克，轻粉、冰片各 5 克，研极细末，浸泡于 75% 酒精 250 毫升中一周后，密封备用。用前先剃去腋毛，腋窝用温水肥皂清洁、拭干，以棉花蘸取上液，每天 3-5 次直接涂擦患处，至狐臭完全消失。

3. Treatment Method: Take 30g each of realgar and litharge, 10g each of exsiccated alum and camphor, and 5g each of calomel and borneol. Grind them into an extremely fine powder and soak them in 250ml of 75% alcohol for a week, then seal and store for later use. Before use, shave off the armpit hair, clean the armpit with warm soapy water, and wipe dry. Dip cotton in the liquid and directly wipe the affected area 3-5 times a day until the body odor completely disappears.

体会：本酊药味芳香，能消除臭味，不污染衣服，局部具有清凉舒适之特点。药源较广，配制简单，治疗方便，疗程短、疗效可靠；对皮肤刺激性少，毒副作用轻。因药物直接、全面地作用在局部，消炎除臭效果迅速确实。

Experience: This tincture has an aromatic smell, can eliminate odor, does not pollute clothes, and has a cool and comfortable feeling locally. The medicinal sources are abundant, the preparation is simple, the treatment is convenient, the course of treatment is short, and the efficacy is reliable. It has little irritation to the skin and mild toxic side effects. Because the medicine acts directly and comprehensively on the local area, the anti-inflammatory and deodorizing effects are rapid and definite.

《中医药信息报》1990 年 7 月 28 日

Chinese Medicine Information News, July 28, 1990

4. 食盐摩擦法：将食盐炒热后，装入纱布袋内，趁热扎好，反复摩擦双腋窝约 5 分钟，每天 1 次，连用 5 天。

4. Salt Rubbing Method: Stir-fry salt until hot, put it into a gauze bag, tie it up while it is still hot, and repeatedly rub both armpits for about 5 minutes. Do this once a day for 5 consecutive days.

5. 生姜外擦法：用干净的生姜切片外擦，每日 2 次，每次擦双腋窝约 5 分钟。

5. Fresh Ginger Wiping Method: Cut clean fresh ginger into slices and wipe the armpits externally twice a day, rubbing both armpits for about 5 minutes each time.

6. 冰片加生姜涂擦法：生姜切碎加白开水挤汁，汁中加适量冰片，用棉球蘸药液涂擦双腋窝，每日 2 次。

6. Borneol and Ginger Wiping Method: Chop fresh ginger, add boiled water, and squeeze out the juice. Add an appropriate amount of borneol to the juice, dip a cotton ball in the medicinal liquid, and wipe both armpits twice a day.

7. 薄荷加白芷外敷：2 味中药各取 30 克研末，每日取 10 克用纱布包敷贴腋窝，次日换之，可连续使用 6 天。

7. Peppermint and Dahurian Angelica Root External Application: Take 30g each of the two herbs, grind them into a powder. Take 10g daily, wrap it in gauze, and apply it to the armpit. Replace it the next day. It can be used continuously for 6 days.

《民族医药报》1998 年 1 月 23 日（虞永水）

Ethnic Medicine News, January 23, 1998 (Yu Yongshui)

8. 取辣味大的红辣椒 5 克，切碎后放入瓶内，加入 30 毫升的 2.5% 的碘酊，密封浸泡 1-2 天，取棉签蘸药液涂擦腋窝，每天 3 次。

8. Take 5g of highly spicy red chili peppers, chop them, and put them in a bottle. Add 30ml of 2.5% iodine tincture, seal and soak for 1-2 days. Dip a cotton swab in the medicinal liquid and wipe the armpits 3 times a day.

9. 取石灰粉 5 克，加陈醋适量，调拌均匀，外涂腋窝，每天 2 次。

9. Take 5g of lime powder, add an appropriate amount of mature vinegar, mix evenly, and apply externally to the armpits twice a day.

10. 洗澡后，取一个已熟但未熟透的西红柿，切开，用切口涂擦腋窝，每天

3次。

10. After taking a bath, take a ripe but not fully ripe tomato, cut it in half, and use the cut surface to wipe the armpits 3 times a day.

《中药科技报》1992年9月26日（黄海平）

Chinese Medicine Science and Technology News, September 26, 1992 (Huang Haiping)

11. 密陀僧酒精液可治腋臭

11. Litharge Alcohol Liquid for Treating Body Odor

腋臭，腋窝部、股内阴部等处，排出的汗液，带有狐臭气味，青春发育期的青年人多见，一年四季皆有，随年龄增长而逐渐减轻。用密陀僧酒精液治疗可获满意效果。

Body odor refers to the foul-smelling sweat discharged from areas such as the armpits and the inner groin. It is common among adolescents during puberty, occurs throughout the year, and gradually alleviates with age. Treating it with litharge alcohol liquid can achieve satisfactory results.

配制方法：密陀僧三十克，研成粉末，然后放入百分之七十五酒精一百毫升中，摇均匀倒入瓶内备用。

Preparation Method: Take 30g of litharge, grind it into a powder, then put it into 100ml of 75% alcohol, shake well, and pour it into a bottle for later use.

用法：用镊子携棉球浸渍在液体中，以棉球涂擦患处，每周涂擦一次。

Usage: Use tweezers to hold a cotton ball, soak it in the liquid, and wipe the affected area with the cotton ball once a week.

《中药科技报》1991年10月26日（祝大中）

Chinese Medicine Science and Technology News, October 26, 1991 (Zhu Dazhong)

12. 醋疗法治狐臭

12. Vinegar Therapy for Body Odor

（用料）：米醋（老陈醋）最佳、石灰粉各适量。

(Ingredients): Rice vinegar (mature vinegar) is the best; take an appropriate amount of it and lime powder.

（制法）：上二味共调匀，将腋下洗净拭干后涂之。

(Preparation): Mix the above two ingredients evenly, wash the armpits, wipe dry, and then apply the mixture.

（功效）：散瘀、杀虫、解毒。用治疗腋下狐臭。

(Efficacy): Promotes blood circulation to remove blood stasis, kills parasites, and detoxifies. Used to treat body odor in the armpits.

《中医药信息报》1992 年 8 月 1 日

Chinese Medicine Information News, August 1, 1992

十五、艾滋病（1 方）
XV. AIDS (1 Prescription)

据最近一则消息报告，我国援外医疗队医生在乌干达金贾市医院用大蒜治疗 98 例艾滋病患者，有 64 例患者的症状出现明显好转。这项研究工作是从 1991 年 9 月起在该市医院艾滋病科进行的。参与这项研究的中国医生说，用大蒜防治艾滋病过程中要克服的问题是：一部分患者（主要是儿童）不能适应大蒜的刺激味，不能长期服用；一部分患者当症状消失后或症状明显改善后就不继续服用；还有的患者后来死于其他并发症。

According to a recent report, doctors from China’s foreign medical aid team treated 98 AIDS patients with garlic at Jinja Regional Referral Hospital in Uganda, with 64 patients showing significant improvement in their symptoms. This research was conducted in the hospital’s AIDS department starting in September 1991. The Chinese doctors involved in the study stated that the challenges to be overcome in using garlic for the prevention and treatment of AIDS include: some patients (mainly children) cannot tolerate the pungent taste of garlic and are unable to take it long-term; some patients stop taking it once their symptoms disappear or significantly improve; and some patients eventually died from other complications.

大蒜能够防治艾滋病其作用机理可能是：一方面，大蒜可增强物质代谢、能量转换和促进血液循环改善体质；大蒜含有硒元素，硒是谷胱甘肽过氧化酶的主要组成成分，它的抗氧化效力比维生素 E 高 500 倍，对细胞膜有保护作用，参与辅酶 A 和辅酶 Q 的合成。艾滋病是一种免疫缺陷病，主要是由于免疫系统中的 T 细胞群大量破坏，而使机体丧失自稳免疫调节能力。实验研究表明，硒元素对细胞免疫反应均有强烈抑制作用，对于恢复和重建艾滋病患者的免疫系统功能大有裨益。另一方面，中国医生用大蒜外涂艾滋病患者淋巴结破溃形成的创面获得痊愈，说明大蒜素具有广谱抗菌和对抗艾滋病病毒的作用。

The possible mechanism of action for garlic in preventing and treating AIDS may be as follows: On the one hand, garlic can enhance substance metabolism and energy conversion, and promote blood circulation to improve physical constitution. Garlic contains selenium, which is a major component of glutathione peroxidase. Its antioxidant efficacy is 500 times higher than that of vitamin E. It protects cell membranes and participates in the synthesis of coenzyme A and coenzyme Q. AIDS is an immunodeficiency disease, primarily caused by the massive destruction of T-cell populations in the immune system, which leads to the loss of the body's homeostatic immune regulation ability. Experimental studies have shown that selenium has a strong inhibitory effect on cellular immune responses, which is highly beneficial for restoring and rebuilding the immune system function of AIDS patients. On the other hand, Chinese doctors achieved complete healing by applying garlic topically to the ulcerated wounds formed by ruptured lymph nodes in AIDS patients, indicating that allicin has broad-spectrum antibacterial and anti-HIV effects.

《中医药信息报》1993 年 4 月 24 日（刘启明）

Chinese Medicine Information News, April 24, 1993 (Liu Qiming)

十六、疝方（3 方）
XVI. Prescriptions for Hernia (3 Prescriptions)

水疝即现代医学所称睾丸鞘膜积液，首见于张子和《儒门事亲》："水疝……囊肿而如水晶。"多因先天不足，肾虚气化不利，加以脾虚积湿内停，或因足厥阴肝经筋聚于阴器，肝失疏泄，复受寒淫，以致气滞，水湿内结而成。此病多见于小儿，1 岁以内可自行消失，1 岁以上则要治疗。现向各位家长推荐两则外洗验方。

Hydrocele, known in modern medicine as testicular tunica vaginalis effusion, was first recorded in Zhang Zihe's Confucian Duties to Parents and Relatives: "Hydrocele... the cyst is as clear as crystal." It is mostly caused by congenital deficiency, kidney deficiency leading to impaired qi transformation, combined with spleen deficiency causing internal accumulation of dampness. Alternatively, because the sinews of the Liver Meridian of Foot-Jueyin converge at the genitalia, liver qi stagnation, combined with exposure to cold, leads to qi stagnation and internal accumulation of water-dampness. This disease is common in children. It can resolve spontaneously within the first year of life, but requires treatment after the age of one. Two proven external washing prescriptions are now recommended to parents.

1. 煅龙骨 20 克，五倍子 15 克，肉桂 10 克，枯矾 15 克（不可用白矾代替）。将四味药用水煎后先熏片刻再坐盆浸泡约 30 分钟，每天 1 次，一般连用 4-5 次。此方疗效好，无副作用，不妨一试。

1. Take 20g of calcined dragon bone (duanlonggu), 15g of Chinese gallnut (wubeizi), 10g of cassia bark (rougui), and 15g of exsiccated alum (kufan) (do not substitute with regular alum). Decoct the four herbs in water. First, fumigate the affected area with the steam for a while, then sit in a basin and soak for about 30 minutes. Do this once a day, generally for 4-5 consecutive times. This prescription has good efficacy and no side effects; it is worth a try.

2. 荔枝核 30-40 枚，打碎，加水煎沸，加食醋小半汤匙，将阴囊浸于水内作热浴。每日 2 次，数天可愈。

2. Take 30-40 lychee seeds, crush them, add water and boil. Add less than half a tablespoon of edible vinegar, and soak the scrotum in the water as a hot bath. Do this twice a day, and it can be cured in a few days.

《民族医药报》1992 年 9 月 4 日（湖南 兰家长）

Ethnic Medicine News, September 4, 1992 (Lan Jiazhang, Hunan)

3. 小肠疝及水疝（鞘膜积液）为婴幼儿多发病常见病，外科以手术治疗。近年来笔者应用民间验方治疗小肠疝、水疝 29 例。均获得满意效果，免于手术之苦。29 例中，小肠疝 8 例（嵌顿性疝 2 例），水疝 21 例。本组年龄为 3 个月龄至 1 周岁。实践表明，1 周岁以上疗效差，所以年龄愈小效果愈好。

3. Inguinal hernia and hydrocele (tunica vaginalis effusion) are common diseases in infants and young children, which are typically treated surgically. In recent years, the author applied folk proven prescriptions to treat 29 cases of inguinal hernia and hydrocele, all achieving satisfactory results and sparing the patients from surgical pain. Among the 29 cases, there were 8 cases of inguinal hernia (including 2 cases of incarcerated hernia) and 21 cases of hydrocele. The patients in this group ranged in age from 3 months to 1 year. Practice has shown that the efficacy is poor for children over 1 year old; therefore, the younger the patient, the better the effect.

验方用药：小茴根 30 克，花椒目 6 克，伙香 12 克，白矾 15 克，水煎熏洗，日 2-3 次，每次约 20-30 分钟。一疗程 3 天，休息 1 天，再行第二疗程，连用 3 个疗程即愈。

Prescription and Usage: Take 30g of fennel root, 6g of Sichuan peppercorn seeds, 12g of fennel fruit (huixiang), and 15g of alum (baifan). Decoct in water for fumigation and washing, 2-3 times a day, about 20-30 minutes each time. One course of treatment is 3 days, followed by 1 day of rest, before starting the second course. Continuous use for 3 courses will result in a cure.

《民族医药报》1993 年 4 月 2 日（青海 刘启明）

Ethnic Medicine News, April 2, 1993 (Liu Qiming, Qinghai)

十七、颈淋巴结肿大（1方）
XVII. Swollen Cervical Lymph Nodes (1 Prescription)

秘方治颈淋巴结肿大

A Secret Recipe for Treating Swollen Cervical Lymph Nodes

笔者祖传有一个专治颈淋巴结肿大的秘方，很有疗效，累试累验，毫无痛苦，无副作用。现介绍如下，有意者不妨一试。

The author has inherited a secret recipe from their ancestors specifically for treating swollen cervical lymph nodes. It is highly effective, has been repeatedly tested and proven, causes no pain, and has no side effects. It is introduced as follows; those who are interested may give it a try.

处方及用法。鲜板蓝根、鲜生地黄各等分，洗净晾干。二药共捣烂如泥作一药饼敷贴脚底涌泉穴，外加一块薄膜，然后用布条包扎固定，24 小时可以除去药饼。敷贴时宜男左女右。一般 2 周后肿大的淋巴结逐渐缩小而痊愈。

Prescription and Usage: Take equal amounts of fresh isatis root (banlangen) and fresh rehmannia root (shengdihuang), wash and air-dry them. Mash the two herbs together into a mud-like paste to form a medicinal cake, and apply it to the Yongquan acupoint on the sole of the foot. Cover it with a plastic film, then bandage and secure it with a cloth strip. The medicinal cake can be removed after 24 hours. When applying, men should use the left foot and women should use the right foot. Generally, after 2 weeks, the swollen lymph nodes will gradually shrink and heal.

《民族医药报》（江苏 顾祥）

Ethnic Medicine News (Gu Xiang, Jiangsu)

十八、治淋巴结核（1方）
XVIII. Treating Scrofula / Tuberculous Lymphadenitis (1 Prescription)

治淋巴结核验方

A Proven Prescription for Treating Scrofula

单用蜈蚣药一味，并备鸭蛋一枚。先从鸭蛋一端打开一小洞，抽出少许蛋清，将一条蜈蚣研成细粉（去头足）从小洞纳入鸭蛋内，用白纸封好，然后把装好蜈蚣的鸭蛋放在文火中烧热为度。每天吃鸭蛋一个（按上法炮制），痊愈为止。一般11（轻者）-44天（最重者）可痊愈。

Use only one ingredient: centipede (wugong), along with one duck egg. First, make a small hole at one end of the duck egg and draw out a little egg white. Grind one centipede into a fine powder (with the head and legs removed), insert the powder into the duck egg through the small hole, and seal it with white paper. Then, heat the duck egg filled with centipede over a gentle fire until it is hot. Eat one duck egg prepared this way every day until fully recovered. Generally, it takes 11 days for mild cases and up to 44 days for the most severe cases to be cured.

《中医药信息报》

Chinese Medicine Information News

十九、治疗顽固性呃逆方（2方）
XIX. Prescriptions for Treating Intractable Hiccups (2 Prescriptions)

1. 治疗顽固性呃逆：给呃逆者服老陈醋20-30毫升，大部分病人服后10-15分钟呃逆开始渐渐减少直至病愈；少部分病人服药后2个小时无好转，可重复服用1次。共治17例，服1次呃逆停止9例；服2次呃逆停止5例；3例服2次仍无好转改其它方法治疗。总有效天82.4%。

1. Treating Intractable Hiccups: Administer 20-30ml of mature vinegar to the patient. For most patients, the hiccups begin to gradually decrease 10-15 minutes after ingestion until they are completely cured. For a small number of patients

who show no improvement 2 hours after taking the medicine, the dose can be repeated once. A total of 17 cases were treated: hiccups stopped after 1 dose in 9 cases, and after 2 doses in 5 cases; 3 cases showed no improvement after 2 doses and were switched to other treatments. The total effective rate was 82.4%.

《民族医药报》

Ethnic Medicine News

2. 治疗呃逆：桂圆干 7 个，放火中烧存性研末，分四次服用，一日 2-3 次。

2. Treating Hiccups: Take 7 dried longan fruits, burn them over a fire until they are charred on the outside but retain their medicinal properties (calcined to retain nature), and grind them into a powder. Divide the powder into four portions and take them 2-3 times a day.

《中药科技报》1992 年 3 月 26 日

Chinese Medicine Science and Technology News, March 26, 1992

二十、治疗鸡眼（8 方）
XX. Treating Corns (8 Prescriptions)

1. 无论生于手部或足部，用蜈蚣粉加 5% 冰片置于鸡眼上，以胶布封固。数日后鸡眼可软化、脱落（胶布必须贴牢、贴紧，否则无效），我们用此方治愈了多人的鸡眼。

1. Whether the corn is on the hand or the foot, apply centipede powder mixed with 5% borneol directly onto the corn, and seal it firmly with adhesive tape. After a few days, the corn will soften and fall off (the tape must be applied securely and tightly, otherwise it will be ineffective). We have used this prescription to cure corns in many people.

《中医药信息报》1992 年 9 月 19 日（安徽 刘大明）

Chinese Medicine Information News, September 19, 1992 (Liu Daming, Anhui)

2. 河南省西峡县田关卫生院李造坤医师等应用蓖麻子外敷法治疗鸡眼，获效满意。取蓖麻籽 1 枚，去外壳，灰火内埋烧，以爆胀为度。患处以热水泡洗，刮去老皮。蓖麻子用手捏软即趁热敷于患处，外以胶布固定，3-5 日换药一次。此法共治疗 160 个鸡眼，其中 1 次治愈 94 个，2 次治愈 52 个，3 次以上治愈 14 个。

2. Dr. Li Zaokun and others at Tianguan Health Center in Xixia County, Henan Province, applied the external application of castor seeds to treat corns with satisfactory results. Take 1 castor seed, remove the outer shell, and bury it in hot ashes to burn until it bursts and expands. Soak the affected area in hot water and scrape off the dead skin. Squeeze the castor seed by hand until soft, and apply it to the affected area while it is still hot. Secure it externally with adhesive tape, and change the dressing once every 3-5 days. This method was used to treat a total of 160 corns: 94 were cured after 1 application, 52 after 2 applications, and 14 after 3 or more applications.

《中医药信息报》（计惠民）

Chinese Medicine Information News (Ji Huimin)

3. 蜂胶外敷法：取与鸡眼或胼胝大小似同薄厚适度的蜂胶一块敷贴于患处面，外用胶布或伤湿止痛膏固定，每隔 3-5 天更换蜂胶一次，换胶时用热水将脚泡洗干净。敷胶期间不要洗脚，一般鸡眼敷胶 2- 3 次即可脱落。

3. Propolis External Application Method: Take a piece of propolis of appropriate thickness, similar in size to the corn or callus, and apply it to the affected area. Secure it externally with adhesive tape or a rheumatism-relieving analgesic plaster. Replace the propolis every 3-5 days. When changing the plaster, soak and wash the foot clean with hot water. Do not wash the foot during the period the plaster is applied. Generally, applying the propolis 2-3 times will cause the corn to fall off.

4. 地红油外涂法：取地骨皮、红花等量、共研细粉，加香油适量调为糊状，于每晚热水烫洗脚后涂于患处，外用无毒塑料薄膜覆盖，再用胶布固定，于次晚烫洗脚时扯去，一般鸡眼 8-10 天即可治愈。

4. Dired Oil External Application Method: Take equal amounts of Chinese wolfberry root bark (digupi) and safflower (honghua), grind them into a fine

powder, and add an appropriate amount of sesame oil to form a paste. After soaking and washing the foot in hot water every night, apply the paste to the affected area. Cover it externally with non-toxic plastic film, and secure it with adhesive tape. Remove it the next evening when soaking the foot in hot water. Generally, corns can be cured in 8-10 days.

5. 鸭仁杨酸外敷法：取鸭蛋子净仁 70-80 粒与水杨酸药粉 10 克共研细，置洁净盒内备用。然后取一块大于鸡眼或胼胝直径 1 厘米的胶布并在胶布中心剪一个与鸡眼或胼胝大小当同的洞，将胶布贴于患处使鸡眼或胼胝从洞中露出，将备用药物敷于鸡眼或胼胝上，外用胶布覆盖固定，待 7-10 天左右将胶布除去，鸡眼即可脱落，若一次未能治愈，可用同法再次敷药治疗，直至愈好，服用药物期间不要洗脚。

5. Brucea Fruit and Salicylic Acid External Application Method: Take 70-80 peeled seeds of Brucea javanica (yadanzi) and 10g of salicylic acid powder, grind them into a fine powder, and store them in a clean container for later use. Then, take a piece of adhesive tape that is 1cm larger in diameter than the corn or callus, and cut a hole in the center of the tape equal in size to the corn or callus. Apply thc tapc to the affected area so that the corn or callus is exposed through the hole. Apply the prepared medicine onto the corn or callus, and cover and secure it with another piece of adhesive tape. Remove the tape after about 7-10 days, and the corn will fall off. If it is not cured in one application, reapply the medicine using the same method until it is completely healed. Do not wash the foot during the medication period.

6. 芦荟外涂法：取芦荟适量用水少许研为糊状，于每晚热水烫洗脚后，将芦荟糊涂于患处，外用无毒塑料薄膜覆盖胶布固定，若次日晚烫洗脚时发现鸡眼或胼胝向上浮起时，可用小刀将浮起部分削去再涂药糊，每日涂药一次，一般鸡眼 5-7 天即可脱落。

6. Aloe External Application Method: Take an appropriate amount of aloe and grind it into a paste with a little water. After soaking and washing the foot in hot water every night, apply the aloe paste to the affected area. Cover it externally

with non-toxic plastic film and secure it with adhesive tape. If the corn or callus floats upward when soaking the foot the next evening, use a small knife to shave off the raised portion before reapplying the paste. Apply the medicine once a day. Generally, the corn will fall off in 5-7 days.

7. 葱膜外贴法：取新鲜青葱根部白色鳞上最外层的薄皮，于每晚热水烫洗脚后，贴于鸡眼患处，外用胶布固定，每日换贴一次，经多次重复贴敷，鸡眼即可自行脱落。

7. Scallion Membrane External Application Method: Take the outermost thin skin of the white bulb at the root of fresh green scallions. After soaking and washing the foot in hot water every night, apply it to the corn. Secure it externally with adhesive tape and change it once a day. After repeated applications, the corn will fall off on its own.

《中药科技报》

Chinese Medicine Science and Technology News

8. 消鸡眼贴。处方及用法：鸦胆子 10 粒，去壳取仁捣烂。先将患鸡眼的脚冷水浸泡 1 小时，待粗皮软化后刮去，拭干净，把上药加老陈醋适量调匀，贴敷患处，胶布固定，2 天后除去，如尚未脱落再如法贴敷 1 次。功效：软坚拔毒。适应症：鸡眼。

8. Corn-Removing Plaster. Prescription and Usage: Take 10 Brucea javanica fruits (yadanzi), remove the shells, take the kernels, and mash them. First, soak the affected foot in cold water for 1 hour. After the thick skin softens, scrape it off and wipe clean. Add an appropriate amount of mature vinegar to the medicine, mix evenly, apply it to the affected area, and secure it with adhesive tape. Remove it after 2 days. If the corn has not yet fallen off, apply it again using the same method. Efficacy: Softens hardness and extracts toxins. Indication: Corns.

《民族医药报》

Ethnic Medicine News

二十一、肺炎（15方）
XXI. Pneumonia (15 Prescriptions)

1. 绣球花叶5-10张，捣烂绞汁，或作煎剂，加食盐或蜂蜜调服，一日数次。

1. Take 5-10 hydrangea leaves, mash them and squeeze out the juice, or decoct them in water. Add salt or honey to mix and take several times a day.

2. 鱼腥草120克，生石膏粉30克。先将鲜鱼腥草捣烂冲开水一碗，后加入石膏粉和匀，分2次服。每次半碗，隔4小时服1次。

2. Take 120g of fresh houttuynia cordata and 30g of raw gypsum powder. First, mash the fresh houttuynia cordata and pour a bowl of boiling water over it. Then add the gypsum powder, mix well, and divide into two doses. Take half a bowl each time, once every 4 hours.

3. 鲜女贞叶500克，鲜芦根30克，加水500毫升，水煎浓缩至200毫升。每次服10毫升，小儿酌减，日服3-4次。

3. Take 500g of fresh glossy privet leaves and 30g of fresh reed rhizome. Add 500ml of water and decoct until concentrated to 200ml. Take 10ml each time (reduce the dose appropriatcly for children), 3-4 times a day.

4. 银花20克，连翘15克，大青叶9克，千里光30克，加水500毫升，水煎浓缩至250毫升，每次服10-15毫升。小儿酌减，日服3-4次。

4. Take 20g of honeysuckle flower, 15g of forsythia fruit, 9g of isatis leaf, and 30g of groundsel. Add 500ml of water and decoct until concentrated to 250ml. Take 10-15ml each time (reduce the dose appropriately for children), 3-4 times a day.

5. 白芥子末、面粉各30克，葱白三根，捣烂，用纱布包后敷贴背部肺俞穴，每天1次，每次约15分钟，出现皮肤发红为止，连用3天。

5. Take 30g each of white mustard seed powder and wheat flour, along with three white scallion stalks. Mash them together, wrap in gauze, and apply to the Feishu acupoint on the back. Do this once a day for about 15 minutes each time, until the skin turns red. Continue for 3 consecutive days.

6. 鱼腥草、桔梗各30克，杏仁9克。先煎桔梗、杏仁半小时，然后加入鱼腥草同煎 10 分钟。每日 1 剂，分 3 次服，连服 3-5 剂。

6. Take 30g each of houttuynia cordata and platycodon root, and 9g of bitter apricot seed. Decoct the platycodon root and bitter apricot seed for half an hour first, then add the houttuynia cordata and decoct together for another 10 minutes. Take one dose daily, divided into three servings. Continue for 3-5 doses.

7. 水芹菜、羊油各 15 克，水煎分数次服，用于治小儿肺炎，连用 3 天。

7. Take 15g each of water celery and sheep fat. Decoct in water and take in several divided doses. This is used to treat pediatric pneumonia. Continue for 3 consecutive days.

8. 石膏 30 克（生用、打碎先煎），知母 6 克，炙枇杷叶（去毛）15 克，五味子 3 克，水煎温服，每日 1 剂，分 3 次服，连用 3-5 天。

8. Take 30g of raw gypsum (crushed and decocted first), 6g of anemarrhena rhizome, 15g of honey-fried loquat leaf (with the fuzz removed), and 3g of schisandra fruit. Decoct in water and take warm. Take one dose daily, divided into three servings. Continue for 3-5 days.

9. 石莲花全草 100 克，加冰糖适量，水煎服，每日 2 次，每日 1 剂。连用 3-5 天。

9. Take 100g of the whole Echeveria plant, add an appropriate amount of rock sugar, and decoct in water. Take one dose daily, divided into two servings. Continue for 3-5 days.

10. 大黄、芒硝、大蒜各 15 克，捣烂后布包敷胸，如皮肤未出现刺激反应，可连用 3-5 天。如出现刺激反应不可再用。

10. Take 15g each of rhubarb, mirabilite, and garlic. Mash them, wrap in cloth, and apply to the chest. If no skin irritation occurs, it can be used continuously for 3-5 days. Discontinue use if skin irritation occurs.

11. 僵蚕、全虫各等分，研成细末，成分每次服 0. 5 克，小儿 0.2 克，日 2 次。开水送服，连用 3-5 天。

11. Take equal amounts of silkworm fungus and scorpion. Grind them into a fine powder. Adults take 0.5g each time, and children take 0.2g each time, twice a

day. Take with boiling water. Continue for 3-5 days.

12. 白果仁 9 克，车前草 30 克，蒲公英 30 克，大青叶 12 克，陈皮 6 克，加水煎煮取浓缩液 300 毫升，加红糖适量。成人每次服 10-15 毫升，小儿每次服 5-10 毫升，日 3 次。

12. Take 9g of ginkgo nut kernels, 30g of plantain herb, 30g of dandelion, 12g of isatis leaf, and 6g of tangerine peel. Add water to decoct and extract 300ml of concentrated liquid, then add an appropriate amount of brown sugar. Adults take 10-15ml each time, and children take 5-10ml each time, 3 times a day.

13. 大青叶、板蓝根各 15 克，草河车 12 克，柴胡、僵蚕各 9 克，水煎服，日 3 次，每日 1 剂，连用 5-10 剂。

13. Take 15g each of isatis leaf and isatis root, 12g of Paris polyphylla (caoheche), and 9g each of bupleurum root and silkworm fungus. Decoct in water. Take one dose daily, divided into three servings. Continue for 5-10 doses.

14. 银花 30 克，当归 15 克，元参、蒲公英各 9 克，水煎服，日 3 次。每日 1 剂。连服 5 天。

14. Take 30g of honeysuckle flower, 15g of angelica root, and 9g each of scrophularia root and dandelion. Decoct in water. Take one dose daily, divided into three servings. Continue for 5 days.

15. 桑白皮、地骨皮各 30 克，知母 12 克，生石膏 15 克，水煎服，日 3 次，每日 1 剂。连用 3-5 天。

15. Take 30g each of mulberry root bark and Chinese wolfberry root bark, 12g of anemarrhena rhizome, and 15g of raw gypsum. Decoct in water. Take one dose daily, divided into three servings. Continue for 3-5 days.

《中药科技报》1992 年 12 月 16 日（青海 刘启明）

Chinese Medicine Science and Technology News, December 16, 1992 (Liu Qiming, Qinghai)

二十二、肺结核（3方）
XXII. Pulmonary Tuberculosis (3 Prescriptions)

1. 抗痨一号。功能：清热泻火，润肺滋阴。症见：午后潮热，夜间盗汗，手足心热，干咳少痰，或痰中带血，胸痛，消瘦乏力。处方：地骨皮15克、麦冬15克、生地15克、百部20克、白薇12克、知母10克、白茅根30克、连翘15克、夏枯草15克、金银花30克、蒲公英15克、黄精15克。服法：每日一剂，水煎两次，早、晚各服一次。

1. Anti-Tuberculosis Formula No. 1. Functions: Clears heat and purges fire, moistens the lungs, and nourishes yin. Symptoms: Afternoon tidal fever, night sweats, heat in the palms and soles, dry cough with little phlegm, or blood-tinged sputum, chest pain, emaciation, and fatigue. Prescription: Take 15g each of Chinese wolfberry root bark (digupi), ophiopogon tuber (maidong), and rehmannia root (shengdi); 20g of stemona root (baibu); 12g of cynanchum root (baiwei); 10g of anemarrhena rhizome (zhimu); 30g of cogongrass rhizome (baimaogen); 15g each of forsythia fruit (lianqiao), selfheal spike (xiakucao), and polygonatum rhizome (huangjing); 30g of honeysuckle flower (jinyinhua); and 15g of dandelion (pugongying). Usage: Take one dose daily, decocted twice in water, and taken once in the morning and once in the evening.

2. 抗痨二号。功能：滋阴降火，补益肺肾。症见：骨蒸潮热，五心烦热，两颧潮红、盗汗，形体消瘦、呛咳少痰、痰黄质稠、经常咯吐鲜血、男子遗精、女子经闭。处方：阿胶15克（烊化）、冬虫夏草10克（先煎）、白芍30克、元参30克、胡黄连10元、大贝母15克、当归15克、白芨粉10克（冲服）、白果10克、侧柏叶15克、石榴皮10克、诃子10克、黄精15克。服法：每日一剂，水煎两次、早、晚各服一次。

2. Anti-Tuberculosis Formula No. 2. Functions: Nourishes yin and reduces fire, tonifies the lungs and kidneys. Symptoms: Bone-steaming tidal fever, vexation and heat in the five centers, flushed cheeks, night sweats, emaciation, choking cough with little phlegm, thick yellow sputum, frequent expectoration of fresh

blood, seminal emission in men, and amenorrhea in women. Prescription: Take 15g of donkey-hide gelatin (ejiao) (melted); 10g of cordyceps (dongchongxiacao) (decocted first); 30g each of white peony root (baishao) and scrophularia root (yuanshen); 10g of picrorhiza rhizome (huhuanglian); 15g of fritillary bulb (dabeimu); 15g of angelica root (danggui); 10g of bletilla powder (baijifen) (taken as a bolus); 10g of ginkgo nut (baiguo); 15g of platycladus leaf (cebaiye); 10g each of pomegranate peel (shiliupi) and chebula fruit (hezi); and 15g of polygonatum rhizome (huangjing). Usage: Take one dose daily, decocted twice in water, and taken once in the morning and once in the evening.

《民族医药报》

Ethnic Medicine News

3. 肺结核: 取中药白芨研末，装瓶备用，每次用开水冲服药粉 6 克，每日 3 次，服药 1 个月为 1 疗程，一般连服 2-3 个疗程可愈，效果显著，无毒性反应。

3. Pulmonary Tuberculosis: Take the Chinese medicine bletilla (baiji), grind it into a powder, and store it in a bottle for later use. Each time, take 6g of the powder and mix it with boiling water to drink, 3 times a day. One month of medication constitutes one course of treatment. Generally, continuous use for 2-3 courses will result in a cure. The effect is remarkable, with no toxic reactions.

二十三、阑尾炎（1 方）
XXIII. Appendicitis (1 Prescription)

白花蛇舌草治疗阑尾炎。白花蛇舌草为清热解毒药。治疗阑尾炎，用鲜草 30-120 克（干品减半）煎服，第一天服 1 剂，第 2 天服 2-3 剂，每剂仅煎 1 次，平均服 3-4 天症状可消失。211 例患者中，痊愈 187 例，基本治愈 15 例，无效转手术 9 例，大大减少了手术率。

Treating Appendicitis with Oldenlandia diffusa. Oldenlandia diffusa is a traditional Chinese medicine used to clear heat and detoxify. To treat appendicitis, take 30-120g of fresh herbs (halve the dosage if using dried herbs) and decoct them for oral administration. Take 1 dose on the first day, and 2-3 doses on the second day. Each dose is decocted only once. On average, the symptoms will disappear after taking the medicine for 3-4 days. Among 211 patients treated, 187 were completely cured, 15 were basically cured, and 9 cases were ineffective and required surgery, significantly reducing the surgical rate.

二十四、荨麻疹（1方）

XXIV. Urticaria (1 Prescription)

马齿苋治疗荨麻疹有良效

Purslane Has Excellent Efficacy in Treating Urticaria

荨麻疹是皮肤科的一种常见病。我院采用具有清热解毒、凉血作用的中草药马齿苋治疗，取得了良好疗效，现介绍如下：

Urticaria is a common disease in dermatology. Our hospital used purslane (machixian), a Chinese herbal medicine with the effects of clearing heat, detoxifying, and cooling the blood, to treat this condition and achieved good therapeutic results. The method is introduced as follows:

取新鲜马齿苋全草 200 克，洗去泥土，加水约 2000 毫升，煎沸后饮汤药，每日 2 次。另外取一纱布蘸上余下药液擦洗红疹处。据临床验证，马齿苋有良好的止痒作用，不妨一试。

Take 200g of fresh whole purslane plant, wash off the dirt, add about 2000ml of water, and boil it. Drink the decoction twice a day. In addition, soak a piece of gauze in the remaining medicinal liquid and wipe the red rash area. Clinical verification has shown that purslane has a good anti-itching effect; it is worth a try.

《中药科技报》1992 年 5 月 6 日（孙扬）

Chinese Medicine Science and Technology News, May 6, 1992 (Sun Yang)

二十五、静脉炎（4 方）
XXV. Phlebitis (4 Prescriptions)

局部的静脉炎症多发于长期反复输液、静脉多次穿刺患者，尤以肿瘤化疗患者更易罹患，此症既增加了患者的痛苦，又影响继续治疗。以往临床上常采用西药局部热敷或封闭等方法治疗，但效果均不尽满意。近年来有报道言，中药治疗效果较佳。现辑录三则如下，供同行选用。

Local venous inflammation is common in patients who receive long-term, repeated intravenous infusions and multiple venipunctures, particularly those undergoing tumor chemotherapy. This condition not only increases the patients' suffering but also affects their continued treatment. In the past, clinical treatments often used Western medicine methods such as local hot compresses or nerve blocks, but the results were not entirely satisfactory. In recent years, reports have indicated that traditional Chinese medicine (TCM) treatments yield better results. Three such prescriptions are compiled below for reference by medical peers.

1. 活血消炎酊局部涂搽

1. Topical Application of Blood-Activating and Anti-Inflammatory Tincture

取具有活血散瘀，消炎止痛的中药，红花、丹参各 10 克，黄柏、黄连、地榆各 6 克，加 75% 乙醇 1000 毫升，浸润一周左右。用其滤液涂抹于患炎静脉，每日 6-8 次。200 例患者治疗观察，治愈率为 87.5%，总有效率达 100%。

Take TCM herbs with the effects of activating blood, dissipating blood stasis, reducing inflammation, and relieving pain: 10g each of safflower (honghua) and salvia root (danshen), and 6g each of amur cork tree bark (huangbai), coptis root (huanglian), and great burnet root (diyu). Add 1000ml of 75% ethanol and soak for about one week. Apply the filtered liquid to the inflamed vein 6-8 times a day. Clinical observation of 200 patients showed a cure rate of 87.5% and a total effective rate of 100%.

2. 新鲜丝瓜叶捣糊外用

2. External Application of Mashed Fresh Luffa Leaves

丝瓜叶属葫芦科植物丝瓜的叶片，内含有皂苷等成分。药理实验提示具有清热解毒、散瘀破结和止痛等作用。民间曾用于治疗疖肿、疮癣，神经性皮炎等疾患。临床用其治疗静脉炎效果比较显著。方法是，摘取新鲜丝瓜叶数片，洗净甩干捣烂成糊状。沿静脉走向，敷于患处，约 0.2-0.3 厘米，范围稍大于患炎处,外用纱布包扎固定,注意保持局部湿润,避免蒸发和外溢,每日换药 1-2 次。

Luffa leaves belong to the gourd family and contain components such as saponins. Pharmacological experiments suggest they have the effects of clearing heat and detoxifying, dissipating blood stasis and resolving nodules, and relieving pain. In folk medicine, they have been used to treat boils, sores, tinea, and neurodermatitis. Clinical use of luffa leaves to treat phlebitis has shown significant results. The method is as follows: Pick several fresh luffa leaves, wash them, shake off the water, and mash them into a paste. Apply the paste along the direction of the vein to the affected area, about 0.2-0.3 cm thick, covering an area slightly larger than the inflamed site. Bandage and secure it with gauze. Keep the area moist to prevent evaporation and leakage, and change the dressing 1-2 times a day.

3. 六神丸、硝酸甘油加陈醋调糊外敷

3. External Application of Paste Made from Liushen Pills, Nitroglycerin, and Mature Vinegar

六神丸乃治咽喉痛之良药，有消炎止痛，散瘀消肿之作用；陈醋活血，促进血液循环；硝酸甘油可扩张局部血管，有利于药物的渗入，三者合用，从而可达到治疗目的。该方是，取六神丸 30-60 粒，硝酸甘油 1 毫克碾碎成粉状。加陈醋 2-4 毫升调成药糊（视患炎静脉多少，按此比例增大用药量），外敷于局部，每次 5-7 小时，每日 2-3 次，一周为一疗程。临床对 53 例 114 处患炎静脉，采用此法治疗，总有效率达 93.4%。

Liushen pills are an excellent remedy for sore throats, with the effects of reducing inflammation, relieving pain, dissipating blood stasis, and reducing swelling. Mature vinegar activates blood and promotes blood circulation. Nitroglycerin dilates local blood vessels, facilitating the penetration of the medication. The combination of these three achieves the therapeutic goal. The prescription is as follows: Take 30-60 Liushen pills and 1mg of nitroglycerin, and crush them into a powder. Add 2-4ml of mature vinegar to form a medicinal paste (adjust the dosage proportionally based on the number of inflamed veins). Apply the paste topically to the affected area for 5-7 hours each time, 2-3 times a day, with one week constituting one course of treatment. Clinically, this method was used to treat 114 inflamed veins in 53 patients, achieving a total effective rate of 93.4%.

上述三法，具有取材方便，调配简单，疗效满意，乐于接受等优点，不妨一试。

The above three methods have the advantages of easily accessible materials, simple preparation, satisfactory efficacy, and high patient acceptance. They are worth a try.

（王洪道）

(Wang Hongdao)

4. 本病是血管病中的常见病，急性期多见四肢或胸腹壁部位局部红肿热痛，可扪及条索状物，触痛拒按，影响患肢活动，或出现恶寒发热，口渴饮水，大便干结，小便发黄，心烦不眠，舌质暗红有瘀班，舌苔白腻，脉细数或弦数。中医辨证属于湿热凝滞血瘀阻络，采用清热化湿，活血通络之法有良效。

4. This disease is a common vascular condition. In the acute phase, patients often present with localized redness, swelling, heat, and pain in the limbs, chest, or abdominal wall. A cord-like mass can be palpated, which is tender to the touch and resists pressure, affecting the movement of the affected limb. Systemic symptoms may include chills and fever, thirst with excessive drinking, dry and hard stools, dark yellow urine, restlessness, and insomnia. The tongue is dark red with petechiae and has a white, greasy coating. The pulse is thready and rapid, or string-taut (wiry) and rapid. In TCM syndrome differentiation, this is classified as damp-heat stagnation with blood stasis obstructing the meridians. The treatment principle of clearing heat, transforming dampness, activating blood, and unblocking the meridians yields good therapeutic effects.

用药：金银花 20 克、连翘 18 克、炒当归 12 克、蒲公英 24 克、元参 18 克、赤芍 12 克、炒丹皮 10 克、红花 6 克、桃仁 10 克、炒延胡索 10 克、甘草 6 克、茵陈 20 克、炒牛膝 10 克 、生薏苡仁 20 克、炒陈皮 10 克，清水煎服，一日 2-3 次。加减：局部条索明显，药后不消者加炙山甲 10 克、三棱 10 克、莪术 10 克；肿胀明显者加车前子 15 克、白术 10 克；患处疼痛加炒川楝 10 克、炙乳没各 8 克；发于胸壁者加桔梗 6 克、升麻 6 克；发于上肢者加桑枝 20 克；发于下肢者去蒲公英加紫花地丁 20 克。如转为慢性，则宜化瘀散结，益气通络。

Prescription: Take 20g of honeysuckle flower (jinyinhua), 18g of forsythia fruit (lianqiao), 12g of stir-baked angelica root (danggui), 24g of dandelion (pugongying), 18g of scrophularia root (yuanshen), 12g of red peony root (chishao), 10g of stir-baked moutan bark (danpi), 6g of safflower (honghua), 10g of peach kernel (taoren), 10g of stir-baked corydalis tuber (yanhusuo), 6g of licorice root (gancao), 20g of capillary wormwood (yinchen), 10g of stir-baked achyranthes root (niuxi), 20g of raw coix seed (shengyiyiren), and 10g of stir-baked tangerine peel (chenpi). Decoct in water and take 2-3 times a day. Modifications: If the local cord-like mass is prominent and does not subside after medication, add 10g of honey-fried pangolin scales (zhishanjia), 10g of sparganium rhizome (sanleng), and 10g of zedoary rhizome (ezhu). If swelling is prominent, add 15g of plantain seeds (cheqianzi) and 10g of atractylodes macrocephala rhizome (baizhu). For pain at the affected site, add 10g of stir-baked chinaberry fruit (chuanlianzi) and 8g each of honey-fried frankincense (ruxiang) and myrrh (moyao). If it occurs on the chest wall, add 6g of platycodon root (jiegeng) and 6g of cimicifuga rhizome (shengma). If it occurs on the upper limbs, add 20g of mulberry twig (sangzhi). If it occurs on the lower limbs, remove dandelion and add 20g of violet herb (zihuadiding). If the condition becomes chronic, the treatment should focus on transforming blood stasis, resolving nodules, tonifying qi, and unblocking the meridians.

《民族医药报》1992 年 4 月 3 日（江苏 袁培春）

Ethnic Medicine News, April 3, 1992 (Yuan Peichun, Jiangsu)

第十五章　单味多效中药

Chapter 15　Single Herbs with Multiple Therapeutic Effects

一、蒲公英

Dandelion (Pu-gong-ying)

1. 主治流行性腮腺炎

1. Indication: Epidemic Parotitis (Mumps)

方药：蒲公英 30 克，板蓝根 20 克。

Prescription: 30g of dandelion and 20g of isatis root.

用法：水煎服，连服三剂，禁忌辛辣食物。

Usage: Decoct in water and take orally. Take 3 consecutive doses. Avoid spicy and pungent foods.

疗效：治疗 150 例，痊愈 100 例，有效 50 例。

Therapeutic Effect: A total of 150 cases were treated, with 100 completely cured and 50 showing effectiveness.

2. 主治急性结膜炎

2. Indication: Acute Conjunctivitis

方药：蒲公英 30 克，菊花 15 克，霜桑叶 10 克。

Prescription: 30g of dandelion, 15g of chrysanthemum flower, and 10g of frost-bitten mulberry leaf.

用法：水煎服三剂，每次煎熬 20 分钟。上述三味药用量加倍煎熬熏洗。

Usage: Decoct in water and take 3 doses, boiling for 20 minutes each time. Double the dosage of the above three herbs, decoct, and use the steam to fumigate and wash the eyes.

疗效：治疗 283 例，有复诊者 83 例，其中痊愈 70 例，显效 9 例，效差 4 例。

Therapeutic Effect: A total of 283 cases were treated, with 83 returning for follow-up. Among them, 70 were completely cured, 9 showed significant improvement, and 4 showed poor response.

3. 主治滴虫性阴道炎

3. Indication: Trichomonas Vaginitis

方药：蒲公英 20 克，苦参、蛇床子、土茯苓各 15 克。

Prescription: 20g of dandelion, and 15g each of sophora flavescens root (kushen), cnidium fruit (shechuangzi), and smilax glabra rhizome (tufuling).

用法：水煎服五剂。局部熏洗加桃树叶 200 克煎水坐浴，同时用棉球或清洁纱巾蘸药水塞阴道内，每晚洗涤一次，连洗五次。

Usage: Decoct in water and take 5 doses. For local fumigation and washing, add 200g of peach leaves, decoct in water, and use for a sitz bath. At the same time, soak a cotton ball or a clean gauze pad in the medicinal liquid and insert it into the vagina. Wash once every night for 5 consecutive nights.

疗效： 治疗 342 例 随访 224 例，治愈 184 例，显效 21 例，效差 19 例。

Therapeutic Effect: A total of 342 cases were treated, with 224 followed up. Among them, 184 were cured, 21 showed significant improvement, and 19 showed poor response.

4. 主治盆腔炎、附件炎

4. Indication: Pelvic Inflammatory Disease (PID) and Adnexitis

方药：蒲公英 40 克，旱莲草 15 克，白花蛇草 20 克，川黄柏 14 克。

Prescription: 40g of dandelion, 15g of eclipta herb (hanliancao), 20g of oldenlandia diffusa (baihuasheshecao), and 14g of Sichuan amur cork tree bark (chuanhuangbai).

用法：连服 14 剂为一疗程。水煎 30 分钟为宜。

Usage: Take 14 consecutive doses as one course of treatment. Decoct in water for 30 minutes.

疗效：治疗 150 例，经随访 133 例，服 3-5 剂即见显效，但患盆腔炎者 14

剂为最长疗期。

Therapeutic Effect: A total of 150 cases were treated, with 133 followed up. Significant improvement was seen after taking 3-5 doses, but for patients with PID, 14 doses were required as the maximum treatment duration.

5. 主治急性乳腺炎

5. Indication: Acute Mastitis

方药：蒲公英 60 克，金银花 30 克，生半夏 9 克，连翘 15 克，白芷 15 克，赤芍 10 克，瓜蒌 10 克，天花粉 10 克。

Prescription: 60g of dandelion, 30g of honeysuckle flower (jinyinhua), 9g of raw pinellia tuber (shengbanxia), 15g of forsythia fruit (lianqiao), 15g of angelica dahurica root (baizhi), 10g of red peony root (chishao), 10g of Chinese trichosanthes fruit (gualou), and 10g of trichosanthes root (tianhuafen).

用法：水煎服 3-7 剂。

Usage: Decoct in water and take 3-7 doses.

疗效：治疗 80 例，一般用药不超过 7 剂即愈。

Therapeutic Effect: A total of 80 cases were treated, and most were cured within no more than 7 doses.

6. 主治急慢性痢疾

6. Indication: Acute and Chronic Dysentery

方药：蒲公英 20 克，鱼腥草 15 克，地锦草、凤尾草各 10 克，川黄连 6 克，酸石榴皮 9 克。

Prescription: 20g of dandelion, 15g of houttuynia cordata (yuxingcao), 10g each of euphorbia humifusa herb (dijincao) and maidenhair fern (fengweicao), 6g of Sichuan coptis root (chuanhuanglian), and 9g of sour pomegranate peel (suanshiliupi).

用法：红糖为引，连服 3-6 剂

Usage: Use brown sugar as a guiding ingredient. Take 3-6 consecutive doses.

疗效：治疗 52 例均有显效。

Therapeutic Effect: All 52 treated cases showed significant improvement.

以上仅是吾临床点滴小结，虽用此药相配得心应手，方能妙用。

The above is merely a brief summary of my clinical experience. Although I am highly proficient in combining this herb, it must still be modified and adjusted according to the specific syndrome to achieve optimal therapeutic effects.

蒲公英外用效果亦佳，如鲜蒲公英洗净捣成泥外用，治疗无名肿毒，腮腺炎、痈疮等外科病，有独特疗效。

Dandelion also has excellent external application effects. For example, washing fresh dandelion, mashing it into a paste, and applying it externally has unique therapeutic effects on surgical conditions such as unexplained swellings and toxic sores, mumps, and carbuncles.

《中药科技报》

Chinese Medicine Science and Technology News

7. 治疗乳腺炎、各种疖肿：全草 30 克与橘核 30 克，煎服；同时用新鲜蒲公英全草捣烂，敷患处。

7. Treating Mastitis and Various Boils: Decoct and take 30g of the whole dandelion plant and 30g of tangerine seeds (juhe). At the same time, mash fresh whole dandelion plants and apply them to the affected area.

8. 内服外洗治疗红眼病：鲜蒲公英 120 克（或干品 60 克），水煎 2 碗，温服一碗，拿一碗趁热熏洗，一般 1-3 次即愈。

8. Treating Pink Eye via Oral Intake and External Washing: Take 120g of fresh dandelion (or 60g of dried dandelion) and decoct it in water to yield 2 bowls. Drink one bowl warm, and use the other bowl while it is still hot to fumigate and wash the eyes. It is generally cured after 1-3 treatments.

9. 治疗上呼吸道感染：蒲公英对金黄色葡萄球菌、肺炎双球菌等病菌有抑制作用，用鲜草 30-60 克煎服，可治疗急性支气管炎。

9. Treating Upper Respiratory Tract Infections: Dandelion has an inhibitory effect on pathogens such as Staphylococcus aureus and Streptococcus pneumoniae. Decocting and taking 30-60g of fresh dandelion can treat acute bronchitis.

10. 治疗胃脘痛：蒲公英含甾醇、胆碱、菊糖和果胶等，对多种细菌均有较好的抑制作用，特别是对幽门弯曲杆菌有较强的杀灭作用，用蒲公英的干品研末冲服可治疗溃疡病或糜烂性胃炎。

10. Treating Epigastric Pain: Dandelion contains sterols, choline, inulin, pectin, and other compounds, which have good inhibitory effects on various bacteria, particularly a strong bactericidal effect against Helicobacter pylori. Grinding dried dandelion into a powder and taking it as a bolus with water can treat peptic ulcers or erosive gastritis.

11. 利尿：中医称蒲公英为"通淋妙品"，对小便频数而涩痛，可取鲜蒲公英 60 克水煎代茶饮，有清热利尿之效。

11. Diuretic Effect: TCM refers to dandelion as a "wonderful remedy for stranguria." For frequent, painful, and astringent urination, taking 60g of fresh dandelion decocted in water as a tea substitute has the effects of clearing heat and promoting diuresis.

12. 治疗粉刺：蒲公英乙醇浸泡剂可作为止痒去屑发露，和薄荷、白芷、樟脑配伍，添加到粉刺露、霜中，对有感染的粉刺及黑头粉刺都有疗效。

12. Treating Acne: Dandelion ethanol extract can be used as an anti-itch and anti-dandruff hair lotion. When combined with mint, angelica dahurica root, and camphor, and added to acne lotions and creams, it is effective against infected acne and blackheads.

13. 用于化妆品：蒲公英水煎剂和水浸剂可用作止痒头油、去屑头油以及发乳、洁白露、清洁露、洁肤露等；又因其含有维生素 C、氨基酸等营养物质，因此也可以添加到营养霜、营养露、增白霜等化妆品中去。

13. Use in Cosmetics: Dandelion aqueous decoctions and infusions can be used as anti-itch and anti-dandruff hair oils, as well as in hair creams, whitening lotions, cleansing lotions, and skin-cleansing lotions. Furthermore, because it contains nutrients such as vitamin C and amino acids, it can also be added to nourishing creams, nourishing lotions, and skin-whitening creams.

《中药科技报》

Chinese Medicine Science and Technology News

二、益母草

2. Leonurus (Motherwort)

益母草是一种妇科良药，为妇人熟悉。祖国医学认为，益母草性微寒、味辛苦，有活血调经，利尿祛痰等功效。

Leonurus (Yimucao / Motherwort) is a well-known and highly effective herb in gynecology. According to Traditional Chinese Medicine (TCM), it is slightly cold in nature, with a bitter and pungent taste. It is known for its effects of promoting blood circulation, regulating menstruation, inducing diuresis, and resolving phlegm.

中医在应用益母草治病方面积累了不少的经验，现撷取几则，以供参考。

TCM has accumulated extensive experience in using Leonurus for treatment. Here are a few practical prescriptions for your reference:

1. 产后恶露不净，小腹胀痛：取益母草 100 克，加水煎取药液服用，或加入大枣 5 枚，红糖适量，以增强活血，养血，健脾的作用。每日一剂，2-3 天为一疗程，有较好的作用。

1. For prolonged postpartum lochia and lower abdominal distension/pain:Take 100g of Leonurus and decoct it in water. Alternatively, add 5 red dates and an appropriate amount of brown sugar to enhance the effects of promoting blood circulation, nourishing blood, and strengthening the spleen. Take one dose daily for 2-3 days as a course of treatment, which usually yields good results.

2. 月经不调、经前腹胀: 用益母草 150 克，当归 100 克，水酒各半同煎取药液，或取益母草 150 克，制香附 50 克，丹参 100 克，共捣为细末炼蜜为丸，每次 10 克，早晚各一次，温开水送服，5-7 天为一疗程。

2. For irregular menstruation and premenstrual abdominal distension:Decoct 150g of Leonurus and 100g of Angelica sinensis (Danggui) in a 50/50 mixture of water and rice wine.Or, pound 150g of Leonurus, 50g of Cyperus rotundus (processed Xiangfu), and 100g of Salvia miltiorrhiza (Danshen) into a fine powder, refine with honey to make pills. Take 10g each time, twice a day (morning and

evening) with warm water. A course of treatment lasts 5-7 days.

3. 闭经：取益母草 50 克，红糖 100 克，加水煎取药液后，趁热加黄酒 100 克，搅匀后服用，每日一剂，连服数剂，有一定疗效。

3. For amenorrhea (absence of menstruation):Decoct 50g of Leonurus and 100g of brown sugar in water. While still hot, stir in 100g of yellow rice wine and drink. Take one dose daily for several consecutive doses; this has shown a certain therapeutic effect.

4. 产后腹痛：用益母草 20 克，生姜 3 片，红糖 50 克，先将益母草、生姜加水煎取汁，再入红糖调匀后趁热服下。

4. For postpartum abdominal pain:Decoct 20g of Leonurus and 3 slices of fresh ginger in water to extract the juice. Stir in 50g of brown sugar and drink while hot.

5. 崩中漏下、产后血晕：取新鲜益母草 120 克，去根洗净，切碎，或干益母草 60 克，煎取浓汁去渣，约 200 毫升，入粳米 50 克，红糖适量，再加水 350 毫升，煮为稀粥，每日 2 次，温热服食。孕妇慎用。

5. For uterine bleeding (metrorrhagia/uterine bleeding) and postpartum blood dizziness:Take 120g of fresh Leonurus (wash and remove the roots, then chop) or 60g of dried Leonurus. Decoct into a concentrated juice, strain out the residue to get about 200ml. Add 50g of japonica rice, an appropriate amount of brown sugar, and 350ml of water, then cook into a thin porridge. Consume warm, twice a day.

《中药科技极》1992 年 5 月 6 日（湖北　徐勤）

Source: May 6, 1992, "Chinese Herbal Medicine Science & Technology" (Author: Xu Qin, Hubei)

三、蓖麻籽

3. Castor Seeds (Bi-ma-zi)

蓖麻仁能消肿拔毒，排脓祛腐，祛风利水，“开道诸窍经络”。其外用亦颇奏奇效，可祛邪祛病痿之功。

Castor kernels can reduce swelling, draw out toxins, discharge pus, remove necrotic tissue, dispel wind, and promote diuresis, as well as "unblock the orifices and meridians." Their external application also yields remarkable effects, achieving the therapeutic goal of eliminating pathogenic factors and curing diseases.

1. 美尼尔氏征：蓖麻仁、生半夏各等份，共捣烂成膏，敷贴百会穴，并以胶布固定同时辅以局部按摩。一般用药后 30 分钟即可获效。

1. Meniere's Disease: Take equal amounts of castor kernels and raw pinellia tuber (shengbanxia), mash them into a paste, apply it to the Baihui acupoint, secure it with medical tape, and assist with local massage. It generally takes effect within 30 minutes after application.

2. 头痛：取蓖麻仁、乳香各等份共捣烂，制成饼状，两侧疼痛者贴太阳穴；前额疼痛者贴印堂；三叉神经痛敷贴相关腧穴亦有显著疗效。

2. Headache: Take equal amounts of castor kernels and frankincense (ruxiang), mash them together, and form them into a cake-like shape. For pain on both sides of the head, apply to the Taiyang acupoints; for pain in the forehead, apply to the Yintang acupoint. Applying to the relevant acupoints for trigeminal neuralgia also yields significant therapeutic effects.

3. 水肿：蓖麻仁 30-40 粒，石蒜 10 个。共捣如泥，外敷双足涌泉穴，1 日换药 1 次，至消肿为度。

3. Edema: Take 30-40 castor kernels and 10 lycoris bulbs (shisuan). Mash them together into a mud-like paste, apply externally to the Yongquan acupoints on both soles, and change the dressing once a day until the swelling subsides.

4. 尿潴留：蓖麻仁 10 粒，田螺 5 个，食盐 9 克，共捣成糊状外敷神阙穴。药后一般 20 分钟即可见效。

4. Urinary Retention: Take 10 castor kernels, 5 river snails (tiansluo), and 9g of salt. Mash them together into a paste and apply externally to the Shenque acupoint (navel). It generally takes effect within 20 minutes after application.

5. 便秘：以蓖麻仁、芒硝2:1量，共捣成饼状，外敷天枢、神阙穴。并辅以按摩，增强疗效。

5. Constipation: Take castor kernels and mirabilite (mangxiao) in a 2:1 ratio, mash them into a cake-like shape, and apply externally to the Tianshu and Shenque acupoints. Assisting with massage can enhance the therapeutic effect.

6. 烫伤：蓖麻仁油 50 克，黄柏、冰片各 10 克（共研细）。将三药调匀后外涂于患处。用药后即可止痛，且无继发感染之忧。起效迅速。

6. Scalds and Burns: Take 50g of castor oil, and 10g each of amur cork tree bark (huangbai) and borneol (bingpian) (grind them into a fine powder together). Mix the three ingredients evenly and apply externally to the affected area. It relieves pain immediately after application and prevents secondary infections. It takes effect rapidly.

7. 内脏下垂：取蓖麻仁、五倍子各等量共捣成膏，外敷百会、神阙穴。胃下垂加中脘穴；子宫下垂加子宫穴；直肠脱垂加石门穴。

7. Visceroptosis: Take equal amounts of castor kernels and Chinese gallnut (wubeizi), mash them into a paste, and apply externally to the Baihui and Shenque acupoints. For gastroptosis, additionally apply to the Zhongwan acupoint; for uterine prolapse, additionally apply to the Zigong acupoint; for rectal prolapse, additionally apply to the Shimen acupoint.

《民族医药报》

Ethnic Medicine News

8. 大家都有这样的体会，手上扎进了竹、木签刺后，既痛苦又难拔，遇到这种情况，可用蓖麻子几粒，捣成泥后敷于患处。用纱布作适度包扎，不能扎得太紧，在刺口处尤宜放松，这样，只需经一夜时间，短刺可完全拔出，长刺也会冒出一截，用手轻拔即可取出。此法屡试屡验、效果极佳。如伤口有感染者，可配合内服消炎药。

8. Many people have experienced the pain and difficulty of extracting bamboo or wooden splinters from their hands. In such cases, you can mash a few castor seeds into a mud-like paste and apply it to the affected area. Bandage

it moderately with gauze; do not wrap it too tightly, and especially keep the splinter entry point relaxed. This way, after just one night, short splinters can be completely drawn out, and long splinters will protrude enough to be easily pulled out by hand. This method has been repeatedly tested and proven highly effective. If the wound is infected, oral anti-inflammatory drugs can be used in combination.

《民族医药报》1992 年 1 月 31 日（贵州 吴彬）

Ethnic Medicine News, January 31, 1992 (Wu Bin, Guizhou)

四、五倍子
4. Chinese Gallnut (Wu-bei-zi)

五倍子味酸、涩、寒，归肺、大肠、肾经，临床外用有解毒、消肿、收湿、敛疮、止血等功效，近年来发现治疗皮肤病有满意效果，特介绍如下。

Chinese gallnut is sour and astringent in flavor, cold in nature, and enters the Lung, Large Intestine, and Kidney meridians. When used externally in clinical practice, it has the effects of detoxifying, reducing swelling, absorbing dampness, promoting the healing of sores, and stopping bleeding. In recent years, it has been found to yield satisfactory results in treating skin diseases. The specific applications are introduced as follows.

1. 治疗口疮：用五倍子、青黛各 30 克共研细末，适量撒在口疮溃疡面上，每日 3 次，一般 3 天见效。

1. Treating Aphthous Ulcers (Canker Sores): Grind 30g each of Chinese gallnut and indigo naturalis (qingdai) into a fine powder. Sprinkle an appropriate amount directly onto the ulcerated surface 3 times a day. It generally takes effect within 3 days.

2. 治疗手足皲裂：用五倍子 10 克，紫草 4 克，甘草 5 克共研细末，将药撒在裂口和周围皮肤上，用胶布固定，3-4 天可愈。

2. Treating Chapped Hands and Feet: Grind 10g of Chinese gallnut, 4g of

arnebia root (zicao), and 5g of licorice root (gancao) into a fine powder. Sprinkle the powder onto the cracks and the surrounding skin, secure it with medical tape, and it can be cured within 3-4 days.

3. 治疗瘢痕疙瘩：用五倍子、红花、蜈蚣、甘草配制成30%的复方五倍子浸剂，进行电导入法治疗瘢痕疙瘩有显著疗效。

3. Treating Keloids: Prepare a 30% compound Chinese gallnut infusion using Chinese gallnut, safflower (honghua), centipede (wugong), and licorice root. Using electro-transfer therapy to treat keloids yields significant therapeutic effects.

4. 治疗肛门病：用五倍子、白矾、白及、花椒共碾粗末，水煎后趁热熏洗，每日1剂洗2次，治疗外痔和肛裂，3-6天可愈。或用五倍子、蛇床子、紫草、土槿皮、白藓皮、石榴皮、黄柏、赤石脂、生甘草煎后熏洗，每日早晚各一次，治疗顽固性肛门湿疹。

4. Treating Anal Diseases: Coarsely grind Chinese gallnut, alum (baifan), bletilla tuber (baiji), and Sichuan pepper (huajiao) together. Decoct in water and use the hot steam to fumigate and wash the area while it is still hot. Use 1 dose daily, washing 2 times a day. External hemorrhoids and anal fissures can be cured within 3-6 days. Alternatively, decoct Chinese gallnut, cnidium fruit (shechuangzi), arnebia root (zicao), pseudolarix bark (tujinpi), dictamnus root bark (baixianpi), pomegranate peel (shiliupi), amur cork tree bark (huangbai), red halloysite (chishizhi), and raw licorice root (shengganscao) for fumigation and washing, once in the morning and once in the evening, to treat stubborn anal eczema.

5. 治疗传染性软疣：用五倍子、乌梅、枯矾、大黄各1份、雄黄2份共研细末，以香醋调成膏涂于软疣上，3日换一次，3-12日可愈。

5. Treating Molluscum Contagiosum: Grind 1 part each of Chinese gallnut, dark plum fruit (wumei), calcined alum (kufan), and rhubarb (dahuang), along with 2 parts of realgar (xionghuang), into a fine powder. Mix with fragrant vinegar to form a paste and apply it to the warts. Change the dressing every 3 days. It can

be cured within 3-12 days.

6. 治疗脓皮病：用五倍子、黄柏、诃子、青果、明矾水煎洗患处，每日 1 剂洗 3 次，5-7 天可愈。

6. Treating Pyoderma: Decoct Chinese gallnut, amur cork tree bark (huangbai), chebula fruit (hezi), Chinese olive fruit (qingguo), and alum (mingfan) in water, and wash the affected area. Use 1 dose daily, washing 3 times a day. It can be cured within 5-7 days.

7. 治疗毛囊炎：用五倍子粉、冰片，以蛋黄油调成膏，外涂于毛囊炎上，每日 1-2 次，至愈为止，2-4 天可愈。

7. Treating Folliculitis: Mix Chinese gallnut powder and borneol (bingpian) with egg yolk oil to form a paste. Apply externally to the folliculitis 1-2 times a day until cured. It can be cured within 2-4 days.

8. 治疗带状疱疹：用五倍子、生大黄、黄柏、芦硝共为细末，加凡士林配成 30% 软膏，敷患处固定，隔日换 1 次，平均 6 天可愈。

8. Treating Herpes Zoster: Grind Chinese gallnut, raw rhubarb (shengdahuang), amur cork tree bark (huangbai), and mirabilite (luniao) into a fine powder. Add petroleum jelly to prepare a 30% ointment. Apply and secure it to the affected area, changing the dressing every other day. On average, it can be cured within 6 days.

9. 治疗淋巴结核溃疡：取蜂蜜 250 克 ，以文火熬熟后加入等量五倍子末成糊状，晾干研末，以米醋调成膏，涂于患处，每日 1 次，1 月可愈。

9. Treating Scrofula Ulcers (Tuberculous Lymphadenitis Ulcers): Take 250g of honey, simmer it over low heat until fully cooked, and add an equal amount of Chinese gallnut powder to form a paste. Air-dry it, grind it into a powder, and mix with rice vinegar to form a paste. Apply to the affected area once a day. It can be cured within 1 month.

10. 治疗皮肤多汗症：用五倍子末 5 克，加水适量调成糊状敷脐，胶布固定，24 小时后取下，每周一次。

10. Treating Hyperhidrosis: Take 5g of Chinese gallnut powder, add an

appropriate amount of water to form a paste, apply it to the navel, and secure it with medical tape. Remove it after 24 hours. Apply once a week.

《中药科技报》1992 年 1 月 6 日

Chinese Medicine Science and Technology News, January 6, 1992

五、韭菜

5. Chinese Chives (Jiu-cai)

1. 小儿误吞玻璃碎片等异物：韭菜 250 克，切成 3-5 厘米小段，煮熟后嚼服。

1. Accidental Ingestion of Foreign Objects (e.g., Glass Fragments) in Children: Take 250g of Chinese chives, cut them into 3-5 cm segments, boil them, and chew and swallow.

2. 身体虚弱盗汗：韭菜根 30 克，加水 200 毫升，煎至 100 毫升，一次服完。

2. Weakness and Night Sweats: Take 30g of Chinese chive roots, add 200ml of water, and decoct until reduced to 100ml. Drink it all at once.

3. 鼻血、便血、尿血：韭菜根洗净捣烂取汁，每次服 10-20 毫升，开水冲服。

3. Epistaxis, Hematochezia, and Hematuria: Wash Chinese chive roots, mash them, and extract the juice. Take 10-20ml each time, mixed with boiling water.

4. 跌打肿痛：韭菜 250 克，生姜 100 克，葱白 50 克，共捣烂，加酒炒热后先烫后敷患处。

4. Swelling and Pain from Falls and Blows: Take 250g of Chinese chives, 100g of fresh ginger, and 50g of white part of green onions. Mash them together, stir-fry with wine until hot, and first scald, then apply to the affected area.

5. 妇女产后血晕、不省人事：韭菜一把，醋一大碗，将韭菜切碎后放入大茶壶中，另将醋煮沸后倒入茶壶内，将茶壶嘴对准患者鼻孔熏鼻。

5. Postpartum Dizziness due to Blood Loss and Unconsciousness in Women: Take a handful of Chinese chives and a large bowl of vinegar. Chop the chives and put them in a large teapot. Boil the vinegar and pour it into the teapot. Point the spout of the teapot at the patient’s nostrils to fumigate.

6. 妇女产后呕清水：韭菜 500 克，洗净捣烂取汁，加姜汁少许服。

6. Vomiting Clear Fluid Postpartum in Women: Take 500g of Chinese chives, wash them, mash them to extract the juice, and add a small amount of ginger juice before drinking.

《中医药信息报》1992 年 3 月 21 日（包心磊）

Chinese Medicine Information News, March 21, 1992 (Bao Xinlei)

7. 新生儿硬肿症：鲜韭菜 1000 克，柚树叶 20 克，加水 2500 毫升，煎煮取药液外洗，注意药液温度适宜为度，每日早中晚各洗 1 次，每次 10-15 分钟，一般 5-7 天可愈。

7. Neonatal Sclerema: Take 1000g of fresh Chinese chives and 20g of pomelo leaves, add 2500ml of water, and decoct to obtain a medicinal liquid for external washing. Ensure the temperature of the liquid is appropriate. Wash 3 times a day (morning, noon, and night) for 10-15 minutes each time. It generally takes 5-7 days to cure.

8. 小儿化脓性中耳炎：将鲜韭菜 250 克洗净捣烂，取汁，按 10 毫升药汁加 0.1 克冰片粉装入干净玻瓶中，每天 1 剂。用法：先用棉签拭净耳内脓液，继之用双氧水反复洗患耳 2-3 次，再用消毒棉签吸干耳内洗液，然后滴入上述药液 2-3 滴，每日 3 次，连治 1 周痊愈。

8. Purulent Otitis Media in Children: Wash 250g of fresh Chinese chives, mash them, and extract the juice. Add 0.1g of borneol powder to every 10ml of juice, and store in a clean glass bottle. Prepare 1 dose per day. Usage: First, use a cotton swab to wipe away the pus in the ear. Next, repeatedly wash the affected ear with hydrogen peroxide 2-3 times. Then, use a sterile cotton swab to absorb the remaining liquid. Finally, drop 2-3 drops of the prepared medicinal liquid into the ear 3 times a day. Continuous treatment for 1 week can cure the condition.

9. 内痔：将鲜韭菜 50 克，捣烂，加 2 克枯矾粉拌匀后用纱布卷成大拇指状的药栓，外涂花生油以作滑润，每晚解净大便，于临睡前轻轻塞入肛内放置，每日 1 次，连用 7-10 天而愈。

9. Internal Hemorrhoids: Mash 50g of fresh Chinese chives, add 2g of calcined

alum powder, and mix well. Roll the mixture into a thumb-sized suppository using gauze, and coat it with peanut oil for lubrication. After completely emptying the bowels every night, gently insert the suppository into the anus before going to bed. Apply once a day for 7-10 consecutive days to achieve a cure.

10. 心绞痛：以往有心绞痛患者，如果突感胸闷不舒，而当时又难以找到应急之西药，可马上将韭菜一大口，慢慢嚼碎并将药汁徐徐吞下，可起到缓解心绞痛的发生。如心绞痛正发作，可一边按上述口嚼韭菜，一边叫家人将一把韭菜捣烂榨取药汁 100 毫升，加上 1 克冰片（无冰片，加麝香粉 0.3 克更好）粉缓缓咽下，片刻可止痛。

10. Angina Pectoris: For patients with a history of angina, if they suddenly feel chest tightness and discomfort and cannot find emergency Western medicine, they can immediately take a large mouthful of Chinese chives, chew them slowly, and gradually swallow the juice to relieve the onset of angina. If an angina attack is occurring, while chewing the chives as mentioned above, ask a family member to mash a handful of chives to extract 100ml of juice, add 1g of borneol powder (or preferably 0.3g of musk powder if borneol is unavailable), and slowly swallow it. This can relieve the pain in a short while.

11. 催乳：每天用猪脚 1 只，按常规配料煮熟后，每 200 毫升汤加 20 毫升新鲜韭菜汁，一天 4-5 次连服 3 天而乳增。

11. Promoting Lactation: Boil 1 pig’s trotter daily with regular seasonings. After boiling, add 20ml of fresh Chinese chive juice to every 200ml of soup. Take this 4-5 times a day for 3 consecutive days to increase milk production.

12. 妇人倒经：（即每次经来鼻衄）鲜韭菜 500 克，捣烂后榨汁 200 毫升，分 2 次服用，每次加锅底黑灰（以烧柴草者）1 克，男童尿 50 毫升，早晚各服 1 次，连服 2-3 天收效。

12. Vicarious Menstruation (i.e., Epistaxis Occurring with Each Menstrual Cycle): Take 500g of fresh Chinese chives, mash them, and extract 200ml of juice. Divide it into 2 doses. For each dose, add 1g of black ash from the bottom of a pot (specifically from burning firewood or straw) and 50ml of urine from a young boy.

Take it once in the morning and once in the evening. Continuous use for 2-3 days will yield therapeutic effects.

13. 阳痿：取鲜韭菜 250 克，榨汁 100 毫升备用。生米 100 克，黑枣 100 克，加水 500 毫升左右煮为粥，韭汁及枣粥混匀后加适量白糖，均分 2 次服用，每日早晚各服 1 次，10 天为 1 疗程，一般轻者一疗程见效，重者 2 个疗程好转，3-4 个疗程可愈。

13. Impotence: Extract 100ml of juice from 250g of fresh Chinese chives and set aside. Boil 100g of raw rice and 100g of black dates in about 500ml of water to make a porridge. Mix the chive juice with the date porridge, add an appropriate amount of white sugar, and divide it into 2 equal portions. Take one portion in the morning and one in the evening. 10 days constitute one course of treatment. Generally, mild cases show effects after one course, severe cases improve after two courses, and 3-4 courses can achieve a cure.

《民族医药报》1998 年 1 月 23 日（龙锦烺）

Ethnic Medicine News, January 23, 1998 (Long Jinlang)

六、丹参

6. Salvia Root (Dan-shen)

1. 治肺痈（肺脓疡）：丹参、白茅根各 30 克，水煎分 2 次服，每日 1 剂。治肺痈 28 例，平均服几剂治愈。在治疗过程中未予任何药物合用，可见丹参抗炎、抑菌、消肿，促进吸收有良好作用。

1. Treating Pulmonary Abscess: Take 30g each of salvia root (danshen) and cogongrass rhizome (baimaogen), decoct in water, and divide into 2 doses. Take 1 dose daily. Twenty-eight cases of pulmonary abscess were treated, and on average, patients were cured after taking several doses. No other medications were used during the treatment, demonstrating that salvia root has good effects in anti-inflammation, bacteriostasis, reducing swelling, and promoting absorption.

2. 治慢性胃炎：每次服丹参粉 3-6 克（重症服 6 克）云南白药 1 克，于饭前半小时用温开水送服，日 2 次，治慢性胃炎 120 例，其中浅表性胃炎 88 例，用药 2 周后胃镜检查胃黏膜恢复正常相。萎缩性胃炎 32 例，用药 4 周后胃镜检查，其中 6 例胃黏膜恢复正常相，显效 23 例，无效 3 例。

2. Treating Chronic Gastritis: Take 3-6g of salvia root powder (6g for severe cases) and 1g of Yunnan Baiyao each time, swallowed with warm water half an hour before meals, twice a day. One hundred and twenty cases of chronic gastritis were treated. Among them, 88 cases of superficial gastritis showed normal gastric mucosa on gastroscopy after 2 weeks of medication. For 32 cases of atrophic gastritis, gastroscopy after 4 weeks of medication showed that 6 cases had normal gastric mucosa, 23 cases showed significant improvement, and 3 cases were ineffective.

3. 用于脾肿大治疗：丹参 600 克，土元 300 克（焙黄），共研成粉末，瓶装备用，每服 9 克，日 2 次。治脾肿大 11 例，药完经 B 超检查，脾脏恢复正常，症状消失。

3. Treating Splenomegaly: Take 600g of salvia root and 300g of ground beetle (tuyuan) (roasted yellow), and grind them together into a powder. Store in a bottle for later use. Take 9g each time, twice a day. Eleven cases of splenomegaly were treated. After finishing the medication, B-ultrasound examination showed that the spleen returned to normal and symptoms disappeared.

4. 治慢性肝炎（活动型和迁延型肝炎）：丹参 15 克，虎杖 20 克，柴胡 6 克，水煎分 2 次服，每日一剂。治疗慢性肝炎 100 余例，经 30 天后肝功能检查各项指数正常。

4. Treating Chronic Hepatitis (Active and Persistent Types): Take 15g of salvia root, 20g of giant knotweed rhizome (huzhang), and 6g of bupleurum root (chaihu). Decoct in water and divide into 2 doses. Take 1 dose daily. Over 100 cases of chronic hepatitis were treated. After 30 days, liver function tests showed that all indicators returned to normal.

5. 治高血压：丹参 15 克，菊花 30 克，水煎分 2 次服，每日 1 剂，治疗原发性高血压 56 例，药用 2 周，血压恢复正常。随访其中 20 例，半年内未见复发。

5. Treating Hypertension: Take 15g of salvia root and 30g of chrysanthemum flower (juhua). Decoct in water and divide into 2 doses. Take 1 dose daily. Fifty-six cases of primary hypertension were treated. After 2 weeks of medication, blood pressure returned to normal. Follow-up of 20 of these cases showed no recurrence within half a year.

6. 治疗紫癜性肾炎: 丹参 15 克，半枝莲 12 克水煎分 2 次服，每日 1 剂，治 8-12 岁儿童紫癜性肾炎 18 例，用药一周，症状消失，尿检正常。

6. Treating Purpuric Nephritis: Take 15g of salvia root and 12g of barbated skullcap herb (banzhilian). Decoct in water and divide into 2 doses. Take 1 dose daily. Eighteen cases of purpuric nephritis in children aged 8-12 were treated. After one week of medication, symptoms disappeared and urine tests returned to normal.

7. 治绝节育术后盆腔瘀血，小腹疼痛：丹参、泽兰、益母草各 15 克，用白酒微炒后，水煎分 2 次服，每日 1 剂。治疗 200 余例，药用 7-10 天即可治愈。

7. Treating Pelvic Blood Stasis and Lower Abdominal Pain Post-Sterilization: Take 15g each of salvia root, lycopus herb (zelan), and motherwort (yimucao). Slightly stir-fry them with white liquor (baijiu), then decoct in water and divide into 2 doses. Take 1 dose daily. Over 200 cases were treated, and they were cured after 7-10 days of medication.

8. 治疗月经痛：丹参 6 克，元胡 3 克，共研成粉末，一次服，日用药 2 次，用黄酒送服，连用 3 天，即可达到一次性治愈。

8. Treating Dysmenorrhea: Grind 6g of salvia root and 3g of corydalis tuber (yuanhu) into a powder. Take it all at once, twice a day, swallowed with yellow rice wine. Continuous use for 3 days can achieve a complete cure.

9. 治急性乳腺炎及疱疡肿毒： 取丹参鲜根及鲜蒲公英全草各等份，加陈醋少许，捣烂敷用，每日用药一次，炎症初期用药 1-3 次即可治愈。

9. Treating Acute Mastitis and Boils/Toxic Sores: Take equal amounts of fresh salvia root and fresh whole dandelion plant. Add a small amount of mature vinegar, mash them, and apply as a poultice. Apply once a day. Using it 1-3 times

in the early stage of inflammation can achieve a cure.

10. 治癣：丹参 30 克，加水 500 毫升文火煎煮，浓缩成 150 毫升，加少许防腐剂，瓶装备用。每次棉签蘸药液涂刷患处，日数次。一般用药 3-5 天见效。

10. Treating Tinea: Take 30g of salvia root, add 500ml of water, and simmer over low heat until concentrated to 150ml. Add a small amount of preservative and store in a bottle. Dip a cotton swab in the medicinal liquid and apply it to the affected area several times a day. It generally takes effect within 3-5 days of medication.

11. 治皮肤瘙痒症：取丹参 60 克，研末浸泡于 60° 白酒或 75% 的酒精 300 毫升，密封，两天后启用，涂擦痒处，每日用药数次。

11. Treating Pruritus (Skin Itching): Take 60g of salvia root, grind it into a powder, and soak it in 300ml of 60-degree white liquor or 75% alcohol. Seal the container. It can be used after two days. Rub it on the itchy areas, applying several times a day.

（青海 刘启明）

(Liu Qiming, Qinghai)

七、补骨脂

7. Psoralea Fruit (Bu-gu-zhi)

补骨脂又名破故纸、胡故子、胡韭子，为豆科植物补骨脂（Psoralea corglifolia L.）的干燥成熟果实。主要含有香豆精类补骨脂素和异补骨脂素、补骨脂乙素、补骨脂酚等成分，本品辛温苦燥，善助命门之火，为壮阳固精，温脾止泻的常用药，传统多用于脾肾阳虚，下元不固之遗精，遗尿，泄泻等症，近年来发展应用于治疗多种皮肤病，有较好效果，兹简介如下，以供参考：

Psoralea fruit, also known as Poguzhi, Huguzi, and Hujiuzi, is the dried mature fruit of the leguminous plant Psoralea corylifolia L. It mainly contains coumarin compounds such as psoralen and isopsoralen, as well as bakuchiol and bavachin. This herb is pungent, warm, bitter, and drying. It is good at assisting the fire of the "Mingmen" (Gate of Life) and is a commonly used medicine for strengthening yang, securing essence, warming the spleen, and stopping diarrhea. Traditionally, it is mostly used for conditions such as seminal emission, enuresis, and diarrhea caused by spleen and kidney yang deficiency and instability of the lower primordial qi. In recent years, it has been increasingly applied to treat various skin diseases with good results. A brief introduction is provided below for reference:

1. 银屑病 可用100%的补骨脂注射液肌注，每天1次，每次4ml。或内服异构补骨脂素，每公斤0.5毫克，同时加黑光照射，其疗效都已被临床肯定。一般认为，银屑病的病理生理特点，是表皮细胞代谢加快，丝状分裂活跃，皮损处表皮细胞过度增生和合成脱氧核糖核酸细胞量增加，已有实验表明，补骨脂素可以影响脱氧核糖核酸的变化，减缓细胞的丝状分裂，并对某些酶的信使脱氧核糖核酸密码的合成及对银屑病表皮细胞的过度增殖，具有明显的抑制作用，从而使皮肤恢复正常。

1. Psoriasis: A 100% psoralea fruit injection can be administered intramuscularly once a day, 4ml each time. Alternatively, oral isopsoralen at a dosage of 0.5mg per kilogram of body weight can be taken, combined with black light irradiation. The therapeutic effects of both methods have been clinically confirmed. Generally, the pathophysiological characteristics of psoriasis include accelerated epidermal cell metabolism, active mitosis, excessive proliferation of epidermal cells in skin lesions, and increased synthesis of deoxyribonucleic acid (DNA). Experiments have shown that psoralen can affect DNA changes, slow down mitosis, and significantly inhibit the synthesis of messenger DNA codes for certain enzymes and the excessive proliferation of psoriatic epidermal cells, thereby restoring the skin to normal.

2. 白癜风 可用100%的补骨脂注射液肌注，同时用紫外线照射，金洪慈等报道用乌梅、补骨脂、毛姜制成消斑酊外用，治疗本病取得较好疗效。补骨脂能够提高皮肤对紫外线的敏感性，紫外线能通过增加酪氨酸酶的活性而刺激黑色素细胞形成较多的黑色素，近年来国外一些临床资料认为本病常和某些自体免疫疾病并存，实验也表明，本药可调整机体的免疫系统，对增高的各型免疫球蛋白有降低的倾向。

2. Vitiligo: A 100% psoralea fruit injection can be administered intramuscularly, combined with ultraviolet (UV) irradiation. Jin Hongci et al. reported that applying a topical depigmentation tincture made of dark plum fruit, psoralea fruit, and hairy ginger achieved good therapeutic effects for this disease. Psoralea fruit can increase the skin' s sensitivity to UV rays. UV irradiation can stimulate melanocytes to produce more melanin by increasing the activity of tyrosinase. In recent years, some foreign clinical data suggest that this disease often coexists with certain autoimmune diseases. Experiments have also shown that this herb can regulate the body' s immune system and tends to reduce elevated levels of various types of immunoglobulins.

3. 外阴白斑 取补骨脂与等量的 95% 酒精浸泡 1 周，将浸出液在文火中煮沸浓缩成膏，于患部均匀涂以浸膏，隔日 1 次，有效，现在多认为外阴白斑是外阴营养障碍所致，有资料报道，补骨脂乙素有扩张动脉血管作用，因此能改善局部组织的营养状况，故其疗效机理可能与此有关。

3. Vulvar Leukoplakia: Soak psoralea fruit in an equal amount of 95% alcohol for one week. Boil and concentrate the extract over low heat into a paste. Apply the paste evenly to the affected area every other day, which is effective. Currently, vulvar leukoplakia is mostly considered to be caused by vulvar nutritional disorders. Reports indicate that bavachin has the effect of dilating arterial blood vessels, thereby improving the nutritional status of local tissues. Therefore, its therapeutic mechanism may be related to this.

4. 斑秃 可用 0.5% 的补骨脂素霜，配合照光，同时口服 8- 甲氧基补骨脂素，疗效确切，肖洪义介绍以补骨脂、旱莲草各 25 克，加 25% 酒精 200 毫升浸泡外搽，同时内服茯苓粉，可在 2 个月内治愈本病。

4. Alopecia Areata: A 0.5% psoralen cream can be used in combination with light therapy, along with oral 8-methoxypsoralen, which yields definite therapeutic effects. Xiao Hongyi introduced a method using 25g each of psoralea

fruit and eclipta herb, soaked in 200ml of 25% alcohol for external application, combined with oral poria cocos powder, which can cure the disease within two months.

5. 汗斑 用补骨脂的酒精浸泡液外搽，一般均可治愈。

5. Tinea Versicolor (Pityriasis Versicolor): External application of the alcohol extract of psoralea fruit can generally cure this condition.

6. 鸡眼 用补骨脂酊 0.2 毫升直接垂直注入鸡眼中心，一次即可取得明显效果，这可能与本药含有的多种香豆精类物质有关，实验表明，补骨脂挥发油和补骨脂乙素对实验性肉瘤有抑制作用。

6. Corns: Directly and vertically inject 0.2ml of psoralea fruit tincture into the center of the corn. Significant effects can be achieved in a single application. This may be related to the various coumarin compounds contained in this herb. Experiments have shown that the volatile oil of psoralea fruit and bavachin have inhibitory effects on experimental sarcomas.

7. 慢性湿疹 可用 10% 的补骨脂馏油酊每日外搽患部 3-4 次，对手、耳、肛周、外耳道、阴囊或全身多发性湿疹皆有效。

7. Chronic Eczema: A 10% psoralea fruit distilled oil tincture can be applied externally to the affected area 3-4 times a day. It is effective for eczema on the hands, ears, perianal area, external auditory canal, scrotum, or multiple systemic eczema.

8. 指、趾甲癣 用补骨脂配合等量菟丝子制成注射液，肌注，每日 1 次 5 毫升，可连续数月而奏效。

8. Onychomycosis (Nail Fungus): Prepare an injection using psoralea fruit combined with an equal amount of dodder seed (tusizi) for intramuscular injection, 5ml once a day. Continuous use for several months can yield therapeutic effects.

9. 黄褐斑 杨烈彪介绍取鲜杏花、鲜桃花、鲜梨花、鲜柿叶各 90 克晒干后，与补骨脂 30 克共研细末，每晚临睡前取药末适量，加香油调糊涂于面部患处，次日早晨洗去，每晚 1 次，连用 6 周，必须晚上用药，如白天用药反而会增加色素沉着，经临床应用统计，有效率可达 89%，也可以药末调入雪花膏中应用，惟疗效稍差于香油调涂。

9. Melasma (Chloasma): Yang Liebiao introduced a method of taking 90g each of fresh apricot blossoms, peach blossoms, pear blossoms, and persimmon leaves, drying them, and grinding them into a fine powder together with 30g of psoralea fruit. Before going to bed every night, take an appropriate amount of the powder, mix it with sesame oil into a paste, and apply it to the affected facial areas. Wash it off the next morning. Apply once a night for 6 consecutive weeks. The medication must be applied at night; applying it during the day will instead increase pigmentation. Clinical application statistics show an effective rate of up to 89%. The powder can also be mixed into cold cream for application, although its therapeutic effect is slightly inferior to mixing it with sesame oil.

《中医药信息报》1990 年 7 月 28 日（南京 徐兆山）

Chinese Medicine Information News, July 28, 1990 (Xu Zhaoshan, Nanjing)

八、凤尾草

8. Phoenix Tail Fern (Feng-wei-cao)

1. 治疗急性菌痢

鲜凤尾草 60 克、蜂蜜 50 克。煎 2 次合并药液分 3 次冲蜂蜜服；或用凤尾草 30 克、红花地桃花根 30 克，水煎，合并药液分 2 次服。

Treating Acute Bacillary Dysentery: Take 60g of fresh phoenix tail fern and 50g of honey. Decoct twice, combine the liquid, and divide it into 3 doses to be mixed with honey. Alternatively, take 30g of phoenix tail fern and 30g of red-flowered ground peach root (honghuaditaohua gen), decoct in water, combine the liquid, and divide it into 2 doses.

2. 治疗胃肠炎

鲜凤尾草 60 克、鲜瓜子菜 60 克，水煎液合并分 2 次服。若有呕吐、腹胀、不发热之症，加莱菔子 10 克、伏龙肝 30 克，同煎，合并药液分 2 次服。

2. Treating Gastroenteritis: Take 60g of fresh phoenix tail fern and 60g of fresh purslane (guazicai), decoct in water, combine the liquid, and divide it into 2 doses. If there are symptoms of vomiting, abdominal distension, and no fever, add 10g of radish seed (laifuzi) and 30g of 灶心土 (fulonggan, earth from the center of a traditional stove), decoct them together, combine the liquid, and divide it into 2 doses.

3. 治疗上感

凤尾草 30 克、一箭球 15 克、枇杷叶 15 克、甘草 10 克水煎服。

3. Treating Upper Respiratory Tract Infections: Take 30g of phoenix tail fern, 15g of yijianqiu (a local herb), 15g of loquat leaf (pipaye), and 10g of licorice root (gancao), and decoct in water to drink.

4. 治疗尿路感染及尿路结石

凤尾草 40 克、金钱草 30 克、粪箕足 30 克、水煎服，若尿路结石位置较上的加入鸡内金 15 克、穿破石 30 克、海金沙藤 30 克，水煎服。

4. Treating Urinary Tract Infections and Urinary Stones: Take 40g of phoenix tail fern, 30g of golden coin grass (jinqiancao), and 30g of ant nest fern (fenjizu), and decoct in water to drink. If the urinary stones are located higher up, add 15g of chicken gizzard lining (jineijin), 30g of chuanposhi (a local herb), and 30g of sea gold fern (haijinsha teng), and decoct in water to drink.

5. 治疗急性咽喉炎、急性扁桃体炎

凤尾草 30 克、一点红 30 克、红花地桃花根 20 克、甘草 10 克，清水煎服，5-7 天一个疗程。

5. Treating Acute Pharyngitis and Acute Tonsillitis: Take 30g of phoenix tail fern, 30g of red flower (yidianhong), 20g of red-flowered ground peach root, and 10g of licorice root. Decoct in clean water to drink. 5-7 days constitute one course of treatment.

6. 治疗急性结膜炎（红眼病）

凤尾草 35 克、犁头草 30 克、半边钱 10 克，水煎，待冷后洗患眼或外敷，一般 3 天可愈。

6. Treating Acute Conjunctivitis (Pink Eye): Take 35g of phoenix tail fern, 30g of 犁头草 (litoucao, a local herb), and 10g of banbianqian (a local herb). Decoct in water, let it cool, and use it to wash the affected eye or apply it externally. It generally takes 3 days to cure.

7. 治疗妇女湿热带下

凤尾草 40 克、鸭脚艾 15 克、一点红 20 克、益母草 10 克、甘草 10 克，每日一剂，清水煎服。阴痒者可去甘草加苦参 30 克、蛇床子 30 克，收集药液，薰洗外阴瘙痒部。

7. Treating Leukorrhea due to Damp-Heat in Women: Take 40g of phoenix tail fern, 15g of yaofeiai (a local herb), 20g of red flower (yidianhong), 10g of motherwort (yimucao), and 10g of licorice root. Take 1 dose daily, decocted in clean water. For patients with vulvar itching, remove the licorice root and add 30g of sophora root (kushen) and 30g of cnidium fruit (shechuangzi). Collect the medicinal liquid to fumigate and wash the itchy vulvar area.

8. 治疗子宫功能性出血：

凤尾草 30 克、红丝线 25 克、海螵蛸 20 克、生地 15 克、煅龙骨 20 克、煅牡蛎 20 克，红枣 10 枚、龙骨牡蛎先煎，再同煎，收液内服，5 天一疗程。

8. Treating Dysfunctional Uterine Bleeding: Take 30g of phoenix tail fern, 25g of red silk thread (hongsixian, a local herb), 20g of cuttlebone (haipiaoxiao), 15g of raw rehmannia root (shengdi), 20g of calcined dragon bone (duanlonggu), 20g of calcined oyster shell (duanmuli), and 10 red dates. Decoct the dragon bone and oyster shell first, then add the remaining ingredients to decoct together. Collect the liquid for oral intake. 5 days constitute one course of treatment.

9. 外伤出血

鲜凤尾草叶冲烂，敷患处可以止血。跌打肿痛，皮下瘀血，用鲜凤尾草、大驳骨叶、红花、归尾、三七、牛膝同冲烂，三花酒同炒热外敷患处，能消肿祛瘀止痛而愈。

9. Traumatic Bleeding: Mash fresh phoenix tail fern leaves and apply them to the affected area to stop bleeding. For swelling and pain from falls and blows, as

well as subcutaneous blood stasis, mash fresh phoenix tail fern, dabo gu leaves (a local herb), safflower (honghua), angelica root tail (guiwei), notoginseng (sanqi), and achyranthes root (niuxi) together. Stir-fry them with Sanhua liquor (a local rice wine) until hot, and apply externally to the affected area. This can reduce swelling, dissipate blood stasis, relieve pain, and achieve a cure.

10. 治流感并高热

凤尾草 30 克、金银花 10 克、地胆头 30 克、甘草 10 克，水煎服。

10. Treating Influenza with High Fever: Take 30g of phoenix tail fern, 10g of honeysuckle flower (jinyinhua), 30g of elephantopus root (didantou), and 10g of licorice root. Decoct in water to drink.

（湖南 彭平建）

(Peng Pingjian, Hunan)

九、黑豆

9. Black Soybean (Hei-dou)

1. 感冒：黑豆 20 克，葱白 10 根煮汁服。可治时令感冒。

1.Common Cold: Boil 20g of black soybeans and 10 white parts of green onions to make a decoction and drink it. It can treat seasonal colds.

2. 头痛：黑豆 16 克，半生半炒，共为末，分 2 次服。淡茶水送下，有效。

2. Headache: Take 16g of black soybeans, half raw and half roasted, grind them into a powder, and divide it into 2 doses. Swallow with light tea, which is effective.

3. 咳嗽：将黄牛胆装满生黑豆，扎严，挂屋檐下，干后每服 7 粒，日 2 次，温水送服。对新久咳嗽均有效。

3. Cough: Fill a yellow cattle gallbladder with raw black soybeans, tie it tightly, and hang it under the eaves. After it dries, take 7 beans each time, twice a day, swallowed with warm water. It is effective for both new and chronic coughs.

4. 哮喘：黑豆 50 克，加水 540 毫升，煎至 360 毫升时，加少量白糖再煎片刻。将其代茶常饮。能预防哮喘发作。

4. Asthma: Take 50g of black soybeans, add 540ml of water, and decoct until reduced to 360ml. Add a small amount of white sugar and decoct for a while. Drink it regularly as a substitute for tea. It can prevent asthma attacks.

5. 气喘：黑豆 20 克，加水 500 毫升，煎至半量，每日分 3 次服，十分有效。

5. Panting: Take 20g of black soybeans, add 500ml of water, and decoct until reduced by half. Divide into 3 doses daily. It is highly effective.

6. 痰喘：梨 1 个，剜空（留盖）装满黑豆扣盖，系住，炭火煨熟，捣做饼每日食之，效果佳。

6. Panting with Phlegm: Hollow out 1 pear (keep the top as a lid), fill it with black soybeans, cover it, and tie it. Simmer it over charcoal fire until cooked, mash it into a cake, and eat it daily. It has excellent effects.

7. 脑出血、脑软化症：取黑豆和海带各等量混合，蒸熟随时服。能强化血管，祛除风邪预防脑出血和脑软化症。

7. Cerebral Hemorrhage and Cerebral Softening: Mix equal amounts of black soybeans and kelp, steam them until cooked, and eat at any time. It can strengthen blood vessels, dispel wind pathogens, and prevent cerebral hemorrhage and cerebral softening.

8. 腹痛：黑豆 50 克，加 1 玻璃杯水，煎至半杯后饮服，即可见效。

8. Abdominal Pain: Take 50g of black soybeans, add 1glass of water, and decoct until reduced to half a glass. Drink it for immediate effects.

9. 水肿：黑豆 100 克，用水煮熟，加入 50 克黄酒煮沸即可。食豆饮汁。

9. Edema: Boil 100g of black soybeans in water until cooked, add 50g of yellow rice wine, and bring to a boil. Eat the beans and drink the broth.

10. 中风不语：黑豆适量煮汁，煎稠如饴，口含片刻再咽下，频服便愈。

10. Aphasia after Stroke: Boil an appropriate amount of black soybeans to make a juice, and simmer until thick like syrup. Hold it in the mouth for a moment before swallowing. Frequent intake will cure the condition.

11. 补脾养肾：黑豆、红枣各适量，先将黑豆放锅内炒出香味，凉后磨成细粉。再将红枣洗净，蒸熟去核，同黑豆共捣烂，捏成丸。每服 15 克，淡盐水或黄酒送服，常服必效。

11. Nourishing the Spleen and Kidneys: Take appropriate amounts of black soybeans and red dates. First, stir-fry the black soybeans in a pan until fragrant, let them cool, and grind them into a fine powder. Then, wash the red dates, steam them until cooked, remove the pits, and mash them together with the black soybean powder. Shape the mixture into pills. Take 15g each time, swallowed with light salt water or yellow rice wine. Regular intake is bound to be effective.

12. 赤白痢：将猪胆囊装满黑豆，在房檐的荫凉处阴干，研末。饭前 30 分钟用姜水服 5 克，日 3 次，获效。

12. Dysentery with Blood and Mucus: Fill a pig gallbladder with black soybeans, air-dry them in a shady place under the eaves, and grind them into a powder. Take 5g with ginger water 30 minutes before meals, 3 times a day, to achieve therapeutic effects.

13. 吐血：将黑豆汤用文火长时间煮稠后饮之即止。

13. Hematemesis (Vomiting Blood): Simmer black soybean soup over low heat for a long time until thick, and drink it to stop the bleeding.

14. 糖尿病：在牛胆囊内装满炒黑豆，阴干研末，日 3 次，饭后服 3 克，疗效佳。

14. Diabetes: Fill a cattle gallbladder with roasted black soybeans, air-dry them, and grind into a powder. Take 3g after meals, 3 times a day, for excellent therapeutic effects.

15. 产后风：黑豆 50 克放锅内炒极焦，冲入热黄酒 100 克，内服立效。

15. Postpartum Wind: Stir-fry 50g of black soybeans in a pan until scorched, pour in 100g of hot yellow rice wine, and take it orally for immediate effects.

16. 月经不调：将黑豆用黄酒煮熟，空腹服 1 匙见效。

16. Irregular Menstruation: Boil black soybeans in yellow rice wine until cooked, and take 1 spoonful on an empty stomach for immediate effects.

17. 产后小腹痛：将黑豆烧焦，研细末，每次用热酒服 10 克，每日 3 次，见效。

17. Postpartum Lower Abdominal Pain: Burn black soybeans until scorched, grind them into a fine powder, and take 10g with hot wine each time, 3 times a day, for effective relief.

18. 妊娠胎动腰痛：取黑豆 100 克用水煮熟用 100 毫升黄酒送服、见效。

18. Fetal Restlessness and Backache during Pregnancy: Boil 100g of black soybeans in water until cooked, and swallow with 100ml of yellow rice wine for effective relief.

19. 虚火牙痛：黑豆、黄酒各适量，共煮，稍烂取其汁漱口多次则止痛。

19. Toothache due to Deficiency-Fire: Take appropriate amounts of black soybeans and yellow rice wine, and boil them together. When slightly softened, take the juice and rinse the mouth multiple times to relieve the pain.

《中药科技报》1993 年 2 月 4 日

Chinese Medicine Science and Technology News, February 4, 1993

黑豆又名乌豆、黑大豆、稆豆。种子和种皮入药。黑豆种子味甘涩，性平。入肝、肾经。有滋阴补血，益肝明目，壮腰健肾之功效。《本草纲目》有云："黑豆者名乌豆，可入药及充食作豉"，"为肾之谷，入肾功多，故能治水消胀下气，制风热而活血解毒"。下面将其食疗用途介绍如下，供大家选用。

Black soybean, also known as Wudou, Heidadou, and Lüdou. Both the seeds and seed coats are used as medicine. Black soybean seeds are sweet and astringent in flavor, and neutral in property. They enter the Liver and Kidney meridians. They have the effects of nourishing Yin and tonifying blood, benefiting the liver and improving vision, and strengthening the waist and kidneys. The Compendium of Materia Medica states: "Black soybean, named Wudou, can be used as medicine and as a food substitute to make fermented beans." "It is the grain of the Kidney, with strong effects on the Kidney, thus it can treat water retention, relieve distension, descend qi, control wind-heat, promote blood circulation, and detoxify." Its dietary therapy uses are introduced below for reference.

20. 治风湿性关节痛：用炒香的黑豆 100 克，生姜 120 克，南蛇皮 120 克，加水 1500 毫升，煮至南蛇皮烂熟即可食用。每日一付，分二次服。

20. Treating Rheumatic Joint Pain: Take 100g of fragrant roasted black soybeans, 120g of fresh ginger, and 120g of nan-she-pi (a local herb). Add 1500ml of water and boil until the nan-she-pi is completely soft. Consume it. Take 1 dose daily, divided into 2 servings.

21. 治妊娠腹痛：用黑豆 100 克，米酒 60 克，置砂锅中，加水慢火煮透吃。日一剂，分二次吃。

21. Treating Abdominal Pain during Pregnancy: Take 100g of black soybeans and 60g of rice wine, place them in a clay pot, add water, and simmer over low heat until thoroughly cooked. Take 1 dose daily, divided into 2 servings.

22. 治肾虚腰痛：取黑豆 60 克，陈皮 3 克，小茴香 3 克，生姜 10 克，猪腰一对，炖烂调味吃，每日一付，分数次吃。

22. Treating Backache due to Kidney Deficiency: Take 60g of black soybeans, 3g of dried tangerine peel (chenpi), 3g of fennel seed (xiaohuixiang), 10g of fresh ginger, and 1 pair of pig kidneys. Stew until tender, season, and eat. Take 1 dose daily, divided into several servings.

23. 治小儿遗尿症：用黑豆 30 克，狗肉 150 克，慢火炖至肉烂，加盐、葱和酒等，当菜吃。

23. Treating Childhood Enuresis: Take 30g of black soybeans and 150g of dog meat. Stew over low heat until the meat is tender, add salt, green onions, and wine, and eat it as a dish.

24. 治老年性耳聋或肾虚耳鸣：用黑豆 60 克，枸杞子 20 克，炒杜仲 10 克，狗肉 300 克，炖烂调味吃。日一付，分数次吃。

24. Treating Senile Deafness or Tinnitus due to Kidney Deficiency: Take 60g of black soybeans, 20g of wolfberry fruit (gouqizi), 10g of roasted eucommia bark (duzhong), and 300g of dog meat. Stew until tender, season, and eat. Take 1 dose daily, divided into several servings.

25. 治脂溢性脱发或产后脱发：用黑豆 500 克，水 1000 毫升，文火熬煮，然后取出晾干，撒少许食盐，贮于瓷瓶内，饭后服，每次 6 克，日服二次。

25. Treating Seborrheic Alopecia or Postpartum Hair Loss: Take 500g of black

soybeans and 1000ml of water. Simmer over low heat, then take them out and air-dry. Sprinkle a little salt, store in a porcelain jar, and take 6g after meals, twice a day.

26. 治阴虚盗汗：用黑豆 100 克，浮小麦 30 克，黄芪 20 克，水煎服。日一剂，分两次服。

26. Treating Night Sweats due to Yin Deficiency: Take 100g of black soybeans, 30g of floating wheat (fuxiaomai), and 20g of astragalus root (huangqi). Decoct in water to drink. Take 1 dose daily, divided into 2 servings.

27. 治酒醉：用黑豆 100 克，水煎后加适量白糖，代茶饮。

27. Treating Alcohol Intoxication: Take 100g of black soybeans, decoct in water, add an appropriate amount of white sugar, and drink as a substitute for tea.

《民族医药报》1992 年 5 月 26 日（广西 朱恩）

Ethnic Medicine News, May 26, 1992 (Zhu En, Guangxi)

28. 黑豆富含蛋白质，其含量高于肉类、蛋品和牛奶，素有食物蛋白之王的称号，而且有广泛的药用价值：

28. Black soybeans are rich in protein, with a content higher than that of meat, eggs, and milk. They are known as the "King of Food Proteins" and have extensive medicinal value:

①抗衰老：《养老书》记载："李守愚每晨水吞黑豆二十七粒，谓五脏谷，到老不衰。"近代研究发现好几种微量元素的缺乏，是导致衰老的重要原因。黑豆含多种微量元素，中年以上的人常吃可防老。

① Anti-aging: The book Yanglao Shu records: "Li Shouyu swallowed 27 black soybeans with water every morning, calling them the grain of the five viscera, remaining vigorous into old age." Modern research has found that the deficiency of several trace elements is an important cause of aging. Black soybeans contain various trace elements, and regular consumption by middle-aged and elderly people can prevent aging.

②治贫血：黑豆含铁质，不仅量多，并且易被人体吸收利用。用黑豆 250-300 克同塘角鱼煲食疗效显著。民间用黑豆 200 克，旱莲草 30 克，塘角鱼适量煎食，是治阴虚出鼻血的验方。

② Treating Anemia: Black soybeans contain iron, which is not only abundant but also easily absorbed and utilized by the body. Stewing 250-300g of black soybeans with Clarias fuscus (tangjiaoyu, a type of catfish) has significant therapeutic effects. A folk remedy using 200g of black soybeans, 30g of eclipta herb (hanliancao), and an appropriate amount of Clarias fuscus is a proven prescription for treating epistaxis (nosebleeds) due to Yin deficiency.

③治白发：民间取黑豆、黑芝麻、黑枣、首乌各 50-100 克同猪瘦肉煲食，可以乌须黑发；若同猪或牛脑（去网膜有效）煲食，治肾虚头晕、妇女血虚眩晕。

③ Treating Premature Graying Hair: Folk remedies use 50-100g each of black soybeans, black sesame seeds, black dates, and fleece-flower root (shouwu), stewed with lean pork to darken hair and beard. If stewed with pig or cow brain (removing the omentum is effective), it treats dizziness due to kidney deficiency and vertigo due to blood deficiency in women.

④治腰痛；民间取黑豆 250 克（炒微爆）、怀牛膝 5 克，杜仲 15 克，与猪肾（腰子）煲食，治肾亏腰痛有良效。

④ Treating Backache: Folk remedies use 250g of black soybeans (roasted until slightly popped), 5g of achyranthes root (huainiuxi), and 15g of eucommia bark (duzhong), stewed with pig kidneys, which has good effects on backache due to kidney deficiency.

⑤治烫伤：《本草纲目》载，用黑豆煮汁饮，可治烫伤。不但能促使创伤面愈合，而且愈合后不留瘢痕。一般用黑豆 250 克，加水煎煮成浓汁，取豆食用，以汁涂伤处，日数次。

⑤ Treating Scalds and Burns: The Compendium of Materia Medica records that drinking black soybean decoction can treat scalds and burns. It not only promotes wound healing but also prevents scarring. Generally, 250g of black soybeans are boiled in water to make a thick decoction. Eat the beans and apply the juice to the wound several times a day.

⑥美容减肥：《延年秘录》云：“服食黑豆，令人长肌肤，益色。”黑豆含有丰富蛋白质和有色脂肪酸、胡萝卜素和维生素 A，以及某些微量元素等，

不仅是皮肤营养的必需之品，还可以减肥，降低血中胆固醇。目前在日本流行的醋豆减肥健美法，即以黑豆为主。在黑豆防美容方中，最佳为黑豆焖猪皮。

⑥ Beauty and Weight Loss: Yannian Milu states: "Consuming black soybeans makes the skin grow and improves complexion." Black soybeans are rich in protein, colored fatty acids, carotene, vitamin A, and certain trace elements. They are not only essential for skin nutrition but can also aid in weight loss and lower blood cholesterol. The vinegar bean diet popular in Japan for weight loss and fitness mainly uses black soybeans. Among black soybean beauty recipes, stewed black soybeans with pig skin are the best.

《民族医药报》1993 年 2 月 26 日（广西 梁庆森）

Ethnic Medicine News, February 26, 1993 (Liang Qingsen, Guangxi)

十、生姜

10. Fresh Ginger (Sheng-jiang)

外用：

External Use:

1. 冻疮：生姜、辣椒、白萝卜各适量，水煎熏洗患处，每日 1-2 次；生姜 60 克，捣烂，加入白酒 100 毫升，浸泡 3 天后，每天 3 次外搽易生冻疮处，冬天可免受冻疮之苦。

Chilblains: Take appropriate amounts of fresh ginger, chili, and white radish, decoct in water, and fumigate and wash the affected area 1-2 times a day. Alternatively, mash 60g of fresh ginger, add 100ml of liquor (baijiu), and soak for 3 days. Apply the mixture externally to areas prone to chilblains 3 times a day to prevent chilblains in winter.

2. 食物中毒：生姜适量，捣烂取汁，加少许温开水滴鼻，每次 2-3 滴，每天 2-3 次。此方还可解生半夏、生南星、生野芋中毒。

2. Food Poisoning: Take an appropriate amount of fresh ginger, mash it to extract the juice, add a small amount of warm boiled water, and instill it into the

nose, 2-3 drops each time, 2-3 times a day. This prescription can also detoxify poisoning from raw Pinellia ternata (Banxia), raw Arisaema (Nanxing), and raw wild taro (Yeyu).

3. 尿闭：生姜 30 克，豆豉 9 克，食盐 6 克，连须葱一棵，捣烂如泥外敷肚脐处。

3. Urinary Retention: Take 30g of fresh ginger, 9g of fermented soybeans (douchi), 6g of salt, and 1green onion with its roots intact. Mash them into a mud-like consistency and apply externally to the navel.

4. 外伤出血：生姜烧焦研末伤口局部消毒后，撒于患处，外敷纱布包扎，可止血止痛。

4. Traumatic Bleeding: Burn fresh ginger until charred and grind it into a powder. After local disinfection of the wound, sprinkle the powder on the affected area, apply gauze, and bandage it to stop bleeding and relieve pain.

5. 烧烫伤：生姜捣烂取汁，用药棉沾姜汁搽患处，可即止痛；若起泡，能消炎除泡，泡破者，可促其结痂。

5. Scalds and Burns: Mash fresh ginger to extract the juice, soak a cotton swab in the juice, and apply it to the affected area for immediate pain relief. If blisters form, it can reduce inflammation and remove blisters; for ruptured blisters, it can promote scabbing.

6. 溃疡久不收口：生姜汁拌干姜粉外敷患处，连续一周。

6. Chronic Non-healing Ulcers: Mix fresh ginger juice with dried ginger powder and apply externally to the affected area continuously for one week.

7. 小儿腹痛：生姜一块，放在文火中烧至皮焦，去皮趁热外敷肚脐。

7. Abdominal Pain in Children: Take a piece of fresh ginger, roast it over low heat until the skin is charred, peel it, and apply it hot to the navel.

8. 晕动症：外出旅游或出差须坐车、船时，可随身携带生姜几片。并贴于太阳穴或肚脐等处，可防止晕车、晕船。

8. Motion Sickness: When traveling or going on business trips by car or boat, carry a few slices of fresh ginger. Apply them to the temples or navel to prevent

motion sickness.

9. 感冒发热：可用 100 毫升白酒放于土碗中，于火上加热，然后用切成片的生姜拌酒涂搽全身，有降温发汗之功用。

9. Cold with Fever: Pour 100ml of liquor (baijiu) into an earthenware bowl and heat it over a fire. Then, mix sliced fresh ginger with the warm liquor and rub it all over the body. This has the effect of reducing fever and inducing sweating.

注意事项：1、本品辛温，故阴虚内热，平素脾胃积热者不宜久服；痔疮、肛裂、便血者忌服。2、烂姜不可用。因烂姜含有黄梓素，可使肝细胞变性、坏死，从而诱发肝癌、食道癌。

Precautions: 1. This herb is pungent and warm; therefore, it should not be taken for a long time by those with Yin deficiency and internal heat, or those with chronic accumulation of heat in the spleen and stomach. It is contraindicated for patients with hemorrhoids, anal fissures, and bloody stools. 2. Rotten ginger must not be used. Rotten ginger contains safrole, which can cause degeneration and necrosis of liver cells, thereby inducing liver cancer and esophageal cancer.

《民族医药报》1992 年 5 月 13 日（云南 董寿琪）

Ethnic Medicine News, May 13, 1992 (Dong Shouqi, Yunnan)

十一、吴茱萸

11. Evodia Fruit (Wu-zhu-yu)

1. 治小儿腮腺炎：吴茱萸 20 克，大黄、黄连各 10 克，胆南星 6 克共研末，以温开水调成糊状，敷涌泉穴。每 4 小时敷换一次药。

1. Treating Pediatric Mumps: Take 20g of evodia fruit, 10g each of rhubarb (dahuang) and coptis root (huanglian), and 6g of Arisaema bile (dannanxing). Grind them into a powder, mix with warm boiled water into a paste, and apply to the Yongquan acupoint. Change the dressing every 4 hours.

2. 治小儿痰鸣、呕吐：吴茱萸研末用醋调糊状，敷涌泉穴，每 6 小时换药一次。

2. Treating Pediatric Phlegm Rattling and Vomiting: Grind evodia fruit into

a powder, mix with vinegar into a paste, and apply to the Yongquan acupoint. Change the dressing every 6 hours.

3. 治腹部气胀：吴茱萸、莱菔子炒盐，纱布包裹，热敷腹部。

3. Treating Abdominal Flatulence: Stir-fry evodia fruit and radish seeds (laifuzi) with salt, wrap them in gauze, and apply as a hot compress to the abdomen.

4. 治痛经：四肢不温，按压喜暖。吴茱萸 10 克，小茴香 10 克，肉桂 5 克研末，用酒炒热，纱布包裹，敷于脐部。

4. Treating Dysmenorrhea: For patients with cold extremities who prefer warmth upon pressure. Take 10g of evodia fruit, 10g of fennel seeds (xiaohuixiang), and 5g of cinnamon bark (rougui), grind into a powder, stir-fry with liquor until hot, wrap in gauze, and apply to the navel.

5. 治口腔溃疡：小儿口舌生疮致口角流涎。吴茱萸研末，用酒、醋或蜜调糊状贴两足心。

5. Treating Oral Ulcers: For children with mouth and tongue sores causing drooling. Grind evodia fruit into a powder, mix with liquor, vinegar, or honey into a paste, and apply to the soles of both feet.

6. 治风热牙痛：吴茱萸、白芷等分，浸水频漱吐延。

6. Treating Wind-Heat Toothache: Take equal amounts of evodia fruit and angelica root (baizhi), soak in water, and frequently rinse the mouth and spit out the liquid.

7. 治高血压：吴茱萸研末，每次取药末 20 克调醋，用布包裹，敷涌泉穴。

7. Treating Hypertension: Grind evodia fruit into a powder. Each time, take 20g of the powder, mix with vinegar, wrap in cloth, and apply to the Yongquan acupoint.

8. 治绣球风（阴囊湿疹）：吴茱萸、蛇床子、艾叶各 30 克，水 3000 毫升煎沸，放盆内加芒硝 15 克，化尽频洗。

8. Treating Scrotal Eczema (Xiuqiufeng): Take 30g each of evodia fruit, cnidium fruit (shechuangzi), and mugwort leaf (aiye). Boil in 3000ml of water,

pour into a basin, add 15g of mirabilite (mangxiao), dissolve completely, and frequently wash the affected area.

9. 治各种癣症：吴茱萸、贯仲、官桂各等分研为细末，醋调擦患处。

9. Treating Various Tinea Infections: Take equal amounts of evodia fruit, male fern (guanzhong), and cinnamon bark (guangui), grind into a fine powder, mix with vinegar, and rub on the affected area.

10. 治痈疽发背：吴茱萸研末，用醋调匀，稀稠适度，摊于纱布上外敷患处。

10. Treating Carbuncles and Back Boils: Grind evodia fruit into a powder, mix evenly with vinegar to a moderate consistency, spread on gauze, and apply externally to the affected area.

11. 治三叉神经痛：吴茱萸研极细末，以浓蜜水调如糊状，敷于痛处，包扎固定。

11. Treating Trigeminal Neuralgia: Grind evodia fruit into an extremely fine powder, mix with thick honey water into a paste, apply to the painful area, and bandage to secure.

12. 治妇女阴部湿痒：吴茱萸 60 克煎水 1000 毫升，频洗取效。

12. Treating Vulvar Pruritus and Dampness in Women: Decoct 60g of evodia fruit in 1000ml of water, and frequently wash the affected area for therapeutic effects.

《中药科技报》1992 年 3 月 11 日

Chinese Medicine Science and Technology News, March 11, 1992

十二、甘蔗

12. Sugarcane (Gan-zhe)

甘蔗汁食疗数则

Several Dietary Therapy Recipes Using Sugarcane Juice

甘蔗的生浆与煎炼之后的熟浆，性能有别功效大不相同。生浆甘寒，能清热去火，清凉生津；蔗汁经煎炼，则变为甘温而助热。我国民间用甘蔗做食疗药用，有不少经验。

Fresh sugarcane juice and the refined syrup have different properties and significantly different effects. Fresh juice is sweet and cold in nature, capable of clearing heat and reducing fire, as well as cooling and generating body fluids. However, when sugarcane juice is boiled and refined, it becomes sweet and warm, and tends to generate heat. There is a wealth of folk experience in China regarding the dietary and medicinal use of sugarcane.

1. 治反胃呕吐、慢性胃炎：青皮蔗汁、葡萄酒各 30 毫升，混合服用。

1. Treating Regurgitation, Vomiting, and Chronic Gastritis: Mix 30ml of green-skinned sugarcane juice with 30ml of grape wine and take the mixture.

2. 治大便秘结：青甘蔗汁、蜂蜜各 30 毫升，混合服用。

2. Treating Constipation: Mix 30ml of green sugarcane juice with 30ml of honey and take the mixture.

3. 治肺热咳嗽，咽干喉痛：甘蔗汁 30 毫升，荸荠汁 15 毫升，温开水送服。

3. Treating Lung-Heat Cough, Dry Throat, and Sore Throat: Take 30ml of sugarcane juice and 15ml of water chestnut juice, swallowed with warm boiled water.

4. 治妊娠恶心呕吐：甘蔗汁一杯，生姜汁数滴，混合服用。

4. Treating Nausea and Vomiting during Pregnancy: Mix one cup of sugarcane juice with a few drops of fresh ginger juice and take the mixture.

5. 治发烧伤津，余热不退：蔗汁杯饮服。

5. Treating Fluid Damage from Fever and Lingering Residual Heat: Drink one cup of sugarcane juice.

6. 治百毒诸疮，痈疽发背：甘蔗捣烂外敷。

6. Treating Various Poisonous Sores, Carbuncles, and Back Boils: Mash sugarcane and apply it externally.

注：由于甘蔗性寒，脾胃虚寒、胃腹寒痛者不宜食用。甘蔗发霉后不能食用。

Note: Because sugarcane is cold in nature, it is not suitable for people with deficiency-cold of the spleen and stomach, or those with cold pain in the stomach and abdomen. Moldy sugarcane must never be consumed.

《民族医药报》（淳 朴）

Ethnic Medicine News (Chun Pu)

十三、虎杖

13. Giant Knotweed (Hu-zhang)

红川七，又名虎杖。虎言其斑，杖言其茎。味苦涩，微寒，无毒。功效利湿退黄，清热解毒，祛痰止咳，活血化瘀。虎杖亭有抑制多种细菌及镇咳作用；黄酮醇配糖体有利尿作用。虎杖干品常用 9-30 克，鲜品 30-60 克，服用过量可引起恶心呕吐，腹泻等胃肠症状，孕妇及经期慎用。

Hongchuanqi, also known as Huzhang (Giant Knotweed). "Hu" (tiger) refers to its spots, and "zhang" (staff) refers to its stem. It is bitter and astringent in flavor, slightly cold in property, and non-toxic. Its effects include promoting diuresis to relieve jaundice, clearing heat and detoxifying, resolving phlegm to stop cough, and promoting blood circulation to dissipate blood stasis. Resveratrol (hu-zhang-ting) has the effect of inhibiting various bacteria and relieving cough; flavonol glycosides have a diuretic effect. The commonly used dosage is 9-30g for the dried herb and 30-60g for the fresh herb. Overdose may cause gastrointestinal symptoms such as nausea, vomiting, and diarrhea. It should be used with caution in pregnant women and during menstruation.

民间验方

Folk Proven Prescriptions

1. 急性黄疸型肝炎：虎杖、茵陈各 30 克，大枣 30 枚。成人一日量，小儿减半。服用法：虎杖、大枣同煎 3-6 小时，茵陈另煎沸后 30 分钟。两药液混合，加糖适量，分 2 次服。

1. Acute Icteric Hepatitis: Take 30g each of giant knotweed and capillary wormwood (yinchen), and 30 red dates. This is the daily dosage for adults; for children, halve the amount. Preparation method: Decoct the giant knotweed and

red dates together for 3-6 hours. Separately, decoct the capillary wormwood for 30 minutes after boiling. Mix the two liquid extracts, add an appropriate amount of sugar, and divide into 2 doses.

2. 烧伤：虎杖叶粉末 100 克，茶叶（细茶）50 克，加水 1000 毫升，煎煮成 500 毫升，用毛笔蘸药液涂布，每日数次，以创面不干为度。如伤口有结痂，改用 100% 的虎杖水溶液进行湿敷，亦可内服，每次 50 毫升，每日 3 次。亦可用虎杖叶粉末调与香油涂布创面。

2. Burns: Take 100g of giant knotweed leaf powder and 50g of tea leaves (fine tea), add 1000ml of water, and decoct to 500ml. Use a brush to dip the liquid and apply it to the wound several times a day, keeping the wound surface moist. If the wound has scabbed, switch to wet compresses with a 100% giant knotweed aqueous solution. It can also be taken orally, 50ml each time, 3 times a day. Alternatively, mix giant knotweed leaf powder with sesame oil and apply it to the wound.

3. 手足麻木、痿软：虎杖 30 克，川牛膝、五加皮、防风、桂枝、当归各 15 克，泡白酒 3 斤，瓶装密封 15 天后启用，每次服 10 毫克，早晚各一次。

3. Numbness and Flaccidity of Hands and Feet: Take 30g of giant knotweed, and 15g each of cyathula root (chuan-niuxi), acanthopanax bark (wujia-pi), saposhnikovia root (fangfeng), cinnamon twig (guizhi), and angelica root (danggui). Soak them in 1.5kg (3 jin) of liquor in a sealed bottle for 15 days before use. Take 10mg each time, once in the morning and once at night.

4. 砂淋、尿闭：虎杖 150 克，加水 500 毫升，煎成 150 毫升，入麝香 0.03 克，分 3 次服下。效速。

4. Urinary Stones and Urinary Retention: Take 150g of giant knotweed, add 500ml of water, and decoct to 150ml. Add 0.03g of musk (shexiang), and divide into 3 doses. It works quickly.

5. 跌打损伤：虎杖 30 克，加水 300 毫升。煎成 150 毫升。每次 50 毫升加米酒 50 毫升服下，每日 2 次。

5. Traumatic Injuries from Falls and Blows: Take 30g of giant knotweed, add

300ml of water, and decoct to 150ml. Each time, take 50ml of the decoction mixed with 50ml of rice wine, twice a day.

6. 风热咳嗽痰多：虎杖 30 克，桔梗、蝉蜕各 10 克，水煎服，日 2 次。服 2 剂即愈。

6. Wind-Heat Cough with Excessive Phlegm: Take 30g of giant knotweed, and 10g each of platycodon root (jiegeng) and cicada slough (chantui). Decoct in water to drink, twice a day. The condition will be cured after taking 2 doses.

7. 经痛：虎杖 30 克，水煎服。连服 3 天即效。连用 3 个周期。

7. Dysmenorrhea (Menstrual Pain): Take 30g of giant knotweed, decoct in water to drink. It will be effective after taking it continuously for 3 days. Use it continuously for 3 menstrual cycles.

《中药科技报》1992 年 7 月 6 日（青海 刘启明）

Chinese Medicine Science and Technology News, July 6, 1992 (Liu Qiming, Qinghai)

十四、车前草

14. Plantain Herb (Che-qian-cao)

车前草性味甘寒，能清热利尿，清肝明目，祛痰止咳，渗湿止泻。常用验方如下：

Plantain herb is sweet and cold in nature. It can clear heat and promote diuresis, clear the liver and improve vision, resolve phlegm to stop cough, and drain dampness to relieve diarrhea. Commonly used proven prescriptions are as follows:

1. 治泌尿系统炎症：车前叶 100 克，淡竹叶 12 克，甘草 10 克。水煎，加冰糖适量，代茶饮，每日一剂，10 天为一疗程。

Treating Urinary System Inflammation: Take 100g of plantain leaves, 12g of lophatherum leaves (dan-zhu-ye), and 10g of licorice root (gan-cao). Decoct in water, add an appropriate amount of rock sugar, and drink as a substitute for tea.

Take 1 dose daily, with 10 days constituting one course of treatment.

2. 治泌尿系统结石：车前叶 500 克，葱白 30 克。水煎，加白糖适量，2 次分服，每日一剂，7 天为一疗程。

2. Treating Urinary System Stones: Take 500g of plantain leaves and 30g of white parts of green onions. Decoct in water, add an appropriate amount of white sugar, and divide into 2 doses. Take 1 dose daily, with 7 days constituting one course of treatment.

3. 治小儿腹泻：车前子炒焦研末，4 个月至 2 周岁每次 0.5-1 克，每日 3 次，以车前叶煎水送服。

3. Treating Childhood Diarrhea: Stir-fry plantain seeds (che-qian-zi) until scorched and grind into a powder. For children aged 4 months to 2 years, take 0.5-1g each time, 3 times a day, swallowed with plantain leaf decoction.

4. 治慢性肝炎：鲜车前叶 30 克，鲜芹菜 100 克，萝卜 100 克。共洗净切碎捣汁，加蜂蜜炖服，每日一剂，分 2 次服。

4. Treating Chronic Hepatitis: Take 30g of fresh plantain leaves, 100g of fresh celery, and 100g of radish. Wash them together, chop them, and mash to extract the juice. Add honey and simmer to drink. Take 1 dose daily, divided into 2 servings.

5. 治湿疹：车前叶 15 克，冬瓜皮 30 克，苡仁 30 克。水煎服，每日一剂，分 2 次服，7 日可愈。

5. Treating Eczema: Take 15g of plantain leaves, 30g of winter melon peel, and 30g of coix seeds (yi-ren). Decoct in water to drink. Take 1 dose daily, divided into 2 servings. It can be cured in 7 days.

（李明）

(Li Ming)

十五、梨的药用
15. Medicinal Uses of Pears

1. 糖尿病：香水梨 5 个，洗净捣烂，加蜂蜜适量，熬成膏。每次食 1 匙，温开水调服，1 日 3 次。

Diabetes: Take 5 fragrant pears, wash them, mash them, add an appropriate amount of honey, and boil into a syrup. Take 1 spoonful each time, mixed with warm boiled water, 3 times a day.

2. 消化不良：将梨去皮，浸入醋中 3 日后食用，每日早晚各服 1 个。

2. Indigestion: Peel the pears, soak them in vinegar for 3 days, and then eat them. Take 1 each in the morning and evening.

3. 便秘腹胀：大梨 1 个，芦根 20 克，蜂蜜适量，水煎，于睡前食梨饮汤。

3. Constipation and Abdominal Distension: Take 1 large pear, 20g of reed rhizome (lu-gen), and an appropriate amount of honey. Decoct in water, and eat the pear and drink the broth before going to bed.

4. 解酒醉：梨汁 30 毫升，加入适量米醋食之。

4. Relieving Alcohol Intoxication: Take 30ml of pear juice, add an appropriate amount of rice vinegar, and consume.

5. 妊娠呕吐：梨 1 个，去核，放入丁香 10 枚，密闭蒸熟，去丁香，食梨。

5. Vomiting during Pregnancy: Take 1 pear, remove the core, put in 10 cloves (ding-xiang), steam in a sealed container until cooked, remove the cloves, and eat the pear.

6. 久咳不愈：雪梨 1 个，银耳 5 克，川贝 3 克，水煎服，1 日 2 次。

6. Chronic Cough: Take 1 snow pear, 5g of white fungus (yin-er), and 3g of Sichuan fritillary bulb (chuan-bei). Decoct in water to drink, twice a day.

7. 烫伤未破：生梨切片敷于患处。

7. Unruptured Scalds and Burns: Slice raw pears and apply them to the affected area.

8. 咳嗽：雪梨 1 个，蜂蜜 50 克，将梨挖去梨核，放入蜂蜜，蒸熟睡前食。

8. Cough: Take 1 snow pear and 50g of honey. Hollow out the pear core, fill it with honey, steam until cooked, and eat before going to bed.

9. 气管炎：大梨 1 个，贝母 8 克研末，冰糖 20 克，梨去皮核，切碎煮熟，汤梨一起吃。

9. Bronchitis: Take 1 large pear, 8g of fritillary bulb (bei-mu) ground into powder, and 20g of rock sugar. Peel and core the pear, chop it, and boil until cooked. Eat both the pear and the broth.

摘自《南方日报》

Excerpted from Nanfang Daily

梨不但醇香宜人，甜酸可口，汁多爽脆，而且营养十分丰富。含有蛋白质、脂肪、糖类、胡萝卜素、钙、磷、铁、维生素 B、C，以及苹果酸、柠檬酸等。

Pears are not only mellow and pleasant, sweet and sour, juicy and crisp, but also highly nutritious. They contain protein, fat, carbohydrates, carotene, calcium, phosphorus, iron, vitamins B and C, as well as malic acid and citric acid.

梨还含有天白冬素，对人体健康及胃脏保健有着特殊功效。

Pears also contain asparagine, which has special effects on human health and stomach care.

祖国医学认为，梨性甘凉，具有生津止渴，润肺清燥，止咳化痰，清热退烧，开胃消食等作用，可治疗多种常见病：

Traditional Chinese medicine believes that pears are sweet and cool in nature, with the effects of generating body fluids to relieve thirst, moistening the lungs and clearing dryness, stopping cough and resolving phlegm, clearing heat and reducing fever, and stimulating appetite and aiding digestion. They can treat various common diseases:

10. 慢性咽炎：雪花梨 500 克，去皮去核，煮至半熟时加入胖大海 3 枚，再以文火煮沸片刻，每日 3 次分服。

10. Chronic Pharyngitis: Take 500g of snow pears, peel and core them. When half-cooked, add 3 malva nuts (pang-da-hai), and simmer over low heat for a while. Divide into 3 doses daily.

11. 感冒发热: 雪花梨1-2只，洗净切片，以凉开水浸泡1天，每日分3次服下。

11. Cold with Fever: Take 1-2 snow pears, wash and slice them, soak in cool boiled water for 1 day, and divide into 3 doses daily.

12. 小儿百日咳: 生梨1只，去皮去核，装入麻黄1.5克，隔水蒸熟后去除药渣，食梨饮汁。

12. Childhood Whooping Cough: Take 1 raw pear, peel and core it, stuff it with 1.5g of ephedra (ma-huang), steam until cooked, remove the herbal residue, and eat the pear while drinking the juice.

13. 支气管哮喘：生梨1只洗净切片，在锅内放入清水2杯，蜂蜜1匙。等水开后，把梨加入煮熟，放凉后日服3次。

13. Bronchial Asthma: Wash and slice 1 raw pear. Put 2 cups of water and 1 spoonful of honey in a pot. After the water boils, add the pear and cook until done. Let it cool and take it 3 times a day.

14. 恶心呕吐：鸭梨1只，去皮去核，加入丁香15枚，煮熟后去丁香吃梨。

14. Nausea and Vomiting: Take 1 Yali pear, peel and core it, add 15 cloves (ding-xiang), boil until cooked, remove the cloves, and eat the pear.

《民族医药报》（江西 陶清华）

Ethnic Medicine News (Tao Qinghua, Jiangxi)

十六、南天竹

16. Nandina (Nan-tian-zhu)

别名：木黄连、天竺子、土黄连、万寿竹、南天竹子。

Aliases: Muhuanglian, Tianzhuzi, Tuhuanglian, Wanshouzhu, Nantianzhuzi.

来源：为小檗科南天竹属植物南天竹的根茎。

Source: The rhizome of Nandina domestica, a plant of the Nandina genus in the Berberidaceae family.

形态：常绿灌木，高约2米。全株无毛。茎直立，幼枝常带红色。叶对生，2-3回奇数羽状复叶，末回小羽片具小叶3-5枚；小叶革质，椭圆状披针形，长3-10

厘米。先端渐尖，基部楔形，全缘，两面光滑无毛，冬季常变红色。圆锥花序顶生，长 20-30 厘米；花白色。浆果球形，鲜红色，含种子 2 颗；种子扁圆形。

Morphology: An evergreen shrub, about 2 meters tall. The entire plant is glabrous (hairless). The stems are erect, and young branches are often reddish. The leaves are opposite, 2-3 times odd-pinnately compound, with the ultimate pinnae having 3-5 leaflets. The leaflets are leathery, elliptic-lanceolate, and 3-10 cm long. The apex is acuminate, the base is cuneate, the margins are entire, and both surfaces are smooth and glabrous, often turning red in winter. The panicles are terminal, 20-30 cm long, with white flowers. The berries are spherical and bright red, containing 2 seeds; the seeds are flattened and round.

生境分布：多生于石山疏林下或灌丛中。分布于云南、贵州、广西、海南、广东、福建、湖南等省区。

Habitat and Distribution: Mostly grows under sparse forests on rocky mountains or in shrub thickets. Distributed in provinces and regions such as Yunnan, Guizhou, Guangxi, Hainan, Guangdong, Fujian, and Hunan.

采集加工：四季可采，洗净，切片，鲜用或晒干备用。

Collection and Processing: Can be harvested in all four seasons. Wash clean, slice, and use fresh or sun-dry for later use.

性味效用：味苦，性平。清热解毒，利湿，止咳，平喘。用于感冒咳嗽，肺结核，支气管炎，哮喘，黄疸型肝炎，痢疾，急性胃肠炎，尿路感染；湿热痹痛。用量：5-10 克。全株含生物碱，有毒，内服宜慎，服过量易引起痉挛和神经麻痹。

Properties, Flavor, and Effects: Bitter in flavor, neutral in property. Clears heat and detoxifies, promotes diuresis, stops cough, and relieves asthma. Used for cold and cough, pulmonary tuberculosis, bronchitis, asthma, icteric hepatitis, dysentery, acute gastroenteritis, urinary tract infections, and arthralgia due to damp-heat. Dosage: 5-10g. The whole plant contains alkaloids and is toxic. It should be used with caution for oral administration; overdose easily causes spasms and nerve paralysis.

附方

Appendix Prescriptions

1. 感冒咳嗽：南天竹根 8 克，枇杷叶（去毛）15 克，冰糖 20 克（后下）。水煎分 3 次服。

Cold and Cough: Take 8g of nandina root, 15g of loquat leaves (with hairs removed), and 20g of rock sugar (added towards the end of decoction). Decoct in water and divide into 3 doses.

2. 黄疸型肝炎：南天竹根 8 克，田基王 20 克，水煎服。

2. Icteric Hepatitis: Take 8g of nandina root and 20g of tianjiwang (Hypericum japonicum). Decoct in water to drink.

3. 急性胃肠炎、痢疾：南天竹根 6 克，古羊藤根 15 克，水煎服。

3. Acute Gastroenteritis and Dysentery: Take 6g of nandina root and 15g of guyangteng root (Streptocaulon griffithii). Decoct in water to drink.

4. 尿路感染：南天竹根 10 克，金钱草 15 克，淡竹叶 10 克，水煎服。

4. Urinary Tract Infections: Take 10g of nandina root, 15g of golden coin grass (jinqiancao), and 10g of lophatherum leaves (dan-zhu-ye). Decoct in water to drink.

（陈孙）

(Chen Sun)

十七、萝卜的药用
17. Medicinal Uses of Radishes

萝卜品种较多，性能相近。药用以肉白辣萝卜为佳。性平，微凉、味甘、辛。有健胃消食，止咳化痰、顺气利尿和清热解毒的功效。用萝卜也可治疗多种疾病。

There are many varieties of radishes with similar properties. For medicinal purposes, the white-fleshed spicy radish is considered the best. It is neutral and slightly cool in property, and sweet and pungent in flavor. It has the effects of invigorating the stomach and aiding digestion, stopping cough and resolving phlegm, regulating qi and promoting diuresis, and clearing heat and detoxifying. Radishes can also be used to treat various diseases.

1. 煤气中毒：生萝卜捣烂取汗，大量服用，一天 3 至 4 次。

Carbon Monoxide Poisoning: Mash raw radishes to extract the juice, take a large amount, 3 to 4 times a day.

2. 冻疮：用萝卜煮水熏洗，每天三次，或将鲜萝卜切成两半、中间放少许盐，再用竹筷子扎住放在火灰里煨半熟，趁热在冻疮部位轻搽，3 天以后可见效。

2. Chilblains: Boil radishes in water to fumigate and wash the affected area, 3 times a day. Alternatively, cut a fresh radish in half, put a little salt in the middle, tie it with bamboo chopsticks, and simmer it in fire ashes until half-cooked. While hot, gently rub it on the chilblains. It will be effective after 3 days.

3. 偏头痛：用萝卜适量捣汁，加少量冰片，缓慢滴入鼻孔，左痛滴右，右痛滴左。

3. Migraine: Mash an appropriate amount of radishes to extract the juice, add a small amount of borneol (bingpian), and slowly instill it into the nostrils. For pain on the left side, instill into the right nostril; for pain on the right side, instill into the left nostril.

4. 痰多咳嗽：取萝卜一个，生姜二片、陈皮二片、白胡椒五粒、煮熟后服用。

4. Cough with Excessive Phlegm: Take 1 radish, 2 slices of fresh ginger, 2 pieces of dried tangerine peel (chenpi), and 5grains of white pepper. Boil until cooked and consume.

5. 咳嗽哮喘：萝卜、生姜，蜂蜜适量，水煎服。

5. Cough and Asthma: Take radishes, fresh ginger, and an appropriate amount of honey. Decoct in water to drink.

6. 吐血、便血：白萝卜汁和藕汁适量混合后使用。

6. Hematemesis (Vomiting Blood) and Hematochezia (Bloody Stools): Mix an appropriate amount of white radish juice and lotus root juice for use.

7. 扁桃体发炎：白萝卜一个，青果十枚，冰糖少许，煎煮代茶饮用。

7. Tonsillitis: Take 1 white radish, 10 Chinese olives (qingguo), and a little rock sugar. Decoct and drink as a substitute for tea.

8. 久咳：萝卜一个，杏仁九克，猪肺半斤，煮熟后喝汤。

8. Chronic Cough: Take 1 radish, 9g of apricot seeds (xingren), and 250g (half a jin) of pig lung. Boil until cooked and drink the broth.

9. 恶心呕吐：萝卜绞汁后，其汁加糖适量，温开水冲服、效果甚佳。

9. Nausea and Vomiting: Extract the juice from radishes, add an appropriate amount of sugar, and mix with warm boiled water to drink. The effect is excellent.

《民族医药报》1991 年 11 月 5 日（开封 荣梦周）

Ethnic Medicine News, November 5, 1991 (Rong Mengzhou, Kaifeng)

十八、马鞭草
18. Verbena (Ma-bian-cao)

马鞭草，又叫龙芽草，风颈草。全草及根皆可入药。本品味甘辛性寒，入肝、脾、膀胱经。具有截疟，清热解毒，活血利尿等功效。可用来治疗下述多种病证。

Verbena, also known as Longyacao and Fengjingcao. Both the whole plant and the roots can be used as medicine. It is sweet and pungent in flavor, cold in property, and enters the Liver, Spleen, and Bladder meridians. It has the effects of arresting malaria, clearing heat and detoxifying, promoting blood circulation, and promoting diuresis. It can be used to treat the following various diseases and syndromes.

1. 治疗疟疾：用马鞭草 30-60 克，酒炖服，日服 2 次，连服 5-7 天。

Treating Malaria: Take 30-60g of verbena, stew with liquor, and take it twice a day continuously for 5-7 days.

2. 治感冒、流行性腮腺炎：用马鞭草 60 克，板蓝根 15 克，水煎，日服 2 次，连服 3 日。

2. Treating Common Cold and Epidemic Parotitis (Mumps): Take 60g of verbena and 15g of isatis root (ban-lan-gen). Decoct in water and take twice a day continuously for 3 days.

3. 治白喉呼吸困难或喘息而欲窒息者，用鲜马鞭草 30 克，洗净，捣汁，加米醋少许，分 2 次服。

3. Treating Diphtheria with Breathing Difficulties or Panting and Near Suffocation: Take 30g of fresh verbena, wash it, mash to extract the juice, add a small amount of rice vinegar, and divide into 2 doses.

4. 治百日咳：用马鞭草 1000 克、白蜂糖 500 克。熬膏，3 岁患儿服 1 匙，日服 3 次，开水送下，可按年龄大小酌情加量或减量服用。

4. Treating Whooping Cough: Take 1000g of verbena and 500g of white honey. Boil into a syrup. For a 3-year-old child, take 1 spoonful, 3 times a day, swallowed with boiled water. The dosage can be increased or decreased according to age.

5. 治痢疾、急性胃肠炎：用马鞭草 30 克，研末，每服 3 克，日服 2 次，连服 4 日。无效，可再服之，并将药量加重。

5. Treating Dysentery and Acute Gastroenteritis: Take 30g of verbena, grind into a powder, take 3g each time, twice a day, continuously for 4 days. If ineffective, continue taking it and increase the dosage.

6. 治黄疸型肝炎：用马鞭草、金钱草、车前草各 15 克，水煎分 2-3 次服，以愈为度。

6. Treating Icteric Hepatitis: Take 15g each of verbena, golden coin grass (jin-qian-cao), and plantain herb (che-qian-cao). Decoct in water and divide into 2-3 doses, continuing until cured.

7. 治急性乳腺炎初期：用马鞭草、丹参各 30 克，水煎分 2 次服，连服 3-5 日。

7. Treating Early-stage Acute Mastitis: Take 30g each of verbena and red sage root (dan-shen). Decoct in water and divide into 2 doses, continuously for 3-5 days.

8. 治阑尾炎：用马鞭草研末，每服 9 克，加甜酒，开水送服，日服 2- 3 次，连服 5-7 天。

8. Treating Appendicitis: Grind verbena into a powder, take 9g each time, add sweet wine, and swallow with boiled water. Take 2-3 times a day continuously for 5-7 days.

9. 治尿路感染、尿结石、毒蛇咬伤：用鲜马鞭草捣汁饮，每次服 50 毫升，口服 2-3 次，以愈为度。

9. Treating Urinary Tract Infections, Urinary Stones, and Venomous Snake Bites: Mash fresh verbena to extract the juice and drink it. Take 50ml each time, orally 2-3 times, continuing until cured.

10. 治疗口疮：用马鞭草叶加蜂蜜捣烂敷患处，每日或隔日换药 1 次。

10. Treating Mouth Ulcers: Mash verbena leaves with honey and apply to the affected area. Change the dressing once a day or every other day.

11. 治手掌疔：用马鞭草根加醋捣烂敷患处，每日 1 换。

11. Treating Palm Boils: Mash verbena roots with vinegar and apply to the affected area. Change the dressing once a day.

12. 治产后发热：用马鞭草、干苋菜各 60 克，水煎，加红糖 1 次炖服，无效，再服，三次一定见效。

12. Treating Postpartum Fever: Take 60g each of verbena and dried amaranth. Decoct in water, add brown sugar, and stew to take in one go. If ineffective, take it again; it will definitely be effective after three doses.

13. 治经闭：用马鞭草 16 克，水煎，加热黄酒 60 克，饭前服，每日 1 剂。

13. Treating Amenorrhea (Absence of Menstruation): Take 16g of verbena, decoct in water, add 60g of warm yellow rice wine, take before meals, 1 dose daily.

14. 治脾脏肿大：用马鞭草根 60 克，捣汁，加酒 2 份，水 1 份，煎开，早晨空腹时服，服后必须卧床 1 小时，连服 30 日。

14. Treating Splenomegaly (Enlarged Spleen): Take 60g of verbena roots, mash to extract the juice, add 2 parts liquor and 1 part water, and boil. Take on an empty stomach in the morning. You must stay in bed for 1 hour after taking it. Continue for 30 days.

15. 治水肿：用马鞭草、地瓜酒各 90 克，红糖 60 克，水煎分 2-3 次服，连服 5 天。若水肿未退尽，可再服之。

15. Treating Edema: Take 90g each of verbena and sweet potato wine, and 60g of brown sugar. Decoct in water and divide into 2-3 doses, continuously for 5 days. If the edema has not completely subsided, continue taking it.

《中药科技报》1993 年 1 月 14 日（惠）

Chinese Medicine Science and Technology News, January 14, 1993 (Hui)

十九、鸡蛋壳
19. Eggshells (Ji-dan-ke)

1. 小儿营养不良、佝偻病、手足抽搐症：将鸡蛋壳适量洗净烤干，研细粉过筛备用。6 个月至 1 岁的患儿每次 0.5 克，1-2 岁患儿每次 1 克，每日 2 次。

Childhood Malnutrition, Rickets, and Tetany: Wash an appropriate amount of eggshells, bake dry, grind into a fine powder, and sift for later use. For infants aged 6 months to 1 year, take 0.5g each time; for children aged 1-2 years, take 1g each time, twice a day.

2. 各种出血症（如咳血、吐血、便血、鼻血）：取鸡蛋壳粉 6 克配合适量食盐及维生素 C，1 日 3 次分服，连服 2-7 日，出鼻血患者可同时用棉球蘸药粉塞鼻。

2. Various Hemorrhagic Conditions (such as hemoptysis, hematemesis, hematochezia, and epistaxis): Take 6g of eggshell powder combined with an appropriate amount of salt and Vitamin C. Divide into 3 doses daily, continuously for 2-7 days. For patients with epistaxis, a cotton ball dipped in the powder can be used to plug the nostril simultaneously.

3. 配合治疗骨折：取鸡蛋壳适量，在锅内炒黄，研为细末，每次服 3 克，用凉开水送服，日服 3 次。

3. Adjunctive Treatment for Bone Fractures: Take an appropriate amount of eggshells, stir-fry in a pan until yellowish, grind into a fine powder, take 3g each time, swallowed with cool boiled water, 3 times a day.

4. 小儿头身患疮疖：取鸡蛋壳适量，炒黄研末，与猪油适量调敷患处，每日换药 1 次。

4. Sores and Boils on the Head and Body in Children: Take an appropriate amount of eggshells, stir-fry until yellowish and grind into a powder, mix with an

appropriate amount of lard, and apply to the affected area. Change the dressing once a day.

5. 过敏性皮疹、荨麻疹：取鸡蛋壳 50 克，洗净烤干研末，每次服 2 克，每日 3 次。

5. Allergic Rashes and Urticaria (Hives): Take 50g of eggshells, wash, bake dry, and grind into a powder. Take 2g each time, 3 times a day.

6. 胃脘疼痛：取鸡蛋壳适量，在锅内炒黄，研成细末（越细越好），每次服 3-5 克，每日 3 次，饭前或饭后用开水送服。

6. Epigastric Pain: Take an appropriate amount of eggshells, stir-fry in a pan until yellowish, and grind into a fine powder (the finer, the better). Take 3-5g each time, 3 times a day, swallowed with boiled water before or after meals.

二十、马兰
20. Indian Calendula (Ma-lan)

马兰，别马齿芽、满地芽、田边菊，既可入药，又可做菜吃。《本草纲目》载“气味辛、平，无毒。破宿血，养新血，解酒疸及诸菌毒。”笔者采撷民间运用马兰验方，兹这介绍于此。

Indian Calendula, also known as Machiya, Mandiya, and Tianbianju, can be used both as a medicinal herb and as a vegetable. The Compendium of Materia Medica (Bencao Gangmu) records that “it is pungent and neutral in property, and non-toxic. It breaks up stagnant blood, nourishes new blood, and relieves alcohol-induced jaundice and various bacterial toxins.” The author has collected some proven folk prescriptions using Indian Calendula and introduces them here.

1. 黄疸：鲜马兰 120 克，雌鸡一只。将雌鸡杀后，去毛、头足，剖开，不见水，去肠杂，用马兰拧成团用线缚住，放鸡肚里，并放适量红糖，将鸡缝好，装入瓦钵内，再放在盛水锅中隔水蒸烂，分四次（鸡药）食，一日二次。

Jaundice: Take 120g of fresh Indian Calendula and one female chicken. After slaughtering the chicken, remove the feathers, head, and feet, and gut it without touching water. Twist the Indian Calendula into a ball, tie it with a thread, and place it inside the chicken' s belly along with an appropriate amount of brown sugar. Sew the chicken closed, place it in an earthenware bowl, and steam it in a water bath until tender. Divide the chicken and herbs into four portions, and consume twice a day.

2. 热淋（泌尿系感染）：鲜马兰 50-100 克，车前草 30 克、玉米须 10 克，加水煎服，一日一剂。5-7 日为一疗程。

2. Heat Strangury (Urinary Tract Infections): Take 50-100g of fresh Indian Calendula, 30g of plantain herb (che-qian-cao), and 10g of corn silk. Decoct in water to drink, 1 dose a day. 5-7 days constitute one course of treatment.

3. 产后胎盘不下（胎盘稽留）：马兰（长流水沟处长为佳）一大把，洗净，用米泔水煎服，片刻即下。

3. Retained Placenta after Childbirth: Take a large handful of Indian Calendula (preferably those grown in flowing ditches), wash them, and decoct in rice-washing water to drink. The placenta will be expelled shortly after.

《中药科技报》1992 年 6 月 26 日（湖北省 徐宏超）

Chinese Medicine Science and Technology News, June 26, 1992 (Xu Hongchao, Hubei Province)

二十一、田螺的药用

21. Medicinal Uses of River Snails (Tian-luo)

1. 治慢性肾炎：大田螺 10 个，去壳取肉捣烂，加入苦荞麦粉 5 克，再捣，平放于布上，贴敷脐部，每日 1 换，10 日为一疗程，间隔 3 日，再做第二个疗程，连治 3 个疗程。

Treating Chronic Nephritis: Take 10 large river snails, remove the shells, mash the meat, add 5g of tartary buckwheat powder, and mash again. Place it flat on a piece of cloth and apply it to the navel. Change the dressing once a day. 10 days constitute one course of treatment. Wait for 3 days before starting the second course. Continue for 3 courses in total.

2. 治肾性水肿：大田螺 10 个去壳，大蒜 5 瓣去皮，车前子 10 克研细，共捣如泥，压成饼状，敷肚脐，胶布固定。对遍身水肿，小便短少者尤佳。

2. Treating Nephrotic Edema: Remove the shells of 10 large river snails, peel 5 cloves of garlic, and grind 10g of plantain seeds (che-qian-zi) into a fine powder. Mash them all together into a mud-like consistency, press into a cake shape, apply to the navel, and secure with medical tape. It is especially effective for generalized edema and oliguria (scanty urination).

3. 治小便不通：田螺 10 个，芭蕉心榨水 250 毫升，水煎冲白糖服食，同时，外用芭蕉根和田螺捣烂敷贴小腹，有化气行水消胀满疗效。

3. Treating Urinary Retention: Take 10 river snails and 250ml of juice squeezed from banana hearts. Decoct in water, mix with white sugar, and consume. At the same time, mash banana roots and river snails and apply them externally to the lower abdomen. This has the effect of transforming qi, promoting diuresis, and relieving distension.

4. 治小儿湿疹：将螺壳置于锅内，煅至黄透不糊，取出放凉，用 15 克加入冰片 1.5 克，共捣研成细末撒患处，有祛湿清热解毒之功效。

4. Treating Childhood Eczema: Place the snail shells in a pan and calcine them until they are completely yellow but not scorched. Take them out and let them cool. Take 15g of the shells, add 1.5g of borneol (bingpian), and grind them together into a fine powder. Sprinkle the powder on the affected area. It has the effects of removing dampness, clearing heat, and detoxifying.

5.治热结便秘：大田螺3-6个，连壳捣烂，加少许食盐，共捣烂如泥，纱布包裹，压成饼状，敷气海穴，胶布固定。

5. Treating Constipation due to Heat Accumulation: Take 3-6 large river snails with their shells, mash them, add a little salt, and mash into a mud-like consistency. Wrap in gauze, press into a cake shape, apply to the Qihai acupoint, and secure with medical tape.

6. 治外痔肿痛：取大田螺若干、去盖，每个田螺入少许冰片，置消毒器皿内，即流水绿色药汁。先将患处以浓茶洗净，蘸取药汁擦患处。每日 6-10 次，连用数日，肿痛可除。

6. Treating Swelling and Pain of External Hemorrhoids: Take several large river snails, remove their opercula (lids), put a little borneol into each snail, and place them in a sterilized container. A green medicinal juice will soon flow out. First, wash the affected area with strong tea, dip the juice, and wipe the affected area. Do this 6-10 times a day for several consecutive days to eliminate the swelling and pain.

7. 治内痔肿痛：取大田螺头（去螺盖截尾）10-15 个，冰片 0.5 克，共捣如泥，消毒纱布包裹。肛门清洗后，将药塞入肛门内。

7. Treating Swelling and Pain of Internal Hemorrhoids: Take 10-15 large river snail heads (with the opercula removed and tails cut off) and 0.5g of borneol. Mash them into a mud-like consistency and wrap in sterilized gauze. After cleaning the anus, insert the medicine into the anal canal.

8. 治子宫脱垂：大田螺 7-10 个，清水中养一夜，黄连 1 克研末，田螺去盖，每个螺中撒入少许黄连，汁流入消毒器皿中，用浓茶清洗患部，再用纱布沾药液，敷在下垂子宫部，然后轻轻托入。

8. Treating Uterine Prolapse: Keep 7-10 large river snails in clean water overnight. Grind 1g of coptis root (huanglian) into a powder. Remove the opercula of the snails, sprinkle a little coptis powder into each snail, and let the juice flow into a sterilized container. Wash the affected area with strong tea, soak a piece of gauze in the medicinal liquid, apply it to the prolapsed uterus, and gently push it back in.

9. 治高热不退：燕窝泥 15-30 克，田螺肉 5-10 个，青黛 3-6 克，加入蛋清适量，（鸡蛋清，共捣如泥，敷肚脐，热退去药。）

9. Treating Persistent High Fever: Take 15-30g of swiftlet nest mud, 5-10 river snail meats, and 3-6g of natural indigo (qingdai). Add an appropriate amount of egg white, and mash them all together into a mud-like consistency. Apply to the navel. Remove the medicine when the fever subsides.

10. 治胃痛：将螺壳焖成黄色，研成细末，每次 3 克，用温开水调酒冲服，每天 3 次，有理气和胃、化瘀止痛疗效。

10. Treating Stomachache: Stew the snail shells until yellow, and grind them into a fine powder. Take 3g each time, mixed with warm boiled water and a little liquor, 3 times a day. It has the effects of regulating qi and harmonizing the stomach, dissipating blood stasis, and relieving pain.

《中药科技报》1992 年 6 月 6 日（胡定绶）

Chinese Medicine Science and Technology News, June 6, 1992 (Hu Dingshou)

二十二、贯众
22. Male Fern (Guan-zhong)

1. 预防流感、麻疹、乙脑：取贯众 50 克，加水 1000 毫升，煎煮 15 分钟，取汁备用，每次服 200 毫升，每日 2 次，儿童减半。

Preventing Influenza, Measles, and Epidemic Encephalitis B: Take 50g of male fern, add 1000ml of water, and decoct for 15 minutes. Set the juice aside. Take 200ml each time, twice a day. The dosage for children should be halved.

2. 治疗外伤出血：取贯众若干，切片或捣碎，置锅中炒黑，研细备用，此粉对外伤出血止血效果较好。

2. Treating Traumatic Bleeding: Take an appropriate amount of male fern, slice or crush it, stir-fry in a pan until blackened, and grind into a fine powder for later use. This powder has a good hemostatic effect on traumatic bleeding.

3. 治疗产后出血或月经过多：用贯众若干，以上等米醋浸泡 4 小时，烘烤干，研末，每次服 10 克，每日 2 次。据现代药理研究证实，贯众有较好的收缩子宫的作用，故服后能止血。

3. Treating Postpartum Hemorrhage or Menorrhagia: Take an appropriate amount of male fern, soak it in high-quality rice vinegar for 4 hours, bake dry, and grind into a powder. Take 10g each time, twice a day. Modern pharmacological

studies have confirmed that male fern has a good uterine-contracting effect, which helps stop bleeding after ingestion.

4. 治疗疮疖：用贯众研末过筛，再加米醋调成糊状，敷于患处（溃后勿用），可对红肿热痛的疮疖起清热解毒作用。此末若加少许六神丸末，调敷腮腺炎，效果很佳。

4. Treating Sores and Boils: Grind male fern into a powder, sift it, and mix it with rice vinegar to form a paste. Apply it to the affected area (do not use after the sores have ruptured). It can clear heat and detoxify sores and boils accompanied by redness, swelling, heat, and pain. If a small amount of Liushen Wan (Six Spirits Pill) powder is added to this powder and applied to mumps, the effect is excellent.

《民族医药报》1992 年 6 月 5 日（江西 文汇）

Ethnic Medicine News, June 5, 1992 (Wen Hui, Jiangxi)

二十三、紫苏
23. Perilla (Zi-su)

据《本草纲目》载，紫苏能“解肌发表，散风寒，行气宽中，消痰利肺；和血温中，止痛定喘”，临床上是常用中药。家庭使用紫苏的范围极广，特介绍便方十则。

According to the Compendium of Materia Medica, perilla can “relieve the exterior and induce diaphoresis, dispel wind-cold, regulate qi and harmonize the middle, resolve phlegm and benefit the lungs; harmonize the blood and warm the middle, relieve pain and calm asthma.” It is a commonly used Chinese medicine in clinical practice. Perilla has a very wide range of household applications. Here are ten convenient home remedies:

1. 感冒：取鲜紫苏叶 30 克，放入熬好的米粥中煮 2-3 分钟，去叶服粥。此粥清香扑鼻，既能散寒止痛，又能养胃护气，对老弱儿童伤风最为相宜。

Common Cold: Take 30g of fresh perilla leaves, add them to freshly cooked rice porridge, and boil for 2-3 minutes. Remove the leaves and eat the porridge.

This porridge is highly fragrant. It can dispel cold and relieve pain, as well as nourish the stomach and protect qi. It is most suitable for the elderly, the weak, and children suffering from colds.

2. 胃痛：取紫苏老梗 30 克，生姜 25 克，花椒 20 粒，放入一猪肚内炖服。此方可治胃气胃寒疼痛，对气郁呃逆、胸胁胀满亦有效。

2. Stomachache: Take 30g of old perilla stems, 25g of fresh ginger, and 20 Sichuan peppercorns. Put them inside a pig' s stomach and stew until cooked. This recipe can treat stomachache caused by stomach qi stagnation and stomach cold. It is also effective for hiccups due to qi stagnation and chest and hypochondriac fullness.

3. 进补：若在炖鸡、炖补药或其它补品时，放入 30 克紫苏根头，煮 5-10 分钟捞起，可防进补所造成的腻滞和消化不良。

3. Tonic Supplementation: When stewing chicken, tonic herbs, or other tonics, add 30g of perilla roots. Boil for 5-10 minutes and then remove them. This can prevent the cloying stagnation and indigestion caused by taking tonics.

4. 痰喘：老年性慢性支气管炎发作时。可用紫苏子 30 克以布包好，炖瘦肉服用，3-5 剂后，可使痰涎减少，气喘获平。

4. Phlegm and Panting: During an attack of senile chronic bronchitis. Take 30g of perilla seeds, wrap them in a piece of cloth, and stew with lean meat. After 3-5 doses, it can reduce phlegm and relieve panting.

5. 头痛：各种头痛，均可取鲜紫苏叶若干，放入茶杯中，用滚开水冲泡，2-5 分钟后取叶滴去水液，贴于太阳穴、大椎穴或头痛处，有止头痛之效。

5. Headache: For various types of headaches, take some fresh perilla leaves, put them in a teacup, and steep with boiling water. After 2-5 minutes, take out the leaves, let the excess water drip off, and apply them to the Taiyang acupoint, Dazhui acupoint, or the painful area. This has the effect of stopping headaches.

6. 虫伤：被虫蛾咬伤或受其毒皮肤发痒时，可用鲜紫苏叶捣烂，或用干紫苏叶研末，调少许食醋，敷于创面，可止痛止痒防感染。

6. Insect Bites: When bitten by insects or moths, or when the skin becomes

itchy due to their venom, mash fresh perilla leaves or grind dry perilla leaves into a powder, mix with a little edible vinegar, and apply to the wound. This can relieve pain and itching, and prevent infection.

7. 解毒：若因食鱼鳖而出现腹痛、呕吐、腹泻时，可立即取紫苏梗 30 克，生姜 15 克，煎水温服，有效。

7. Detoxification: If abdominal pain, vomiting, and diarrhea occur after eating fish or soft-shelled turtles, immediately take 30g of perilla stems and 15g of fresh ginger, decoct in water, and drink it warm. It is effective.

8. 防腐蛀：在腌制品中加适量紫苏梗细末，可防腐及防生虫；在泡菜罐中放几节紫苏梗，可防罐水生花，还可增味；在衣橱中放一些紫苏（用布包好），可防蛀；在冰箱中放紫苏，可除异味。

8. Preserving and Preventing Moths: Adding an appropriate amount of finely ground perilla stems to pickled products can prevent spoilage and insect infestation. Putting a few pieces of perilla stems in a pickle jar can prevent a white film from forming on the brine and enhance the flavor. Placing some perilla (wrapped in cloth) in a wardrobe can prevent moth damage. Putting perilla in the refrigerator can eliminate odors.

9. 止孕吐：妊娠呕吐不止，取鲜紫苏 20 克，或干紫苏 10 克，煎水加少许食糖服，有较好的止吐效果。

9. Stopping Morning Sickness: For persistent vomiting during pregnancy, take 20g of fresh perilla or 10g of dry perilla, decoct in water, add a little sugar, and drink. It has a good antiemetic effect.

（四川 陈永）

(Chen Yong, Sichuan)

二十四、柳枝的药用

24. Medicinal Uses of Willow Twigs (Liu-zhi)

柳树不仅是美化环境、供人观赏、用途广泛的优质树种，还是治疗疾病的良药。我国民间流传着不少用柳治病的有效验方，现介绍如下，供大家对症选用。

The willow tree is not only a high-quality tree species widely used for beautifying the environment and providing ornamental value, but also a good medicine for treating diseases. Many effective proven prescriptions using willow to treat diseases have been passed down among the Chinese people. They are introduced below for people to choose according to their symptoms.

1. 治急性膀胱炎：柳根须一把，血余炭（人发烧得炭）十克，水煎服。

Treating Acute Cystitis: Take a handful of willow rootlets and 10g of hair charcoal (carbonized human hair). Decoct in water to drink.

2. 治风火牙痛：柳枝嫩尖一把，栀子十克，大枣（去核）五枚，混合煎汤，兑白糖内服。

2. Treating Wind-Fire Toothache: Take a handful of tender willow twig tips, 10g of gardenia fruit (zhi-zi), and 5 pitted red dates. Boil them together in water, mix in white sugar, and take orally.

3. 治口舌生疮：细柳枝一段，剥去表面青皮，取中间白皮在口中嚼碎，咽下苦水，治口舌生疮，甚效。

3. Treating Mouth and Tongue Ulcers: Take a piece of thin willow twig, peel off the green outer bark, and chew the white inner bark in your mouth until crushed. Swallow the bitter juice. This is highly effective for treating mouth and tongue ulcers.

4. 治慢性气管炎：柳枝一百二十克切碎洗净，加水五百克，每日一次水煎服。

4. Treating Chronic Bronchitis: Take 120g of willow twigs, chop them into pieces, and wash them. Add 500g of water and decoct once a day.

5. 治小便白浊：取清明节前后的柳枝，煎汤代茶饮。

5. Treating Cloudy Urine: Take willow twigs gathered around the Qingming Festival, decoct them in water, and drink as a substitute for tea.

6. 治眉毛脱落、瘙痒：垂柳嫩叶适量，阴干，用姜汁在铁器中调和，涂敷患处。

6. Treating Eyebrow Loss and Itching: Take an appropriate amount of tender weeping willow leaves, shade-dry them, mix them with ginger juice in an iron

utensil, and apply the mixture to the affected area.

7. 治疗吐血：柳絮一百克，焙干研粉，每日三次，每次五克，温米汤送服。

7. Treating Hematemesis (Vomiting Blood): Take 100g of willow catkins, roast dry, and grind into a powder. Take 5g each time, 3 times a day, swallowed with warm rice soup.

8. 治黄水疮：柳条白皮适量，焙黄研面，香油调涂患处。

8. Treating Impetigo: Take an appropriate amount of white bark from willow twigs, roast until yellow, and grind into a powder. Mix with sesame oil and apply to the affected area.

9. 治风火烂眼：柳根须一百克，研粉，加面粉焙焦饼吃。

9. Treating Wind-Fire Conjunctivitis (Red Eyes): Take 100g of willow rootlets, grind into a powder, add flour, and bake into a scorched cake to eat.

10. 治关节炎：炒柳叶十克，炒柏叶十克，桂皮五克，水煎服。

10. Treating Arthritis: Take 10g of stir-fried willow leaves, 10g of stir-fried arborvitae leaves (bai-ye), and 5g of cinnamon bark (gui-pi). Decoct in water to drink.

《民族医药报》（孟庆荣）

Ethnic Medicine News (Meng Qingrong)

二十五、蜂蜜的药用

25. Medicinal Uses of Honey (Feng-mi)

蜂蜜治病，源远流长，作用甚广。东汉张仲景用治大便燥结，创蜜煎导法：而明代李时珍盛称其功，认为能补中，润燥、解毒、止痛、能清热、调和诸药，与甘草同功。据现代药理研究：蜂蜜含有东菌剂，抑制素，吸水性极强有利于水肿吸收，清洁伤口，组织修复。实验室培养表明：受绿脓杆菌，化脓球菌感染的伤口，经蜂蜜治疗一周后，从伤口拭子作细菌培养，没有微生物生长。随着人们的认识不断提高，更拓宽了蜂蜜运用范围。现仅就其在五官科疾病中的运用简介如下，以窥一斑

The use of honey to treat diseases has a long history and a wide range of applications. Zhang Zhongjing of the Eastern Han Dynasty used it to treat dry and hard stools, creating the honey enema method. Li Shizhen of the Ming Dynasty highly praised its effects, believing it can tonify the middle, moisten dryness, detoxify, relieve pain, clear heat, and harmonize various medicines, sharing the same merits as licorice root. Modern pharmacological studies show that honey contains antibacterial agents and inhibitors. Its strong water-absorbing property helps absorb edema, clean wounds, and promote tissue repair. Laboratory cultures show that wounds infected with Pseudomonas aeruginosa and pyogenic cocci, after one week of honey treatment, show no microbial growth in bacterial cultures from wound swabs. As people' s understanding continues to deepen, the scope of honey' s application has been further broadened. The following is a brief introduction to its application in ENT (Ear, Nose, and Throat) and ophthalmology diseases, just to give a glimpse:

1. 青光眼（高眼压期）：蜂蜜 100 克加开水约 300 毫升，搅拌至蜜融化，待温，一次饮下每日 1-2 次，糖尿病人禁用。

Glaucoma (High Intraocular Pressure Stage): Add 100g of honey to about 300ml of boiling water, stir until dissolved, wait until warm, and drink at once, 1-2 times a day. Contraindicated for diabetic patients.

2. 电光性眼炎：蜂蜜 50 克，盐酸可卡因 0. 5 克，盐酸麻黄素 0.5 克。滴眼，每日 3-4 次，每次 1-2 滴。

2. Photokeratitis (Electric Ophthalmia): Take 50g of honey, 0.5g of cocaine hydrochloride, and 0.5g of ephedrine hydrochloride. Use as eye drops, 3-4 times a day, 1-2 drops each time.

3. 急性结膜炎：用活蚂蝗 3 条，置 6 毫升生蜂蜜中 6 小时后，将浸出液倒入清洁瓶内每日滴眼 2 次，每次 1-2 滴。

3. Acute Conjunctivitis: Take 3 live leeches and place them in 6ml of raw honey. After 6 hours, pour the extract into a clean bottle. Use as eye drops 2 times a day, 1-2 drops each time.

4. 急性咽炎：取适量茶叶用纱布包好，置于杯中，用沸水泡出较浓的茶汁，待凉后加蜂蜜适量搅匀，每隔半小时用此液漱喉并咽下。

4. Acute Pharyngitis: Wrap an appropriate amount of tea leaves in gauze, place them in a cup, and steep with boiling water to make a strong tea. After it cools, add an appropriate amount of honey and stir well. Gargle the throat with this liquid and swallow it every half hour.

5. 化脓性中耳炎：生蜂蜜 6 毫升，另加胆矾、冰片少许，先用 3% 双氧水洗尽外耳道脓性分泌物，再用此液滴耳，每日 3 次，每次 2 滴，滴后头歪三分钟，以免药液流出，影响疗效。

5. Suppurative Otitis Media: Take 6ml of raw honey, and add a small amount of blue vitriol (dan-fan) and borneol (bing-pian). First, wash away the purulent secretions in the external auditory canal with 3% hydrogen peroxide, then use this liquid as ear drops, 3 times a day, 2 drops each time. After instilling the drops, tilt the head to one side for 3 minutes to prevent the liquid from flowing out and affecting the efficacy.

6. 萎缩性鼻炎：生蜂蜜 4 毫升，芝麻油 2 毫升，另加冰片少许，先清除鼻腔脓痂，再用其液滴鼻。每日 3 次，每次每侧 2 滴。

6. Atrophic Rhinitis: Take 4ml of raw honey, 2ml of sesame oil, and a small amount of borneol. First, clear the purulent crusts in the nasal cavity, then use this liquid as nasal drops. 3 times a day, 2 drops in each nostril each time.

《中医药信息报》1992 年 5 月 9 日（湖北洪湖市中医医院 郑运发）

Chinese Medicine Information News, May 9, 1992 (Zheng Yunfa, Honghu City Hospital of Traditional Chinese Medicine, Hubei Province)

二十六、薏米

26. Coix Seed (Yi-mi)

苡仁，即薏苡仁。又叫苡米、沟子米、薏珠子。本品既可食用，又可入药。其性味甘淡微寒，入脾、胃、肺、大肠经，具有清热排脓，健脾除湿之功效，以苡仁为主组成的偏方较多，治病也广。现选十款介绍如下。

Coix seed, also known as Yi-ren, Yi-mi, Gouzi-mi, and Yi-zhu-zi. It can be used both as food and as medicine. It is sweet and bland in flavor, slightly cold in property, and enters the Spleen, Stomach, Lung, and Large Intestine meridians. It has the effects of clearing heat and expelling pus, strengthening the spleen, and removing dampness. There are many folk remedies mainly composed of coix seed, and it is widely used to treat various diseases. Ten of them are selected and introduced below.

1. 治肺痈：用苡仁 60 克，冬瓜子 30 克，苇茎 15 克，桃仁 12 克，水煎，分 3 次服，服 10 剂。

Treating Pulmonary Abscess: Take 60g of coix seed, 30g of winter melon seeds, 15g of reed stems, and 12g of peach seeds. Decoct in water, divide into 3 doses, and take 10 doses in total.

2. 治急性阑尾炎：用苡仁、银花藤各 30 克，瓜蒌仁 15 克，桃仁 12 克，水煎，分 2-3 次服，以愈为度。

2. Treating Acute Appendicitis: Take 30g each of coix seed and honeysuckle stem, 15g of trichosanthes seeds, and 12g of peach seeds. Decoct in water, divide into 2-3 doses, continuing until cured.

3. 治慢性肾炎：用生黄芪 18 克，苡仁、炙龟板各 60 克。先将龟板捣碎煮 1 小时，再入余药煎 1 小时，分 2 次服，久服。

3. Treating Chronic Nephritis: Take 18g of raw astragalus root (huang-qi), and 60g each of coix seed and honey-fried tortoise shell. First, crush the tortoise shell and boil it for 1 hour, then add the remaining herbs and decoct for another 1 hour. Divide into 2 doses and take it continuously for a long period.

4. 治传染性肝炎：用苡仁 60 克，苡仁根 45 克，水煎，分 3 次服，服半月有效。

4. Treating Infectious Hepatitis: Take 60g of coix seed and 45g of coix seed root. Decoct in water, divide into 3 doses. It will be effective after taking it for half a month.

5. 治腰腿痛：用苡仁、黄芪各 60 克，核桃树皮 30 克，水煎，分 2 次服，服时加白酒少许。3 剂即效。

5. Treating Lower Back and Leg Pain: Take 60g each of coix seed and astragalus root, and 30g of walnut tree bark. Decoct in water, divide into 2 doses, and add a little liquor when taking. It will be effective after 3 doses.

6. 治白带过多：用苡仁 50 克，苍术 15 克，黄柏 12 克，车前子 9 克，水煎，分 2 次服，连服 1-2 周。

6. Treating Excessive Leucorrhea: Take 50g of coix seed, 15g of atractylodes rhizome (cang-zhu), 12g of phellodendron bark (huang-bai), and 9g of plantain seeds (che-qian-zi). Decoct in water, divide into 2 doses, and take continuously for 1-2 weeks.

7. 治烦渴引饮者：用苡仁煮粥食，久服必验。

7. Treating Restlessness, Thirst, and Excessive Drinking: Boil coix seed into porridge and eat it. Long-term consumption will definitely be effective.

8. 治乳糜尿：用苡仁 30 克，厚朴、茯苓各 15 克，鹅不食草 12 克，水煎，分 2 次服，连服 1 月。

8. Treating Chyluria: Take 30g of coix seed, 15g each of magnolia bark (hou-po) and poria (fu-ling), and 12g of small centipeda (e-bu-shi-cao). Decoct in water, divide into 2 doses, and take continuously for 1 month.

9. 治风湿身痛：用苡仁 60 克，桑枝 30 克，水煎，分 2 次服。

9. Treating Rheumatic Body Pain: Take 60g of coix seed and 30g of mulberry twigs (sang-zhi). Decoct in water, divide into 2 doses.

10. 治沙石热淋：用淋：用苡仁、苡仁根、苡仁叶各 45 克，水煎分 3 次服，其效甚佳。

10. Treating Heat Strangury with Sand and Stones: Take 45g each of coix seed, coix seed root, and coix seed leaves. Decoct in water, divide into 3 doses. The effect is excellent.

《民族医药报》1992 年 9 月 11 日（四川 陈国华）

Ethnic Medicine News, September 11, 1992 (Chen Guohua, Sichuan)

二十七、西瓜的药用

27. Medicinal Uses of Watermelon (Xi-gua)

1. 治急、慢性肾炎：取全西瓜洗净切碎，浓煮成膏状，每日以开水调服两汤匙，连服一个月为一个疗程。

Treating Acute and Chronic Nephritis: Wash a whole watermelon, chop it into pieces, and boil it down into a thick paste. Mix 2 tablespoons of it with boiling water and drink daily. Taking it continuously for one month constitutes one course of treatment.

2. 治糖尿病口渴：取西瓜皮、冬瓜皮各 20 克，天花粉 15 克。水煎服，每日一剂，连服 10-15 天。

2. Treating Thirst in Diabetes: Take 20g each of watermelon rind and winter melon rind, and 15g of trichosanthes root (tian-hua-fen). Decoct in water to drink, 1 dose a day, continuously for 10-15 days.

3. 治高血压：取西瓜皮 30 克，决明子 15 克，煎汤代茶饮，每日一剂，连服 10-15 天。

3. Treating Hypertension: Take 30g of watermelon rind and 15g of cassia seeds (jue-ming-zi). Decoct in water and drink as a substitute for tea, 1 dose a day, continuously for 10-15 days.

4. 治夏季感冒发热，口渴，烦躁，食欲不振：先将西瓜取瓤，去籽，用洁净纱布绞挤汁液，再将番茄用沸水冲烫、剥皮、去籽，用纱布绞挤汁液，然后二液混合，制成西瓜番茄汁，随量饮用。每日三次，一般连饮 3-5 次可愈。

4. Treating Summer Cold with Fever, Thirst, Restlessness, and Loss of Appetite: First, scoop out the watermelon flesh, remove the seeds, and squeeze out the juice with clean gauze. Then, scald tomatoes with boiling water, peel and deseed them, and squeeze out the juice with gauze. Mix the two juices to make watermelon-tomato juice, and drink as much as desired. Drink 3 times a day; it can generally be cured after drinking 3-5 times continuously.

5. 治目赤、口疮及热病消渴：先将西瓜取瓤去籽，切成条，曝晒成干，再加入白糖少许即可，制成糖渍西瓜肉，随量食用，每日三次，一般5-7次可愈。

5. Treating Red Eyes, Mouth Ulcers, and Thirst due to Febrile Diseases: First, scoop out the watermelon flesh, remove the seeds, cut into strips, and sun-dry them. Then, add a little white sugar to make candied watermelon flesh. Eat as much as desired, 3 times a day; it can generally be cured after 5-7 times.

6. 治水肿、小便不利：先将西瓜取瓤，去籽，用洁净纱布绞挤汁液，先以武火，后以文火煎煮成膏，停火冷却，加入白糖适量将汁膏混匀，晒干，再压碎，装瓶备用。每次15克，以沸水冲化，制成西瓜速溶饮，每日饮三次。

6. Treating Edema and Dysuria: First, scoop out the watermelon flesh, remove the seeds, and squeeze out the juice with clean gauze. Boil it over high heat first, then over low heat until it becomes a paste. Remove from heat, let it cool, add an appropriate amount of white sugar, and mix well. Sun-dry it, crush it, and store it in a bottle for later use. Take 15g each time, dissolve it in boiling water to make instant watermelon drink, and drink 3 times a day.

7. 治风火牙痛：取经日晒夜露的西瓜皮适量，研成细末，以少许涂擦风火牙痛处，疗效甚佳。

7. Treating Wind-Fire Toothache: Take an appropriate amount of watermelon rind that has been exposed to the sun by day and dew by night, grind it into a fine powder, and apply a small amount to the painful area. The effect is excellent.

8. 治烫伤：取西瓜皮晒干烧灰，加冰片少许，研成细末混匀，用菜油适量调敷。

8. Treating Scalds and Burns: Sun-dry watermelon rinds and burn them into ash. Add a little borneol (bing-pian), grind into a fine powder, and mix well. Mix with an appropriate amount of rapeseed oil and apply to the affected area.

9. 醉酒：饮西瓜汁一碗有醒酒的功效。

9. Drunkenness: Drinking a bowl of watermelon juice has the effect of sobering up.

10. 咽喉肿痛：取西瓜皮适量，加水两碗煎成一碗，代茶饮，有较好的疗效。

10. Sore and Swollen Throat: Take an appropriate amount of watermelon rind, add 2 bowls of water, and decoct to 1 bowl. Drink it as a substitute for tea. It

has a good therapeutic effect.

《中药科技报》1992 年 6 月 26 日（李子云）

Chinese Medicine Science and Technology News, June 26, 1992 (Li Ziyun)

二十八、虎耳草的药用

28. Medicinal Uses of Saxifrage (Hu-er-cao)

虎耳草为虎耳草科植物虎耳草的全草内服，煎汤，9-15 克。外用：捣汁液或煎水熏洗。

Saxifrage is the whole plant of Saxifraga stolonifera (Saxifragaceae). For internal use, decoct 9-15g in water. For external use, mash to extract the juice or decoct in water for fumigation and washing.

处方：

Prescriptions:

1. 治中耳炎：取鲜虎耳草捣汁滴入耳内。

Treating Otitis Media: Mash fresh saxifrage to extract the juice and drop it into the ear.

2. 治化脓性中耳炎：取虎耳草鲜叶数片，捣汁，纱布滤过，加入适量冰片，装入滴眼瓶中备用。用时先用百分之三双氧水洗涤外耳道，将脓性分泌物清除干净。然后取虎耳草液滴耳，每次一至二滴，每日三次，疗效显著。

2. Treating Suppurative Otitis Media: Take several fresh saxifrage leaves, mash to extract the juice, filter through gauze, add an appropriate amount of borneol (bing-pian), and store in an eye-drop bottle for later use. When using, first wash the external auditory canal with 3% hydrogen peroxide to completely remove purulent secretions. Then, drop the saxifrage liquid into the ear, 1-2 drops each time, 3 times a day. The effect is significant.

3. 治荨麻疹：虎耳草、青黛煎服。

3. Treating Urticaria: Decoct saxifrage and natural indigo (qing-dai) in water to drink.

4. 治风丹热毒、风火牙痛：鲜虎耳草一两，水煎服。

4. Treating Wind-Dan Heat Toxin and Wind-Fire Toothache: Take 30g (one liang) of fresh saxifrage, decoct in water to drink.

5. 治湿疹、皮肤瘙痒：鲜虎耳草一斤，切碎，加百分之九十五酒精拌湿，再加百分之三十酒精一千毫升浸泡一周，去渣，外敷患处。

5. Treating Eczema and Skin Pruritus: Take 500g (one jin) of fresh saxifrage, chop it into pieces, add 95% alcohol to moisten it, then add 1000ml of 30% alcohol and soak for one week. Remove the residue and apply externally to the affected area.

6. 治风疹瘙痒、湿疹：鲜虎耳草十五至三十克。煎服。

6. Treating Rubella Pruritus and Eczema: Take 15-30g of fresh saxifrage, decoct in water to drink.

7. 治肺热咳嗽气逆：虎耳草九至十八克，冰糖十五克，水煎服。

7. Treating Lung-Heat Cough with Panting: Take 9-18g of saxifrage and 15g of rock sugar, decoct in water to drink.

8. 治百日咳：虎耳草三至九克，冰糖九克，煎服。

8. Treating Whooping Cough: Take 3-9g of saxifrage and 9g of rock sugar, decoct in water to drink.

9. 治肺痈吐臭脓：虎耳草十二克，忍冬叶三十克。水煎二次，分服。

9. Treating Pulmonary Abscess with Foul-Smelling Pus: Take 12g of saxifrage and 30g of honeysuckle leaves. Decoct in water twice, divide into portions, and drink.

10. 治吐血：虎耳草十克，瘦猪肉四两。混同剁烂，做成肉饼，加水蒸熟食。

11. Treating Hematemesis (Vomiting Blood): Take 10g of saxifrage and 120g (four liang) of lean pork. Chop them together into a mince, make into a meat patty, add water, and steam until cooked to eat.

11. 治血崩：鲜虎耳草三十克至六十克，加黄酒、水各半煎服。

11. Treating Metrorrhagia (Uterine Bleeding): Take 30-60g of fresh saxifrage, add half yellow rice wine and half water, and decoct to drink.

12. 治痔疮：虎耳草三十克，水煎，加食盐少许，放罐内，坐熏，一日二次。

12. Treating Hemorrhoids: Take 30g of saxifrage, decoct in water, add a little salt, pour into a pot, and sit over it for fumigation, twice a day.

13. 治冻疮溃烂：鲜虎耳草叶捣烂敷患处。

13. Treating Ulcerated Chilblains: Mash fresh saxifrage leaves and apply to the affected area.

《中药科技报》1993 年 1 月 14 日（湖北 刘金茂）

Chinese Medicine Science and Technology News, January 14, 1993 (Liu Jinmao, Hubei)

二十九、荸荠的药用
29. Medicinal Uses of Water Chestnut (Bi-qi)

荸荠，又名马蹄、地栗、乌芋。性味甘微寒，具有清热利胆，化痰消积，开胃化食，解铜毒，降血压之功效。中医古籍《本草备药》一书中说："荸荠甘微寒滑，益气安中，开胃消食、除胸中实热、治五种噎嗝、消渴、黄疸、血症、蛊毒、能毁铜。"据现代药理分析，荸荠中含有丰富的淀粉，还含有蛋白质、钙、磷、铁和维生素 A、B1、B2、C 等多种成分。近年来还发现荸荠种含有抑菌、抗癌、降低血压的有效成分。其抗菌成分——荸荠英，对金黄色葡萄球菌、大肠杆菌等有抑制作用。笔者在临床上常用荸荠治病。疗效颇佳，现介绍如下。

Water chestnut, also known as Ma-ti, Di-piao, and Wu-yu. It is sweet in flavor, slightly cold in property, and has the effects of clearing heat and benefiting the gallbladder, resolving phlegm and relieving food retention, invigorating the stomach and aiding digestion, detoxifying copper, and lowering blood pressure. The ancient TCM book Bencao Beiyao states: "Water chestnut is sweet, slightly cold, and slippery. It tonifies qi, harmonizes the middle, invigorates the stomach and relieves food retention, clears excess heat in the chest, treats five types of dysphagia, diabetes, jaundice, blood diseases, parasitic toxins, and can destroy copper." Modern pharmacological analysis shows that water chestnut is rich in starch and also contains protein, calcium, phosphorus, iron, and various vitamins such as A, B1, B2, and C. In recent years, it has also been found to contain effective components with antibacterial, anti-cancer, and blood-pressure-lowering properties. Its antibacterial component, puchiin, has an inhibitory effect on Staphylococcus aureus, Escherichia coli, etc. The author frequently uses water chestnut to treat diseases in clinical practice with good efficacy. The following are introduced below.

1. 治黄疸湿热，小便不利（急慢性胆囊炎、胆石症、肝炎）：用荸荠适量，洗净切片，煎水代茶饮服。

Treating Jaundice with Damp-Heat and Dysuria (Acute and Chronic Cholecystitis, Cholelithiasis, Hepatitis): Take an appropriate amount of water chestnuts, wash, slice, decoct in water, and drink as a substitute for tea.

2. 治尿路结石，小便不畅，尿道刺痛：用荸荠五百克，冬瓜皮、芥菜各一百克，洗净切片，煎水代茶饮服。

2. Treating Urinary Stones, Poor Urination, and Urethral Stinging Pain: Take 500g of water chestnuts, 100g each of winter melon rind and mustard greens. Wash, slice, decoct in water, and drink as a substitute for tea.

3. 治小儿麻疹透发不快：用荸荠一百克，洗净切片，西河柳十五克，水煎，分二次服。

3. Treating Poor Eruption of Measles in Children: Take 100g of water chestnuts, wash, slice, and add 15g of tamarisk twigs (xi-he-liu). Decoct in water, divide into 2 doses, and drink.

4. 治流鼻血：用荸荠二百五十克，生藕一百五十克，白萝卜一百克，洗净切片，煎水代茶饮服。

4. Treating Epistaxis (Nosebleed): Take 250g of water chestnuts, 150g of fresh lotus root, and 100g of white radish. Wash, slice, decoct in water, and drink as a substitute for tea.

5. 治咽喉肿痛：用荸荠一百五十克，洗净去皮绞汁频服。

5. Treating Sore and Swollen Throat: Take 150g of water chestnuts, wash, peel, squeeze out the juice, and drink frequently.

6. 治高血压：用荸荠一百克，洗净切片，海蜇皮六十克，浸洗去盐，煎汤，每日服二次。

6. Treating Hypertension: Take 100g of water chestnuts, wash, slice, and add 60g of jellyfish skin. Soak and wash to remove the salt, decoct in water to make a soup, and drink twice a day.

7. 治痔疮出血：用荸荠五百克，洗净打碎，加入红糖一百五十克，煎煮一小时，饮汤，每日一次，一般连服三天可愈。

7. Treating Hemorrhoidal Bleeding: Take 500g of water chestnuts, wash, crush, add 150g of brown sugar, and boil for one hour. Drink the soup once a day. It can generally be cured after taking it continuously for three days.

8. 治妇女乳头裂痛：用荸荠五枚，洗净去皮捣汁，涂擦患处。如在汁中加入冰片少许调敷，止痛效果更佳。

8. Treating Cracked and Painful Nipples in Women: Take 5 water chestnuts, wash, peel, mash to extract the juice, and apply to the affected area. If a small amount of borneol (bing-pian) is added to the juice and applied, the analgesic effect is even better.

（李子云）

(Li Ziyun)

三十、荷叶
30. Lotus Leaf (He-ye)

荷叶，来源于睡莲科植物莲的叶，性平，味苦、涩，具有清暑利湿、升发清阳，止血等功效。现辑验方六则，供临症选用。

Lotus leaf comes from the leaves of the lotus plant (Nymphaeaceae). It is neutral in property, and bitter and astringent in flavor. It has the effects of clearing summer heat and promoting diuresis, raising clear yang, and stopping bleeding. Six proven prescriptions are compiled here for clinical use.

1. 减肥：取干荷叶 20 克或鲜荷叶 50 克左右，切成丝或块放入茶杯中，用开水冲泡代茶饮，至味淡为止。

Weight Loss: Take 20g of dried lotus leaves or about 50g of fresh lotus leaves, cut them into shreds or pieces, and put them in a teacup. Steep with boiling water and drink as a substitute for tea until the flavor becomes light.

2. 防治小儿痱子：取干荷叶 10-20 克或鲜荷叶 30 克，加绿豆 50 克，加水熬汤，常给小儿饮用。

2. Preventing and Treating Prickly Heat in Children: Take 10-20g of dried lotus leaves or 30g of fresh lotus leaves, add 50g of mung beans, and boil in water to make a soup. Give it to children to drink regularly.

3. 止血：外伤出血时取本品适量烧炭存性或焙干研粉，敷于出血处，包好，可止血。鼻衄、咯血、便血、牙龈出血等出血症可配合艾叶、生地、侧柏叶同用。

3. Stopping Bleeding: For traumatic bleeding, take an appropriate amount of this product, burn it into charcoal (carbonize it without burning it to ash) or bake it dry, grind into a powder, apply it to the bleeding site, and bandage it to stop the bleeding. For epistaxis, hemoptysis, hematochezia, and bleeding gums, it can be used in combination with mugwort leaves (ai-ye), rehmannia root (sheng-di), and arborvitae leaves (ce-bai-ye).

4. 治梦遗滑精：荷叶 30 克研末。每次服 3 克，早晚各服 1 次，热米汤送服。

4. Treating Nocturnal Emission and Spermatorrhea: Grind 30g of lotus leaves into a powder. Take 3g each time, once in the morning and once at night, swallowed with warm rice soup.

5. 止泻：用 10-20 克干荷叶煮汤饮或煮粥吃，有止泻作用。

5. Stopping Diarrhea: Boil 10-20g of dried lotus leaves in water to make a soup to drink, or cook it into porridge to eat. It has the effect of stopping diarrhea.

6. 防治中暑：取荷叶焙干研粉，调入稀粥中，加适量冰糖食用。也可采摘鲜荷叶洗净后撕成粗片放入粥中同煮，或整张荷叶当锅盖盖在粥上熬。用于因感受暑热而出现的头胀、头晕、胸闷、口渴、小便短赤等症。

6. Preventing and Treating Heatstroke: Bake lotus leaves dry, grind into a powder, mix it into thin porridge, and add an appropriate amount of rock sugar to

eat. Alternatively, pick fresh lotus leaves, wash them, tear them into coarse pieces, and cook them together with the porridge; or use a whole lotus leaf as a lid to cover the porridge while boiling. It is used for symptoms caused by summer heat, such as head swelling, dizziness, chest tightness, thirst, and short, dark urine.

《民族医药报》（魏永泉）

Ethnic Medicine News (Wei Yongquan)

三十一、鸡内金

31. Chicken Gizzard Lining (Ji-nei-jin)

1. 治小儿消化不良：鸡内金炒焦研粉，取 1 克加奶粉、红糖少许，开水冲服，每日二次。

Treating Pediatric Indigestion: Stir-fry chicken gizzard lining until scorched and grind into a powder. Take 1g, add a little milk powder and brown sugar, steep with boiling water to drink, twice a day.

2. 治小儿营养不良：取鸡内金 10 克，红薯叶 30 克，将红薯叶洗净后加鸡内金煎汤，调味服。

2. Treating Pediatric Malnutrition: Take 10g of chicken gizzard lining and 30g of sweet potato leaves. Wash the sweet potato leaves, add the chicken gizzard lining, and decoct in water to make a soup. Season and drink.

3. 治小儿遗尿：鸡内金 10 个，鸡肠 1 副（洗净），炙后研末，每次服 3-6 克，每日 3 次，饭后服，或取鸡内金 10 克，桑螵蛸 10 克，水煎后服汤。

3. Treating Pediatric Enuresis (Bedwetting): Take 10 chicken gizzard linings and 1 set of chicken intestines (washed). Roast them, grind into a powder, take 3-6g each time, 3 times a day, after meals. Alternatively, take 10g of chicken gizzard lining and 10g of mantis egg cases (sang-piao-xiao), decoct in water, and drink the soup.

4. 治小儿流涎：取鸡内金 1 克，穿山甲 0.1 克，鸡蛋 1 个。在鸡蛋大头处打一小孔备用。将内金、山甲烘干研末，装入鸡蛋内搅匀，用纸糊住鸡蛋小孔，立在饭上蒸热。每日吃 3 次，一般 5-7 天可愈。

4. Treating Pediatric Drooling: Take 1g of chicken gizzard lining, 0.1g of pangolin scales (chuan-shan-jia), and 1 egg. Make a small hole at the larger end of the egg for later use. Dry and grind the gizzard lining and pangolin scales into a powder, put them into the egg, and stir well. Seal the small hole with paper, stand the egg upright on top of rice, and steam it. Eat 3 times a day; it can generally be cured in 5-7 days.

5. 治慢性肠炎、腹泻：炒鸡内金、炒白术各 90 克，研末，每次 6 克，每日 2 次。

5. Treating Chronic Enteritis and Diarrhea: Take 90g each of stir-fried chicken gizzard lining and stir-fried atractylodes macrocephala (bai-zhu). Grind into a powder, take 6g each time, twice a day.

6. 治食积腹胀：取麦芽 15 克，莱菔子 8 克，鸡内金 10 克。加水煮汤，调味服。

6. Treating Food Retention and Abdominal Distension: Take 15g of malt (mai-ya), 8g of radish seeds (lai-fu-zi), and 10g of chicken gizzard lining. Boil in water to make a soup, season, and drink.

7. 治遗精：鸡内金 18 克，炒干后研末，每次 3 克，每日早晚各服一次，睡前可冲热黄酒半杯，加入药，温开水送服。

7. Treating Spermatorrhea: Take 18g of chicken gizzard lining, stir-fry dry, and grind into a powder. Take 3g each time, once in the morning and once at night. Before going to bed, you can steep half a cup of warm yellow rice wine, add the powder, and swallow it with warm water.

8. 治反胃呕吐：鸡内金炒焦研末，酒冲服，每次 3 克。

8. Treating Regurgitation and Vomiting: Stir-fry chicken gizzard lining until scorched, grind into a powder, and steep with wine to drink, 3g each time.

9. 治痉夏：用鸡内金粉装胶囊，早中晚各 2 粒，车前草 30 克，煎汤送服。

9. Treating Summer Spasm: Put chicken gizzard lining powder into capsules, take 2 capsules in the morning, noon, and evening, and use 30g of plantain (che-qian-cao) decocted in water as a soup to swallow the capsules.

10. 治骨结核、肠结核：鸡内金炒焦研末，每次 9 克，日服 3 次，空腹温酒送下。

10. Treating Bone Tuberculosis and Intestinal Tuberculosis: Stir-fry chicken gizzard lining until scorched, grind into a powder, take 9g each time, 3 times a day, swallowed with warm wine on an empty stomach.

《中药科技报》1992 年 7 月 26 日（郑俊芝）

Chinese Medicine Science and Technology News, July 26, 1992 (Zheng Junzhi)

三十二、百草霜

32. Stove Soot (Bai-cao-shuang)

百草霜，俗名锅底墨。即柴草燃烧积在锅底的墨状物质。黔东北务川一带的仡佬族群众善用它治多种疾病。

Stove soot, commonly known as "pot-bottom ink," is an ink-like substance accumulated at the bottom of a pot from burning firewood and grass. The Gelao ethnic people in the Wuchuan area of northeastern Guizhou are good at using it to treat various diseases.

1. 吐血、咯血：百草霜 10 克，调米汤服，很快可止血。用量可视病情而定。

Hematemesis and Hemoptysis (Vomiting and Coughing up Blood): Take 10g of stove soot, mix it with rice soup, and take it. It can stop bleeding quickly. The dosage can be adjusted according to the condition.

2. 妇女崩漏：百草霜 15 克，槐花（炒焦研末）50 克，二味混合，白酒冲服，一服即止。宜再服 2-5 次，以稳定疗效。

2. Metrorrhagia and Uterine Bleeding: Take 15g of stove soot and 50g of sophora flowers (stir-fried until scorched and ground into powder). Mix the two ingredients, steep with liquor to drink, and it will stop bleeding after one dose. It is advisable to take it 2-5 more times to stabilize the effect.

3. 产后大出血：百草霜 20 克，赭石粉 2 克，二药研末开水冲服。

3. Postpartum Hemorrhage: Take 20g of stove soot and 2g of ochre powder. Grind both into a powder and steep with boiling water to drink.

4. 胃痛：百草霜 10 克，儿童小便冲服即愈。

4. Stomachache: Take 10g of stove soot and steep it with children’s urine to drink. It will be cured.

5. 痢疾腹痛：百草霜 10 克，白酒冲服，1 日 3 次。

5. Dysentery and Abdominal Pain: Take 10g of stove soot, steep with liquor to drink, 3 times a day.

6. 咳嗽痰稀薄：百草霜 5 克，桃树脂 150 克，烘干为末，二味混合，蜜调服。1 日 3 次，连服数日可愈。愈后宜再服 15 日，以巩固疗效。

6. Cough with Thin Phlegm: Take 5g of stove soot and 150g of peach resin. Dry and grind into a powder, mix the two ingredients, and blend with honey to take. Take it 3 times a day for several days to be cured. After recovery, it is advisable to take it for another 15 days to consolidate the effect.

7. 跌打肿痛：百草霜 15 克，白酒冲服，1 日 3 次，7 日可愈。

7. Swelling and Pain from Falls and Blows: Take 15g of stove soot, steep with liquor to drink, 3 times a day. It can be cured in 7 days.

8. 口疮、喉痛：百草霜 0.5 克，含于口中 10-20 分钟，几次可愈。

8. Mouth Ulcers and Sore Throat: Take 0.5g of stove soot, hold it in the mouth for 10-20 minutes. It can be cured after a few times.

9. 创伤小出血：百草霜适量，撒于伤口，按压片刻即止。大出血无效。

9. Minor Bleeding from Wounds: Take an appropriate amount of stove soot, sprinkle it on the wound, and press for a moment to stop the bleeding. It is ineffective for massive bleeding.

注意事项：一定要取草木燃烧形成的百草霜。服药前后不宜喝浓茶。

Precautions: You must use stove soot formed by burning plants. Drinking strong tea before and after taking the medicine is not advisable.

《民族医药报》（贵州 谢众力 谢草芳）

Ethnic Medicine News (Xie Zhongli, Xie Caofang, Guizhou)

三十三、芋头
33. Taro (Yu-tou)

1. 淋巴结核：芋头粉，加入适量生姜汁烘热，用水做成绿豆大小的药丸。每服 9 克，日 3 次，用海蜇皮、荸荠煎汤送服。

Scrofula (Tuberculous Lymphadenitis): Take taro powder, add an appropriate amount of ginger juice, and heat it. Use water to make pills the size of mung beans. Take 9g each time, 3 times a day, swallowed with a soup decocted from jellyfish skin and water chestnuts.

2. 慢性胃痛：嫩芋头切片，拌上白糖佐饭适量服食。

2. Chronic Stomachache: Slice tender taro, mix it with white sugar, and eat an appropriate amount as a side dish with rice.

3. 慢性肾炎：鲜芋头 1000 克，红糖 250 克。芋头洗净切片，放锅炒成炭，研末，与红糖拌匀，1 日 3 次，每服 30-50 克。

3. Chronic Nephritis: Take 1000g of fresh taro and 250g of brown sugar. Wash and slice the taro, stir-fry it in a pan until carbonized, and grind into a powder. Mix evenly with brown sugar. Take 30-50g each time, 3 times a day.

4. 火烫伤未破：可将鲜芋头捣烂敷患处。

4. Unbroken Burns and Scalds: Mash fresh taro and apply it to the affected area.

5. 跌打损伤、扭伤、腰肌劳损、腰痛、肢体关节痛等：鲜芋头、生姜各适量，捣烂，再以适量面粉拌匀，制成芋姜糊外敷患处。1 日 2 次。

5. Falls, Blows, Sprains, Lumbar Muscle Strain, Lower Back Pain, and Joint Pain: Take an appropriate amount of fresh taro and ginger, mash them, and mix evenly with an appropriate amount of flour to make a taro-ginger paste. Apply it externally to the affected area, twice a day.

6. 大便秘结：鲜芋头 200 克，剥皮切块，加大米 50 克及油盐适量，煲粥服食。

6. Severe Constipation: Take 200g of fresh taro, peel and cut into pieces, add

50g of rice and an appropriate amount of oil and salt, and cook into porridge to eat.

7. 牛皮癣：芋头、大蒜各适量，共捣烂如泥敷患处。

7. Psoriasis: Take an appropriate amount of taro and garlic, mash them together into a mud-like paste, and apply to the affected area.

8. 毒虫蜇伤：鲜芋叶捣烂敷患处。

8. Venomous Insect Stings: Mash fresh taro leaves and apply to the affected area.

9. 吐血：芋头花 30 克，炖猪肉服食。

9. Hematemesis (Vomiting Blood): Take 30g of taro flowers, stew them with pork, and eat.

10. 子宫脱垂、小儿脱肛：鲜芋头花 6 朵与陈腊肉炖服。

10. Uterine Prolapse and Pediatric Rectal Prolapse: Take 6 fresh taro flowers and stew them with aged cured meat to eat.

11. 荨麻疹：芋头干茎 60 克，洗净，酌量配猪排骨炖服。

11. Urticaria: Take 60g of dried taro stems, wash them, and stew them with an appropriate amount of pork ribs to eat.

12. 脾胃虚弱、虚劳乏力：鲜芋头 250 克，鲫鱼或鲤鱼 500 克，加水同煮至烂熟，放调味料服食。

12. Spleen and Stomach Deficiency, and Debility from Overwork: Take 250g of fresh taro and 500g of crucian carp or common carp. Boil them together in water until soft and thoroughly cooked, add seasonings, and eat.

《民族医药报》（李俊杰）

Ethnic Medicine News (Li Junjie)

三十四、苦参

34. Sophora flavescens

苦参，味苦，性寒，功能清热凉血，燥湿杀虫，多用于医治热毒血痢、肠风下血等。近来，在临床上依其作用，应用于皮肤诸病，效果良好兹介绍数方，供参考使用。

Sophora flavescens (Ku Shen) has a bitter taste and a cold nature. Its functions include clearing heat, cooling the blood, drying dampness, and killing parasites. It is frequently used to treat conditions such as toxic-heat dysentery with bloody stools and intestinal wind with bloody stools. Recently, based on its pharmacological effects, it has been successfully applied in clinical practice to treat various skin diseases. Here are a few prescriptions for reference:

1. 治面黑粉刺：苦参 500 克，赤芍药、冬瓜仁各 120 克，玄参 60 克。共为细粉，每天早晚取少许搽面，也可用蛋清调敷。

1. For dark facial complexion and acne:Take 500g of Sophora flavescens, 120g each of Paeonia lactiflora (Chi Shao) and winter melon seeds, and 60g of Scrophularia ningpoensis (Xuan Shen). Grind them together into a fine powder. Apply a small amount to the face every morning and evening. Alternatively, it can be mixed with egg white to form a facial mask.

2. 治白癜风：苦参 1500 克、露蜂房、松香、附子、防风各 90 克，栀子仁 150 克，乌蛇脯 120 克，木兰皮 60 克。捣研为末，每服一匙，以温酒调下。宜常吃萝卜菜，勿食鸡肉、猪肉、冷水、热面、生菜。

2. For vitiligo:Take 1500g of Sophora flavescens, 90g each of Polistes japonicus (Lu Feng Fang), rosin, Aconitum carmichaelii (Zhi Fu Zi), and Saposhnikovia divaricata (Fang Feng), 150g of gardenia seeds (Zhi Zi Ren), 120g of dried black snake meat (Wu She Fu), and 60g of magnolia bark (Mu Lan Pi). Pound and grind these into a fine powder. Take one spoonful per dose, mixed with warm wine.Dietary advice: It is advisable to regularly consume radish greens. Avoid eating chicken, pork, cold water, hot noodles, and raw vegetables.

3. 治酒渣鼻：苦参 120 克，当归 60 克，用酒糊丸，如梧桐子大，每服八九十丸，食后热茶送服。

3. For rosacea:Take 120g of Sophora flavescens and 60g of Angelica sinensis (Dang Gui). Make them into pills the size of Chinese parasol tree seeds using wine and starch paste. Take 80 to 90 pills per dose after meals, washed down with hot tea.

4. 治麻疯病：苦参 750 克，生地黄 300 克，乳香 15 克，丹砂 35 克，共研匀，过筛，炼蜜为丸，如梧桐子大。每日空腹夜卧前以温水下 20 丸，渐加至 30 丸。

4. For leprosy:Take 750g of Sophora flavescens, 300g of fresh Rehmannia glutinosa (Sheng Di Huang), 15g of frankincense (Ru Xiang), and 35g of cinnabar (Dan Sha). Grind them evenly, sift the powder, and refine with honey to make pills the size of Chinese parasol tree seeds. Take 20 pills on an empty stomach before bedtime with warm water. Gradually increase the dosage to 30 pills.

5. 治扁平疣：用苦参、板蓝根，大青叶、鱼腥草各 30 克，桃仁、红花各 10 克，每日 1 剂，煎汤取浓汁分 2 次治疗，用棉球蘸药液反复敷搽患处，每次 15-20 分钟；然后取冰片、玄明粉各 10 克研极细末，适量加水调成糊状，反复搽患处 15-20 分钟，5 日 1 疗程。

5. For flat warts:Take 30g each of Sophora flavescens, Isatis indigotica (Ban Lan Gen), Isatis tinctoria (Da Qing Ye), and Houttuynia cordata (Yu Xing Cao), and 10g each of peach kernels (Tao Ren) and safflower (Hong Hua). Take one dose daily, decocted into a concentrated liquid and divided into two treatments. Soak a cotton ball in the liquid and repeatedly apply it to the affected area for 15-20 minutes. Then, grind 10g each of borneol (Bing Pian) and mirabilite (Xuan Ming Fen) into an extremely fine powder, add an appropriate amount of water to form a paste, and repeatedly apply it to the affected area for 15-20 minutes. A course of treatment lasts 5 days.

6. 治白发、头痒：苦参 15 克，青黛 30 克，生盐 30 克，共煎汤，沐浴头发，保留 20 分钟后再洗去。

6. For premature gray hair and itchy scalp:Take 15g of Sophora flavescens, 30g of natural indigo (Qing Dai), and 30g of raw salt. Decoct them in water to make a herbal bath for the hair. Leave it on for 20 minutes before washing it off.

《中医药信息报》1993 年 12 月 11 日（宁在兰）

Source: December 11, 1993, China Traditional Chinese Medicine Information News (Author: Ning Zailan)

三十五、白花丹的药用
35. Medicinal Uses of Plumbago zeylanica

白花丹别名白雪花、铁茉莉、猛老虎、天槟榔、一见消等。味辛苦涩，性温，有小毒。白花丹具有散瘀消肿，祛风杀虫之功，笔者对白花丹应用已有二十余年，现介绍如下：

Plumbago zeylanica, also known as Bai Xue Hua (White Snow Flower), Tie Mo Li (Iron Jasmine), Meng Lao Hu (Fierce Tiger), Tian Bing Lang (Sky Betel Nut), and Yi Jian Xiao (Instant Relief), has a pungent, bitter, and astringent taste, and a warm nature. It is slightly toxic. This herb is known for its effects of dissipating blood stasis, reducing swelling, dispelling wind, and killing parasites. Having used Plumbago zeylanica in clinical practice for over twenty years, I would like to share the following applications:

1. 治慢性肝炎肝肿大：鲜白花丹叶 30 张，鲜柚果刺 100 条，猪胰腺 1 条，前二味捣烂，同猪胰腺煎熟，食肉喝汤，每日一剂，连服 15 天。

1. For chronic hepatitis with hepatomegaly (liver enlargement):Take 30 fresh leaves of Plumbago zcylanica and 100 fresh thorns from pomelo fruit. Pound the first two ingredients into a paste, then boil them together with one pig pancreas until cooked. Eat the meat and drink the broth. Take one dose daily for 15 consecutive days.

2. 治结膜炎、角膜炎、角膜白斑：取鲜白花丹叶 4-6 张，茴茴蒜（广西药用植物名录，72 页，药用全草，杀虫，外用治疥疮，有毒）全草适量，共捣烂，用二层布包好挂于患侧，2-4 天可愈。

2. For conjunctivitis, keratitis, and corneal leukoma:Take 4-6 fresh leaves of Plumbago zeylanica and an appropriate amount of whole Ranunculus cantoniensis (Hui Hui Suan - a medicinal plant in Guangxi used as an insecticide and externally for scabies; toxic). Pound them together into a paste, wrap it in two layers of cloth, and hang it over the affected side. It can heal within 2-4 days.

3. 治陈年跌打损伤：鲜白花丹叶 30-40 张，切细，瘦猪肉 50 克，调食油，米酒各适量炒熟一次服完，每日一剂，连用 2-3 天。

3. For old traumatic injuries:Take 30-40 fresh leaves of Plumbago zeylanica, chop them finely, and stir-fry them with 50g of lean pork, an appropriate amount of cooking oil, and rice wine until cooked. Consume it all at once. Take one dose daily for 2-3 consecutive days.

4. 治乳腺炎: 取鲜白花丹叶 10-15 张捣烂用布包好挂于患侧，连挂 2-3 天可愈。

4. For mastitis:Pound 10-15 fresh leaves of Plumbago zeylanica into a paste, wrap it in cloth, and hang it over the affected side. It can heal within 2-3 consecutive days of application.

5. 治牛皮癣：鲜白花丹适量与红糖少许，捣烂外敷至皮肤热辣后除药，待皮癣脱落结痂后，再如法敷用 2-3 次即可。

5. For psoriasis:Take an appropriate amount of fresh Plumbago zeylanica and a small amount of brown sugar, pound them into a paste, and apply it externally. Remove the medicine once the skin feels hot and stinging. After the psoriatic scales fall off and form scabs, apply it again in the same manner for 2-3 times to achieve a cure.

《民族医药报》1992 年 1 月 31 日（广西 韦昭聪）

Source: January 31, 1992, "National Minority Medicine News" (Author: Wei Zhaocong, Guangxi)

三十六、丁香的药用

36. Medicinal Uses of Clove (Ding-xiang)

1. 治急性胃肠炎：丁香 10 克，取马的酸奶 100 毫升，将丁香倒入，浸泡 24 小时，每晚空腹服 15 毫升，连服 7-9 天。治疗期间勿需服用其它药物，一般 7 天可治愈。

Treating Acute Gastroenteritis: Take 10g of cloves and pour them into 100ml of mare’s yogurt. Soak for 24 hours. Take 15ml on an empty stomach every night, continuously for 7-9 days. No other medications are needed during the treatment period, and it can generally be cured in 7 days.

2. 治阳痿：鸡蛋黄 20 个晒干，除虫菊根、丁香、肉桂、干姜、良姜各 120 克，上药共研细粉，每晚服一次，每次服 3 克，用温开水送服。

2. Treating Impotence (Erectile Dysfunction): Sun-dry 20 egg yolks. Take 120g each of pyrethrum root (chu-chong-ju-gen), cloves, cinnamon bark (rou-gui), dried ginger (gan-jiang), and galangal (liang-jiang). Grind all the above herbs into a fine powder. Take 3g once every night, swallowed with warm water.

3. 治偏瘫：牛膝、丁香、麻黄、广木香各 20 克，黄母鸡 1 只。先取出母鸡内脏，洗净，再将药物放入鸡腹内炖熟，食肉饮汤，每日分 2-3 次吃完。服药期间忌盐。

3. Treating Hemiplegia: Take 20g each of achyranthes root (niu-xi), cloves, ephedra (ma-huang), and costus root (guang-mu-xiang), along with 1 yellow hen. First, remove the internal organs of the hen and wash it clean. Then, put the herbs into the hen’s belly and stew until cooked. Eat the meat and drink the soup, finishing it in 2-3 portions a day. Avoid salt during the medication period.

4. 治顽癣：丁香 5 克，斑蝥 7 个，红娘 7 个，广木香 3 克，米醋适量。先将前四味共研粗末，再用醋浸泡 7 日备用，然后每日取适量涂搽患处 1-2 次。

4. Treating Stubborn Tinea (Ringworm): Take 5g of cloves, 7 blister beetles (ban-mao), 7 red-winged locusts (hong-niang), 3g of costus root, and an appropriate amount of rice vinegar. First, grind the first four ingredients into a coarse powder, then soak them in vinegar for 7 days for later use. After that, take an appropriate amount and apply it to the affected area 1-2 times daily.

《民族医药报》1993 年 1 月 1 日（内蒙古蒙药厂 贺喜格图）

Ethnic Medicine News, January 1, 1993 (Hexige Tu, Inner Mongolia Mongolian Medicine Factory)

三十七、黄荆

37. Negundo Chastetree (Huang-jing)

1. 止咳喘：取黄荆根 120 克，水煎 2 小时以上，滤渣，加 20% 的红糖收膏，每次服 2 匙，每日 2 次，亦可取黄荆子若干，研粉过筛，每日取 3 克蒸鸭蛋服。

Relieving Cough and Panting: Take 120g of negundo chastetree roots, decoct in water for over 2 hours, filter out the residue, add 20% brown sugar to make a paste. Take 2 spoonfuls each time, twice a day. Alternatively, take an appropriate amount of negundo chastetree seeds, grind into a powder and sift. Take 3g daily, steamed with duck eggs to eat.

2. 消饱胀：取黄荆子（炒黄）、半夏粬等量，研末去渣过筛，每取此粉 4-6 克调白糖服，儿童酌减。此方对小儿消化不良效佳。

2. Relieving Fullness and Distension: Take equal amounts of negundo chastetree seeds (stir-fried until yellow) and pinellia yeast (ban-xia-qu). Grind into a powder, remove the residue, and sift. Take 4-6g of this powder each time, mixed with white sugar to take. Reduce the dosage appropriately for children. This prescription has good efficacy for pediatric indigestion.

3. 止疼痛：取黄荆根 30 克煎水服治腹痛；取黄荆子 30 克入猪肚炖服，止胃疼；取黄荆子过筛粉 6 克调蜜服，能缓解腹部术后粘连疼痛；取黄荆叶若干置杯中，开水冲浸 1-2 分钟，取叶贴太阳穴、印堂穴，止头痛。

3. Relieving Pain: Decoct 30g of negundo chastetree roots in water to drink for abdominal pain; stew 30g of negundo chastetree seeds inside a pig's stomach to eat for stomachache; take 6g of sifted negundo chastetree seed powder, mixed with honey to take, to relieve postoperative abdominal adhesion pain; put an appropriate amount of negundo chastetree leaves in a cup, steep with boiling water for 1-2 minutes, take the leaves and apply them to the Taiyang and Yintang acupoints to relieve headaches.

4. 治疮疖：取黄荆叶捣烂，敷痈疮可消；取黄荆全草煎水洗澡，可治痱子；取黄荆子叶粉调醋敷疖，可散。

4. Treating Sores and Boils: Mash negundo chastetree leaves and apply them to carbuncles and sores to dissipate them; decoct the whole plant of negundo chastetree in water to wash the body, which can treat prickly heat; mix negundo chastetree seed and leaf powder with vinegar and apply it to boils to dissipate

them.

5. 治失眠：取黄荆子做枕芯，可明目、祛风、醒脑，治失眠多梦。

5. Treating Insomnia: Use negundo chastetree seeds as a pillow filling. It can brighten the eyes, dispel wind, refresh the brain, and treat insomnia with excessive dreaming.

6. 疗脚癣：取鲜黄荆叶 500 克，水煎 5 分钟，渣液共置盆中，洗脚，并用脚互擦叶，5-10 分钟后，擦干，勿清洗。

6. Treating Athlete' s Foot (Tinea Pedis): Take 500g of fresh negundo chastetree leaves, decoct in water for 5 minutes, and put both the residue and the liquid into a basin. Wash the feet, and rub the feet against the leaves with each other. After 5-10 minutes, wipe dry and do not wash with clean water.

7. 灭蚊蛆：取半干黄荆叶若干，混适量干草助燃，闭门窗，其烟可灭蚊；取黄荆全株切碎，加水浸 8-12 小时，连液倒入粪坑，蛆虫尽灭。

7. Eradicating Mosquitoes and Maggots: Take an appropriate amount of semi-dried negundo chastetree leaves, mix with an appropriate amount of dry grass to help combustion, close the doors and windows, and the smoke can eradicate mosquitoes; chop the whole plant of negundo chastetree, soak in water for 8-12 hours, and pour the liquid into a cesspool to completely eradicate maggots.

《中药科技报》1992 年 4 月 17 日（陈 永）

Chinese Medicine Science and Technology News, April 17, 1992 (Chen Yong)

三十八、无花果的药用

38. Medicinal Uses of Fig (Wu-hua-guo)

无花果性甘、酸、平，无毒。有清热、解毒、止泻、润肠的功效。清代王士雄《随息居饮食谱》对此果有“清热，疗痔，润肠，上利咽喉”的记载。在湘西苗族民间流传有不少无花果疗疾的验方，兹录数方如下。

Fig is sweet and sour in flavor, neutral in property, and non-toxic. It has the effects of clearing heat and detoxifying, stopping diarrhea, and moistening the intestines. In the Qing Dynasty, Wang Shixiong recorded in Sui Xi Ju Yin Shi Pu (Dietary Materia Medica of Sui Xi Ju) that this fruit can "clear heat, treat hemorrhoids, moisten the intestines, and benefit the throat." Among the Miao people in western Hunan, there are many proven prescriptions for treating diseases with figs. Several of them are recorded below.

1. 慢性腹泻：对慢性腹泻久治不愈者，用无花果枝叶 60 克洗净切碎煎汤服，1 日 1 剂，分 3 次服，连服数剂痼疾可愈。

Chronic Diarrhea: For patients with chronic diarrhea that has been difficult to cure for a long time, take 60g of fig branches and leaves, wash, chop, and decoct in water to drink. Take 1 dose a day, divided into 3 portions. Taking several consecutive doses can cure the chronic disease.

2. 肺热咳嗽、咽喉痛：无花果 2 枚切碎水煎加冰糖服，1 日 3 次，有良效。

2. Lung-Heat Cough and Sore Throat: Chop 2 figs, decoct in water, add rock sugar, and drink. Take it 3 times a day with good efficacy.

3. 痔疮、脱肛、便秘：每日生食无花果 3-5 枚，痔疾者配合用其叶煎汤坐浴，疗效更佳。

3. Hemorrhoids, Rectal Prolapse, and Constipation: Eat 3-5 raw figs daily. For patients with hemorrhoids, combining this with a sitz bath using a decoction of fig leaves will yield better results.

4. 消化不良：取无花果干果适量切成小块，炒至半焦，加白糖适量，用开水冲泡代茶饮，有很好的助消化之功。

4. Indigestion: Take an appropriate amount of dried figs, cut them into small pieces, and stir-fry until half-scroched. Add an appropriate amount of white sugar, steep with boiling water, and drink as a substitute for tea. It has a very good effect of aiding digestion.

《民族医药报》1992 年 7 月 10 日（湖南 兰家长）

Ethnic Medicine News, July 10, 1992 (Lan Jiazhang, Hunan)

三十九、青蒿的药用

39. Medicinal Uses of Sweet Wormwood (Qing-hao)

1. 治秋季泻：青蒿20-30克，水煎2次，分3次温服（不可热服，否则易致恶心、呕吐），平均3天痊愈。

Treating Autumn Diarrhea: Take 20-30g of sweet wormwood, decoct in water twice, and divide into 3 portions to drink warm (do not drink it hot, otherwise it easily causes nausea and vomiting). It takes an average of 3 days to cure.

2. 治皮肤瘙痒：用青蒿鲜品2斤，切碎、水煎（加水没过药即可）煎至约剩药液200ml左右，倒出，加入冰片2克（先用酒精将其溶化），用药液涂患处，每日3-5次。此法兼治荨麻疹。

2. Treating Skin Pruritus: Take 500g (two jin) of fresh sweet wormwood, chop it, and decoct in water (just add enough water to cover the herbs) until about 200ml of liquid remains. Pour it out, add 2g of borneol (bing-pian) (dissolve it in alcohol first), and apply the liquid to the affected area 3-5 times a day. This method also treats urticaria.

3. 治心动过速：青蒿30克、炙甘草30克，水煎服，每日一剂，分2次服（小儿酌减，冠心病患者酌用）。

3. Treating Tachycardia: Take 30g of sweet wormwood and 30g of honey-fried licorice root (zhi-gan-cao), decoct in water to drink. Take 1 dose daily, divided into 2 portions (reduce the dosage appropriately for children, and use with caution for patients with coronary heart disease).

4. 治急性黄胆型肝炎：青蒿30克、车前草30克、龙胆草20克，水煎服。每日一剂，疗程3-4周。

4. Treating Acute Icteric Hepatitis: Take 30g of sweet wormwood, 30g of plantain (che-qian-cao), and 20g of gentian root (long-dan-cao), decoct in water to drink. Take 1 dose daily, with a course of treatment of 3-4 weeks.

《中医药信息报》1990年10月6日（周国民）

Chinese Medicine Information News, October 6, 1990 (Zhou Guomin)

四十、辣椒的药用
40. Medicinal Uses of Chili Pepper (La-jiao)

辣椒性味辛温，有温中下气，驱寒祛湿，活血祛风的功效，据营养学资料报道获悉：一只生辣椒内含维生素 C 可达 300-500 毫克，还含有丰富的维生素 B1、B2 以及碳水化合物和人体所需的微量氨基酸元素，能预防和控制心脏病及冠状动脉硬化的发生。下面介绍辣椒的几种用途：

Chili pepper is pungent in flavor and warm in property. It has the effects of warming the middle and descending qi, dispelling cold and eliminating dampness, promoting blood circulation and dispelling wind. According to nutritional data, a single raw chili pepper can contain 300-500mg of vitamin C, and is also rich in vitamins B1 and B2, carbohydrates, and trace amino acids and elements needed by the human body. It can prevent and control the occurrence of heart disease and coronary atherosclerosis. Several uses of chili peppers are introduced below:

1. 感冒：用生辣椒三只、生姜 30g、红糖 60g 煎水服，能治伤风感冒。

Common Cold: Decoct 3 raw chili peppers, 30g of fresh ginger, and 60g of brown sugar in water to drink. It can treat the common cold.

2. 神经性头痛：用生辣椒一只捣烂、贴于太阳穴位能立即止痛。

2. Neurological Headache: Mash 1 raw chili pepper and apply it to the Taiyang acupoint. It can relieve pain immediately.

3. 冻疮：用辣椒粉 15 克冲开水三市斤浸泡冻疮患处。

3. Chilblains: Use 15g of chili pepper powder steeped in 1500g (three shi-jin) of boiling water to soak the chilblain-affected area.

4. 风湿性关节炎：用生辣椒五只、蒜头一只共捣烂，隔布敷于痛处，片刻即起到止痛的神效。

4. Rheumatoid Arthritis: Mash 5 raw chili peppers and 1 clove of garlic together, apply them to the painful area through a piece of cloth. It will have a miraculous analgesic effect in a moment.

《民族医药报》1992年1月31日（谭荣登）

Ethnic Medicine News, January 31, 1992 (Tan Rongdeng)

四十一、大枣的药用

41. Medicinal Uses of Jujube (Da-zao)

1. 治小儿湿疹：红枣适量，去核后在枣中加入少许明矾，焙干，研末，撒于患处，每日2次。

Treating Pediatric Eczema: Take an appropriate amount of red dates, remove the pits, add a small amount of alum to the dates, bake them dry, and grind into a powder. Sprinkle the powder on the affected area twice a day.

2. 治过敏性紫癜：食用洗净的生红枣，每次10粒，一日3次。可使紫癜消退。

2. Treating Allergic Purpura: Eat 10 washed raw red dates each time, 3 times a day. It can make the purpura subside.

3. 治血小板减少：红枣100克，浓煎，吃枣喝汤，每日2次。

3. Treating Thrombocytopenia: Take 100g of red dates, decoct them into a concentrated soup, eat the dates and drink the soup, twice a day.

4. 治贫血：红枣100克，浓煎，食枣饮汁，每日3次。

4. Treating Anemia: Take 100g of red dates, decoct them into a concentrated soup, eat the dates and drink the juice, 3 times a day.

5. 治肝炎：红枣200克，茵陈90克，水煎，食枣饮汤，早晚分服。

5. Treating Hepatitis: Take 200g of red dates and 90g of capillary wormwood (yin-chen), decoct in water, eat the dates and drink the soup, divided into morning and evening doses.

6. 治血友病：红枣30克，鲜猪皮100克，洗净，加水共煮至稀烂，每日一剂，疗程不限。

6. Treating Hemophilia: Take 30g of red dates and 100g of fresh pig skin. Wash them, add water, and boil together until soft and mushy. Take 1 dose daily, with no limit on the course of treatment.

《中药科技报》1991 年 2 月 6 日（李明）

Chinese Medicine Science and Technology News, February 6, 1991 (Li Ming)

四十二、西红柿的药用

42. Medicinal Uses of Tomato (Xi-hong-shi)

1. 治胃热口苦：取西红柿汁、甘蔗汁各半杯，混匀服下，每日 2-3 次。

Treating Stomach Heat and Bitter Taste in the Mouth: Take half a cup each of tomato juice and sugarcane juice, mix them well, and drink. Take it 2-3 times a day.

2. 治口疮：取西红柿汁适量，含在口里待 3-5 分钟，每日数次。

2. Treating Mouth Ulcers: Take an appropriate amount of tomato juice, hold it in the mouth for 3-5 minutes, several times a day.

3. 治胃溃疡：取西红柿汁、土豆汁各半杯，混合服下，每日早晚各一次。

3. Treating Gastric Ulcers: Take half a cup each of tomato juice and potato juice, mix them and drink, once in the morning and once at night.

4. 治腋臭：先洗澡，后在一盆加有 500 毫升西红柿汁的温水中浸泡 15 分钟，每日 1 次。

4. Treating Bromhidrosis (Body Odor): Take a bath first, then soak in a basin of warm water with 500ml of tomato juice added for 15 minutes, once a day.

5. 治高血压：每日早晨空腹生吃西红柿 1-2 只，坚持吃一段时间后，就能起到降血压作用。

5. Treating Hypertension: Eat 1-2 raw tomatoes on an empty stomach every morning. After persisting for a period of time, it can have the effect of lowering blood pressure.

（山东 李明）

(Shandong, Li Ming)

四十三、鸡胆治病便方

43. Simple Prescriptions for Treating Diseases with Chicken Gallbladder (Ji-dan)

1. 小儿百日咳：取鸡胆 1 个，红枣 5 枚，水煎服。每日一次，连用 5 天。

Pediatric Whooping Cough: Take 1 chicken gallbladder and 5 red dates, decoct in water to drink. Take it once a day, continuously for 5 days.

2. 老年性气管炎：取鸡胆 3 个，百合 10 克，川贝 10 克，水煎服。每日 1 次，连服 5-10 天。

2. Senile Bronchitis: Take 3 chicken gallbladders, 10g of lily bulbs (bai-he), and 10g of Fritillaria cirrhosa (chuan-bei), decoct in water to drink. Take it once a day, continuously for 5-10 days.

3. 急慢性肝炎：取鸡胆 3 个，车前草 50 克，满天星 50 克，水煎服，每日 1 次，连服一周。

3. Acute and Chronic Hepatitis: Take 3 chicken gallbladders, 50g of plantain (che-qian-cao), and 50g of Speranskia tuberculata (man-tian-xing), decoct in water to drink. Take it once a day, continuously for one week.

4. 高血压：取鸡胆 3 个，夏枯草 50 克，水煎服。每日 1 次，连服 1 周。待血压稳定后，隔 2 天服 1 次，再服 1 周，以巩固疗效。

4. Hypertension: Take 3 chicken gallbladders and 50g of common selfheal fruit spike (xia-ku-cao), decoct in water to drink. Take it once a day, continuously for one week. After the blood pressure stabilizes, take it once every 2 days for another week to consolidate the effect.

5. 牙痛：取鸡胆 1 个，晒干研为细末，白酒适量混合，用棉花蘸药液点牙痛患处，每日 3 次，连点 1 周。

5. Toothache: Take 1 chicken gallbladder, sun-dry and grind into a fine powder, mix with an appropriate amount of liquor. Dip a piece of cotton in the liquid and apply it to the painful tooth area, 3 times a day, continuously for one week.

《民族医药报》（陕西 绪林）

Ethnic Medicine News (Xu Lin, Shaanxi)

第十六章　其他疗法
Chapter 16　Other Therapies

一、食疗（28方）
I. Dietary Therapy (28 Prescriptions)

月经不调食疗验方：

Proven Dietary Prescriptions for Irregular Menstruation:

1.木耳：月经过少患者，用黑木耳五十克、核桃肉五十克，加红糖每日炖一次，有效。

Wood Ear Mushroom: For patients with hypomenorrhea (scanty menstruation), stew 50g of black wood ear mushrooms and 50g of walnut kernels with brown sugar once a day. It is effective.

2. 月季花：月经后延患者，每日用月季花十二朵煎水做饮料，如经色淡少，可加当归六克同煎；如经色紫而又腹胀者，可加三棱、莪术各六克同煎。

2. Chinese Rose Flower: For patients with delayed menstruation, decoct 12 Chinese rose flowers in water daily to drink as a beverage. If the menstrual blood is pale and scanty, add 6g of angelica root (dang-gui) to decoct together. If the menstrual blood is purple accompanied by abdominal distension, add 6g each of sparganium stem (san-leng) and zedoary rhizome (e-zhu) to decoct together.

3. 艾叶：月经过多患者，用醋炒艾叶六克，鸡蛋黄二枚，先将艾叶煎汤，饭前冲蛋黄吃，有效。

3. Mugwort Leaf: For patients with menorrhagia (excessive menstruation), stir-fry 6g of mugwort leaves with vinegar. Take 2 egg yolks. First, decoct the mugwort leaves in water, then mix the egg yolks into the hot soup and consume it

before meals. It is effective.

4. 芹菜：月经超前患者，可用干芹菜五十克，加水二杯煎成一杯，温服有效。

4. Celery: For patients with premature menstruation, take 50g of dried celery, add 2 cups of water, and decoct until 1 cup remains. Drink it warm. It is effective.

痛经食疗验方：

Proven Dietary Prescriptions for Dysmenorrhea:

5. 生姜：经痛有寒性症状，如四肢发冷，面青唇白时，可用生姜加红糖煎服。

5. Fresh Ginger: For dysmenorrhea with cold symptoms, such as cold extremities and a pale face and lips, decoct fresh ginger with brown sugar and drink.

6. 牡丹花根：月经不调又有痛经者，可用红牡丹花根煮甜酒糟吃，每日一次。

6. Red Peony Root: For irregular menstruation accompanied by dysmenorrhea, boil red peony roots with sweet fermented glutinous rice (jiu-zao) and eat it once a day.

7. 益母膏：经前后腹痛，均可用益母草二斤煎成膏，于行经前三天起每次吃一匙，每日二次，早晚空腹吃。

7. Motherwort Paste: For abdominal pain before or after menstruation, decoct 500g (two jin) of motherwort into a paste. Starting 3 days before menstruation, take 1 spoonful each time, twice a day, on an empty stomach in the morning and evening.

8. 玉簪花：不论何种痛经，可用玉簪花十二克，红糖十五克，煮鸡蛋三个吃，每日一次。

8. Fragrant Hosta Flower: For any type of dysmenorrhea, take 12g of fragrant hosta flowers and 15g of brown sugar, boil them with 3 eggs, and eat. Take it once a day.

眩是眼花，晕是头晕，常同时并见，通称眩晕。现代医学中的内耳性眩晕症，脑动脉硬化、高血压、贫血、神经衰弱，以及某些脑部疾患，常以眩晕为主症，可参考本法治疗。

“Xuan” refers to blurred vision, and “Yun” refers to dizziness.

They often occur simultaneously and are collectively referred to as vertigo. In modern medicine, conditions such as inner ear vertigo, cerebral arteriosclerosis, hypertension, anemia, neurasthenia, and certain brain diseases often present with vertigo as the main symptom. The following methods can be used for reference in treatment.

9. 肝阳上亢型：症见眩晕耳鸣，头痛且胀。面色潮红，急躁易怒。口苦、舌质红、脉眩。

9. Hyperactive Liver-Yang Type: Symptoms include vertigo, tinnitus, headache with a distending sensation, flushed face, irritability, bitter taste in the mouth, red tongue, and string-taut (wiry) pulse.

菊花粥 粳米 50 克，冰糖适量煮粥，煮至粥米稠时，加入菊花 10 克（纱布包好），再煮至粥稠，有清肝明目、疏风散热之效。

Chrysanthemum Porridge: Boil 50g of japonica rice and an appropriate amount of rock sugar into porridge. When the rice becomes thick, add 10g of chrysanthemum flowers (wrapped in gauze) and continue boiling until the porridge is thick. It has the effects of clearing the liver, brightening the eyes, dispelling wind, and clearing heat.

白木耳粥 白木耳 10 克，大枣 10 枚、桑叶 10 克（炒布包）粳米 50 克共煮粥，有清肝明目、滋阴润肺之效。

White Wood Ear Porridge: Boil 10g of white wood ear mushrooms, 10 red dates, 10g of mulberry leaves (stir-fried and wrapped in cloth), and 50g of japonica rice together into porridge. It has the effects of clearing the liver, brightening the eyes, nourishing yin, and moistening the lungs.

10. 气血亏虚型：眩晕动则加剧，劳累即发，面色唇淡，心悸失眠，神疲食少、舌质淡，脉细微且弱。

10. Qi and Blood Deficiency Type: Vertigo worsens with movement and is triggered by fatigue, with a pale face and lips, palpitations, insomnia, fatigue, poor appetite, pale tongue, and a thready and weak pulse.

人参粥 人参 3 克，粳米 50 克，冰糖适量，加水入砂锅内煮粥，每日晨起服之，有大补元气补充脾胃之效，久服能抗衰老延年益寿。

Ginseng Porridge: Add 3g of ginseng, 50g of japonica rice, and an appropriate amount of rock sugar into a casserole with water to make porridge. Take it every morning upon waking. It has the effects of greatly tonifying primordial qi and supplementing the spleen and stomach. Long-term consumption can resist aging and prolong life.

大枣花生粥 大枣 10 枚、花生米 15 克、粳米或小米 50 克共煮粥，有补益脾胃养血止血之功。

Red Date and Peanut Porridge: Boil 10 red dates, 15g of peanuts, and 50g of japonica rice or millet together into porridge. It has the effects of tonifying the spleen and stomach, nourishing the blood, and stopping bleeding.

11. 肾精不足型：眩晕神疲健忘，腰膝酸软，遗精耳鸣。偏阴虚者，五心烦热，舌红脉弦细；偏阳虚者，四肢不温，舌淡脉沉细。

11. Kidney Essence Deficiency Type: Vertigo, fatigue, poor memory, soreness and weakness of the lower back and knees, seminal emission, and tinnitus. For those with yin deficiency, there is heat in the palms, soles, and chest, with a red tonguc and a thready and wiry pulse. For those with yang deficiency, there are cold extremities, with a pale tongue and a deep and thready pulse.

浮小麦、黑大豆，水煎服，有心肾双补之效，治眩晕有自汗表现者。

Boil floating wheat and black soybeans in water to drink. It has the effect of tonifying both the heart and kidneys, and is used to treat vertigo accompanied by spontaneous sweating.

黑芝麻、胡桃肉、桑叶各 60 克，研末制成蜜丸，每日 6-9 克，分二次服。

Take 60g each of black sesame seeds, walnut kernels, and mulberry leaves. Grind them into a powder and make into honey pills. Take 6-9g daily, divided into two doses.

猪脑一具，淮山药 50 克，枸杞子 15 克，加适量调味品炖烧，吃猪脑，有滋补肝肾之功。

Stew 1 pig brain with 50g of Chinese yam (huai-shan-yao) and 15g of wolfberry fruits (gou-qi-zi), adding appropriate seasonings. Eat the pig brain. It has the effect of tonifying the liver and kidneys.

枸杞子 30 克，羊脑一具，加调味品炖食，有补养肝肾与壮阳之效，偏肾阳虚者更为适用。

Stew 30g of wolfberry fruits with 1 sheep brain, adding appropriate seasonings, and eat. It has the effects of tonifying the liver and kidneys and strengthening yang. It is especially suitable for those with kidney-yang deficiency.

12. 痰湿中阻型：眩晕头重，蒙、胸闷恶心，少食多寐，舌淡苔白腻，脉濡滑。

12. Phlegm-Dampness Obstructing the Middle Type: Vertigo with a heavy and clouded head, chest tightness, nausea, poor appetite, excessive sleepiness, pale tongue with a white and greasy coating, and a soggy and slippery pulse.

石菖蒲粥 石菖蒲 45 克，研末备用。用粳米 50 克、冰糖适量，在砂锅内煮粥，粥稠前调入石菖蒲末即可，有和中开胃化痰开窍之效。

Grassleaf Sweetflag Porridge: Grind 45g of grassleaf sweetflag (shi-chang-pu) into a powder and set aside. Boil 50g of japonica rice and an appropriate amount of rock sugar in a casserole to make porridge. Stir in the sweetflag powder just before the porridge becomes thick. It has the effects of harmonizing the middle, stimulating the appetite, resolving phlegm, and opening the orifices.

《中药科技报》1992 年 7 月 26 日（昌 永）

Chinese Medicine Science and Technology News, July 26, 1992 (Chang Yong)

冬春季，由于气候寒冷，呼吸道疾病及心、脑血管疾病的发病率均有明显的提高。在此季节中，如能及时正确地应用食物防治，可以有效地预防疾病的发生和帮助疾病的康复。现介绍几种食疗方法如下：

In winter and spring, due to the cold climate, the incidence of respiratory diseases and cardiovascular and cerebrovascular diseases significantly increases. During this season, timely and correct application of dietary prevention and treatment can effectively prevent the occurrence of diseases and aid in recovery. Several dietary therapy methods are introduced below:

13. 支气管哮喘

13. Bronchial Asthma

羊骨粥 羊骨1000克左右，粳米100克，葱白2根，生姜3-5片。先将羊骨洗净打碎，加水煎汤，然后取汤与米煮成粥，待粥将成时，加入细盐、生姜、葱白、稍煮片刻即成。早晚温热空腹食用，10-15天为一疗程。

Sheep Bone Porridge: Take about 1000g of sheep bones, 100g of japonica rice, 2 scallion whites, and 3-5 slices of fresh ginger. First, wash and crush the sheep bones, decoct them in water to make a soup. Then, use the soup to boil the rice into porridge. When the porridge is almost done, add fine salt, fresh ginger, and scallion whites, and boil for a moment. Eat it warm on an empty stomach in the morning and evening. 10-15 days constitute one course of treatment.

14. 慢性支气管炎

14. Chronic Bronchitis

花生粥 花生仁45克（不去衣），白莲子30克，粳米100克，冰糖适量。先将花生、莲子洗净后打碎，加入粳米，同煮为粥，待粥将成时，放入冰糖稍煮片刻即可食用。

Peanut Porridge: Take 45g of peanut kernels (with the red skins intact), 30g of white lotus seeds, 100g of japonica rice, and an appropriate amount of rock sugar. First, wash and crush the peanuts and lotus seeds, add the japonica rice, and boil them together into porridge. When the porridge is almost done, add the rock sugar and boil for a moment before eating.

核桃生姜粥 核桃肉4-5个，生姜5片，粳米50-100克，共煮成粥。分1-2天服完。

Walnut and Ginger Porridge: Take 4-5 walnut kernels, 5 slices of fresh ginger, and 50-100g of japonica rice, and boil them together into porridge. Finish it within 1-2 days.

15. 心血管病

15. Cardiovascular Diseases

双耳汤 黑木耳、白木耳各10克，红枣15个，以温水泡发后洗净，放入小碗中，加水和少量冰糖，隔水蒸一小时，连汤服食，每日两次。

Double Ear Soup: Take 10g each of black wood ear mushrooms and white wood ear mushrooms, and 15 red dates. Soak them in warm water until expanded, wash them clean, and put them in a small bowl. Add water and a small amount of rock sugar, and steam over boiling water for one hour. Eat the soup and the ingredients, twice a day.

莲子百合炖瘦肉 莲子、百合各 50 克，瘦肉 250 克，文火炖熟食用。

Stewed Lean Meat with Lotus Seeds and Lily Bulbs: Take 50g each of lotus seeds and lily bulbs, and 250g of lean meat. Stew over low heat until cooked and eat.

16. 高血压病

16. Hypertension

黑木耳柿饼汤 取黑木耳 6 克，冰糖少许，柿饼 50 克，同煮烂食之。此为一日量。

Black Wood Ear and Dried Persimmon Soup: Take 6g of black wood ear mushrooms, a small amount of rock sugar, and 50g of dried persimmons. Boil them together until soft and eat. This is the daily dosage.

《现代中医药报》1998 年 2 月 1 日（小宇）

Modern Chinese Medicine News, February 1, 1998 (Xiao Yu)

冠心病药粥疗法

Medicinal Porridge Therapy for Coronary Heart Disease

17. 薤白粥：用薤白 12 克、葱头二个，同粳米 100 克煮粥，温热服食。薤白功能宽胸通阳，李时珍谓：“温补，助阳道，心病宜食之。”用薤白煮粥，可增强它的温补力量，适用于冠心病，心阳不振，胸部闷痛。

17. Macrostem Onion Porridge: Take 12g of macrostem onion bulbs (xie-bai) and 2 scallion heads, and boil them with 100g of japonica rice into porridge. Eat it warm. Macrostem onion has the function of relieving chest tightness and unblocking yang. Li Shizhen said, “It is warming and tonifying, assists the yang channels, and is suitable for heart diseases.” Boiling it into porridge can enhance its warming and tonifying power. It is suitable for coronary heart disease, poor heart-yang activity, and chest stuffiness and pain.

18. 桃仁粥：用桃仁 10 克捣烂加水后去渣，入粳米 100 克同煮为粥。桃仁有活血祛瘀的功效。适用于冠心病，血行不畅，胸脘疼痛，心痛彻背。又因桃仁尚有润燥滑肠的作用，所以对便秘者尤其适宜。

18. Peach Kernel Porridge: Mash 10g of peach kernels (tao-ren), add water, filter out the residue, and add 100g of japonica rice to boil into porridge. Peach kernels have the effect of promoting blood circulation and removing blood stasis. It is suitable for coronary heart disease, poor blood circulation, chest and epigastric pain, and heart pain radiating to the back. Because peach kernels also have the effect of moistening dryness and lubricating the intestines, it is especially suitable for patients with constipation.

19. 山楂粥：用山楂 15-20 克捣碎煎汤取汁，以粳米二两煮粥，待粥半熟，加入山楂汁和冰糖适量，同煮为粥。山楂功能活血散瘀，现代药理试验证明，有扩张冠状动脉，增加血流量，降血脂，减轻血管内膜粥样硬化的作用。可用作冠心病，心血瘀阻的辅助治疗，尤其适用于体质肥胖者。

19. Hawthorn Porridge: Crush 15-20g of hawthorn fruits (shan-zha), decoct in water to extract the juice, and use 100g (two liang) of japonica rice to make porridge. When the porridge is half cooked, add the hawthorn juice and an appropriate amount of rock sugar, and boil them together. Hawthorn has the function of promoting blood circulation and dissipating blood stasis. Modern pharmacological tests have proven that it can dilate coronary arteries, increase blood flow, lower blood lipids, and alleviate atherosclerosis of the vascular endothelium. It can be used as an auxiliary treatment for coronary heart disease and blood stasis blocking the heart, especially suitable for obese patients.

20. 葛根粉粥：先将新葛根洗净切片，经水磨石磨取淀粉，晒干备用。每次以葛根粉 30 克，与粳米 50 克共同煮成稀粥。近代药理试验报道，葛根有扩张脑及冠状动脉的作用，增加脑及冠状动脉的血流量，用于治疗冠心病有较好效果，对缓解心绞痛和改善心电图有一定疗效。

20. Kudzu Root Starch Porridge: First, wash and slice fresh kudzu roots (ge-gen), grind them with a stone mill to extract the starch, and sun-dry for later use.

Each time, take 30g of kudzu root starch and 50g of japonica rice to boil into thin porridge. Recent pharmacological tests have reported that kudzu root can dilate cerebral and coronary arteries, increase blood flow to the brain and coronary arteries, and has good effects in treating coronary heart disease, with certain efficacy in relieving angina pectoris and improving electrocardiograms.

21. 玉米粉粥：先以玉米粉适量，冷水溶和，待粳米粥煮沸后，调入玉米粉同煮为粥。玉米中所含的玉米油是一种富含多个不饱和链脂酸的油脂，有降低血脂和抑制胆固醇吸收的作用，对动脉硬化、冠心病等心血管疾病有一定的防治作用，尤其适宜于年龄较轻而血浆胆固醇浓度已较高的中年冠心病患者。

21. Cornmeal Porridge: First, dissolve an appropriate amount of cornmeal in cold water. After the japonica rice porridge boils, stir in the cornmeal and boil together. The corn oil contained in corn is a fat rich in polyunsaturated fatty acids, which can lower blood lipids and inhibit cholesterol absorption. It has a certain preventive and therapeutic effect on cardiovascular diseases such as arteriosclerosis and coronary heart disease, and is especially suitable for middle-aged coronary heart disease patients who are relatively young but already have high plasma cholesterol levels.

22. 菊花粥：秋季霜降前，将菊花去蒂烘干或蒸后晒干，然后磨粉备用。先用粳米 100 克煮粥，待粥将熟时，调入菊花末 12 克，稍煮一二沸即可。菊花功能清肝火，清热明目，前人称其“久服得血气，轻身耐老延年。”现代菊理研究证明，菊花能降血压，扩张冠状动脉，增强心肌收缩力，故可用于防治高血压、冠心病等属于肝火旺盛者。

22. Chrysanthemum Porridge: Before the Frost’s Descent solar term in autumn, remove the calyxes from chrysanthemum flowers, bake or steam them dry, and then grind them into powder for later use. First, boil 100g of japonica rice into porridge. When the porridge is almost cooked, stir in 12g of chrysanthemum powder and boil for a moment. Chrysanthemum has the function of clearing liver fire, clearing heat, and brightening the eyes. The ancients said, “Long-term consumption can nourish qi and blood, lighten the body, resist aging, and

prolong life." Modern research has proven that chrysanthemum can lower blood pressure, dilate coronary arteries, and enhance myocardial contractility. Therefore, it can be used to prevent and treat hypertension and coronary heart disease caused by hyperactive liver fire.

23. 甜浆粥：用黄豆浸泡后磨取豆腐浆，取豆浆适量同粳米 100 克煮粥，粥成后，加入白糖少许，供早餐温热服食。黄豆营养价值更高，有很好的滋润补虚作用，科学研究表明，黄豆有很好的降低血清胆固醇的效果，对于冠心病、高血脂症、动脉血管硬化症，均有一定的防治作用，尤其适用于体质虚弱者。

23. Sweet Soybean Milk Porridge: Soak soybeans, grind them to extract soy milk, and take an appropriate amount of soy milk to boil with 100g of japonica rice into porridge. After the porridge is done, add a little white sugar and eat it warm for breakfast. Soybeans have high nutritional value and a good effect of moistening and tonifying deficiency. Scientific research shows that soybeans are very effective in lowering serum cholesterol. They have a certain preventive and therapeutic effect on coronary heart disease, hyperlipidemia, and arteriosclerosis, and are especially suitable for patients with weak constitutions.

《中药科技报》1993 年 1 月 14 日（广东 王绵年）

Chinese Medicine Science and Technology News, January 14, 1993 (Wang Mian-nian, Guangdong)

产后病药粥疗法

Medicinal Porridge Therapy for Postpartum Diseases

分娩以后，有的产妇经常出现大便秘结、恶露不尽、乳汁过少、虚寒腹痛和自汗等病症。笔者在临床上常采用中医的药粥疗法加以调治，既可健脾养胃，增加食欲，促进气血恢复，又能祛病邪，解除病痛。方法简便易行，疗效显著。现笔者将药粥疗法介绍如下：

After childbirth, some parturients often suffer from constipation, prolonged lochia, insufficient breast milk, abdominal pain due to deficiency-cold, and spontaneous sweating. In clinical practice, the author often uses the traditional Chinese medicinal porridge therapy to treat these conditions. It can not only invigorate the spleen and nourish the stomach, increase appetite, and promote the recovery of qi and blood, but also dispel pathogenic factors and relieve pain. This method is simple and easy to apply, with remarkable efficacy. The author now introduces the medicinal porridge therapy as follows:

24. 大便秘结 黑芝麻粥 取黑芝麻 50 克，碾细，加粳米 100 克，同煮粥，分早晚二次空腹食用。黑芝麻富含脂肪、蛋白质和多种脂溶性维生素及钙、磷、铁等微量元素，是一味补益佳品。中医认为，其性味甘平，具有滋补五脏、润汤通便的功效。故对产后气血耗损、津亏肠燥所致的大便干结疗效颇佳。同时因其营养丰富、能增加乳汁，对兼有乳汁缺少者更为适宜。

24. Constipation - Black Sesame Porridge: Take 50g of black sesame seeds, grind them finely, add 100g of japonica rice, and boil into porridge. Eat it on an empty stomach twice a day, in the morning and evening. Black sesame seeds are rich in fat, protein, various fat-soluble vitamins, and trace elements such as calcium, phosphorus, and iron, making them an excellent tonic. Traditional Chinese medicine believes that they are sweet and neutral in nature, with the effects of nourishing the five zang-organs, moistening the intestines, and relieving constipation. Therefore, they have good efficacy for dry stools caused by postpartum qi and blood consumption, and fluid deficiency leading to intestinal dryness. At the same time, because they are highly nutritious and can increase breast milk, they are especially suitable for those with insufficient lactation.

25. 恶露不尽 山楂粥 取鲜山楂 50 克（干品 30 克），浓煎去渣留汁，加粳米 100 克，煮粥，熟后拌入红糖适量，早晚空腹时温食。山楂功能消食化积，活血散瘀，是人们日常喜爱食用的佳品。现代医学证实，山楂能增加消化液分泌，并可加强子宫收缩，促使恶露排除，帮助产后子宫复原。故对产后子宫收缩不良、恶露不尽者疗效显著，对伴有食欲不振者尤为合适。

25. Prolonged Lochia - Hawthorn Porridge: Take 50g of fresh hawthorn fruits (or 30g of dried ones), decoct them into a concentrated liquid, filter out the residue, add 100g of japonica rice, and boil into porridge. After cooking, mix in an appropriate amount of brown sugar and eat it warm on an empty

stomach in the morning and evening. Hawthorn has the functions of promoting digestion, eliminating food accumulation, promoting blood circulation, and dissipating blood stasis, and is a favorite daily food. Modern medicine has confirmed that hawthorn can increase the secretion of digestive juices, strengthen uterine contractions, promote the discharge of lochia, and help the postpartum uterus recover. Therefore, it has significant efficacy for poor postpartum uterine contractions and prolonged lochia, and is especially suitable for those accompanied by poor appetite.

26. 缺乳 猪蹄粥 取猪蹄 1 只，切成小块，与花生仁 60 克，粳米 200 克同煮粥，于临熟时放入适量食盐、葱末以调味，供餐食用。猪蹄、花生仁均有补营血、通乳汁的作用，对产后乳汁缺乏者疗效显著。

26. Insufficient Lactation - Pig’s Trotter Porridge: Take 1 pig’s trotter, cut it into small pieces, and boil it with 60g of peanut kernels and 200g of japonica rice into porridge. When it is almost cooked, add an appropriate amount of salt and chopped scallions for seasoning, and serve as a meal. Both pig’s trotters and peanut kernels have the effects of nourishing nutrient blood and promoting lactation, with significant efficacy for postpartum lactation deficiency.

27. 虚寒腹痛 羊肉粥 取精羊肉 150 克切碎，加粳米 100 克同煮粥，临熟时加适量食盐、生姜等佐料，再煮至熟，供早晚温食。羊肉性味甘温，功能益气养血，温中暖下。对产后气血亏虚、小腹虚寒而绵绵作痛者颇宜；具有补益气血、散寒止痛之效验，并能促进乳汁分泌。

27. Abdominal Pain due to Deficiency-Cold - Mutton Porridge: Take 150g of lean mutton, chop it, and boil it with 100g of japonica rice into porridge. When it is almost cooked, add appropriate seasonings such as salt and fresh ginger, and continue boiling until fully cooked. Eat it warm in the morning and evening. Mutton is sweet and warm in nature, with the functions of tonifying qi and nourishing blood, and warming the middle and lower body. It is very suitable for postpartum qi and blood deficiency, and continuous dull pain in the lower abdomen due to deficiency-cold. It has the effects of tonifying qi and blood,

dispelling cold, and relieving pain, and can also promote lactation.

28. 自汗 黄芪粥 取生黄芪 50 克，水煎后去渣留汁，加粳米 100 克同煮粥，待微温时顿食。一日三次。黄芪有较强的补气健脾、固表止汗的功效。产妇因气虚、外表不固而致自汗出者，食用黄芪粥可补气固表、收缩汗孔而敛汗，并能消除疲乏。

28. Spontaneous Sweating - Astragalus Porridge: Take 50g of raw astragalus root (huang-qi), decoct in water, filter out the residue, add 100g of japonica rice, and boil into porridge. Wait until it is slightly warm and eat it all at once. Take it 3 times a day. Astragalus root has strong effects of tonifying qi, invigorating the spleen, stabilizing the exterior, and stopping sweating. For parturients who experience spontaneous sweating due to qi deficiency and an unconsolidated exterior, eating astragalus porridge can tonify qi, stabilize the exterior, constrict the sweat pores to stop sweating, and eliminate fatigue.

《中药科技报》1992 年 3 月 6 日（广西 李子云）

Chinese Medicine Science and Technology News, March 6, 1992 (Li Zi-yun, Guangxi)

二、涌泉穴敷药法（14 方）

II. Herbal Plaster Therapy on the Yongquan Acupoint (14 Prescriptions)

涌泉穴位于足底（去趾）前 1/3，踡足时呈凹陷处，俗称足心，为足少阴肾经之“井”穴，具有开窍、宁神功能。近年来，采用涌泉敷药治疗儿科常见病，疗效显著，且具有方便、无副作用、患儿较之服药易于接受等优点，据有关报道，将小儿五种常见病（症）的敷药方法介绍如下。

The Yongquan acupoint is located on the anterior one-third of the sole (excluding the toes), in the depression formed when the foot is curled. Commonly known as the center of the sole, it is the “Jing-Well” point of the Kidney Meridian of Foot-Shaoyin, possessing the functions of opening the orifices and calming the mind. In recent years, applying herbal plasters to the Yongquan acupoint has shown remarkable efficacy in treating common pediatric diseases. It is convenient, has no side effects, and is more acceptable to children than taking oral medications. Based on relevant reports, the plaster methods for five common pediatric diseases (symptoms) are introduced below.

1. 高热：王忠明介绍，用生栀子粉 10 克和蛋清调成稠糊状，做成药饼，按男左女右敷于涌泉穴，如发热伴见抽搐者，加敷内关穴，治疗小儿因流感、腮腺炎、风疹等病引起的高热及夏季热，疗效颇佳。邵金阶介绍，用生绿豆粉 50 克研细过 80 月筛，加蛋清调成糊状敷两涌泉穴，治疗流感等引起的高热，疗效亦好。

High Fever: Wang Zhongming introduced using 10g of raw gardenia powder mixed with egg white into a thick paste, made into a medicinal cake, and applied to the Yongquan acupoint on the left foot for boys and the right foot for girls. If the fever is accompanied by convulsions, apply an additional plaster to the Neiguan acupoint. This method has excellent efficacy for high fever and summer heat in children caused by influenza, mumps, rubella, etc. Shao Jinjie introduced grinding 50g of raw mung bean powder finely (passing through an 80-mesh sieve), mixing it with egg white into a paste, and applying it to both Yongquan acupoints. This also has good efficacy for high fever caused by influenza.

2. 鹅口疮：杨迎民介绍，取蓖麻籽 30 克，吴萸 30 克，大黄 6 克，制南星 6 克，共研细末，用鸡蛋清调成糊状，每晚睡前贴于涌泉穴上，外用胶布固定，次晨取去。上药共分 5 次贴完，共治疗 34 例，结果痊愈 19 例，好转 12 例，无效 3 例。曾令德介绍，用吴茱萸 10 克研末，用陈醋调成糊状敷于涌泉穴，外敷一层塑料布，以绷布包裹，每日换药一次，共治疗 2 例，效果满意。

2. Oral Thrush: Yang Yingmin introduced taking 30g of castor seeds, 30g of evodia fruit (wu-zhu-yu), 6g of rhubarb (da-huang), and 6g of processed arisaema (zhi-nan-xing). Grind them into a fine powder, mix with egg white into a paste, apply to the Yongquan acupoint before bed every night, fix it with medical tape, and remove it the next morning. The above medicine is applied in 5 sessions. A total of 34 cases were treated, with 19 cured, 12 improved, and 3 ineffective. Zeng Lingde introduced grinding 10g of evodia fruit into a powder, mixing it with aged

vinegar into a paste, applying it to the Yongquan acupoint, covering it with a layer of plastic film, and wrapping it with a bandage. Change the medicine once a day. Two cases were treated with satisfactory results.

3. 口舌糜烂：文钊介绍，用附片 10 克，吴茱萸 6 克共研末，醋调敷涌泉穴，效果良好。

3. Oral and Tongue Ulcers: Wen Zhao introduced grinding 10g of aconite root slices (fu-pian) and 6g of evodia fruit into a powder, mixing it with vinegar, and applying it to the Yongquan acupoint, which has good effects.

4. 流涎：褚成炎介绍，用制南星 30 克，生蒲黄 12 克，共为细末，米醋适量调制成饼，包涌泉穴，男左女右，12 小时换药 1 次，经治 132 例，结果痊愈 118 例，好转 11 例，无效 3 例。总有效率为 97.7%。

4. Drooling: Chu Chengyan introduced taking 30g of processed arisaema and 12g of raw cattail pollen (pu-huang), grinding them into a fine powder, mixing with an appropriate amount of rice vinegar to make a cake, and wrapping it around the Yongquan acupoint (left foot for boys, right foot for girls). Change the medicine once every 12 hours. A total of 132 cases were treated, with 118 cured, 11 improved, and 3 ineffective. The total effective rate was 97.7%.

5. 遗尿：陈尔明介绍，取白芍、白及各 10 克，白术 12 克，白矾 3 克，共研细末，用葱汁适量调成药饼，外敷涌泉、关元穴，以塑料薄膜覆盖，胶布固定，每晚睡前敷药。次晚再换药，连用 5 次，治疗本病效果满意。

5. Enuresis: Chen Erming introduced taking 10g each of white peony root (bai-shao) and bletilla tuber (bai-ji), 12g of atractylodes macrocephala (bai-zhu), and 3g of alum (bai-fan). Grind them into a fine powder, mix with an appropriate amount of scallion juice to make a medicinal cake, and apply it externally to the Yongquan and Guanyuan acupoints. Cover with plastic film and fix with medical tape. Apply the medicine before bed every night, change the medicine the next night, and use it continuously for 5 times. The treatment effect for this disease is satisfactory.

6. 缩泉贴 处方及用法：生硫磺末 5 克，葱白 10 克。一起捣烂，分 2 份，每晚睡前贴敷两侧涌泉穴，次日换药，连贴敷 3-5 次，每次 1 剂。功效：温肾壮阳，固摄止泻。适应症：小儿肾阳虚遗尿，老人肾虚夜尿频数，脾肾阳虚泄泻。

6. Suoquan Plaster. Prescription and Usage: 5g of raw sulfur powder and 10g of scallion whites. Mash them together, divide into 2 portions, and apply to both Yongquan acupoints before bed every night. Change the medicine the next day, and apply continuously for 3-5 times, 1 dose each time. Effects: Warming the kidneys, strengthening yang, securing astringency, and stopping diarrhea. Indications: Enuresis in children due to kidney-yang deficiency, frequent nocturia in the elderly due to kidney deficiency, and diarrhea due to spleen-kidney yang deficiency.

7. 小儿流涎：取吴茱萸 12 克、胆南星 4 克共研末备用。临睡前将两脚洗净，以陈醋将上药调敷涌泉穴包扎固定，12 小时后取下。

7. Pediatric Drooling: Take 12g of evodia fruit and 4g of arisaema with bile (dan-nan-xing), grind them into a powder, and set aside. Wash both feet before bed, mix the medicine with aged vinegar, apply it to the Yongquan acupoint, bandage and fix it, and remove it after 12 hours.

8. 小儿百日咳：将鲜紫皮大蒜瓣 5 枚捣烂成泥，敷贴涌泉穴，包扎固定，每日一次。

8. Pediatric Whooping Cough: Mash 5 cloves of fresh purple-skinned garlic into a mud, apply it to the Yongquan acupoint, bandage and fix it, and apply once a day.

9. 小儿厌食症：炒神曲、炒麦芽、焦山楂、炒鸡内金、炒莱菔子等量共研末，开水调成糊状，于临睡前敷脐部并以布带固定，次早取下，每日一次。

9. Pediatric Anorexia: Take equal amounts of stir-fried medicated leaven (shen-qu), stir-fried malt (mai-ya), scorched hawthorn (jiao-shan-zha), stir-fried chicken gizzard lining (ji-nei-jin), and stir-fried radish seeds (lai-fu-zi). Grind them into a powder, mix with boiling water into a paste, apply it to the navel before bed, fix it with a cloth band, remove it the next morning, and apply once a day.

10. 小儿泄泻：将丁香、木香各5-10克、肉桂4-6克，研末装袋内，置脐上一夜，绷带固定。

10. Pediatric Diarrhea: Take 5-10g each of clove (ding-xiang) and costus root (mu-xiang), and 4-6g of cinnamon bark (rou-gui). Grind them into a powder, put them in a small bag, place it on the navel overnight, and fix it with a bandage.

11. 小儿疳积：取大黄、山栀、杏仁、桃仁各 6 克，皮硝 9 克，研末，用蛋清、葱白汁、酒少许混合后调药末，敷脐部每日一次。

11. Pediatric Infantile Malnutrition: Take 6g each of rhubarb (da-huang), gardenia fruit (shan-zhi), apricot kernel (xing-ren), and peach kernel (tao-ren), and 9g of mirabilite (pi-xiao). Grind them into a powder, mix with egg white, scallion juice, and a little liquor to blend the powder, and apply it to the navel once a day.

12. 小儿遗尿：以连须葱白 3 克和硫磺 30 克共捣如泥，外敷脐部，纱布固定，8-10 小时。

12. Pediatric Enuresis: Take 3g of scallion whites with roots intact and 30g of sulfur, mash them into a mud, apply it externally to the navel, fix it with gauze, and leave it for 8-10 hours.

13. 小儿夜喘：取朱砂 0.5 克、五倍子 1.5 克共研末，与茶叶少许（捣烂）拌匀加水制成小饼状，敷于脐部，胶布固定，每晚换药一次。

13. Pediatric Nocturnal Asthma: Take 0.5g of cinnabar (zhu-sha) and 1.5g of Chinese gallnut (wu-bei-zi), grind them into a powder, mix evenly with a small amount of tea leaves (mashed), add water to make a small cake, apply it to the navel, fix it with medical tape, and change the medicine once every night.

14. 茶虎贴 处方及用法：茶辣（吴茱萸）9 克、虎杖、紫花地丁各 6 克，胆南星 3 克。共研细来。每次取药末 12 克，酸醋调软，分 2 份，捏成饼状，贴双足底涌泉穴，固定，12 小时除去，每日 1 次，连贴 2 天。功效：解毒消肿，软坚散结。适应症：痄腮（腮腺炎），老鼠疬（颌下淋巴结炎）。

14. Chahu Plaster. Prescription and Usage: 9g of evodia fruit (cha-la/wu-zhu-yu), 6g each of giant knotweed rhizome (hu-zhang) and common violet herb (zi-

hua-di-ding), and 3g of arisaema with bile (dan-nan-xing). Grind them into a fine powder. Each time, take 12g of the powder, soften it with sour vinegar, divide it into 2 portions, pinch them into cakes, apply them to the Yongquan acupoints on both soles, fix them, remove them after 12 hours, apply once a day, and continue for 2 days. Effects: Detoxifying, reducing swelling, softening hardness, and dissipating nodules. Indications: Mumps (zha-sai) and submandibular lymphadenitis (lao-shu-li).

《中药科技报》1991 年 11 月 26 日（王廷兆）

Chinese Medicine Science and Technology News, November 26, 1991 (Wang Ting-zhao)

三、药兜疗法（11 方）

III. Herbal Abdominal Binder Therapy (11 Prescriptions)

中药兜肚疗法，是将一些中草药碾成细末，以柔软的棉布摺成大小能覆盖脐腹部的兜肚形，内铺少许药棉，把药末均匀撒上，再覆以稍厚普通棉花，经过纵横缝纫，使药末固定在网状小格中以免堆积，戴在脐腹部即可。下面介绍男科疾病的中药兜肚疗法。

The herbal abdominal binder therapy involves grinding various Chinese herbal medicines into a fine powder. A soft cotton cloth is folded into a binder shape large enough to cover the navel and abdominal area. A small amount of medical cotton is laid inside, and the herbal powder is sprinkled evenly over it. A slightly thicker layer of ordinary cotton is then placed on top. The binder is sewn in a grid pattern (vertically and horizontally) to fix the powder in small compartments, preventing it from clumping. The binder is then worn over the navel and abdomen. Below is an introduction to this therapy for treating andrological diseases.

1. 治阳痿：将巴戟天、淫羊藿、金樱子、葫芦巴各 10 克，阳起石 12 克，柴胡 6 克碾为细末，做成兜肚长久佩戴，每 10 天换药 1 次，每晚用热水袋热敷药兜 15-30 分钟。

Treating Impotence (Erectile Dysfunction): Grind 10g each of morinda root (ba-ji-tian), epimedium (yin-yang-huo), Chinese rose fruit (jin-ying-zi), and fenugreek seeds (hu-lu-ba), 12g of actinolite (yang-qi-shi), and 6g of bupleurum root (chai-hu) into a fine powder. Make it into an abdominal binder and wear it continuously. Change the medicine once every 10 days. Apply a hot water bottle to the binder for 15-30 minutes every night.

2. 治早泄：把金樱子、芡实、莲子肉、益智仁各 12 克，生牡蛎、白蒺藜各 12 克碾为细末，做成兜肚经常佩戴，10 日换药 1 次，每晚用热水袋热敷药兜 15-30 分钟。

2. Treating Premature Ejaculation: Grind 12g each of Chinese rose fruit (jin-ying-zi), Gordon euryale seeds (qian-shi), lotus seeds (lian-zi-rou), and alpinia fruit (yi-zhi-ren), as well as 12g each of raw oyster shell (sheng-mu-li) and white tribulus fruit (bai-ji-li) into a fine powder. Make it into an abdominal binder and wear it regularly. Change the medicine once every 10 days. Apply a hot water bottle to the binder for 15-30 minutes every night.

3. 治慢性前列腺炎：取红花、桃红、乌药、萆薢各 15 克，车前子、金钱草、败酱草各 20 克，刘寄奴、白花蛇舌草各 30 克，制香附 18 克碾为细末，做成药兜长久佩戴，每 15 天换药 1 次，每晚用热水袋热敷药兜 15-30 分钟。

3. Treating Chronic Prostatitis: Take 15g each of safflower (hong-hua), peach flower (tao-hong), lindera root (wu-yao), and dioscorea rhizome (bi-xie), 20g each of plantain seeds (che-qian-zi), golden grass (jin-qian-cao), and patrinia herb (bai-jiang-cao), 30g each of herba patriniae (liu-ji-nu) and oldenlandia herb (bai-hua-she-she-cao), and 18g of processed cyperus rhizome (zhi-xiang-fu). Grind them into a fine powder, make an abdominal binder, and wear it continuously. Change the medicine once every 15 days. Apply a hot water bottle to the binder for 15-30 minutes every night.

4. 治遗精：把金樱子 20 克，芡实 15 克，煅牡蛎 30 克，刺猬皮 25 克，硫磺 10 克，龟板、女贞子各 12 克，旱莲草 28 克碾为细末，制成药兜经常佩戴，每10日换药1次。

4. Treating Spermatorrhea: Grind 20g of Chinese rose fruit (jin-ying-zi), 15g of Gordon euryale seeds (qian-shi), 30g of baked oyster shell (wei-mu-li), 25g of hedgehog skin (ci-wei-pi), 10g of sulfur (liu-huang), 12g each of tortoise plastron (gui-ban) and glossy privet fruit (nv-zhen-zi), and 28g of eclipta herb (han-lian-cao) into a fine powder. Make it into an abdominal binder and wear it regularly. Change the medicine once every 10 days.

5. 治前列腺肥大：把肉桂30克，升麻15克碾为细末，与麝香0.3克混匀，制成药兜经常佩戴小腹部，每5日换药1次，每晚用热水袋热敷药兜15-30分钟。

5. Treating Prostatic Hypertrophy: Grind 30g of cinnamon bark (rou-gui) and 15g of cimicifuga rhizome (sheng-ma) into a fine powder, mix evenly with 0.3g of musk (she-xiang), and make it into an abdominal binder. Wear it over the lower abdomen regularly. Change the medicine once every 5 days. Apply a hot water bottle to the binder for 15-30 minutes every night.

《民族医药报》（刘健英）

National Ethnic Medicine News (Liu Jian-ying)

壮医药兜疗法是流行在广西壮族地区的一种民间疗法，此法对小儿常见病有较好的疗效。药兜的制作方法是：将中草药研成细末，用绸布或柔软而薄、透气良好的棉布制成10X15厘米能覆盖胃脘和脐腹部的兜肚形，内层铺少许干净棉花，把药末均匀撒上，再覆以稍厚的一层棉花，经纵横缝好，使药末固定在网形小格中以免堆积，佩戴在胃脘或脐腹部即可。现精选一些治小儿常见病的药兜疗法验方介绍如下。

The Zhuang herbal abdominal binder therapy is a folk remedy popular in the Zhuang ethnic areas of Guangxi. This method has good efficacy for common pediatric diseases. The binder is made by grinding Chinese herbal medicines into a fine powder. A silk cloth or a soft, thin, and breathable cotton cloth is used to make a 10x15 cm binder that covers the epigastrium and the navel/abdomen. A small amount of clean cotton is laid inside, and the herbal powder is sprinkled evenly over it. A slightly thicker layer of cotton is then placed on top. The binder is sewn in a grid pattern (vertically and horizontally) to fix the powder in small compartments, preventing it from clumping. It is then worn over the epigastrium or the navel/abdomen. Below are some selected proven prescriptions of this therapy for treating common pediatric diseases.

6. 治小儿厌食药兜：黄芪、焦山楂、焦白术、砂仁各 10 克，炒鸡内金、皮硝各 6 克，共研成细末，加麝香 0.2 克，制成药兜，盖在脐部，10 天换药 1 次。

6. Herbal Binder for Pediatric Anorexia: Take 10g each of astragalus root (huang-qi), scorched hawthorn (jiao-shan-zha), scorched atractylodes macrocephala (jiao-bai-zhu), and cardamom (sha-ren), and 6g each of stir-fried chicken gizzard lining (chao-ji-nei-jin) and mirabilite (pi-xiao). Grind them into a fine powder, add 0.2g of musk (she-xiang), and make it into an abdominal binder. Place it over the navel and change the medicine once every 10 days.

7. 治小儿疳症药兜：五谷虫、使君子、胡黄连、麦芽、神曲、党参、苍术、炒鸡内金、槟榔、莪术、陈皮、砂仁、白蔻仁各 6 克，冰片 3 克，共研成细末，制成药兜，佩戴于胃脘部，15 天换药 1 次。

7. Herbal Binder for Pediatric Infantile Malnutrition: Take 6g each of blowfly larvae (wu-gu-chong), rangoon creeper fruit (shi-jun-zi), pseudostellaria rhizome (hu-huang-lian), malt (mai-ya), medicated leaven (shen-qu), codonopsis root (dang-shen), atractylodes lancea (cang-zhu), stir-fried chicken gizzard lining (chao-ji-nei-jin), betel nut (bin-lang), zedoary rhizome (e-zhu), dried tangerine peel (chen-pi), cardamom (sha-ren), and white cardamom (bai-dou-kou), along with 3g of borneol (bing-pian). Grind them into a fine powder, make it into an abdominal binder, wear it over the epigastrium, and change the medicine once every 15 days.

8. 治小儿慢性腹泻药兜：苍术、木香、党参、诃子、茯苓、神曲、炒淮山、炒扁豆各 6 克，熟附子 3 克，共研成细末，制成药兜，佩戴于脐腹部，10 天换药 1 次。

8. Herbal Binder for Pediatric Chronic Diarrhea: Take 6g each of atractylodes lancea (cang-zhu), costus root (mu-xiang), codonopsis root (dang-shen), chebula

fruit (he-zi), poria (fu-ling), medicated leaven (shen-qu), stir-fried Chinese yam (chao-huai-shan), and stir-fried hyacinth bean (chao-bian-dou), along with 3g of processed aconite root (shu-fu-zi). Grind them into a fine powder, make it into an abdominal binder, wear it over the navel and abdomen, and change the medicine once every 10 days.

9. 治小儿慢性痢疾药兜：人参 5 克，白术 12 克，肉桂 6 克，赤石脂 15 克，枯矾 10 克，共研成细末，制成药兜，佩戴于脐腹部，10 天换药 1 次。

9. Herbal Binder for Pediatric Chronic Dysentery: Take 5g of ginseng root (ren-shen), 12g of atractylodes macrocephala (bai-zhu), 6g of cinnamon bark (rou-gui), 15g of red halloysite (chi-shi-zhi), and 10g of calcined alum (ku-fan). Grind them into a fine powder, make it into an abdominal binder, wear it over the navel and abdomen, and change the medicine once every 10 days.

10. 治小儿哮喘药兜：麻黄 6 克，苏子、款冬花、杏仁各 10 克，葶苈子 8 克，生石膏 15 克，甘草 4 克，共研成细末，制成药兜，佩戴于脐腹部，10 天换药 1 次。

10. Herbal Binder for Pediatric Asthma: Take 6g of ephedra herb (ma-huang), 10g each of perilla fruit (su-zi), coltsfoot flower (kuan-dong-hua), and apricot kernel (xing-ren), 8g of descurainia seeds (ting-li-zi), 15g of raw gypsum (sheng-shi-gao), and 4g of licorice root (gan-cao). Grind them into a fine powder, make it into an abdominal binder, wear it over the navel and abdomen, and change the medicine once every 10 days.

11. 治小儿慢惊风药兜：全蝎、白僵蚕、公丁香、白蔻仁、胡椒、人参、白术、茯神、天麻、琥珀、防风、地龙、胆南星各 3 克，石菖蒲、艾叶各 10 克，加麝香 0.2 克，共研成细末，制成药兜，佩戴于脐腹部，15 天换药 1 次。

11. Herbal Binder for Pediatric Chronic Infantile Convulsions: Take 3g each of scorpion (quan-xie), white silkworm (bai-jiang-can), clove (gong-ding-xiang), white cardamom (bai-dou-kou), black pepper (hu-jiao), ginseng root (ren-shen), atractylodes macrocephala (bai-zhu), poria with hostwood (fu-shen), gastrodia rhizome (tian-ma), amber (hu-po), saposhnikovia root (fang-feng), earthworm (di-long), and arisaema with bile (dan-nan-xing), along with 10g each of grassleaf

sweetflag (shi-chang-pu) and mugwort leaf (ai-ye). Add 0.2g of musk (she-xiang), grind them into a fine powder, make it into an abdominal binder, wear it over the navel and abdomen, and change the medicine once every 15 days.

《民族医药报》（李子云）

National Ethnic Medicine News (Li Zi-yun)

四、脐疗（30 方）

IV. Umbilical Therapy (30 Prescriptions)

脐疗是将中药敷于脐窝而达治病的目的。这种疗法是我国自古至今的传统治病方法。具有疗效好无副作用，方法简便，容易掌握运用等特点。今介绍几种疾病脐疗法，请试用。

Umbilical therapy involves applying Chinese herbal medicines to the navel (umbilicus) to treat diseases. This therapy is a traditional medical method in China that has been used since ancient times. It is characterized by good efficacy, no side effects, simplicity, and ease of use. Below are several umbilical therapies for different diseases for you to try.

1. 肝硬化腹水：方药和用法：甘遂 3 克研末（无甘遂可用商陆 6 克代替），连头葱白 5 根（如患者伴有畏寒症状加肉桂粉 6 克），上药共捣烂备用。先将肚脐间和周围用陈醋涂搽（防感染），然后将药适量敷上，再用纱布覆盖，胶布固定即妥，日 1 剂。

Liver Cirrhosis with Ascites. Prescription and Usage: Grind 3g of kansui root (gan-sui) into a powder (if unavailable, substitute with 6g of pokeweed root/shang-lu). Mash 5 scallion whites with roots together with the above medicine and set aside. First, apply aged vinegar around and inside the navel to prevent infection. Then, apply an appropriate amount of the mashed medicine to the navel, cover it with gauze, and fix it with medical tape. Use 1 dose per day.

2. 慢性气管炎：将苍耳、苍尤、细辛、白芥子各 5 份、公丁香、肉桂、半夏各 3 份、麻黄 10 份，人造麝香 1 份，共研极细末，每次 5 克填入脐中，外用纱布固定，隔 48 小时换药一次，10 次为一疗程，一般三个疗程可愈。

2. Chronic Bronchitis: Take 5 parts each of cocklebur fruit (cang-er), atractylodes lancea (cang-zhu), asarum herb (xi-xin), and white mustard seed (bai-jie-zi), 3 parts each of clove (gong-ding-xiang), cinnamon bark (rou-gui), and pinellia tuber (ban-xia), 10 parts of ephedra herb (ma-huang), and 1 part of artificial musk (ren-zao-she-xiang). Grind them into an extremely fine powder. Fill 5g into the navel each time, fix it with gauze, and change the medicine every 48 hours. 10 times make up one course of treatment. It is generally cured after three courses.

3. 治尿床（遗尿）：鲜葱白 7 段，硫磺适量。共捣泥，每晚睡前将脐部洗净，将药泥敷于脐部，纱布覆盖，胶布固定，次晨除去，连敷 5 日，遗尿即止。以后改为隔日晚间敷药一次，以巩固疗效。主治较大年龄的遗尿儿童。

3. Treating Bedwetting (Enuresis): Take 7 pieces of fresh scallion whites and an appropriate amount of sulfur. Mash them into a mud. Wash the navel clean before bed every night, apply the medicinal mud to the navel, cover it with gauze, and fix it with medical tape. Remove it the next morning. Apply continuously for 5 days, and the enuresis will stop. Afterwards, change to applying the medicine once every other night to consolidate the efficacy. It is mainly used for older children with enuresis.

4. 高血压病：将胆制吴茱萸 500 克、龙胆草 6 克、硫磺、朱砂各 50 克，醋制白矾 100 克、环戊甲噻嗪 175 毫克，共研极细末，每次用 200 毫克左右，倒入脐窝，敷盖棉球，胶布固定，每周更换 1 次，1 个月为一疗程。

4. Hypertension: Take 500g of bile-processed evodia fruit (dan-zhi-wu-zhu-yu), 6g of gentian root (long-dan-cao), 50g each of sulfur (liu-huang) and cinnabar (zhu-sha), 100g of vinegar-processed alum (cu-zhi-bai-fan), and 175mg of cyclopenthiazide. Grind them into an extremely fine powder. Each time, use about 200mg, pour it into the navel, cover it with a cotton ball, and fix it with medical tape. Change the medicine once a week, with 1 month making up one course of treatment.

5. 小儿肾虚遗尿：煅龙骨、五倍子各等份，研细末，以冷开水调成厚糊状，涂满肚脐，外用小红布膏药或“肤疾宁”贴紧，两天换药 1 次，两周一个疗程。主治小儿肾虚、膀胱失约、夜间遗尿，亦治大人遗精、自汗、盗汗等症。

5. Pediatric Enuresis due to Kidney Deficiency: Take equal amounts of calcined dragon bone (duan-long-gu) and Chinese gallnut (wu-bei-zi), grind them into a fine powder, and mix with cold boiled water into a thick paste. Apply it to fill the navel, and stick a small red cloth plaster or "Fu-ji-ning" plaster tightly over it. Change the medicine once every two days, with two weeks making up one course of treatment. It is mainly used for pediatric enuresis at night caused by kidney deficiency and loss of bladder control. It also treats spermatorrhea, spontaneous sweating, and night sweats in adults.

6. 胃下垂：蓖麻仁 1 份、五倍子 1 份，共捣烂，敷于脐外周围，用关节镇痛膏 6-8 张固定，每日早、中、晚用热水袋热敷 1 次，第 4 天取掉，一般敷 6 次见效。

6. Gastroptosis: Take 1 part of castor seeds (bi-ma-ren) and 1 part of Chinese gallnut (wu-bei-zi), mash them together, and apply them around the outside of the navel. Fix it with 6-8 pieces of joint analgesic plasters. Apply a hot water bottle to the area once in the morning, noon, and evening every day. Remove it on the 4th day. It generally takes effect after 6 applications.

7. 心绞痛：将山楂 100 克、白芍 150 克，厚朴 100 克、葛根 10 克、甘草 5 克，共烘干研面，加入鸡矢藤挥发油 2 毫升、鸡矢藤挥发油 2 毫升、冰片少许混合，每次 200 毫升，用黄酒调糊敷于脐部，3 天换药 1 次。尤其对气滞血淤型效果好。

7. Angina Pectoris: Dry and grind 100g of hawthorn (shan-zha), 150g of white peony root (bai-shao), 100g of magnolia bark (hou-po), 10g of kudzu root (ge-gen), and 5g of licorice root (gan-cao) into a powder. Add 2ml of paederia vine volatile oil (ji-shi-teng-hui-fa-you) and a little borneol (bing-pian), and mix well. Each time, take 200mg (Note: The original text says 200ml, which is likely a typo for 200mg), mix it with yellow rice wine into a paste, and apply it to the navel. Change the medicine once every 3 days. It is especially effective for the type

caused by qi stagnation and blood stasis.

8. 老年性前列腺肥大：将白矾、生白盐各 7.5 克，共研末，以纸圈围脐，填药在内，药上滴数滴冷水，小便即通，此为通关法。

8. Senile Prostatic Hypertrophy: Grind 7.5g each of alum (bai-fan) and raw white salt (sheng-bai-yan) into a powder. Encircle the navel with a paper ring, fill the medicine inside, and drop a few drops of cold water on the medicine. Urination will be unblocked immediately. This is called the "Unblocking Pass Method".

9. 治寒痢：吃冷凉食物或受寒邪所致。取胡椒适量，研末，放入肚脐中，胶布固定。3 岁以下日 1 粒，3 岁以上日 1.5-2 粒，成年人 2. 5-3 粒，分 3 次用。

9. Treating Cold Dysentery: Caused by eating cold food or exposure to cold pathogens. Take an appropriate amount of black pepper (hu-jiao), grind it into a powder, put it into the navel, and fix it with medical tape. For children under 3 years old, use 1grain per day; for those over 3, use 1.5-2grains per day; for adults, use 2.5-3grains per day, divided into 3 doses.

10. 小腹冷痛：胡椒适量研末以少许水调涂肚脐，用胶布固定，每日 1 次，另取红糖 15 克、干姜 3 片研末，以开水冲服。内外夹攻，冷痛很快痊愈。

10. Cold Pain in the Lower Abdomen: Grind an appropriate amount of black pepper into a powder, mix it with a little water, and apply it to the navel. Fix it with medical tape, once a day. In addition, grind 15g of brown sugar and 3 slices of dried ginger into a powder, and brew it with boiling water to drink. The combined internal and external treatment can quickly cure the cold pain.

《民族医药报》（河北 张金声）

National Ethnic Medicine News (Zhang Jin-sheng, Hebei)

11. 治心绞痛：用人参 10 克，寸冬 15 克，五味子 8 克，当归 12 克，五灵脂 10 克研为细末，与麝香 0.3 克混匀，用黄酒调成糊状，纳入脐中，外用胶布固定。5 天换约 1 次，每天用热水袋热敷 15-30 分钟。

11. Treating Angina Pectoris: Grind 10g of ginseng root (ren-shen), 15g of dwarf lilyturf tuber (cun-dong), 8g of schisandra fruit (wu-wei-zi), 12g of angelica

root (dang-gui), and 10g of flying squirrel feces (wu-ling-zhi) into a fine powder. Mix evenly with 0.3g of musk (she-xiang), blend with yellow rice wine into a paste, put it into the navel, and fix it with medical tape. Change the medicine once every 5 days, and apply a hot water bottle to the area for 15-30 minutes daily.

12. 治中风后遗症：用黄芪、羌活、威灵仙各 90 克、乳香、没药、琥珀各 40 克，肉桂 10 克共研细末混匀。取上述药末 6 克用黄酒调成糊状，炒温热，敷入脐中，加麝香风湿膏固定。每周换药 1 次。

12. Treating Sequelae of Stroke: Grind 90g each of astragalus root (huang-qi), incised notopterygium root (qiang-huo), and clematis root (wei-ling-xian), 40g each of frankincense (ru-xiang), myrrh (mo-yao), and amber (hu-po), and 10g of cinnamon bark (rou-gui) into a fine powder and mix well. Take 6g of the powder, mix it with yellow rice wine into a paste, stir-fry until warm, apply it into the navel, and fix it with a musk rheumatism plaster. Change the medicine once a week.

13. 治老人癫痫：用胆南星、雄黄各 3 克，醋芫花 50 克，白胡椒挥发油 0.05 毫升，制成细末，每次用 150 毫克敷脐，15 天换药 1 次。

13. Treating Epilepsy in the Elderly: Take 3g each of arisaema with bile (dan-nan-xing) and realgar (xiong-huang), 50g of vinegar-processed lilac flower (cu-yuan-hua), and 0.05ml of white pepper volatile oil (bai-hu-jiao-hui-fa-you). Make them into a fine powder. Each time, use 150mg to apply to the navel, and change the medicine once every 15 days.

《中药科技报》1992 年 2 月 16 日（河北省 刘健英）

Chinese Medicine Science and Technology News, February 16, 1992 (Liu Jian-ying, Hebei Province)

14. 温脐贴 处方及用法：吴茱萸、木香各 5 克，公丁香、地榆各 4 克。共研细末，用生姜汁调润贴敷脐部，固定，48 小时换药，每次 1 剂。功效：温中行气，收涩止泻。适应症：小儿脾胃虚寒泄泻、久痢、腹胀。

14. Wenqi (Warming Navel) Plaster. Prescription and Usage: Take 5g each of evodia fruit (wu-zhu-yu) and costus root (mu-xiang), and 4g each of clove (gong-

ding-xiang) and great burnet root (di-yu). Grind them into a fine powder, moisten with fresh ginger juice, and apply it to the navel. Fix it and change the medicine every 48 hours, using 1 dose each time. Effects: Warming the middle jiao, promoting qi circulation, astringing, and stopping diarrhea. Indications: Diarrhea, chronic dysentery, and abdominal distension in children due to deficiency-cold of the spleen and stomach.

敷脐疗法是把鲜的植物药捣烂或用干药碾末，加酒、蜜、醋等汁调和，敷于脐部从而达到治疗疾病目的的传统外治法。由于小儿口服中药有一定困难，加之某些中药对小儿有一定的毒、副作用，所以敷脐疗法扩大了儿科疾病中新的给药途径，越来越受到医药界的重视。下面辑录采用敷脐疗法治疗儿科几种疾病的数则验方供读者参考选用。

Umbilical plaster therapy is a traditional external treatment method that involves mashing fresh herbal medicines or grinding dry medicines into a powder, mixing them with liquids such as wine, honey, or vinegar, and applying them to the navel to treat diseases. Because it is somewhat difficult for children to take oral Chinese medicines, and some Chinese medicines have certain toxic or side effects on children, umbilical therapy has expanded new drug administration routes for pediatric diseases and is receiving increasing attention from the medical community. Below are several proven prescriptions using umbilical therapy for pediatric diseases for readers’ reference.

15. 夜啼：取牵牛子 2 克，米砂 0.5 克，共研为细末，混匀后调成糊状，于睡前用湿毛巾将脐孔擦净，将药敷于脐孔上。

15. Night Crying: Take 2g of morning glory seeds (qian-niu-zi) and 0.5g of cinnabar (mi-sha), grind them into a fine powder, mix evenly, and blend into a paste. Before bed, wipe the navel clean with a wet towel, and apply the medicine to the navel.

16. 遗尿症：取硫磺 50 克，五倍子 15 克，葱白 5 根共捣烂如泥状敷脐，每日换药 1 次。1-2 次可愈。

16. Enuresis: Take 50g of sulfur (liu-huang), 15g of Chinese gallnut (wu-bei-

zi), and 5 scallion whites. Mash them into a mud-like consistency and apply to the navel. Change the medicine once a day. It can be cured after 1-2 applications.

17. 泄泻：将胡椒 1.5 克，米壳 1.5 克，共研为细末，混匀调合成糊状，于睡前用湿毛巾擦净脐孔，将药敷上。

17. Diarrhea: Grind 1.5g of black pepper (hu-jiao) and 1.5g of poppy capsule (mi-qiao) into a fine powder, mix evenly, and blend into a paste. Before bed, wipe the navel clean with a wet towel, and apply the medicine.

18. 急惊风：用芙蓉花嫩叶 6 片，切碎捣烂，鸡蛋 1 个，和匀煎作薄饼，敷小儿脐部，治急惊风可缓解症状。

18. Acute Infantile Convulsions: Take 6 tender leaves of cotton rose flower (fu-rong-hua), chop and mash them. Mix evenly with 1 egg, and pan-fry into a thin pancake. Apply it to the child’ s navel. It can relieve the symptoms of acute infantile convulsions.

19. 支气管炎：生麻黄 3 克，苍耳子 3 克，半夏 2 克，公丁香 0.5 克，肉桂 3 克。将上药共研为细粉，温水调成糊状，敷于脐孔。每日换药 1 次。对慢性支气管炎总有效率在 90% 以上。

19. Bronchitis: Take 3g of raw ephedra herb (sheng-ma-huang), 3g of cocklebur fruit (cang-er-zi), 2g of pinellia tuber (ban-xia), 0.5g of clove (gong-ding-xiang), and 3g of cinnamon bark (rou-gui). Grind the above medicines into a fine powder, mix with warm water into a paste, and apply it to the navel. Change the medicine once a day. The total effective rate for chronic bronchitis is over 90%.

20. 口腔溃疡：细辛 5 克，黄连 3 克，共研细粉，用陈醋调成糊状敷脐，每日换药 1 次，3-4 次可愈。

20. Oral Ulcers: Grind 5g of asarum herb (xi-xin) and 3g of coptis root (huang-lian) into a fine powder, mix with aged vinegar into a paste, and apply it to the navel. Change the medicine once a day. It can be cured after 3-4 applications.

21. 急性肾炎：用商陆、大戟、芝芪、甘遂、二丑各 3 克，冰片 2 克，共研为细末，葱白 2 根，共捣匀敷脐，12 小时后取下，连用 3 天。

21. Acute Nephritis: Take 3g each of pokeweed root (shang-lu), kansui root

(da-ji), astragalus root (zhi-qi), gansui root (gan-sui), and morning glory seeds (er-chou), along with 2g of borneol (bing-pian). Grind them into a fine powder. Mash them evenly with 2 scallion whites and apply to the navel. Remove it after 12 hours, and use it continuously for 3 days.

22. 急性腹泻：苦参末 1-2 克，温水调敷脐部，以伤湿止痛膏固定，24 小时换 1 次，治急性热性腹泻；丁香、肉桂各等分，研极细末，每取 0.5-1 克敷脐，方法同上，治虚寒腹泻。

22. Acute Diarrhea: Take 1-2g of sophora root powder (ku-shen-mo), mix with warm water, and apply to the navel. Fix it with a rheumatism analgesic plaster and change it once every 24 hours to treat acute febrile diarrhea. For deficiency-cold diarrhea, take equal parts of clove (ding-xiang) and cinnamon bark (rou-gui), grind them into an extremely fine powder, take 0.5-1g each time to apply to the navel using the same method.

23. 急性传染性肝炎：甜瓜蒂、秦艽各 60 克，青皮、紫草、黄芩、丹参各 30 克，铜绿 15 克，冰片 6 克，共研极细，过 60 目筛，密封备用，每次用 0.1 克，填脐窝，外用胶布密封，每 48 小时换药 1 次。

23. Acute Infectious Hepatitis: Take 60g each of muskmelon pedicel (tian-gua-di) and gentian root (qin-jiao), 30g each of unripe tangerine peel (qing-pi), gromwell root (zi-cao), scutellaria root (huang-qin), and salvia root (dan-shen), 15g of copper green (tong-lv), and 6g of borneol (bing-pian). Grind them extremely fine, pass through a 60-mesh sieve, and seal for later use. Each time, use 0.1g to fill the navel, seal it with medical tape, and change the medicine once every 48 hours.

《民族医药报》1992 年 5 月 13 日（江苏 郑俊芝）

National Ethnic Medicine News, May 13, 1992 (Zheng Jun-zhi, Jiangsu)

24. 胡椒粉敷脐治腹泻

24. Applying Black Pepper Powder to the Navel to Treat Diarrhea

婴幼儿常因受寒引起腹泻，大便稀薄或呈蛋花样，一天数次不止，体温又多正常，此症可用胡椒粉贴敷脐眼，疗效甚佳。其法：先用温水洗净脐眼周围的灰垢，然后将数粒胡椒研成细粉，放满肚脐眼，再把伤湿止痛膏剪成圆形，对着肚脐眼贴上，二至三天换一次，病愈后两天停用，一般 1-2 次即可止泻。

Infants and young children often suffer from diarrhea due to catching a cold, with thin or egg-drop-like stools occurring several times a day, mostly with normal body temperature. Applying black pepper powder to the navel has excellent efficacy for this condition. Method: First, wash away the dirt around the navel with warm water. Then, grind several black pepper grains into a fine powder and fill the navel. Cut a rheumatism analgesic plaster into a circle and stick it over the navel. Change the plaster once every two to three days, and stop using it two days after recovery. Generally, 1-2 applications can stop the diarrhea.

《中药科技报》1992 年 4 月 17 日（湘喆）

Chinese Medicine Science and Technology News, April 17, 1992 (Xiang Zhe)

25. 小儿脐疮验方 取川黄连、煅龙骨各 20 克，乌贼骨 10 克，共研成细末，瓶装备用。使用时，先用 3% 双氧水清洗脐部并用消毒药棉揩干，再将本品均匀地撒于疮面，用干净柔软的纱布包扎固定好，每日换 1 次，连用 3-5 日可愈。近来，笔者用此方治疗小儿脐疮 18 例，效果显著。

25. Proven Prescription for Pediatric Umbilical Ulcers: Take 20g each of Sichuan coptis root (chuan-huang-lian) and calcined dragon bone (duan-long-gu), and 10g of cuttlebone (wu-zei-gu). Grind them into a fine powder and store in a bottle for later use. When using, first clean the umbilical area with 3% hydrogen peroxide and wipe it dry with sterilized cotton. Then, sprinkle the powder evenly over the ulcerated surface, and bandage it securely with clean, soft gauze. Change the dressing once a day, and it can be cured after 3-5 consecutive days of use. Recently, the author used this prescription to treat 18 cases of pediatric umbilical ulcers with significant effects.

《民族医药报》1992 年 1 月 31 日（江西 钟久春）

National Ethnic Medicine News, January 31, 1992 (Zhong Jiu-chun, Jiangxi)

在广西苗族聚居地区的民间贴敷疗法，对不少常见病有较好的疗效。现将常用方法介绍如下。

The folk plaster therapy in the Miao ethnic areas of Guangxi has good efficacy for many common diseases. The commonly used methods are introduced below.

26. 姜葱散寒贴 处方及用法：生姜 20 克，葱白 15 克。捣碎炒热制成饼状。婴幼儿患者贴于前囟上，儿童及成人患者贴两侧太阳穴，盖上纱布固定，一般 8-12 小时，最长不超过 24 小时除药。每日 1 次，最多不超过 4 天。功效：祛风散寒、解表通窍。适应症：风寒感冒、鼻炎。

26. Ginger and Scallion Cold-Dispersing Plaster. Prescription and Usage: Take 20g of fresh ginger and 15g of scallion whites. Mash them, stir-fry until hot, and make them into a cake. For infants, apply it to the anterior fontanelle. For children and adults, apply it to both Taiyang acupoints. Cover it with gauze to fix it. Generally, remove the medicine after 8-12 hours, with a maximum of 24 hours. Use once a day, for no more than 4 days. Effects: Dispelling wind and cold, relieving exterior syndromes, and unblocking the orifices. Indications: Wind-cold common cold and rhinitis.

27. 蒜蓉贴 处方及用法：大蒜头米 8 瓣，苏子末 2 克，蒜米剥去衣捣碎与苏子末调匀。每晚睡前贴涌泉穴，或背部肺俞穴（第 3 胸椎下凹陷向外 1.5 厘米处），治腹胀贴脐部，固定，次晨除去，每晚 1 次，每次 1 剂。功效：温肺散寒、理气化痰。适应症：百日咳、慢性支气管炎、腹胀。

27. Garlic Paste Plaster. Prescription and Usage: Take 8 cloves of peeled garlic and 2g of perilla fruit powder. Peel the garlic, mash it, and mix evenly with the perilla fruit powder. Apply it to the Yongquan acupoint or the Feishu acupoint on the back (1.5 cm lateral to the depression below the 3rd thoracic vertebra) before bed every night. For abdominal distension, apply it to the navel. Fix it and remove it the next morning. Use once a night, 1 dose each time. Effects: Warming the lungs and dispelling cold, regulating qi and resolving phlegm. Indications: Whooping cough, chronic bronchitis, and abdominal distension.

28. 固喘贴 处方及用法：白芥子 15 克，甘遂 10 克，延胡索 8 克，细辛 6 克。共研为细末，分为 3 份。哮喘缓解后，每隔 10 天取一份，生姜汁或开水调润后压成小饼状，睡前贴两侧肺俞穴，伤湿膏固定，次日晨除去，10天1次，连贴3次。功效：温肺除痰、理气宽胸。适应症：小儿哮喘。

28. Asthma-Stabilizing Plaster. Prescription and Usage: Take 15g of white mustard seed (bai-jie-zi), 10g of kansui root (gan-sui), 8g of corydalis rhizome (yan-hu-suo), and 6g of asarum herb (xi-xin). Grind them into a fine powder and divide into 3 portions. After asthma is relieved, take one portion every 10 days, moisten it with fresh ginger juice or boiling water, and press it into a small cake. Apply it to both Feishu acupoints before bed, fix it with a rheumatism analgesic plaster, and remove it the next morning. Apply once every 10 days, for 3 consecutive times. Effects: Warming the lungs and eliminating phlegm, regulating qi and relieving chest tightness. Indications: Pediatric asthma.

29. 温中止泻贴 处方及用法：苍术、吴茱萸、公丁香、胡椒各等分，研细末。每次取药末 3 克，植物油调润贴敷脐部，每日 1 次。功效：温中止泻。适应症：婴幼儿脾胃虚寒泄泻。

29. Warming the Middle and Stopping Diarrhea Plaster. Prescription and Usage: Take equal amounts of atractylodes lancea (cang-zhu), evodia fruit (wu-zhu-yu), clove (gong-ding-xiang), and black pepper (hu-jiao), and grind them into a fine powder. Each time, take 3g of the powder, moisten it with vegetable oil, and apply it to the navel. Use once a day. Effects: Warming the middle jiao and stopping diarrhea. Indications: Diarrhea in infants and young children due to deficiency-cold of the spleen and stomach.

30. 消积贴（内关穴贴） 处方及用法：桃仁、杏仁、栀子各 30 克，冰片、樟脑各 2 克。先将前 3 味共研细末，入后 2 味研调匀。每次取药末 15 克，鸡蛋清调润后分为 2 份，贴敷两侧内关穴（前臂内侧腕关节横纹向上 3 横指处中点），固定，24 小时换药，最多不超过 3 次。功效：消食去积，行气消胀。适应症：小儿食积，气滞腹胀。

30. Digestive Stagnation-Relieving Plaster (Neiguan Acupoint Plaster). Prescription and Usage: Take 30g each of peach kernel (tao-ren), apricot kernel (xing-ren), and gardenia fruit (zhi-zi), and 2g each of borneol (bing-pian) and

camphor (zhang-nao). First, grind the first three ingredients into a fine powder, then add the last two ingredients and grind to mix evenly. Each time, take 15g of the powder, moisten it with egg white, and divide it into 2 portions. Apply them to both Neiguan acupoints (the midpoint on the inner forearm, 3 finger-widths above the wrist crease). Fix it and change the medicine after 24 hours, for a maximum of 3 times. Effects: Promoting digestion, eliminating food accumulation, regulating qi, and relieving distension. Indications: Pediatric food retention and abdominal distension due to qi stagnation.

《民族医药报》1991 年 11 月 25 日（广西 李子云）

National Ethnic Medicine News, November 25, 1991 (Li Zi-yun, Guangxi)

五、发泡疗法（2 方）

V. Blistering Therapy (2 Prescriptions)

发泡疗法是根据祖国医学中的经络、穴位学说的机理而采取的一种刺激性疗法。具有用药简单。使用方便，疗效迅速，费用低廉等特点。现介绍如下：

Blistering therapy is a stimulating treatment based on the principles of meridians and acupoints in traditional Chinese medicine. It is characterized by simple medication, convenient application, rapid efficacy, and low cost. The details are introduced below:

药物：鲜朝天辣椒（以将成熟时呈紫红色者为佳）、野薄荷、鲜毛茛、白芥子、鲜辣蓼草（以嫩枝叶取药用）、紫皮大蒜籽。

Medicines: Fresh 朝 天 chili peppers (preferably those that are purplish-red when nearly ripe), wild mint, fresh buttercup, white mustard seeds, fresh 辣 蓼 (Polygonum hydropiper) grass (using tender branches and leaves), and purple-skinned garlic cloves.

制法：根据不同病症，选择适宜药物、同大蒜籽（比例为 3:1）共捣烂为泥状，做成五分硬币大小的药饼，以用时配制为宜。

Preparation: Depending on the specific disease, select the appropriate medicine and mash it together with garlic cloves (at a ratio of 3:1) into a mud-like consistency. Make it into a medicinal cake the size of a five-cent coin. It is best prepared right before use.

用法：根据不同病症选用不同穴位。

Usage: Select different acupoints according to the specific disease.

1. 疟疾

Malaria

选穴：大椎、内关。

Acupoints: Dazhui (GV14) and Neiguan (PC6).

方法: 以野薄荷配大蒜籽，在疟疾发作前患者略有寒意时将药饼贴于穴位上，外以胶布固定。至局部有灼热疼痛感除药。弃药时应小心揭下，以免碰破水泡；泡不宜弄破，任其自行吸收消失；如不慎破溃，以龙胆紫液外除，以防感染。

Method: Mix wild mint with garlic cloves. When the patient feels a slight chill before a malaria attack, apply the medicinal cake to the acupoints and fix it with medical tape. Remove the medicine when the local area feels a burning pain. When removing the medicine, peel it off carefully to avoid breaking the blisters. Do not intentionally break the blisters; allow them to absorb and disappear naturally. If they accidentally rupture, apply gentian violet solution topically to prevent infection.

备注：以发泡疗法治疗疟疾，可明显减轻各种症状，但不能根治，故应配合其他抗疟药以杀灭疤原虫而根治疟疾。

Note: Blistering therapy for malaria can significantly alleviate various symptoms, but it cannot cure the disease fundamentally. Therefore, it should be combined with other antimalarial drugs to kill the Plasmodium parasites and achieve a radical cure.

2. 胃痛（各种胃炎、胃溃疡、饮食不当及受凉引起的胃脘部疼痛）

2. Stomachache (Epigastric pain caused by various gastritis, gastric ulcers, improper diet, and catching a cold)

选穴：胃俞、脾俞、中脘。

Acupoints: Weishu (BL21), Pishu (BL20), and Zhongwan (CV12).

方法：以鲜毛茛同大蒜籽（比例为 2:1）相配，制成药饼后贴穴，外以胶布固定，弃药时间如上。

Method: Mix fresh buttercup with garlic cloves (at a ratio of 2:1). After making the medicinal cake, apply it to the acupoints and fix it with medical tape. The timing for removing the medicine is the same as above.

《民族医药报》（江西 俞瑜）

National Ethnic Medicine News (Yu Yu, Jiangxi)

六、放血疗法（4 方）

VI. Bloodletting Therapy (4 Prescriptions)

放血疗法是指在人体外表某一部位或穴位，用针刺入一定的深度，或用刀片轻轻割破皮肉后，压出数滴血液治疗疾病的方法。它的机理是疏通经络，引邪毒外出。放血疗法历史悠久，效果显著，尤其是高热，惊风抽搦。头痛等一些急症，运用得当，常收到立竿见影的效果。

Bloodletting therapy is a method of treating diseases by inserting a needle to a certain depth at a specific part or acupoint on the body surface, or gently cutting the skin and flesh with a blade, and then pressing out a few drops of blood. Its mechanism is to unblock meridians and collaterals and draw out pathogenic toxins. Bloodletting therapy has a long history and remarkable effects. When used properly for acute conditions such as high fever, convulsions, and headaches, it often yields immediate results.

1. 唐高宗李治有一天处理繁杂的朝政后，下朝回宫，突感头昏目眩，视物不清，皇后武则天急命太监召御医秦鹤鸣进宫为皇治病。秦鹤鸣经过细心诊察认为皇上乃劳心过度，并风毒上攻头目，经络闭阻所致暴盲。在高宗恩准后，秦鹤鸣在高宗的百会穴和脑户穴施行放血疗法，一个多钟头后，高宗高兴地叫道："联眼明矣！联眼明矣！神医！神医！"秦鹤鸣除治好唐高宗外，还用同样的方法治好一些平民百姓的暴盲病。

One day, after handling complicated state affairs, Emperor Gaozong of the Tang Dynasty, Li Zhi, returned to the palace and suddenly felt dizzy with blurred vision. Empress Wu Zetian urgently ordered a eunuch to summon the imperial physician Qin Heming to treat the emperor. After careful diagnosis, Qin Heming believed that the emperor's sudden blindness was caused by overexertion of the mind, combined with wind toxins attacking the head and eyes, leading to the blockage of meridians and collaterals. With Emperor Gaozong's permission, Qin Heming performed bloodletting therapy at the Baihui and Naohu acupoints. Over an hour later, the emperor happily exclaimed, "My eyes are clear! My eyes are clear! Divine physician! Divine physician!" Besides curing Emperor Gaozong, Qin Heming used the same method to cure sudden blindness in some common people.

2. 高热是小儿常见的急症，有的体温达 40C，笔者常用针刺中冲穴（中指指端）放血，取得良好的效果。亦有针刺少商穴、十宣穴放血的。

2. High fever is a common pediatric emergency, with some body temperatures reaching 40° C. The author often uses bloodletting by needling the Zhongchong acupoint (the tip of the middle finger), achieving good results. Bloodletting by needling the Shaoshang and Shixuan acupoints is also effective.

3. 高血压头痛难忍，可在耳背耳廓沟处，用针沿耳背静脉斜针放血，或针耳垂放血。有良好的降压止痛效果。

3. For unbearable headaches caused by hypertension, bloodletting can be performed by needling obliquely along the auricular veins in the posterior auricular groove, or by needling the earlobe. This has a good effect on lowering blood pressure and relieving pain.

4. 感冒发热头痛，针刺两侧太阳穴放血；疟疾，用锋利的小刀片，轻轻浅割印堂穴，压出血数滴等，均有良效。

4. For headaches with fever due to the common cold, bloodletting by needling the Taiyang acupoints on both sides is effective; for malaria, gently and superficially cutting the Yintang acupoint with a sharp small blade and pressing

out a few drops of blood also yields good results.

放血时，要选择准确的穴位（部位），针刺穴位及用具应注意消毒，以防感染。放血量一般为 3-5 滴，不要放得太多。

When performing bloodletting, it is important to select accurate acupoints (locations). The acupoints and instruments must be disinfected to prevent infection. The amount of bloodletting is generally 3-5 drops; do not let out too much.

《民族医药报》1992 年 4 月 17 日（广西中医学院 玉振熹）

National Ethnic Medicine News, April 17, 1992 (Yu Zhen-xi, Guangxi College of Traditional Chinese Medicine)

七、药枕疗法（2 方）

VII. Herbal Pillow Therapy (2 Prescriptions)

药枕疗法：高血压病由于病程长，且常易波动不稳，药枕使用比较方便，而且作用持久，是较为理想的外治方法。

Herbal Pillow Therapy: Because hypertension has a long disease course and is often prone to fluctuations and instability, using herbal pillows is quite convenient and has a lasting effect, making it a relatively ideal external treatment method.

1. 用冬桑叶，白菊花，夏枯草，黄芩，晚蚕砂，丹皮，白芷，薄荷，川牛膝，决明子，明矾，冰片为基本方，并随症加减，伴头晕耳鸣加灵磁石、五味子；心悸失眠加炒枣仁、夜交藤；健忘加远志、石菖蒲等。上药共研粗末，装入约 50cmX25cm 布袋内，中间用线缝扎，使药物平整均匀，挪动不致堆积，放于枕头上铺上枕巾即可。一般枕用 3 个月，血压即可降至正常水平。

Basic Formula: Winter mulberry leaves, white chrysanthemum, common selfheal fruit spike, scutellaria root, late silkworm excrement, moutan bark, angelica dahurica root, mint, achyranthes bidentata root, cassia seed, alum, and borneol. Modify the formula according to symptoms: add magnetite and schisandra fruit for dizziness and tinnitus; add stir-fried sour jujube seeds and polygonum multiflorum vine for palpitations and insomnia; add polygala root and acorus tatarinowii rhizome for poor memory. Grind the above herbs into a coarse powder, put them into a cloth bag of about 50cm x 25cm, and stitch the middle with thread to keep the herbs flat and even, preventing them from clumping when moved. Place it on top of a pillow and cover it with a pillowcase. Generally, after using it as a pillow for 3 months, blood pressure can drop to normal levels.

2. 选用杭菊花、冬桑叶、野菊花、辛夷花各 500g，薄荷、红花各 150g。研末后加入冰片 50g，装入布袋中做枕头使用，每剂药用 3-6 个月（使用过程中可取出常晒）。用杭菊花 1000g，配牡丹皮、香白芷、川芎各 250g，研末做枕用亦可。

2. Take 500g each of Hangzhou chrysanthemum, winter mulberry leaves, wild chrysanthemum, and flos magnoliae, and 150g each of mint and safflower. After grinding them into a powder, add 50g of borneol, put them into a cloth bag to be used as a pillow. Each dose can be used for 3-6 months (it can be taken out and sun-dried frequently during use). Alternatively, use 1000g of Hangzhou chrysanthemum combined with 250g each of moutan bark, angelica dahurica root, and ligusticum wallichii rhizome, ground into a powder to make a pillow.

八、药烟疗法（3 方）

VIII. Herbal Smoke Therapy (3 Prescriptions)

准备：烟斗 1 支或烟纸若干张。

Preparation: 1 smoking pipe or several pieces of rolling paper.

适应证及选方：本法多适用于呼吸道疾病，举例如下。

Indications and Prescription Selection: This method is mostly applicable to respiratory diseases. Examples are as follows.

1. 久咳：

Chronic Cough:

①向日葵花瓣适量。

① An appropriate amount of sunflower petals.

②款冬花、木鳖子各 31 克。

② 31g each of coltsfoot flower and woody gourd seed.

2. 哮喘：

2. Asthma:

①闹羊花（曼陀罗花）1 份，烟叶 5-10 份

① 1 part of datura flower (yangjinhua), 5-10 parts of tobacco leaves.

②蓖麻叶（烤干）1 份，草烟 10 份。

② 1 part of castor leaves (roasted dry), 10 parts of grass tobacco.

3. 呃逆：手指甲、香烟各适量。

3. Hiccups: An appropriate amount of human fingernails and cigarettes.

使用方法：将药物分别切丝、和匀，装入烟斗或用烟纸卷成香烟状，当烟抽，每次 1 支卷烟量，每日 1-3 次。

Usage: Shred the medicines separately, mix them evenly, load them into a smoking pipe, or roll them into a cigarette shape using rolling paper. Smoke it like a regular cigarette. The dosage is 1 rolled cigarette each time, 1-3 times a day.

注意事项：对药烟过敏者，热毒症者禁用；吸入药烟治疗咳嗽时，若吸药烟后咳嗽加重，也不要中断治疗，而应适当休息，并忌食酸、辣等刺激性食物。

Precautions: Contraindicated for those allergic to herbal smoke and those with heat-toxin syndromes. When inhaling herbal smoke to treat cough, if the cough worsens after inhalation, do not interrupt the treatment. Instead, you should rest appropriately and avoid eating irritating foods such as sour and spicy ones.

《民族医药报》（李凤珍）

National Ethnic Medicine News (Li Feng-zhen)

九、隔姜疗法（1方）

IX. Ginger-Separated Moxibustion Therapy (1 Prescription)

隔姜灸治疗腱鞘炎：

Ginger-Separated Moxibustion for Tenosynovitis:

腱鞘炎是由手指和手腕活动过度或兼感受寒湿而致。属中医学“伤筋”“筋痹”范畴。本病临床除可用针灸、封闭、敷贴、推拿等法治疗外，还可用丁桂散隔姜灸治疗。

Tenosynovitis is caused by excessive movement of the fingers and wrists, or combined exposure to cold and dampness. It belongs to the categories of “tendon injury” and “tendon arthralgia” in traditional Chinese medicine. Clinically, besides treatments such as acupuncture, local injection (block therapy), plaster application, and massage, it can also be treated with ginger-separated moxibustion using Dinggui Powder.

具体方法：上等肉桂，公丁香各等份研成细末，鲜生姜洗净切成如一分硬币样厚度的薄片，中间用针刺六七个小孔备用，先在患者疼痛部位撒丁桂散少许，然后放上姜片，将艾绒做成艾炷在姜片上点燃灸之，待患者感觉有灼热感时取下换另一壮，连灸3-5壮，使局部生红晕为度，大多数患者灸治5-10壮，病即告愈。

Specific Method: Grind equal amounts of high-quality cinnamon bark and cloves into a fine powder. Wash fresh ginger and cut it into thin slices as thick as a one-cent coin, and prick 6-7 small holes in the middle with a needle for later use. First, sprinkle a little Dinggui Powder on the patient’s painful area, then place the ginger slice on it. Make mugwort floss into moxa cones, place them on the ginger slice, and ignite them for moxibustion. When the patient feels a burning sensation, remove the cone and replace it with another one. Continuously apply 3-5 cones until the local skin turns red. For most patients, the disease will be cured after 5-10 cones of moxibustion.

病案举例：韩先生，男53岁，某单位会计，1986年5月27日初诊，主诉右腕部酸痛无力半年，曾行封闭及推拿，效果不理想。经查：右侧桡骨茎突处稍肿，局部压痛；并可推及捻发音，屈伸活动受限，诊为“右侥骨基突狭窄性腱鞘炎”，遂在阳溪，列缺两穴加丁桂散隔姜各灸 3 壮，每日 1 次，并属其注意休息，右腕制动，共治 7 次痊愈。

Case Example: Mr. Han, male, 53 years old, an accountant at a certain unit, had his first visit on May 27, 1986. He complained of aching and weakness in his right wrist for half a year. He had previously received local injections and massage therapy with unsatisfactory results. Examination showed slight swelling and local tenderness at the right radial styloid process; crepitus could be felt upon palpation, and flexion and extension were limited. He was diagnosed with “right radial styloid stenosing tenosynovitis”. Therefore, ginger-separated moxibustion with Dinggui Powder was applied to the Yangxi and Lieque acupoints, 3 cones each, once a day. He was also advised to rest and immobilize his right wrist. He was completely cured after a total of 7 treatments.

（江苏 钱焕祥）

(Qian Huan-xiang, Jiangsu)

www.ingramcontent.com/pod-product-compliance
Lightning Source LLC
LaVergne TN
LVHW062033101126
852251LV00025B/323
* 9 7 8 1 6 8 3 7 2 8 7 4 0 *